FOUNDATIONS OF CRIMINAL JUSTICE

A TREATISE ON POISONS

BY

SIR ROBERT CHRISTISON

with a new introduction by

Brian Parker

AMS PRESS INC.
NEW YORK
LONDON   TORONTO
1973

FOUNDATIONS OF CRIMINAL JUSTICE

A

TREATISE

ON

P O I S O N S

IN RELATION TO

MEDICAL JURISPRUDENCE, PHYSIOLOGY, AND THE PRACTICE OF PHYSIC.

BY

ROBERT CHRISTISON, M.D., F.R.S.E.,

Professor of Materia Medica in the University of Edinburgh,
Fellow of the Royal College of Physicians, &c.,
Member of the American Philosophical Society, — of the Royal Acad. of Med. of Paris, — of the Imp.
Soc. of Physicians of Vienna, — of the Imp. Med. Chir. Acad. of St. Petersburg, — of the
Med. Chir. Soc. of Berlin, — of the Med. Chir. Assoc. of Hamburg, — of the Soc.
of Nat. and Phys. of Heidelberg, — of the Philadelphia Coll. of Pharm.

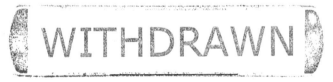
FIRST AMERICAN, FROM THE FOURTH EDINBURGH EDITION.

PHILADELPHIA:
ED. BARRINGTON & GEO. D. HASWELL.
1845.

Library of Congress Cataloging in Publication Data

Christison, Sir Robert, bart., 1797-1882.
    A treatise on poisons in relation to medical juris-
prudence, physiology, and the practice of physic.

    (Foundations of criminal justice)
    Original ed. issued in series: The Select medical
library (new series) and bulletin of medical science.
    1. Toxicology. 2. Medical jurisprudence.
I. Title. II. Series. III. Series: The Select
medical library (new series) and bulletin of medical
science.
RA1211.C56   1973   615.9   79-156011
ISBN 0-404-09111-3

Foundations of Criminal Justice Series, General
Editors: Richard H. Ward and Austin Fowler, John Jay
College of Criminal Justice

International Standard Book Number: 0-404-09111-3

Manufactured in the United States of America

An Introduction to the New Edition of

A TREATISE ON POISONS

Sir Robert Christison's *A Treatise on Poisons* was the
first English language compilation of the principles and
practices of scientific toxicology. The first edition appeared
in 1829 and found an immediate acceptance by the medico-
legal community of that era. To the literature of medical
jurisdprudence, it added a taxonomy based on a rich blend
of knowledge assembled from medical and legal sources in
France, Germany, and England. Christison's dual command
of experimental method and concise statement produced a
book of great practical value for his contempories. Moreov-
er, his discussion on the integration of information regarding biological symptoms, pathological findings, and toxicological investigations (with other information in the specific
instance at hand) is still pertinent to current inquiries. The
Treatise was translated into the German language in 1831;
three more English language editions, with Christison's
careful supervision and changes, were forthcoming in 1832,
1835, and 1845. An American edition was based on the
fourth edition of 1845.

The success of this book is to be found in the
development of Christison the man. As the son of a
professor of the humanities, his early education was guided
into a broad contact with the states of the arts and the
sciences at that time in history. Born July 18, 1797, in
Edinburgh, he completed his basic studies at the not
unusual age of fourteen and his university classes by
eighteen. Christison's first inclination seems to have been
towards engineering as a career, but his final choice was
medicine. During the next four years, he acquired not only
an understanding of medicine and surgery but also a fine
grasp of botany and chemistry. In the former two subjects,
he was afforded much practical experience as the result of
his selection as resident assistant in the Royal Infirmary at
the end of his sophomore year. In the latter subjects,
especially chemistry, he and a few fellow students formed a
group devoted to repeating and expanding the formal
lecture experiments. This activity resulted not only in some
humorous episodes later described in his autobiography[1]

but provided him opportunities to master manual manipulations of chemical appartus.

On his graduation as a Doctor of Medicine in 1819, Christison sought to expand his knowledge by studies in London and, later, in Paris. In London, he studied under a prominent surgeon, John Abernethy, and Sir William Lawrence for the several months he was in residence at St. Bartholomew's Hospital. The rapidly evolving field of chemistry and its preeminent status in Paris attracted Christison to that city. There, he worked in the laboratory of the chemist Pierre J. Robiquet, who isolated narcotine (noscapine) in 1807 and codeine in 1832. For six days a week over a five-month period, Christison diligently pursued the practice of chemistry. His previous activities stood him in good stead, and his joy in careful and precise experimentation resulted in a thorough training in the state of art for that field. Indeed, he later wrote that one of the important lessons he learned was "in any nice investigations [I would make] use only of jars and tubes graduated with my own hands."[2] Christison attended, among a number of lectures, those given by Louis N. Vauquelin on chemistry and Mathieu J. B. Orfila on toxicology. Vauquelin was professor of chemistry to the Medical Faculty in Paris and a prodigious writer of chemical papers. This chemist had discovered two elements and a number of organic compounds. Orfila had been a student of Vauquelin's and was, when Christison heard him, a professor of medical jurisprudence in the French capital. The publication in 1813 by Orfila of his *Traite des poisons* established the field of scientific toxicology. In Christison's own words Orfila "studied with untiring energy the action of poisons, the details of their several effects, the mode of detecting them in all varying circumstances, and their antidotes and treatment — till he erected Toxicology on a solid foundation as a science."[3]

While Christison was in Paris, the Chair of Medical Jurisprudence in the Institutes of Medicine, Edinburgh University, became vacant, and his friends proposed him as a candidate. On January 3, 1822, in his twenty-fourth year, Robert Christison became the third man appointed to hold this Chair. Dr. Andrew Duncan, Sr., who introduced forensic medicine as a subject for medical students in Great Britain at Edinburgh in 1791, was instrumental in the creation of the Chair of Medical Jurisprudence in 1807 by royal decree.[4] Christison was an excellent choice for the position; he had acquired a good background in the practical knowledge of disease, was well versed in the theory and practice of chemistry, and had the most recent information on toxicology at hand. Aware of "a vast mine of medico-legal facts" in the German literature, he quickly absorbed that language and added that knowledge to his repertoire in preparation for his new duties. Determined to advance the status of medical jurisprudence and bring honor to the Chair, he decided that toxicology was the subject that would accomplish his purpose. Christison began an earnest course of action that involved experimental studies of the chemistry of poisons and extensive searches into the literature on the physiology, pathology, and symptomatology of poisoning. In the span of eleven years, his abilities in systematizing information succeeded in increasing his class numbers from twelve to ninety and earning him the reputation as the leading medical jurist in Scotland.

The circumstances leading to the appearance of the *Treatise* are explained best by the author himself, along with his evaluation of the work written sometime between 1870 and 1879. "My materials accumulated far beyond what could be used for my lectures. I therefore determined to gratify mine enemy by writing a book; but the *Treatise on Poisons*, first published in 1829, met with no enemy. In my own opinion, the best part of the book is the summation of my whole toxicological studies in the introductory dissertation on General Poisoning. This is the view of the medico-legal relations of poisoning in the abstract — a new inquiry, comprising all the various ways in which, in criminal trials, the history of the symptoms during life, the appearances after death, and the chemical investigation, may bear, not merely on the discovery of poison, but likewise on all branches of the general evidence, or, as it is usually called, the moral evidence. I do not think there is any statement in that dissertation which does not stand good to the present day."[5]

The scope of his knowledge and his appointment as a professor in medical jurisprudence quickly involved him in the law courts. One of the first cases Christison took part in was the trial of William Burke and Helen M'Cougal. He was one of the doctors who performed the postmortem examination on a victim of Burke and William Hare. The case was notorious for the fact that Burke and Hare murdered by strangulation for the profit in selling the corpses for medical studies. Christison's testimony in that case[6] was to prove to be the deliberate statement of medical opinion in the clear and impartial language that characterized his demeanor in many criminal cases to follow. Often his examinations of the medical aspects of a case brought the proceedings to a halt before trial by showing proof of innocence on the suspect's part or demonstrating inadequate proof of guilt from the criminal investigation. In time the respect for both nonpartisan conduct and thorough professional examination by Christison resulted in a steady decrease in the cross examination of his testimony. His desire to improve the status of medical jurisprudence led him to draw up instructions for the examination of dead bodies which became the accepted format in such proceedings.

Soon after the second edition of the *Treatise*, Christison resigned the Chair of Medical Jurisprudence to accept the Chair of Materia Medica in 1833. In the next forty-five years, he gained a reputation in this field equal to that he had established for himself in medical jurisprudence. His abilities to combine the strengths of several sciences gave a distinct flavor to his teaching and work on medical agents. As he had heard of toxicology from the pioneer Orfila in Paris, he had heard of pharmaceutics from the pioneers Pierre J. Pelletier and Joseph B. Caventou. Christison became the first pharmaceutical chemist in Scotland and published a work in 1842 representing contemporary advancements in chemistry, pharmacy, and therapeutics. Its attributes were distinctly Christison — clear and precise exposition, considered generalization, and extensive empirical knowledge. He was still concerned with the questions of poisoning and investigated doses in excess of therapeutic amounts among the more active substances in the medicinal agents. His interest in the physiological concepts of Francois Magendie and Magendie's pupil, Claude Bernard, was expressed in public and before an academic commission. Several of his students were the first in Scotland to begin investigations in the emerging field of pharmacology.

It was Christison's intent to advance the study of therapeutics to as high a level as he had taken the study of toxicology. The success of the Medical Faculty of the University of Edinburgh unfortunately intervened. Students, attracted from abroad to this center of learning, returned to their own countries and established effective teaching centers. Gradually this resulted in diminished income and Christison, among others, found it necessary to engage in private practice. His position as a physician increased to a leading role and forced him to reduce and then withdraw from teaching. A publication in 1838 on kidney disease along with a number of papers in the *Edinburgh Medical Journal* added to his reputation. At the age of seventy he finally ceased his consulting practice, which had become the largest and most remunerative in Scotland.

Throughout his long career he displayed an ingenious ability in conducting experimental investigations and in designing appartus. Typical of Christison's attention to chemical and pharmacological phenomena in toxicological investigations is his paper on "On the poisonous properties of Hemlock, and its alkaloid Conia."[7] He replicated the German work on isolation of the active principle and confirmed many facts concerning the chemical and the physiological nature of the product. Christison experimented with higher forms of animals in seeking to explain the poisonous effects of hemlock. His results led him to conclude that the soluble salts of conia were as poisonous as the base in accordance with physiological laws of absorption. He was intrigued by the question of how the rapid action of this substance was promulgated but confounded by an inability to measure the distribution of the poison in the blood. Part of Christison's paper summarized the existing knowledge in his usual style of integrating available information. One remark of his alludes to the difficult problem of human response facing every investigator: "I wish I could have added to these observations on the poisonous effects of conia and hemlock, some account of their physiological properties in small doses. This branch of the inquiry into their action I have not been able to investigate. It cannot be pursued with any accuracy by experiments on the lower animals. The phenomena must be ascertained in the human subject chiefly, which I have not hitherto been able to accomplish."[8]

The accomplishments of Christison brought him honors and distinctions from many countries as well as from Scotland. The University of Edinburgh took the unprecedented step, while he was still a professor, of conferring upon him the degree of LL.D. which required the setting aside of an academic order prohibiting such action. He was an honorary member of several foreign scientific and medical societies, such as the Royal Academy of Medicine of Paris and the Hufelandian Medico-Chirurgical Society of Berlin. On two occasions he presided over the Royal College of Physicians of Edinburgh. From 1868 to 1873 Christison held the Presidency of the Royal Society of Edinburgh. The British Medical Association elected him to the Presidentship in 1875. On the recommendation of Prime Minister Gladstone the highest distinction accorded a member of his profession was conferred — a baronetcy.

A physically robust man, Christison delighted in athletic activity. His endurance remained at a high level through most of his life. Mountain climbing was a pastime till his eightieth year although he continued thereafter a walking exercise on level ground. In the last year of his life, physical impairment advanced rapidly, yet his mental faculties seemed little affected. Death occurred on January 27, 1882.

Brian Parker
Stanford Research
Institute
Menlo Park, Calif.

NOTES

1. *The Life of Sir Robert Christison, Bart.*, Ed. by His Sons, Blackwood, Edinburgh vol. 1 *Autobiography* (1885) vol. 2 *Memoirs* (1886)

2. *Ibid*, vol. 1, p. 269

3. *Ibid*, vol. 1, p. 241

4. Littlejohn, Henry H., "Deparment of Forensic Medicine, University of Edinburgh, Edinburgh, Scotland" in *Methods and Problems of Medical Education* The Rockefeller Foundation New York 1928 (Reprinted in the International Microfilm Journal of Legal Medicine *1* (1) cards 3, 5 (Fall 1965)).

5. *Life*, vol. 1, p. 298

6. "The crimes and trial of Burke and Hare," *International Microfilm Journal of Legal Medicine 5* (4) cards 8-14 (1970); Christison, R. "Cases and observations in medical jurisprudence . . . IV Murder by Strangling, with some remarks on the effects of external violence on the human body soon after death," *Edinburgh Medical and Surgical Journal 31* 229 (1829)

7. *Transactions of the Royal Society of Edinburgh, 13*:383 (1836)

8. *Ibid* p. 398

PREFACE

TO THE FOURTH EDITION.

THE author regrets that circumstances beyond his con-
trol have delayed the re-appearance of the present work
beyond the period at which it was called for by the favourable reception of the last edition. He has endeavoured to
take advantage of the numerous investigations which have
been carried on during the interval into the several depart-
ments of Toxicology in the leading countries of Europe;
and has in consequence been led to enlarge the work materially.

He trusts it may be allowed him to express his satisfaction at finding, that the rapid progress made by Toxicological
science during the last eight years, while it has been pro-
ductive of many important additions to our knowledge, has
nevertheless not rendered any important alterations necessary either in the general principles formerly laid down in
this work, or in what had been there stated as well ascertained general facts.

EDINBURGH COLLEGE,
November, 1844.

CONTENTS.

PART FIRST.

OF GENERAL POISONING.

~~~~~~~~~~

CHAPTER I.

ON THE PHYSIOLOGICAL ACTION OF POISONS.

I SHALL discuss this subject by considering first the mode in which poisons act, and secondly, the causes by which their action is liable to be modified.

SECTION I. — *On the Mode of Action of Poisons.*

On attending to the effects which follow the application of a poison to the body, we perceive that they are sometimes confined to the part where it is applied, and at other times extend to distant organs. Hence the action of poisons may be naturally considered as *local* and *remote*.

The local effects of poisons are of three kinds. Some decompose chemically or corrode the part to which they are applied. Others, without immediately injuring its organization, inflame or irritate it. Others neither corrode nor irritate, but make a peculiar impression on the sentient extremities of the nerves, unaccompanied by any visible change of structure.

We have examples of local *corrosion* or chemical decomposition in the effects of the concentrated mineral acids or alkalis on the skin, and in the effects of strong oxalic acid, lunar caustic, or corrosive sublimate on the stomach. In all of these instances the part to which the poison is applied undergoes chemical changes, and the poison itself sometimes undergoes chemical changes also. Thus oxalic acid dissolves the gelatin of the animal textures; and in the instance of corrosive sublimate, the elements of the poison unite with the albumen, fibrin, and other principles of the tissues.

Of local *irritation* and its various consequences we have many examples, from redness, its slightest, to ulceration and gangrene, its most severe effect. Thus externally, alcohol reddens the skin; cantharides irritates the surface of the true skin and causes vesication; tartar-emetic causes deep-seated inflammation of the true skin and a

3

pustular eruption; the juice of manchineel* spreading inflammation of the subcutaneous cellular tissue; arsenic inflammation of all these textures, and also death of the part and subsequent sloughing. Internally, alcohol reddens the stomach, as it does the skin,—but more permanently; while other substances, such as the diluted mineral acids, arsenic, cantharides, euphorbium, and the like, may cause all the phenomena of inflammation in the stomach and intestines, namely, extravasation of blood, effusion of lymph, ulcers, gangrene. Many of these irritants, such as arsenic, are in common speech called corrosives; but they have not any power of causing chemical decomposition: if they produce a breach in the texture of an organ, it is merely through the medium of inflammation and its effects.

Of *nervous impressions*, without any visible organic change, few well authenticated and unequivocal instances are known. A good example has been mentioned by Sir B. Brodie in the effect of monkshood on the lips when chewed,† an effect which I have also often experienced: it causes a sense of numbness and tingling in the lips and tongue, lasting for some hours, and quite unconnected with any affection of the general nervous system. Another instance, first mentioned to me by M. Robiquet, and which I have verified, occurs in the effects of the strong hydrocyanic acid: when this acid is confined in a glass tube with a finger on its open end, the point of the finger becomes benumbed, exactly as from the local action of great cold. These are undoubted instances of a purely nervous local impression on the external surface of the body. The most unequivocal instance I know of a similar impression on internal parts is a fact related by Dr. W. Philip with regard to opium.‡ When this poison was applied to the inner coat of the intestines of a rabbit during life, the muscular contractions of the gut were immediately paralyzed, without the general system being for some time affected. The same effect has been observed by Messrs. Morgan and Addison to follow the application of ticunas to the intestine:§ an instant and complete suspension of the peristaltic movement took place as soon as it touched the gut. A parallel fact has also been described by Dr. Monro, *secundus:*‖ when an infusion of opium was injected between the skin and muscles of the leg of a frog, that leg soon became palsied, while the animal was able to leap briskly on the other three. Analogous results have farther been obtained with the prussic acid by M. Coullon.¶ He remarked, that when one hind-leg of a frog was plunged in the acid, it became palsied in thirty-five minutes, while the other hind-leg continued perfectly sensible and irritable. Acetate of lead probably possesses the same property.

These facts are important, because some physiologists have doubted whether any local impressions of a purely nervous nature, uncon-

* Orfila and Ollivier, Archives Générales de Médecine, x. 360.
† Philosophical Transactions, 1811, 186.
‡ Experiments on Opium, 1795, reprinted in his Treatise on Fevers, iv. 697.
§ Essay on the Operation of poisonous agents on the living body, 1829, p. 63.
‖ Edin. Phys. and Lit. Essays, iii. 311.
¶ Researches sur l'Acide Hydrocyanique, 1819, p. 179.

nected with appreciable organic change, may arise from the action of poisons. Yet the existence of impressions of the kind is essential to the stability of the doctrine of the sympathetic operation of poisons,—that is, of the transmission of their influence from organ to organ along the nerves. Nay, in the instance of many poisons supposed to act in that manner, we must still farther believe in the existence of primary nervous impressions, which are not only unconnected with organic change, but likewise undistinguishable by any local sign whatsoever.

Of the three varieties in the local effects of poisons—corrosion, irritation, and nervous impressions,—the first two may take place in any tissue or organ; for example, they have been observed on the skin, on the mucous membrane of the stomach, intestines, windpipe, air tubes, bladder, and vagina, in the cellular tissue, in the serous membranes of the chest and abdomen, in the muscular fibre. We are not so well acquainted with the nature of local nervous impressions on different tissues; but it is probable that in some textures of the body they are very indistinct.

So much for the local effects of poisons.

On tracing the phenomena which follow more remotely, we observe that the affected part sometimes recovers without any visible change, sometimes undergoes the usual processes consequent on inflammation, sometimes perishes at once and is thrown off; and if the organ is one whose function is necessary to life, death may gradually ensue, in consequence of that function being irrecoverably injured. The purest example of the last train of phenomena is to be seen in the occasional effects of the mineral acids or alkalis: death may take place simply from starvation, because the inner surface of the stomach and intestines is so much injured that a sufficient quantity of nutriment cannot be assimilated.

But death and its antecedents can seldom be accounted for in this way. For symptoms are often witnessed, which bear no direct relation to the local injury: death is generally too rapid to have arisen from the function of the part having been annihilated: and the rapidity of the poisoning is not proportional in different cases to the local injury produced. Even the mineral acids and alkalis seldom kill by impeding or annihilating digestion, because they often prove fatal in a few hours; and among other poisons there are few which ever cause death simply by disturbing the function of the part primarily acted on. Death and the symptoms preceding it arise from an injury of some other organ, to which they are not and cannot be directly applied. We are thus led to consider their remote action.

The term *remote* is here used in preference to the common phrase *general* action, because the latter implies an action on the general system or whole body; whereas it appears that an action of such a kind is rare, and that most poisons which have an indirect action exert it on one or more of the important organs only, and not on the general system.

There is not a better instance of the remote action of poisons than oxalic acid.   It has been already mentioned that concentrated oxalic acid is a corrosive: yet it never kills by destroying the function of the stomach.   Man, as well as the lower animals, will live several days or weeks without nutriment.   Now this poison has been known to kill a man in ten minutes, and a dog in three minutes only.   Neither does it always induce, when swallowed, symptoms of an injury of the stomach; for death is often preceded by tetanus, or apoplexy, or mortal faintness.   Nor is the violence of the poisoning proportional to the extent of the local injury : in fact, death is most rapid under circumstances in which the stomach is least injured, namely, when the acid is considerably diluted.*

Let us now proceed to enquire, then, in what way the influence of a poison is conveyed from one organ to another.

Here it will at once be perceived that the conveyance can be accomplished in one of two ways only.   Either the local impression passes along the nerves to the organ secondarily affected ; or the poison enters the bibulous vessels, mingles with the blood, and passes through the medium of the circulation.   In the former way poisons are said to act through *sympathy*, in the latter, through *absorption*.

1. *On the Action of Poisons through Sympathy.*   In the infancy of toxicology all poisons were believed to act through sympathy.   Since Magendie's discoveries on venous absorption in 1809, the favourite doctrine has on the other hand been, that most, if not all, act through the medium of the blood.   And a recent theory, combining both views, represents that, although many poisons do enter the blood, the operation even of these nevertheless consists of an impression made on the sentient extremities of the nerves of the blood-vessels and conveyed thence along their filaments to the brain or other organs.

The nerves certainly possess the power of conveying from one organ to another various impressions besides those of the external senses.   This is shown by many familiar phenomena ; and in reference to the present subject, is aptly illustrated by the remote or sympathetic effects of mere mechanical injury and natural disease of the stomach.   Acute inflammation of the stomach generally proves fatal long before death can arise from digestion being stopped ; and it is accompaned with constitutional symptoms, neither attributable to injury of that function, nor developed in so marked a degree during inflammation in other organs.   These symptoms and the rapid death which succeeds them are vaguely imputed to the general system sympathizing with the affected part; but it is more probable that one organ only is thus, at least in the first instance, acted on sympathetically, namely, the heart.   The effects of mechanical injuries are still more in point.   Wounds of the stomach may prove fatal before inflammation can begin ; rupture from over-distension may cause instant death ; and in either case without material hemorrhage.

* Experimental Inquiry on poisoning with oxalic acid. By Dr. Coindet and my‑ self. — Edin. Med. and Surg. Journal, xix. *passim.*

These observations being held in view, it is impossible to doubt, that some organs sympathize with certain impressions made on others at a distance; nor can we imagine any other mode of conveyance for these impressions except along the nerves. The question, then, comes to be what are the impressions that may be so transmitted?

The statements already made will prepare us to expect a sympathetic action in the case of poisons that manifestly injure the structure of the organ to which they are applied. In the instance of the pure corrosives its existence may be presumed from the identity of the phenomena of their remote action with those of natural disease or mechanical injury. It was stated above that the mineral acids when swallowed often prove fatal in a very short space of time; and here, as in mere injury from disease or violence, the symptoms are an imperceptible pulse, fainting, and mortal weakness. Remote organs therefore must be injured; and from the identity of the phenomena with those of idiopathic affections of the stomach, even if there were no other proof, it might be presumed that the primary impression is conveyed along the nerves. We are not restricted, however, to such an argument: The presumptive inference is turned to certainty by the effect of dilution on the activity of these poisons. Dilution materially lessens or even takes away altogether the remote action of the mineral acids. Now dilution facilitates, instead of impeding their absorption: consequently they do not act on remote organs through that channel. There is no other way left by which we can conceive them to act, except by conveyance of the local impression along the nerves. — As to the irritants that are not corrosive, it can hardly be doubted, since they inflame the stomach, that the usual remote effects of inflammation will ensue, namely, a sympathetic injury of distant organs.

But it remains to be considered, whether distant organs may sympathize also with the peculiar local impressions called nervous, — which are not accompanied by any visible derangement of structure. This variety of action by sympathy is the one which has chiefly engaged the attention of toxicologists; and it has been freely resorted to for explaining the effects of many poisons. Nevertheless its existence is doubtful.

The only important arguments in support of the sympathetic action of poisons are, that unequivocal instances exist of local nervous impressions being conveyed to a limited extent along the nerves, — and that the rapidity of the effects of some poisons is so great as to be incompatible with any other medium of action except the nervous system.

In the first place it is maintained, that a limited nervous transmission, that is, the conveyance of a local impression, purely functional in its nature, to parts at a short distance from the texture acted on directly, must occur in some instances, — as, for example, in the action of belladonna in dilating the pupil when applied to the conjunctiva of the eye, and in the effect of opium in allaying deep-seated pain when applied to the integuments over the affected part. It is by no means

4

clear, however, that nervous transmission is in such circumstances the only possible medium of action ; and that the phenomena may not as well be owing to the agent being conveyed in substance, by imbibition or absorption, to the parts ultimately acted on.   It is not unworthy of remark too, that in the case of hydrocyanic acid, — a poison, which, more perhaps than any other, has been held to act by sympathy, and which produces on the integuments a direct local impression of a peculiar and unequivocal kind, — there is positive evidence of the direct impression not being conveyed along the nerves, even to the most limited distance ; for I have not been able to observe the slightest effect beyond the abrupt line on the skin which defines the spot with which the acid had been in contact.

Secondly, it is thought that certain poisons, such as hydrocyanic acid, strychnia, alcohol, conia, and some others, produce their remote effects with a velocity, which is incompatible with any conceivable mode of action except the transmission of a primary local impulse along the nerves, and more especially incompatible with the poison having followed the circuitous route of the circulation to the organs which are affected by it remotely.   Thus in regard to the hydrocyanic acid, Sir B. Brodie has stated,* that a drop of the essential oil of bitter almonds, which owes its power to this acid, caused convulsions instantly when applied to the tongue of a cat ; and that happening once to taste it himself, he had scarcely applied it to his tongue, when he felt a sudden momentary feebleness of his limbs, so that he could scarcely stand.   Magendie,† speaking of the pure hydrocyanic acid, compares it in point of swiftness of action to the cannon ball or thunderbolt.   In the course of certain experiments made not long ago with the diluted acid by Dr. Freer, Mr. Macaulay and others,‡ to decide the true rapidity of this poison, several dogs were brought under its influence in ten, eight, five, and even three seconds ; during an experimental inquiry I afterwards undertook for the same purpose,§ I remarked on one occasion that a rabbit was killed outright in four seconds ; and Mr. Taylor has more recently stated, that he has seen the effects induced so quickly in cats, that there was no sensible interval of time between the application of the poison to the tongue and the first signs of poisoning.‖   Strychnia, the active principle of nux-vomica, acts sometimes with a speed little inferior to that of hydrocyanic acid ; for Pelletier and Caventou have seen its effects begin in fifteen seconds.¶   Alcohol, according to Sir B. Brodie,** also acts on animals with equal celerity ; for when he introduced it into the stomach of a rabbit, its effects began when the injection was hardly completed.   Conia, the active principle of hem-

* Philosophical Transactions, 1811, p. 184.
† Annales de Chimie et de Physique, vi. 349.
‡ Report of the Trial of Freeman for the murder of Judith Buswell, London MedicalGazette, viii. 796-8.
§ See subsequently the chapter on Hydrocyanic acid.
‖ Taylor's Medical Jurisprudence. p. 18.
¶ Annales de Chim. et de Phys. xxvi. 54.
** Philosophical Transactions, 1811, p. 182.

lock, is not less prompt in its operation: when it was injected in the form of muriate into the femoral vein of a dog, I was unable, with my watch in my hand, to observe an appreciable interval between the moment it was injected and that in which the animal died;[*] certainly the interval did not exceed three or at most four seconds.

Facts such as these have been long held adequate to prove that some poisons must act on remote organs by sympathy or transmission of a local impulse along the nerves; and in the last edition of this work they were acknowledged to warrant such a conclusion. It was thought difficult to account for the phenomena on the supposition that the poison was conveyed in substance with the blood to the organ remotely affected by it; for it appeared impossible that, in so short a space of time as elapsed in some of the instances now referred to, the poison could enter the veins of the texture to which it was applied, pass into the right side of the heart, follow the circle of the pulmonary circulation into the left side of the heart, and thence be transmitted by the arterial system to the capillaries of the organ ultimately affected. But the progress of physiological discovery has lately brought the soundness of these views into question. Some years ago Dr. Hering of Stuttgardt showed that the round of the circulation may be accomplished by the blood much more speedily than had been conceived before; for the ferrocyanide of potassium, injected into the jugular vein of a horse, was discovered by him throughout the venous system at large in the short space of twenty or thirty seconds, and consequently must have passed in that period throughout the whole double circle of the pulmonary and systemic circulation.[†] This discovery at once shook the validity of many, though not all, of the facts which had been previously referred to the agency of nervous transmission on the ground of the celerity with which the effects of poisons are manifested. More recently an attempt has been made by Mr. Blake to prove, that the circulation is so rapid as to admit even of the swiftest cases of poisoning being referred to the agency of absorption. Mr. Blake, who is altogether opposed to the occurrence of nervous transmission in the instance of any poison, has found that ammonia, injected into the jugular vein of a dog, was indicated in its breath in four seconds; and that chloride of barium or nitrate of baryta, introduced into the same vessel, could be detected in the blood of the carotid artery in about sixteen seconds in the horse, in less than seven seconds in the dog, in six seconds in the fowl, and in four seconds in the rabbit.[‡] These interesting discoveries, however, will not absolutely destroy the conclusiveness of all the facts quoted above in support of the existence of a sympathetic action. For example they do not shake the validity of those observations, in which it appeared that an interval inappreciable, or barely appreciable, elapsed between the application and action of hydrocyanic acid and of conia. Mr. Blake indeed denies the accuracy of

[*] Trans. Royal Soc. of Edinburgh, xiii. 393.
[†] Zeitschrift für die Physiologie, iii. i. 81.
[‡] Edin. Med. and Surg. Journal, liii. 35, and lvi. 412.

these observations, insisting that, in those he made himself with the
most potent poisons, he never failed to witness, before the poison
began to act, an interval considerably longer' than what had been
observed by others, and longer also than what he had found sufficient
for the blood to complete the round of the circulation ; that, for example, the wourali poison injected into the femoral or jugular vein
did not begin to act for twenty seconds, conia and tobacco for fifteen
seconds, and extract of nux vomica for twelve seconds ; and that
hydrocyanic acid dropped on the tongue did not act for eleven seconds if the animal was allowed to inhale its vapour, and not for
sixteen seconds, if direct access to the lungs was prevented by making
the animal breathe through a tube in the windpipe.   But Mr. Blake
cannot rid himself thus summarily of the positive facts which stand
in his way.   Duly weighed, the balance of testimony is in favour of
those whose accuracy he impugns.   For in the first place, they had
not, like him, a theory to build up with their results, but were observing, most of them at least, the simple fact of the celerity of action.
Then, their result is an affirmation or positive statement, and his
merely a negative one : They may perfectly well have observed
what he was not so fortunate as to witness.   And lastly, it is not
unreasonable to claim for Sir B. Brodie, Dr. Freer, Mr. Macaulay,
and Mr. Taylor, all of them practitioners of experience, the faculty
of noting time as accurately as Mr. Blake himself.   As for my own
observations, I feel confident they could not have been made more
carefully, and that I had at the moment no preconceived views
which the results upheld, but, if anything, rather the reverse.

It is impossible therefore to concede, that Mr. Blake's inquiries,
merely because they are at variance with prior results, apparently
not less precise and exact than his own, put an end to the argument
which has been drawn, in favour of the existence of a sympathetic
action, from the extreme swiftness of the operation of some poisons.
At the same time, on a dispassionate view of the whole investigation,
it must be granted to be doubtful, whether this argument can be now
appealed to in its present shape with the confidence which is desirable.   And on the whole, the velocity of the circulation on the one
hand, and the celerity of the action of certain poisons on the other,
are both of them so very great, and the comparative observation of
the time occupied by the two phenomena respectively becomes in
consequence so difficult and precarious, that it seems unsafe to found
upon such an inquiry a confident deduction on either side of so important a physiological question as the existence or non-existence of
an action of poisons by sympathy.

In concluding these statements it is necessary to notice certain
positive arguments which have been brought against the doctrine of
nervous transmission.

It is alleged to be contrary to nature's rule to adopt two ways of
attaining the same end ; and therefore, that, since many poisons undoubtedly act through absorption, it is unphilosophical to hold that
others act by sympathy.   There seems no sound reason, however, for

thus imposing arbitrary limits on the functional powers conferred by nature on the organs of the animal body. And besides, the presumption thus derived is counterbalanced by the equally plausible supposition, that, — since nature has clearly established an action on remote organs through the medium of the nerves in the case of poisons which cause destruction or inflammation of the tissues to which they are applied, — the same medium of action may also exist in the instance of poisons which produce merely a peculiar nervous impression where they are applied.

But it is farther alleged, that poisons of the most energetic action have no effect, when they are applied to a part, the connection of which with the general system is maintained by nerves only. It is true that poisons seem to have no effect whatever when the circulation of the part to which they are applied has been arrested, or when every connecting tissue has been severed except the nerves. Thus Emmert found that the wourali poison does not act on an animal when introduced into a limb connected with the body by nerves alone.* And I have ascertained that in the same circumstances no effect is produced on the dog by pure hydrocyanic acid dropped into the cellular tissue of the paw. But it cannot be inferred absolutely from these facts, that the wourali poison and hydrocyanic acid do not act through sympathy; because it has been urged that the integrity of the functions of the sentient extremities of the nerves, more especially their capability of receiving those nervous impressions which are held to be communicated backwards along their course, may be interrupted by arresting the circulation of the part. Still, as the function of sensation is maintained for some time in a severed limb connected with the trunk by nerves only, there is a probability, that all other functions of the nerves must be retained for a time also. And the presumption thus arising is strengthened by an imperfect experiment performed by Mr. Blake, which tends to show, although it does not absolutely prove, that a poison, introduced into the severed limb whose nervous connection with the trunk is entire, will not act, even if the blood be allowed to enter the limb by its artery and to escape from a wound in its vein, so that local circulation is in some measure maintained, without the blood returning to the trunk and general system.†

On considering impartially all the facts that have been adduced in this inquiry, an impression must be felt that the doctrine of the sympathetic action of those poisons which produce merely a nervous local impression is insecurely founded. But an *experimentum crucis* is still wanted to decide the question.

2. *Of the Action of Poisons through Absorption.* — If doubts may be entertained whether poisons ever act by the transmission of local impulses, from the part to which they are applied, along the nerves to the organ upon which they act, no reasonable doubt can be enter-

* Archiv. für Anatomie und Physiologie, iv. 192.
† Ed. Med. and Surg. Journ. liii. 46

tained that many poisons act through the medium of absorption into
the blood.

Poisons are believed to act through the blood for the following
reasons. First, they disappear during life from the shut cavities or
other situations into which they have been introduced; that is, they
are absorbed. Several clear examples to this effect have been related by Dr. Coindet and myself in our paper on oxalic acid. In
one experiment four ounces of a solution of oxalic acid were injected
into the peritoneal sac of a cat, and killed it in fourteen minutes;
yet, on opening the animal, although none of the fluid had escaped
by the wound, we found scarcely a drachm remaining.* In recent
times Professor Orfila has proved that various poisons, such as arsenic,
tartar-emetic, and acetate of lead, disappear in part or wholly from
wounds into which they had been introduced.† Next, many poisons
act with unimpaired rapidity, when the nerves supplying the part to
which they are applied have been previously divided, or even when
the part is attached to the body by arteries and veins only. Dr.
Monro, *secundus*, proved this in regard to opium;‡ and the same
fact has been since extended by Sir B. Brodie and Professor Emmert
to wourali,§ by Magendie to nux vomica,‖ by Coullon to hydrocyanic acid,¶ by Charret to opium,** and by Dr. Coindet and myself
to diluted oxalic acid.†† Magendie's experiment was the most precise of all: for, besides the communication with the poisoned part
being kept up by a vein and an artery only, these vessels were also
severed and reconnected by two quills. Farther, many poisons will
not act when they are applied to a part of which the circulation has
been arrested, even although all its other connections with the body
have been left entire. This has been shown distinctly by Emmert
in regard to the hydrocyanic acid; which, when introduced into the
hind-leg of an animal after the abdominal aorta has been tied, produces no effect till the ligature be removed, but then acts with
rapidity.‡‡ An experiment of a similar nature performed by Mr.
Blake with the wourali poison yielded the same result.§§ Again,
many poisons act with a force proportional to the absorbing power
of the texture with which they are placed in contact. This is the
criterion which has been commonly resorted to for discovering whether a poison acts through the medium of the blood. It is applicable,
however, only when the poison acts sensibly in small doses; for
those which act but in large doses cannot be applied in the same
space of time over equal surfaces of different textures. The difference
in the absorbing power of the different tissues has been well ascer-

* Ed. Med. and Surg. Journ. xix. 335.
† Bull. de l'Acad. Roy. de Méd. iii. 426, et *passim*.
‡ Edin. Phys. and Lit. Essays, iii. 334.
§ Philosophical Transactions, 1811, 198; and Archiv. für Anatomie und Physiologie,
iv. 192.
‖ Sur le Mechanisme de l'Absorption, 1809; republished, in Journ. de Physiol. i. 26.
¶ Recherches sur l'Acide Hydrocyanique, 180.
** Revue Médicale, 1827, i. 515.
†† Edin. Med. and Surg. Journal, xix. 173.
‡‡ Diss. Inaug. de Venenatis acidi Borussici effectibus. Tubingæ, 1805.
§§ Edin. Med. and Surg. Journal, liii. 45.

tained in respect to a few of them only. The most rapid channel of absorption is by a wound, or by immediate injection into a vein ; the surface of the serous membranes is a less rapid medium, and the mucous membrane of the alimentary canal is still less rapid. Now it is proved of many poisons that, when applied in similar circumstances to these several parts or tissues, their activity is proportional to the order now laid down. Lastly, it has been proved of nux-vomica, that if the extract be thrust into the paw of an animal after a ligature has been tightened round the leg so as to stop the venous, but not the arterial circulation of the limb, blood drawn from an orifice in a vein between the wound and the ligature, and transfused into the vein of another animal, will excite in the latter the usual effects of the poison, so as even to cause death ; while, on the contrary, the animal from which the blood has been taken will not be affected at all, if a sufficient quantity be withdrawn before the removal of the ligature. These interesting facts, which are capable of important practical applications, were ascertained by M. Vernière.*

On weighing attentively the arguments here brought forward, it seems impossible to doubt, that some poisons are absorbed into the blood before they act, and that their entrance into the blood is not a mere fortuitous antecedent, but a condition essential to their action.

But it is farther held that poisons which act through absorption, do so by being conveyed in substance along with the blood to the part where their action is developed, — that their action eventually depends on the organ, whose functions are thrown into disorder, becoming impregnated with poisoned blood. Now, the arguments detailed above do not absolutely prove this conveyance and impregnation. They show that poisons enter the blood, and act somehow in consequence of entering it ; but they do not prove in what manner the action subsequently takes place.

It was at one time indeed supposed that the same facts, which prove their admission into the blood, proved also their transmission in substance to the organs acted on by them. But Dr. Addison and Mr. Morgan have shown that this is not a legitimate conclusion, and that a different theoretical view may be taken of the facts, — namely, that the action may really take place by the poison producing on the sentient extremities of the nerves of the inner membrane of the blood-vessels a peculiar impression which is conveyed through the nerves to the part ultimately affected.† They have endeavoured to found this theory upon evidence, that the poison is not carried beyond the venous system ; or that, if conveyed farther, it is carried incidentally, and not for the purpose of impregnating the textures of the organ which suffers. The evidence they have brought forward on this head is chiefly the following. 1. Poisons which act on a particular organ at a distance do not act more quickly when introduced into the artery which supplies it, than when introduced into its vein, or even into the principal artery of a distant part of the body.‡ 2.

* Journal des Progrès des Sciences Méd. 1827, iii. 121.
† Essay on the Operation of Poisonous Agents on the Living Body.
‡ Essay, &c. pp. 75, 76.

If a poison be introduced into a great vein with a provision for pre-venting its passage towards the heart, it will act with as great ra-pidity, as if no obstacle of the kind existed. Thus, if the jugular vein, secured by two temporary ligatures, be divided between them and re-connected by a tube containing wourali, the animal will not be affected more quickly on the removal of both ligatures, than on removing only the ligature farthest from the heart.[*]   3. The arterial blood of a poisoned anmal is incapable of affecting another animal. Thus, if the carotid artery and jugular vein of one dog be divided, and both ends of each reciprocally connected by tubes with the di-vided ends of the corresponding vessels of another dog, and extract of nux-vomica be introduced into a wound in the face of one of them, — the animal directly poisoned alone perishes, and the other remains unharmed to the last.[†]

These are at first view strong arguments against the transmission of poisons with the blood to the organs remotely acted on ; and the facts on which they are founded are on the other hand easily explained under the new theory advanced by the authors, that the medium of action is the nerves which supply the inner membrane of the blood-vessels.   But their inquiries, however ingenious and plausible, have not stood the test of physiological scrutiny.   Their first experimen-tal fact has been contradicted by Mr. Blake ; who has found that the wourali poison, which does not begin to act for twenty seconds when injected into a vein, will produce obvious effects in seven seconds only if injected into the aorta through the axillary artery.[‡]   The second experiment, showing that poison confined in a vein will act although prevented by a ligature from reaching the heart, is held by the op-ponents of Dr. Addison and Mr. Morgan to be fallacious, in as much as the blood behind the ligature may be carried backwards till it meets with an anastomosing vein and is so carried by a collateral vessel to the heart.   To the third experiment it may be objected, that there was, in the mode in which they conducted it, no satisfac-tory evidence that the reciprocal circulation was kept up by the carotid artery and jugular vein.   And this will appear an important objection to every one practically acquainted with experiments of transfusion.   For on the one hand it is exceedingly difficult, in such complicated experiments, to prevent coagulation of the blood in one vessel or another, before the connection of all the arteries and veins is established ; and on the other, it may be urged, as Mr. Blake has done, that the pressure of the blood in the distal end of the carotid artery in the animal not directly poisoned may be equal, or even superior, to the pressure in the proximal end of the same vessel in the other animal, — so that the blood may not pass from the latter into the former, although it should continue fluid.

In opposition to the theory of Dr. Addison and Mr. Morgan, and in support of the doctrine, that poisons act by being carried in sub-stance with the blood into the tissues of the remote organs on which they act, a variety of important experimental evidence has been

* Essay, &c. pp. 69, 71.   † Ibidem, pp. 81, 87.
‡ Edin. Med. and Surg. Journal, liii. 35.

brought forward since the publications of the Essay of these gentlemen.   In the first place, the concurrent testimony of a great number
of recent chemical inquirers establishes undeniably, that poisons absorbed into the veins of the part to which they are applied are to be
detected throughout many of the tissues of distant organs.   This fact
will be enlarged on and illustrated presently.   Secondly, on the authority of Mr. Blake, and in contradiction of the experiments of Dr.
Addison and Mr. Morgan, it appears that, as already stated, poisons
act more quickly when injected into the aorta than into the venous
system ; a fact which is easily understood, on considering that when
injected into the aorta they reach their destination directly, whereas,
if injected into a vein they must first arrive at the right side of the
heart, and then be transmitted through the circle of the pulmonary
circulation before reaching even the aorta.   Thirdly, the relative rapidity with which poisons act on different animals follows the ratio of
the velocity of the circulation in each.   Thus, Mr. Blake found, that
in the horse nitrate of baryta is conveyed by the circulation from the
jugular vein to the carotid artery in sixteen seconds, and that strychnia
injected into the jugular vein begins to act on the nervous system
after exactly the same interval : That in the dog chloride of barium
passes from the vein to the artery in seven seconds, and extract of
nux-vomica begins to act as a poison in twelve seconds : That in the
fowl the passage of the blood seems to take place in six seconds,
and the nitrate of strychnia to act in six seconds and a half : And that
in the rabbit the passage of the blood is effected in four seconds only,
and the first signs of the action of strychnia occur in four seconds
and a half.*

On the whole, then, it may be considered as well established,
that probably all, but certainly some, poisons, — of the kind whose
topical action does not consist in causing destruction or inflammation
of the textures to which they are applied, — produce their remote
effects solely by entering the blood, and through its means impregnating the organs which are acted on at a distance.   And farther,
if this doctrine be admitted as established, it may also be allowed,
that many poisons which do cause topically destruction or inflammation, and remotely the usual sympathetic effects of these changes of
structure, also possess the power of affecting distant organs through
the medium of the blood.

Of the discovery of Poisons in the Blood. — Such being the case,
it becomes an object of paramount interest, with reference both to
the practice of medical jurisprudence, to inquire whether poisons
can be detected in the circulating fluids, or generally in parts of the
body remote from the place where they are introduced.

A variety of circumstances long rendered it impossible to determine satisfactorily the question, whether poisons could be detected
in the blood, the secretions, and the soft textures of the body.   In
the first place, we now know that the quantity of the more active
poisons, which is required to occasion death, is so small, that, con-

* Ed. Med. and Surg. Journal, lvi. 412.

5*

sidering the crude methods of analysis formerly trusted to, and the obstacles opposed to the successful application of them by the presence of organic matter, there can be no wonder that chemists, even but a few years ago, could not satisfy themselves whether the objects they were in search of had been detected or not. Then, it was partly known before, and is now fully established, that various poisons are removed beyond the reach of analysis before death, in consequence of passing off with the secretions, particularly the urine. Farther, it seems probable that, of the poisons which act through absorption, several do not remain or at least do not accumulate, in the blood; and that they are not distributed with it throughout the textures indifferently, but are deposited, as absorption goes on, in particular organs, such as the liver, — which it was not much the practice to examine in former investigations. And lastly, some poisons are speedily decomposed on entering the blood: They either cause obvious changes in the constitution of the blood, and themselves undergo alteration likewise; or without the blood becoming appreciably different in its properties from the healthy state, the poison undergoes a rapid change in the molecular affinities of its elements, and so disappears. Of the former course of things distinct illustrations are furnished by nitric oxide gas and sulphuretted-hydrogen gas when injected into a vein in a living animal: of the latter an equally unequivocal example occurs in oxalic acid, which Dr. Coindet and I found to be undiscoverable in the blood of the vena cava of a dog killed in thirty seconds by the injection of eight grains and a half of it into the femoral vein.

But the improvements that have been lately made in the methods of analysis for the detection of poisons in a state of complex mixture with organic substances have done away with a great part of the obstacles which prevented a thorough inquiry as to the existence of poisons in the blood and textures of the body. Some important researches of this kind were referred to in the last edition of the present work; and since then many additional facts, of equal variety and precision, have been communicated by different observers, but especially by Professor Orfila. Under the head of each poison an account will be given hereafter of the evidence in support of the discovery of it by chemical analysis in the blood, textures, and excretions. In the present place it is sufficient to state in general terms that the evidence is quite satisfactory in the instances of iodine, sal-ammoniac, oxalic acid, nitre, sulphuret of potassium, arsenic, mercury, copper, antimony, tin, silver, zinc, bismuth, lead, hydrocyanic acid, cyanide of potassium, carbazotic acid, sulphuretted-hydrogen, camphor, and alcohol.

Of the Organs affected by the remote action of Poisons. — Having now taken a general view of the mode in which poisons act on distant parts, I shall next consider what organs are thus brought under their operation. Poisons have been often, but erroneously, said to affect remotely the general system. A few of them, such as arsenic and mercury, do indeed appear to affect very many organs of the body. But by much the larger proportion seem on the contrary to act on one or more organs only, not on the general system.

Of the poisons which act remotely through a sympathy of distant parts with an organic injury of the textures directly acted on, many appear to act sympathetically on the heart alone. Taking the mineral acids as the purest examples of poisons that act independently of absorption into the blood-vessels, it will be seen on inquiry that all the symptoms they produce, in addition to the direct effects of the local injury, are those of depressed action of the heart, — great feebleness, fainting, imperceptible pulse, cold extremities. Even the less prominent of the secondary symptoms are almost all referrible to a depressed state of the circulation. In particular, they are not necessarily, and indeed are seldom actually, blended with any material symptom of disorder in the brain ; which certainly could not be the case if the general or whole system suffered.

With respect to that more numerous class, which act remotely either through the medium of the blood or by the transmission along the nerves of an undiscernible impression made on their sentient extremities, some certainly possess a very extended influence over the great organs of the body ; but the greater number are much more limited in their sphere of action. Some act chiefly by enfeebling or paralyzing the heart, others principally by obstructing the pulmonary capillaries, others by obstructing the capillaries of the general system, others by stimulating or depressing the functions of the brain or of the spinal cord, others by irritating the alimentary canal, others by stimulating one or another of the glandular organs, such as the salivary glands, the liver, the kidneys, or the lymphatic glands.

Some poisons of this kind act chiefly, if not solely, on the *heart*. The best examples are infusion of tobacco, and upas antiar. Sir B. Brodie observed, that when the infusion of tobacco was injected into any part of the body, it speedily caused great faintness and sinking of the pulse ; and on examining the body instantly after death, he found the heart distended and paralyzed, not excitable even by galvanism, and its aortal cavities filled not with black, but with florid blood, while the voluntary muscles were as irritable as after other kinds of death.* The upas antiar he found to be similarly circumstanced.† Arsenic and oxalic acid are also of this kind. In an animal killed by arsenic, and in which the gullet and voluntary muscles continued long contractile, Dr. Campbell found the heart immediately after death containing arterial blood in its aortal cavities, and insensible to galvanism.‡ Dr. Coindet and I frequently witnessed the same facts in animals killed with oxalic acid : When the heart at the moment of death was completely palsied and deprived of irritability, we saw the intestines moving, and the voluntary muscles contracting long and vigorously from the mere contact of the air.§

* Philosophical Transactions, 1841, p. 186. When death begins with any other organ but the heart, the heart remains irritable for some time after, and contains black blood in all its cavities.

† Ib. p. 196.   ‡ Diss. Inaug. de Venenis Mineralibus. Edinburgi, 1813.
§ Edin. Med. and Surg. Journal, xix. *passim.*

An interesting series of investigations has been lately made by Mr. Blake, relative to the influence of poisons on the heart, when they are directly introduced into the great veins. It does not absolutely follow that an action on the heart manifested in this way proves the occurrence of a similar action when the substance is admitted into the body through more ordinary channels, such as the stomach, intestines or cellular tissue. For on the one hand, some of the substances used by this physiologist cannot be admitted into the blood through ordinary channels in the quantity necessary for developing that action on the heart, which is excited when they are injected at once into the blood-vessels. And on the other hand, the results at which he thus arrives are not always in conformity with what have been obtained by prior observers, who resorted to the ordinary channels for introducing poisons into the body. It is possible, therefore, that Mr. Blake's researches may not have the extensive bearings, which might at first sight appear, on the physiology of poisons and remedies. Nevertheless they are in themselves full of interest. They show that the salts of magnesia, zinc, copper, lime, strontia, baryta, lead, silver, ammonia, and potash, also oxalic acid, and digitalis, if injected into the jugular vein, produce a powerful and permanent depression of the heart's action ; which is evinced by the hæmadynamometer,* indicating diminution of pressure in the great arteries, by the heart becoming motionless or nearly so before the breathing ceases, by its muscular structure presenting little or no irritability when stimulated immediately after death, and by the left cavities being found full of florid arterial blood.*

Other poisons act on the *lungs ;* but probably few, perhaps none, act on them alone. Magendie found that in poisoning with tartaremetic the lungs are commonly inflamed and sometimes even hepatized.† Mr. Smith and M. Orfila both remarked similar signs of pulmonary inflammation in animals poisoned with corrosive sublimate.‡ But these poisons produce important effects on other organs likewise.

A set of novel and important facts setting forth the frequent operation of poisons on the lungs when they are admitted directly into the blood, has been recently brought to light by the researches of Mr. Blake. Many of the poisons mentioned above as acting powerfully on the heart were found by him not to exert any influence upon the lungs, such as oxalic acid and the salts of magnesia, lime, zinc, copper, ammonia, potash, and strychnia. Others, however, such as the salts of strontia, baryta, lead, and silver, as well as digitalis, all of which powerfully affect the heart, and, in addition to these, the salts of soda, which have no action at all on the heart, and hydrocyanic acid, tobacco, and euphorbium, which influence it feebly, or even

---

* Edin. Med. and Surg. Journal, li. 330 ; liv. 339 ; lvi. 104. The Hæmadynamometer is an instrument invented by M. Poiseulle, which, when communicating with the interior of a blood-vessel, indicates the force of the circulation by the pressure of the blood on a column of mercury.

† Mémoire sur l'Emétique — Bulletins de la Société Philomatique, 1812-13, p. 361.

‡ Orfila, Toxicologie Générale, i. 258.

dubiously, — produce, when injected into the jugular vein, obstruction of the capillaries of the pulmonary circulation, and consequently asphyxia. This is proved by the hæmadynamometer introduced into a vein indicating great increase of pressure in the venous circulation a few seconds after the introduction of the poison ; by this instrument introduced into the femoral artery indicating great diminution of arterial pressure, although the heart continues to beat vigorously; by the breathing becoming at the same time laborious, without the heart suffering ; by these symptoms preceding any signs of action on the nervous system ; by the heart pulsating for some time after death ; and in many instances by frothy mucus having accumulated in the air-passages, and congestion and extravasation having taken place in the lungs themselves.*

A great number of the poisons whose action is remote, operate on the *brain*. The most decided proof of such an action is the nature of the symptoms ; which are, giddiness, delirium, insensibility, convulsions, palsy, coma. Some physiologists have also sought for evidence in the body after death, and have imagined they found it in congestion of the vessels in the brain, and even extravasation of blood there ; but it will be seen under the head of Narcotic Poisons that such appearances are far from being essential, and indeed are seldom witnessed. All narcotic poisons act on the brain, and most narcotico-acrids too ; but very frequently other organs are affected at the same time, and in particular the spine and heart.

The influence of poisons on the brain seems to be sometimes induced, not immediately, but indirectly through the intervention of a more direct influence on the pulmonary circulation. Thus Mr. Blake appears to have succeeded in proving that the insensibility and tetanic convulsions which immediately precede death, when certain substances, such as the salts of soda, are injected into the veins, depend simply on the obstruction directly produced in the pulmonary circulation causing increased pressure in the systemic veins, and consequently upon the brain and nervous centre generally. For when the jugular vein was opened after the development of tetanic convulsions, and blood was allowed to flow out, the nervous symptoms ceased, and the animal continued for two hours sensible and without any return of convulsions, dying eventually of hemorrhage.† But more generally the effect produced on the brain is direct and specific. Thus opium and its active principle morphia suspend the functions of external relation, which are peculiarly dependent on the brain ; while for a long time the respiration and circulation are little affected. Even when the poison is admitted directly into the veins, the pulmonary capillaries are not obstructed, and the heart is only somewhat enfeebled in its contractions ;‡ and in ordinary cases of poisoning with these substances the heart continues to pulsate, and the lungs also discharge their office, long after sensibility is extinguished and voluntary motion arrested, — until at length the circulation and re-

* Edin. Med. and Surg. Journal, lvi. 104, and other papers there quoted above.
† Ibid. liv. 121.   ‡ Ibid. li. 344.

spiration become affected consecutively by the depressed state of the
nervous system.

Some poisons act specifically on the *spinal cord*. Those which
are best known to possess such an action are nux-vomica, the other
species of plants which, like it, contain strychnia, and also conia and
the wourali poison. The tribe of poisons of which nux-vomica may
be taken as the type excite violent fits of tetanus, during the intervals
of which the mind and external senses are quite entire ; and death
takes place during a paroxysm, apparently from suffocation caused
by spasmodic fixing of the chest. Their action on the spine is quite
independent of any action on the brain ; if indeed such action exist
at all. For when the spinal cord is separated from the brain by
dividing the medulla oblongata, the effects on the muscles supplied
by the spinal cord are produced as usual.* Conia, the active principle of hemlock, according to my own researches, produces in the
lower animals, howsoever introduced, gradually increasing paralysis,
without insensibility or delirium, and without the circulation or
respiration being for some time affected, till at length death takes
place from stoppage of the breathing by palsy of the respiratory
muscles ; and after death the heart continues beating vigorously,
the muscles contract when irritated, and arterialization of the blood
in the lungs may be kept up long by maintaining artificial respiration. In this instance it would appear, that the first effect is arrestment of the functions of the spinal cord ; that the paralysis does not
depend upon a direct action on the muscles ; and that neither the
brain, heart, nor lungs can be influenced, except secondarily through
the consequences of general muscular paralysis.† Many poisons
which act on the brain also act on the spinal cord.

Other poisons apparently possess the singular property of impeding
or arresting the *general capillary circulation*, and produce their tan-
gible effects more or less through the medium of this operation.
Such at least are the inferences which seem to flow from the researches of Mr. Blake ; who found that many substances, soon after
they are injected backwards by the axillary artery into the aorta,
produce increased pressure in the arterial system indicated by the
hæmadynamometer during life, and frequently congestion of the membranous textures as observed after death. Some substances have no
effect of this kind. Others act on the general capillaries in concurrence with a similar action on the capillaries of the pulmonary circulation, such as the salts of strontia, baryta, lead, silver, and soda,
euphorbium, tobacco and digitalis. But a few, such as potash and
ammonia, with their salts, seem to influence the capillaries of the
general circulation only.‡ These are important conclusions, if legitimate ; but it cannot be denied, that the facts on which they are
based must be very difficult to isolate and observe with accuracy and
without bias.

* Emmert, Archiv. für Anatomie und Physiologie, i. l. 180. See also the Article
False Angustura.
† Transactions of the Roy. Soc. of Edinburgh. xiii.
‡ Edin. Med. and Surg. Journal, li. 330, liv. 339, lvi. 104.

The organs not immediately necessary to life may be likewise all acted on by poisons indirectly. On this subject details are not called for at present. It may be sufficient to remark that there is hardly a considerable organ in the body, except perhaps the spleen and pancreas, which is not acted on by one poison or another. Arsenic inflames the alimentary mucous membrane, mercury the salivary organs and mouth, cantharides the urinary organs, chromate of potass the conjunctiva of the eyes, manganese the liver; iodine acts on the lymphatic glands; lead on the muscles; and spurred rye causes gangrene of the limbs.

Some poisons, as was already mentioned, may act on one important organ only, every other being left undisturbed: thus nux-vomica in general acts only on the spine. But much more commonly they act on several organs at once; and the action of some of them is complicated in an extreme degree. I may instance oxalic acid and arsenic. Oxalic acid when swallowed irritates and inflames the stomach directly, and acts indirectly on the brain, the spine, and the heart. A large dose causes sudden death by paralyzing the heart; if the dose is somewhat less, the leading symptom is violent tetanic spasm, indicating an action on the spine, and death takes place during a paroxysm, the heart continuing to contract for some time after; if the dose is still less, the spasms, at first distinct, become by degrees fainter and fainter, while the sensibility in the intervals, at first unimpaired, becomes gradually clouded, till at length pure coma is formed without convulsions, — thus indicating an action on the brain. As for arsenic, coupling together the symptoms during life and the appearances in the dead body, it will be seen afterwards to have the power of acting on the brain, heart, and lungs, — the throat, gullet, stomach, and intestines, — the lining membrane of the nostrils and eyelids, — the kidneys, bladder, and vagina; and, what is remarkable, proofs of an action on all these parts may be witnessed in the course of a single case. The effects of mercury are hardly less multifarious.

SECTION II. — *On the Causes which modify the Actions of Poisons.*

By a variety of causes the action of poisons may be modified both in degree and in kind. The most important of them are — quantity; state of aggregation; state of chemical combination; mixture; difference in tissue; difference in organ; habit; idiosyncrasy; and lastly, certain states of disease.

1. *Quantity* affects their action materially. Not only do they produce their effects more rapidly in large doses; it is sometimes even quite altered in kind. A striking example has just been related in the case of oxalic acid; which, according to the dose, may corrode the stomach, or act on the heart, or on the spine, or on the brain. In like manner arsenic in a small dose may cause gastritis of several days' duration; while a large dose may prove fatal in two or three hours by affecting the action of the heart. White hellebore in small doses excites inflammation in the stomach and bowels, in larger doses giddiness, convulsions, coma; and in either way it may prove fatal.

2. *As to state of aggregation,* — poisons act the more energetically the more minutely they are divided, and hence most energetically when in solution. Some which are very energetic in the fluid state, hardly act at all when undissolved. Morphia, the alkaloid of opium, may be given in powder to a dog without injury in a dose, which, if dissolved in oil or alcohol, would soon kill several. Previously dissolving poisons favours their action in two ways, — by diffusing them quickly over a large surface, and by fitting them for entering the bibulous vessels. Poisons, before being absorbed, must be dissolved ; and hence, those which act though solid and insoluble in water, must, as a preliminary step, be dissolved by the animal fluids at the mouths of the vessels. In this way the poisonous effects of carbonate of baryta and arsenite of copper are explained ; for though insoluble in water, they are soluble in the juices of the stomach.

Differences in aggregation, like differences in quantity, may affect the kind as well as the degree of action. Camphor in fragments commonly causes inflammation of the stomach ; dissolved in spirit or olive oil, it causes delirium or tetanus and coma.

The reduction of certain poisons to the state of vapour serves the same end as dissolving them. When poisons are to be introduced by the skin, no previous operation is more effectual than that of converting them into vapour.

3. The next modifying cause is *chemical combination.* This is sometimes nothing more than a variety of the last. If a poison, in combining with another substance, acquire greater solubility, it also generally acquires greater activity, and *vice versa :* Morphia, itself almost inert, because insoluble, becomes active by uniting with acids, for they render it very soluble : Baryta as a very active poison, becomes quite inert by uniting with sulphuric acid, for the sulphate of baryta is altogether insoluble.

In regard to the influence of chemical combination two general laws may be laid down. One is, that *poisons which only act locally, have their action much impaired or even neutralized, in their chemical combinations.* Sulphuric acid and muriatic acid on the one hand, and the two fixed alkalis on the other, possess a violent local action ; but if they are united so as to form sulphates or muriates, although still very soluble, they become merely gentle laxatives. But the case is altered if either of the combining poisons also act by entering the blood. For the second general law is, that *the action of poisons which operate by entering the blood, although it may be somewhat lessened, cannot be destroyed or altered in their chemical combinations.* Morphia acts like opium if dissolved in alcohol or fixed oil ; if an acid be substituted as the solvent, a salt is formed which is endowed with the same properties : The sulphate, muriate, nitrate, acetate of morphia all act like opium. Strychnia, arsenic, hydrocyanic acid, oxalic acid, and many more come under the same denomination : Each produces its peculiar effects, with whatever substance it is combined, provided it do not become insoluble.

Mr. Blake has recently laid down what may be considered a branch or corollary of the second of these general propositions, and has confirmed it by many appropriate experimental facts,—namely, that *the salts of the same base produce the same actions, independently of the acids with which they are combined.** The law, however, is a more general one, as given above, and was stated in former editions of the present work. It applies not only to bases, but likewise to acids, such as the hydrocyanic, oxalic, arsenious, and arsenic acids, and also to neutral organic principles which act through the blood, such as picrotoxin, colocynthin, elaterin, and narcotin.

The same author considers it to be also a probable conclusion from a variety of experiments on the salts of various bases, that *those salts which are isomorphous, or possess the same crystalline form, are closely allied in action.*†

4. The effect of *mixture* depends partly on the poisons being diluted. Dilution, by prolonging the time necessary for their being absorbed, commonly lessens their activity; yet not always; for if a poison which acts through the blood is also a powerful irritant, moderate dilution will enable it to enter the vessels more easily: a small dose of concentrated oxalic acid acts feebly as an irritant or corrosive; moderately diluted, it quickly enters the blood and causes speedy death.‡ The effect of mixture may depend also in part on the mere mechanical impediment interposed between, the poison and the animal membranes. This is particularly obvious when the mass containing the poison is solid or pulpy; for then the first portions of the poison that touch the membrane may cause an effort of the organ to discharge the rest beyond the sphere of action,—if, for example, it is the stomach,—by vomiting. The effect of mixture in interposing a mechanical impediment is also well illustrated where the substance mixed with the poison is a fine, insoluble powder, capable of enveloping its several particles. Thus it is that small, yet poisonous doses of arsenic may be swallowed and retained with impunity, if mixed with finely powdered charcoal, magnesia, and probably cinchona-bark, or the like. Besides diluting and mechanically obstructing their application, the admixture of other substances may alter the chemical nature of poisons, and so change their action.

It is important to keep in view, that the influence of mixture may be exerted in consequence of the cavity into which a poison is introduced being at the time filled with contents. Some of the most powerful and unerring poisons may in such circumstances altogether fail to produce their usual effect, if speedily vomited. Thus Wibmer notices the case of a man, who swallowed an ounce and a half of arsenic after a very hearty meal, had merely a severe attack of vomiting with subsequent colic, and got quite well in four days.§ And a still more pointed instance has been briefly mentioned by Dr. Booth of Birmingham, where an ounce of corrosive sublimate was swallowed after a full meal without any material ill consequence, vomiting having been speedily induced.||

* Archives Gén. de Med. Nov. 1839, and Edin. Med. and Surg. Journal, lvi. 106.
† Ibidem, lvi. 123 and 422.　　　　　‡ Ibid. xix. 326, 327.
§ Die Wirkung der Arzneimittel und Gifte, i. 278. || London Med. Gazette, xiv. 63.

5. *Difference of tissue* is an interesting modifying power in a physiological point of view, but does not bear so directly on medico-legal
practice as the rest, and may therefore be passed over cursorily.

On the corrosives and irritants a difference of tissue acts but indirectly: their effects vary not so much with the tissue as with the
organ of which it forms part. But as to poisons which act through
the blood, their energy must evidently depend on the activity of absorption in each texture.

The cutaneous absorption is slow, on account of the obstacle presented by the cuticle, and by the intricate capillaries of the true skin.
Accordingly many active poisons are quite inert when applied to the
unbroken skin, or even to the skin deprived of the cuticle. Hydrocyanic acid, perhaps the most subtle of all poisons, was found by
Coullon to have no effect when dropped on the skin of a dog.* Some
authors have even gone so far as to deny that poisons can be absorbed at all through the skin, unless they are pressed by friction
through the cuticle. But this is an error ; most gaseous poisons, such
as carbonic acid and sulphuretted hydrogen, and some solid poisons
when volatilized, such as the vapours of cinnabar, will act though
simply placed in contact with the skin ; and there is distinct evidence
that corrosive sublimate will bring on mercurial action in the form of
warm bath, or when used as a liniment.

On the mucous membrane of the stomach and intestines, poisons
act much more energetically than on the skin ; which clearly depends
in a great measure on the superior rapidity of absorption there, — or,
according to some, on the facility with which poisons come in contact with the sentient extremities of nerves.

The serous membranes possess an activity of absorption which
hardly any other unbroken texture can equal. Accordingly many
poisons act much more rapidly through the peritonæum than through
the stomach. When oxalic acid is introduced under the same
collateral circumstances into the stomach of one dog and the peritonæum of another, the dose may be so apportioned, that the same
quantity, which does not prove fatal to the former, kills the latter in
fourteen minutes.†

While the preceding modes in which poisons enter the blood are
indirect, they may be introduced directly by a wound in the vein.
There is no way in which poisons, that act through the blood, prove
more rapidly fatal. Some which act very slowly through the stomach cause instant death when injected into a vein. A peculiar variety of this mode of introducing poisons deserves to be distinguished,
namely, the application of them to a wound. If the surface bleeds
freely, they may not act at all, because they are washed away. But
if they adhere, they soon enter the divided veins. Hence, if they act
in small doses, this mode of applying them is hardly less direct than
if they were at once injected into a vein.

So far the effect of difference in tissue has been determined.

* Recherches sur l'Acide Hydrocyanique, 140.
† Edin. Med. and Surg. Journal, xix. 330.

Poisons that act through the blood act least energetically on the skin, more actively on the alimentary mucous membrane, still more so on serous membranes, and most powerfully of all when introduced directly into a vessel. There are other textures, however, which merit notice, although their place in the scale of activity has not been exactly settled.

On the mucous membrane of the pulmonary air-cells and tubes, poisons act with a rapidity which is scarcely surpassed by their direct introduction into a vein. This is plainly owing to the exceeding delicacy and wide surface of the membrane. Hence three or four inspirations of carbonic oxide gas will cause instant coma. A single inspiration of the noxious gas of privies has caused instant extinction of sense and motion. Nay, liquid poisons have been known to act through the same channel with almost equal swiftness. For M. Ségalas found that a solution of extract of nux-vomica caused death in a few seconds when injected in sufficient quantity into the windpipe; and that half a grain will thus kill a dog in two minutes, while two grains will rarely prove fatal when injected into the stomach, peritonæum, or chest.*

As to the nervous tissue, it is a fact worthy of mention, that the poisons which appear to act on the sentient extremities of the nerves, do not act at all on the cut surface of the brain and nerves, or upon any part of the course of the latter. This has been proved with respect to most active narcotics.

The power of the cellular tissue as a medium of absorption, has not been, and cannot easily be, ascertained. On the one hand it is difficult to apply poisons to it, without also applying them to the mouths of divided vessels; and, on the other hand, it is difficult to make a set of experiments for comparison with others on the stomach, pleura, or peritonæum, as the cellular tissue does not form an expanded cavity, and consequently, the extent of surface to which a poison is applied cannot be made the same in each experiment of a series. It is a ready medium, however, for admitting poisons into the blood, especially if an artificial cavity be made where the tissue is loose, as, for example, by separating the skin from the muscles of the back with the finger introduced through a small incision in the integuments.

The variations caused by difference of tissue in the activity of poisons have been viewed in the previous remarks as depending chiefly on the relative quickness with which absorption goes on. But in this way it is impossible to explain the whole amount of the differences sometimes observed. Some poisons cause death when applied to a wound in the minutest quantity, but are quite harmless when swallowed in large doses: Others are diminished a little in activity, but still remain powerful and fatal poisons. There is not much difference in the power of arsenic when it is applied to different textures, the skin excepted. But oxalic acid injected into the peritonæum will act eight or ten times more rapidly than when swallowed?

* Journal de Physiologie, iv. 285.

and the poison of the viper may prove fatal to a man through a wound in almost invisible doses, while the whole poison of six vipers may be swallowed by so small a creature as a blackbird, with complete impunity.* Differences in the absorbing power of the tissues cannot explain these facts.

The only rational way of accounting for them is by supposing that a part of the poison is decomposed, — the change being greatest where absorption is slowest and the power of assimilation strongest, namely, in the stomach, — and least where absorption is quickest and assimilation almost wanting, namely, in a wound. This explanation derives support from the different effects of change of tissue on poisons of the different kingdoms. Mineral poisons are least, and animal poisons are most, affected in their action by differences of tissue, while vegetable poisons hold the middle place : — an arrangement which coincides with the respective difficulty of decomposition among mineral, vegetable, and animal substances generally, whether under physical or under vital processes.†

6. With respect to differences arising from *difference of organ*, these will, of course, be partly attributable to differences in tissue, but not altogether. For example, in the case of the pure corrosives or irritants, the injury caused will depend for its danger on the importance of the organ to the general economy of the body : Inflammation caused by a local poison in the stomach will be more quickly fatal than that excited in the intestines only; and such a poison may act violently on the external parts without materially impairing the general health.

7. *Habit and Idiosyncrasy.* — The remarks to be made under the present head are important in a medico-legal point of view: for they show how one man may be poisoned by a substance generally harmless, and another not harmed by a substance usually poisonous.

The tendency of *idiosyncrasy* is generally to increase the activity of poisons, or even to render some substances deleterious which are commonly harmless.

The effect of opium in medicinal doses is commonly pleasant and salutary; but in some individuals it produces disagreeable and even dangerous effects. Calomel, which in moderate doses is for the most part a mild laxative or sialagogue, will cause in some people, even in the dose of a few grains, violent salivation, ulceration of the mouth, nay, fatal gangrene. On the other hand, a few substances, which to most people are actively poisonous, have on some individuals comparatively little effect. There are extremely few poisons, however, in regard to which this kind of idiosyncrasy is well-established and prominent. Mercury and alcohol are examples. The compounds of mercury, which in moderate quantity are mildly laxative or sialagogue to most people, but to some persons dangerously poisonous in very small doses, would, on the contrary, appear in

* Giornale di Fisica, ix. 458.

† These views regarding the decomposition of poisons, were suggested to me in 1823 by my friend Dr. Coindet, Junior, of Geneva.

other constitutions to be extremely inactive ; for it has occasionally been found impossible to bring on the peculiar constitutional action of mercury by continuing the use of its preparations for months toge-ther. In general children are not easily affected by calomel as a sialagogue, but easily by its laxative action. As to alcohol, it is a familiar fact, that independently of the effects of habit, there are some constitutions which cannot be brought under the influence of intoxi-cating liquors without an extraordinary quantity of them and a long-continued debauch, while others are overpowered in a short space of time, and by very moderate excess ; and there is no reason to doubt that very great constitutional differences also prevail in regard to the operation of a single large dose. A rarer idiosyncrasy is unusual in-sensibility to the action of opium. I am acquainted with a gentleman unaccustomed to the use of opium who has taken without injury nearly an ounce of good laudanum, — a dose which would certainly prove fatal to most people.

But not only does idiosyncrasy modify the action of poisons : Through its means, too, some substances are actually poisonous to certain individuals, which to mankind in general are unhurtful, nay, even nutritive.

With some people all kinds of red fish, trout, salmon, and even the richer white fish, herring, mackerel, turbot, or holibut, disagree as it is called — that is, act after the manner of poisons : They produce fainting, sickness, pain of the stomach ; and if they were not speedily evacuated by vomiting, dangerous consequences might ensue. The same is often the case with mushrooms. The esculent mushrooms act on some people nearly in the same way as the poisonous varieties. Bitter almonds and other vegetable substances that contain hydrocyanic acid, sometimes produce stupor or nettle-rash in the small quantities used for seasoning food. In like manner many flowers, which to most persons are agreeable and not injurious, cannot be kept in the same room with some people on account of the severe nervous affec-tions that are developed.

This idiosyncrasy may even be acquired. One of my relations, who was for many years violently affected by very small quantities of the richer kinds of fish, used at a previous period to eat them, and can now again do so, with impunity. Many people have acquired a simi-lar idiosyncrasy with respect to eggs ; instances of the same kind will be afterwards mentioned in respect to shell-fish, particularly muscles ; indeed there are probably few articles of food in regard to which such idiosyncrasies may not in a few rare instances be met with, if we ex-cept the grains and common kinds of butcher-meat. I may add, that from facts which have come under my notice, I have sometimes suspected that a similar idiosyncrasy may be acquired in a slight degree, and for a short time only, in regard even to some kinds of butcher-meat, especially the flesh of young animals and pork. On this subject some illustrations will be found at the close of the chapter on dis-eased and decayed animal matter.

It does not appear well ascertained, that the effect of idiosyncrasy
6*

is ever to impair materially the energy of poisons, except in the instances of mercury, alcohol, and opium.

On the contrary, the tendency of *habit* when it does affect their energy, is, with a few exceptions, to lessen it. By the force of habit a person may take without immediate harm such enormous quantities of some poisons as would infallibly kill an unpractised person or himself when he began. There have been opium-eaters in this country who took for days together ten or even seventeen ounces of laudanum daily.

The influence of habit has been ascertained precisely in the case of a few common poisons only. On the whole, it would appear that more change is effected by habit in the action of the organic than in that of the inorganic poisons; and that of the former, those which act on the brain and nervous system, and produce *narcotism*, are altered in the most eminent degree. The best examples of the influence of habit are opium and vinous spirits. The action of such poisons is not always, however, entirely thrown away; they still produce some immediate effect; and farther, by being frequently taken, they may slowly bring on certain disease, or engender a predisposition to disease. A very singular exception to this rule prevails in the instance of tobacco ; which, under the influence of habit, may be smoked daily to a considerable amount, and, so far as yet appears, without any cumulative effect on the constitution, like that of opium-eating or drinking spirits.

The inorganic poisons are most of them little impaired in activity by the force of habit. The pure irritants, indeed, do lose a little of their energy : for it seems that persons have acquired the power of swallowing with impunity considerable doses of the mineral acids. But as to inorganic poisons that enter the blood, habit certainly does not diminish, probably rather increases, their power. There is no satisfactory evidence, that a person by taking gradually-increasing doses of arsenic may acquire the power of enduring a considerably larger dose than when he began : On the contrary, the stomach rather becomes more tender to the subsequent dose by each repetition. I have little hesitation in avowing my disbelief of the alleged cases of arsenic-eaters and corrosive-sublimate-eaters, who could swallow whole drachms at once with impunity. Some have expressed surprise at this statement having been made in former editions of the present work, when there is such authority as Byron, Pouqueville, &c., for the hacknied story of Soleyman, the sublimate-eater of Constantinople, who lived to the age of a hundred, eating a drachm of corrosive sublimate daily. I must avow, however, that such reporters of a feat so very extraordinary, and where deception was so highly probable, are to me no authority at all.

In the relative influence of habit on poisons of the three kingdoms of nature, a new argument will be discovered for the opinion given above respecting the partial decomposition of organic poisons in some of the tissues. In fact this partial decomposition accounts very well for the effect of habit : The effect of habit is probably nothing more than an increased power acquired by the stomach of decomposing the poison,— just as it gradually acquires an increased facility in digesting some alimentary substances which are at first very indigestible.

8. The last modifying cause to be mentioned comprehends certain *diseased states of the body.* The effect of disease, like that of habit, is in general to impair the activity of poisons. But it is only in the instance of a few diseases that this diminution is so strongly marked as to be important in relation to medical jurisprudence. — In the continued fever of this country there is a diminished susceptibility of the constitutional action of mercury ; and this peculiarity is very strongly marked in the yellow fever, as well as in the bilious fevers generally of tropical climates. In some varieties of typhoid fever there is obviously a diminished sensibility to the action of wine and other spirituous liquors ; but this diminution in a great majority of cases is much inferior to what some physicians have represented. — In severe dysentery the susceptibility of the narcotic action of opium is so much impaired, that a person unaccustomed to the use of that drug, may continue to take daily, for several days together, a quantity which might prove fatal to him in a state of health. In the severe form which dysentery occasionally puts on in this coontry I have known a patient take from twenty-four to thirty grains of opium daily, and retain it all, without experiencing more than a mild narcotic action. — In epidemic cholera the same insensibility has been remarked to the operation of opium. — It also occurs in the instance of excessive hemorrhagy. — According to the doctrines and practice of the present dominant school in Italy, there is an unusual insensibility during inflammatory dropsy to the irritant action of gamboge, so that sixty or eighty grains may be taken without harm. — There is no disease, however, in which the power of mitigating the action of poisons is more remarkably exhibited, than in tetanus : It is often scarcely possible to bring on the narcotic action of opium by any doses which can be administered ; calomel, too, acts with much less energy than usual ; and even common purgatives must be administered in doses considerably larger than those required in most other disorders. — Mania is similarly circumstanced : almost all remedies must be given in increased doses, narcotic remedies in particular. But there is good reason for believing that the impaired susceptibility of the action of poisons remarked in this disorder is far from being always so great as some have alleged. — Another disease allied to the last, where the diminution of susceptibility is often great, is delirium tremens. It has in particular been often found, that to produce sleep in this disease opium must be given in frequent large doses, — so large indeed, that they would undoubtedly prove fatal to a person in health. At the same time it is worthy of remark, that in some cases of delirium tremens, even violent in degree, the peculiarity now specified, as I have myself several times witnessed, is far from being strongly marked. — Hydrophobia always, and hysteria sometimes, impair the activity of poisons. I have seen cases of hysteria, more particularly those assuming the form of tetanus, where very large doses of opium were required to produce a calmative effect and sleep ; and in hy-

drophobia it is well shown that the narcotic action of opium is not produced even by large doses often repeated. — The same state occurs in excessive hemorrhage.

In the operation of this class of modifying agents it is a general law, to which there are probably few exceptions, that they chiefly affect poisons of the organic kingdoms, and the narcotics above all. At least in the instance of most mineral poisons their influence is very inferior. Their operation may be accounted for in various ways. Sometimes, as in dysentery and cholera, the poison is carried with unusual rapidity through the alimentary canal. Sometimes again it remains comparatively inert, because on account of the impaired activity of absorption, it is not taken up with the usual quickness by the absorbent vessels. And sometimes, as in the instance of tetanus, mania, and rabies, the nervous system is in a state of peculiar excitement, by which the customary action of the poison is in a great measure, if not entirely, counteracted.

In a few diseased states of the system there is an increased susceptibility of the action of poisons: and it is important that the medical jurist should attend to this circumstance. When a poison has a tendency to bring on a peculiar pathological state of the system, or of a particular organ, which state is also produced by a disease existing at the time or impending, violent and even fatal consequences may ensue from doses of poisons which in ordinary circumstances are innocuous or beneficial. Thus in persons affected with apoplexy an ordinary dose of opium may accelerate death; and in people even with a mere tendency to apoplexy, if it is strongly marked, or appears from what are called warning symptoms to be on the point of developing itself, a common dose of such narcotics as occasion determination to the brain may excite the apoplectic attack. Thus, too, in cases of inflammatory disorders of the alimentary canal, irritating substances, in doses not otherwise injurious, may produce dangerous impressions on the tender membrane with which they come in contact. But in respect to this last example, it must be remarked, that the improvements or the caprice of medical practice have gone directly in face of the rule, by suggesting that some internal inflammations of the alimentary canal may be successfully treated with irritating remedies.

I might here perhaps have added among the causes which modify the action of poisons, sleep, and the administration of other poisons. The latter subject, however, will be better considered at the end of the Individual Poisons, under the title of Compound Poisoning. The former agent is of doubtful effect. Some observations on its influence will be found in the chapter on the Evidence of General Poisoning, p. 41.

Application of the preceding remarks to the Treatment of Poisoning. As an appendix to what has been said respecting the physiological action of poisons, and the causes by which it is liable to be modified, I shall here state shortly certain applications to the treatment of poisoning.

In the instance of internal poisoning, the great object of the physician is to administer an antidote or counter-poison. Antidotes are of two kinds. One kind takes away the deleterious qualities of the poison before it comes within its sphere of action, by altering its chemical nature. The other controls the poisonous action after it has begun, by exciting a contrary action in the system. In the early ages of medicine almost all antidotes were believed to be of the latter description, but in fact very few antidotes of the kind are known.

Chemical antidotes operate in several ways, according to the mode of action of the poison for which they are given. If the poison is a pure corrosive, such as a mineral acid, it will be sufficient that the antidote destroy its corrosive quality : Thus the addition of an alkali or earth will neutralize sulphuric acid, and destroy or at least prodigiously lessen its poisonous properties. In applying this rule care must be taken to choose an antidote which is either inert in itself, or, if poisonous, is, like the poison for which it is given, a pure corrosive or local irritant, and one whose properties are reciprocally neutralized.

If the poison, on the other hand, besides possessing a local action, likewise acts remotely through absorption, or by an impression on the inner coat of the vessels, mere neutralization of its chemical properties is not sufficient ; for we have seen above that such poisons act throughout all their chemical combinations which are soluble. Here, therefore, it is necessary that the chemical antidote render the poison insoluble or nearly so ; and insoluble not only in water, but likewise in the animal fluids, more particularly the juices of the stomach. The same quality is desirable even in the antidotes for the pure corrosives ; for it often happens that in their soluble combinations these substances retain some irritating, though not any corrosive power. When we try by the foregoing criterions many of the antidotes which have been proposed for various poisons, they will be found defective ; and precise experiments have in recent times actually proved them to be so.

The other kind of antidote operates not by altering the form of the poison, but by exciting in the system an action contrary to that established by the poison. On considering attentively, however, the phenomena of the action of individual poisons, it will be found exceedingly difficult to say what is the essence of a contrary action, and still more how that counter-action is to be brought about. Accordingly, few antidotes of the kind are known. Physiology or experience has not yet brought to light any mode of inducing an action counter to that caused by arsenic and most of the irritant class of poisons. It appears probable that the remote operation of lead may be sometimes corrected by mercury given to salivation, and that the violent salivation caused by mercury may be occasionally corrected by nauseating doses of antimony. But these are the only instances which occur to me at present of antidotes for irritant poisoning which operate by counter-action, unless we choose to designate by the name of antidote the conjunction of remedial means which constitute the

antiphlogistic method of cure.   In the class of narcotics we are acquainted with equally few constitutional antidotes, although the nature
of the action of these poisons seems better to admit of them.   Ammonia is to a certain extent an antidote for hydrocyanic acid, but by
no means so powerful as some persons believe ; and I am not sure
that in this class of poisons we can with any propriety mention another
antidote of the constitutional kind.

On the whole, then, it is chiefly among the changes induced by
chemical affinities that the practitioner must look for counter-poisons ;
and the ingenuity of the toxicologists has thence supplied the materia
medica with many of singular efficacy.   When given in time, magnesia
or chalk is an antidote for the mineral acids and oxalic acid, albumen
for corrosive sublimate and verdigris, bark for tartar-emetic, common
salt for lunar caustic, sulphate of soda or magnesia for sugar of lead
and muriate of baryta, chloride of lime or soda for liver of sulphur,
vinegar or oil for the fixed alkalis ; and these substances act either
by neutralizing the corrosive power of the poison, or by forming with
it an insoluble compound.

In recent times a new object in the treatment of poisoning has
been pointed out by the discoveries made in its physiology.   As it
has been proved that many of the most deadly poisons enter the blood,
and in all probability act by circulating with that fluid, so it has been
inferred that an important object in the treatment is to promote their
discharge by the natural secretions.   In support of this reasonable inference it has been lately rendered probable by Orfila, as will be seen
under the head of the treatment of the effects of arsenic, that it is of
great advantage in some forms of poisoning to increase the discharge
of urine.

In the instance of external poisoning the main object of the treatment is to prevent the poison from entering the blood, or to remove
it from the local vessels which it has entered.

One mode, which has been known to the profession from early
times, and after being long in disuse was lately revived by Sir D.
Barry, and applied with success to man, is the application of cupping
glasses to the part where the poison has been introduced.*   This
method may act in various ways.   It certainly prevents the farther
absorption of the poison by suspending for a time the absorbing
power of the vessels of the part covered by the cup.   It also sucks
the blood out of the wound, and may consequently wash the poison
away with it.   Possibly it likewise compresses the nerves around,
and prevents the impression made by the poison on their sentient
extremities from being transmitted along their filaments.

* It is not any part of the object of this work to enter into the history of toxico-
ogy, more especially in early times.   But it may be well here to state, that the claim
which has been made by some for Dr. Barry, of having discovered this mode of
treatment, is groundless.   It is distinctly laid down by Nicander, Celsus, Dioscarides,
Galen, and others who lived in their times ; and among the moderns who have mentioned it, Gräter, in 1767, notices it in his thesis, " de venenis in genere," printed at
Frankfort.   On the ancient history of toxicology the reader will find an excellent
summary by Mr. Adams in the Edinburgh Medical and Surgical Journal, xxxiii. 315,
and a full exposition in Professor Marx's elaborate work, " die Lehre von den Giften."

Another mode is by the application of a ligature between the injured part and the trunk, so as to check the circulation. This is a very ancient practice in the case of poisoned wounds, and is known even to savages. But as usually practised it is only a temporary cure : As soon as the ligature is removed the effects of the poison begin. It may be employed, however, for many kinds of poisoning through wounds, so as to effect a radical cure. We have seen that most poisons of the organic kingdom are in no long time either thrown off by the system or decomposed in the blood. Hence if the quantity given has not been too large, recovery will take place. Now, by means of a ligature, which is removed for a short time at moderately distant intervals, a poison, which has been introduced into a wound beyond the reach of extraction, may be gradually admitted into the system in successive quantities, each too small to cause death or serious mischief, and be thus in the end entirely removed and destroyed. Such is a practical application which may be made of some ingenious experiments performed not long ago by M. Bouillaud with strychnia, the poisonous principle of nux-vomica.*

The last mode to be mentioned is by a combination of the ligature with venesection, deduced by M. Vernière from his experimental researches formerly noticed (p. 19). Suppose a fatal dose of extract of nux-vomica has been thrust into the paw of a dog ; M. Vernière applies a tight ligature round the limb, next injects slowly as much warm water into the jugular vein as the animal can safely bear, and then slackens the ligature. The state of venous *plethora* thus induced completely suspends absorption. The ligature is next tied so as to compress the veins without compressing the arteries of the limb, and a vein is opened between the wound and the ligature in such a situation, that the blood which flows out must previously pass through, or at least near the poisoned wound. When a moderate quantity has been withdrawn, the ligature may be removed with safety ; and the extraction of the poison may be farther proved by the blood that has been drawn being injected into the veins of another animal ; for rapid death by tetanus will be the result.† It is not improbable that in this plan the preliminary production of venous plethora may be dispensed with ; and then the treatment may be easily and safely applied to the human subject.

CHAPTER II.

ON THE EVIDENCE OF GENERAL POISONING.

THIS subject is purely medico-legal. It comprehends an account of the various kinds of evidence by which the medical jurist is enabled to pronounce whether poisoning in a general sense (that is,

* Archives Générales de Médecine, Nov. 1826.
† Journal des Progrès des Sciences Médicales, 1827, iii. 121.

without reference to a particular poison), is impossible, improbable, possible, probable, or certain. It likewise comprises an appreciation of the circumstances which usually lead the unprofessional, as well as the professional, to infer correctly or erroneously a suspicion of such poisoning.

Under the present head might likewise be included the history of poisoning, the art of secret poisoning, and some other topics of the like kind. But the want of proper documents, and the unmeasured credulity which has prevailed on the subject of poisoning throughout all ages down to very recent times, has entangled these subjects in so intricate a maze of fable, that a notice of them, sufficiently detailed to interest the reader, would be quite misplaced in this work.

On the art of secret poisoning, however, as having been once an important object of medical jurisprudence, it might be expected that some comments should here be offered. But really I do not see any good reason for wading through the mass of credulous conjectures and questionable facts, which have been collected on the subject, and which have been copied into one modern work after another, for no other cause than that they are of classic origin, or feed our appetite for the mysterious. No one now seriously believes that Henry the Sixth was killed by a pair of poisoned gloves, or Pope Clement the Seventh by a poisoned torch carried before him in a procession, or Hercules by a poisoned robe, or that the operation of poisons can be so predetermined as to commence or prove fatal on a fixed day, and after the lapse of a definite and remote interval. With regard to the noted instances of secret poisoning, which occurred towards the close of the seventeenth century in Italy and France, it is plain to every modern toxicologist, from the only certain knowledge handed down to us of these events, that the actors in them owed thir success rather to the ignorance of the age, than to their own dexterity. And as to the refined secrets believed to have been possessed by them, it is sufficient here to say, that although we are now acquainted with ten times as many and ten times as subtile poisons as were known in those days, yet none exist which are endowed with the hidden qualities once so universally dreaded.

The crime of poisoning, from its nature, must always be a secret one. But little apprehension need be entertained of the art of secret poisoning as understood by Toffana or Brinvilliers,* or as it might be improved by a modern imitator. It seems to have escaped the attention of those who have written on the subject, that the practice of such an art requires the knowledge not only of a dexterous toxicologist, but also of a skilful physician ; for success must depend on the exact imitation of some natural disease. It is only among medical men, therefore, and among the higher orders of them, that a Saint-Croix can arise now-a-days. How little is to be dreaded on that head is apparent from the domestic history of the European kingdoms for the last half century, compared with their history some centuries

* See the Chapter on Arsenic for some remarks on this subject. — Also Beckman's History of Inventions.

ago. Few medical men have even been suspected, and those few only upon visionary grounds, and under the impulse of violent political feeling.* In one late instance only, so far as I am aware, has it been proved that the physician's art was actually prostituted to so fearful a purpose ; and the detection of the crime in that case shows how difficult concealment will always be wherever justice is administered rigorously, and medico-legal investigations skilfully conducted.†

Two extraordinary incidents which happened lately in Germany may appear at first sight at variance with these views. I allude to the cases of Anna Margaretha Zwanziger and Margaretha Gottfried, which justly excited much interest where they occurred, and are notorious to continental toxicologists. Zwanziger, while serving as housekeeper in various families in the territory of Bayreuth in Bavaria- during the years 1808 and 1809, contrived to administer poison, — sometimes under the instigation of mere revenge or spite, sometimes for the purpose of clearing the way for her schemes of marriage with her masters, — to no fewer than seventeen individuals in the course of nine months ; and of these three died.‡ Gottfried, a woman in affluent circumstances and tolerable station in the town of Bremen, was even more successful. For she pursued her criminal career undiscovered for fifteen years ; and when detected in 1828 had murdered actually fourteen persons, and administered poison unsuccessfully to several others. Her motive, as in the case of Zwanziger, was the mere gratification of a malevolent temper, or the removal of supposed obstacles to her matrimonial dreams. In neither of these instances, however, did the criminal possess any particular skill, or observe much measure in her proceedings. The cases of poisoning were of the common kind, — produced by arsenic, — proving in general quickly fatal, — and presenting the ordinary phenomena. I cannot help thinking, therefore, that the events now alluded to prove rather the ineffectiveness of the police where they happened, than the adroitness of the actors by whom they were brought about; and that they constitute no sound objection to the statement, that the art of secret poisoning is now unknown, and is not likely to be again revived.

It must be granted, indeed, that the late discoveries in chemistry and toxicology have made poisons known which might be employed in such a way as to render suspicion unlikely, and to baffle inquiry. But the methods now alluded to are hitherto very little known ; they cannot easily be attempted on account of the rarity and difficult preparation of the poisons ; they can never be practised except by a person conversant with the minute phenomena of natural disease ; and it is no part of the object of this work to make them public.

* See subsequently the cases of the Crown Prince of Sweden, in the first section of the present chapter, and that of General Hoche, Part II. Chap. ii. Sect. 2.

† I allude to the case of Castaing. See Opium.

‡ Feuerbach. Actenmässige Darstellung Merkwürdiger Verbrechen, i. l. For some observations on the three fatal cases, see the Chapter en Arsenic, under the head of the effects of that poison as an antiseptic.

7

The evidence, by which the medical jurist is enabled to pronounce on the existence or non-existence of poisoning in general, and to determine the subordinate questions that relate to it, is derived from five sources, — 1, the symptoms during life ; 2, the appearances in the dead body ; 3, the chemical analysis ; 4, experiments and observations on animals ; and 5, certain moral circumstances, which are either inseparably interwoven with the medical proof, or cannot be accurately appreciated without medical knowledge.

SECTION I. — *Of the Evidence from Symptoms.*

Not many years ago it was the custom to decide questions of poisoning from the symptoms only. Till the close of last century, indeed, no other evidence was accounted so infallible : and for the simple reason, that in reality the other branches of evidence were even more imperfectly understood. So lately as 1763, and even in Germany, the solemn opinions of whole colleges were sometimes grounded almost exclusively on the symptoms.* About that time, however, doubts began to be entertained of the infallibility of such evidence ; these doubts have since assumed gradually a more substantial form ; and it is now laid down by every esteemed author in Medical Jurisprudence, that the symptoms, however exquisitely developed, can never justify an opinion in favour of more than high probability.† In laying down this doctrine medical jurists appear to me to have injudiciously confounded together actual symptoms with their general characteristics. If the doctrine is to be held as applying to the evidence from symptoms, only so far as they are viewed in questions of general poisoning, — that is, as applying to the general characters merely of the symptoms, — it is deduced from accurate principles. But if it is likewise to be applied, as recent authors have done, to the actual symptoms produced by particular poisons, and in all cases whatever of their action, then it is a rule clearly liable to several important exceptions. These exceptions will be noticed under the heads of the mineral acids, oxalic acid, arsenic, corrosive sublimate, nux vomica, &c. At present it is only the general characters of the symptoms, and the points in which they differ from the general characters of the symptoms of natural disease, that I propose to consider.

The chief characteristics usually ascribed to the symptoms of poisoning considered generally, are, that they commence suddenly and prove rapidly fatal, — that they increase steadily, — that they are uniform in nature throughout their course, — that they begin soon after a meal, — and that they appear while the body is in a state of perfect health.

* See an opinion of the Berlin College in Pyl's Repertorium für die gerichtlichen Arzneikunde. i 244.
† Orfila. Médecine-Légale, ii. 360.
  Henke. Lehrbuch der gerichtlichen Medizin, 448.
  Tortosa. Istituzioni di Medicina Forense, ii. 86.
  Beck's Medical Jurisprudence, 419.

1. The first characteristic is the *suddenness of their appearance and the rapidity of their progress* towards a fatal termination. Some of them act instantaneously, and the effects of most of them are in general fully developed within an hour or little more. But this character is by no means uniform. The most violent may be made to act, so as to bring on their peculiar symptoms slowly, or even by imperceptible degrees. Thus arsenic, which usually causes violent symptoms from the very beginning, may be so administered as to occasion at first nothing more than slight nausea and general feebleness ; and afterwards in slow succession its more customary effects. In like manner corrosive sublimate may be given in such a way as to cause at first mild salivation, and finally gangrene of the mouth. Even many vegetable poisons might be administered in the same way. The well-known consequences of digitalis in medicinal doses will serve as a familiar instance. A still better illustration is supplied by the medicinal effects of the alkaloid of nux-vomica, whose action in other circumstances is most rapid and violent : Strychnia in a moderate dose will cause death by violent tetanus in two or three minutes ; but when given in frequent small doses as a remedy in palsy, it has been known to bring on first starting of the limbs, then stiffness of the jaw, afterwards pain and rigidity of the neck ; and these effects might be increased so gradually, that the patient would seem to die under ordinary tetanus. Nevertheless, the foregoing considerations being kept always in mind, it still remains true, that the effects of poisons for the most part begin suddenly, when the dose is large. This is an important circumstance in regard to certain active poisons, such as the mineral acids, oxalic acid, arsenic, strychnia, &c. For when it is considered that in criminal cases they are given for the most part in unnecessarily large doses, it follows that if the effect ascribed to these poisons in such doses have not begun suddenly, the suspicion is probably incorrect.

The same remarks may be applied to the sudden termination of the symptoms. Poison is for the most part given criminally in doses so large that it proves rapidly fatal. Yet this is not always the case ; the diseased state occasioned by poisons has often been prolonged, as will be seen hereafter, for several weeks, sometimes for several months ; nay, a person may be carried off by a malady, the seeds of which have been sown by the operation of poison years before.

The present would be the proper place for noticing the important question regarding the interval of time, after which, if death supervenes, it cannot be laid to the charge of the person who administered the poison. It is unnecessary, however, to say much on the subject. According to the English law, death must take place within a year. As to the Scottish law, it may be inferred from what has been said by the late Baron Hume on the subject of homicide generally, that a charge of poisoning is relevant although the person should die at a period indefinitely remote, and that it will infer the pains of law, provided the operation of the poison can be distinctly traced, unmodified by extraneous circumstances, from the commencement of the symptoms to the fatal termination.* Of course the influence of these modifying circumstances in lessening the criminal's responsibility will increase with the interval. The question for the medical jurist to determine in such a case would therefore be, the distance of time to which death may be delayed in the case of poisoning generally, and in that of the particular poison. This question cannot be answered even with an approach to precision, except in the instance of a few common poisons. Most vegetable and animal poisons prove fatal either in a few days or not at all; but some mineral poisons may cause death after an interval of many days. It appears probable that arsenic may cause death after an interval of several months, and it is well ascertained that the symptoms of poisoning with the mineral acids have continued uninterruptedly and without modification for eight months, and then terminated fatally.

2. The next general characteristic of the symptoms of poisoning is *regularity in their increase.* It is clear, however, that even this character cannot be universal. For in all cases of slow poisoning by repeated small doses there must be remissions and exacerbations, just as in natural diseases. Besides, as we can seldom watch the symptoms advancing in their simple form, but must endeavour to remove them by remedies, remissions may thus be produced and their tendency to increase steadily counteracted. Farther, some poisons admit of exacerbations and remissions, even when given in one large dose; and there are others, the very essence of whose action is to produce violent symptoms in frequent paroxysms. Of the latter kind are nux vomica, and the other substances that contain strychnia. Of the former kind is arsenic: in cases of poisoning with arsenic it often happens, that after the first five or six hours have been passed in great agony, the symptoms undergo a striking remission for as many hours, and then return with equal or increased violence. Still it is true that on the whole the symptoms of poisoning are steady in their progress; so that this should always be attended to as one of the general characters. In the case of slow poisoning, too, when the most remarkable deviations from it are observed, the very occurrence of exacerbations and remissions, combined with certain points of moral proof, may furnish the strongest evidence possible. Thus, on the trial of Miss Blandy at Oxford in 1752, for the murder of her father, one of the strongest circumstances in proof was, that repeatedly after she gave the deceased a bowl of gruel, suspected to be poisoned, his illness was much increased in violence.†

As connected with the present subject, a question might here be noticed that has been discussed on the occasion of various trials, namely, whether the symptoms of poisoning are susceptible of a complete intermission. It cannot be answered satisfactorily, however, except with reference to particular poisons. The property alluded to has been ascribed to several poisons, even to mercury, arsenic, and opium; but oftener, I believe, in consequence of an improper desire

* Hume on Crimes, i. 178.   † Howell's State Trials, xviii. 1135.

on the part of the witness to prove or to perfect their view of the case, than through legitimate induction from facts.

3. Another characteristic is *uniformity in the nature of the symptoms* throughout their whole progress. This character is the least invariable of them all; for many poisons cause very different symptoms towards the close from those which they cause at the beginning. Arsenic may induce at first inflammation of the alimentary canal, and afterwards palsy or epilepsy; nux-vomica may excite at first violent tetanus, and afterwards inflammation of the stomach and bowels; and corrosive sublimate, after exciting in the first instance inflammation, may prove eventually fatal by inducing excessive ptyalism. In truth, certain changes of this kind in the nature of the symptoms will, in special cases, afford strong presumption, perhaps absolute proof, not only of general poisoning, but even also of the particular poison given. The reason for mentioning so uncertain a character as uniformity in the nature of the symptoms among their characteristics will appear presently.—[pp. 47 & 50.]

4. The fourth characteristic is, that *the symptoms begin soon after a meal*, or rather, soon after food, drink, or medicine has been taken. The occasions on which we eat and drink are so numerous and so near one another, that unless the poison suspected is one which acts with rapidity, it may be difficult to attach any weight to this circumstance. Some poisons rarely produce their effects till a considerable time after they are swallowed; the poisonous mushrooms, for example, may remain in the alimentary canal for several hours or even an entire day and more, before their effects begin; poisonous cheese in like manner may not act for five or six hours,[*] or even a whole day;[†] and that kind of cholera, which is caused in some people by putrid, diseased, and new-killed meat, seldom begins, so far as I have observed, till twelve hours or more after the noxious meal. With regard to the commoner poisons, such as arsenic, corrosive sublimate, the mineral acids, oxalic acid, nux-vomica, and the like, it is a good general rule, that the symptoms, if violent from the beginning, must have begun soon after food, drink, or medicine has been taken.

In making inquiries respecting this point, however, care must be taken not to lose sight of certain circumstances which may cause a deviation from the general rule.

In the first place, it should be remembered that poisons may be administered in many other ways besides mixing them with articles of food or drink, or substituting them for medicines. They may be introduced into the anus; they have been introduced into the vagina; they have also been introduced by inhalation in the form of vapour; and there can be no difficulty in introducing some of them through wounds.

Secondly, another circumstance which may be kept in view is, that, if a person falls asleep very soon after swallowing a poison, es-

* Hünefeld in Horn's Archiv, 1827, i. 203.
† Weiss in Revue Médicale, Janv. 1826.

7*

pecially one of the irritants, the commencement of the symptoms may be considerably retarded, provided it be not one of the powerful corrosives. This statement is not so fully supported by facts as to admit of its being laid down with confidence as a general rule. But from various incidents which have come under my notice it appears not improbable, that sleep does possess the power of putting off for a while the action of some poisons. In particular some instances have occurred to me where arsenic taken at night did not begin to act for several hours, the individual having in the meantime been asleep.[*] The occurrence of so long an interval between its administration and the first appearance of the symptoms is so contrary to what generally happens, that some cause or another must be in activity; and the insensibility of the system during sleep to most sources of excitement seems to supply a sufficient explanation. The slow operation of laxatives during sleep compared with their effects during one's waking hours, is an analogical fact.

A third consideration to be attended to is, that poison may be secretly administered during sleep to a person who lies habitually with his mouth open. This is fully proved by an interesting case which will be noticed under the head of the moral evidence of poisoning. In that particular case the individual immediately awoke, because the poison was concentrated sulphuric acid; but it may admit of question whether a sound sleeper might not swallow less irritating poisons without being awakened. In such circumstances no connexion of course could be traced between the taking of a suspected article and the first appearance of the symptoms.

5. Lastly, *the symptoms appear during a state of perfect health.* This is an important character, yet not universal; for it cannot be expected to apply to cases of slow poisoning, and poisons may be given while the person is actually labouring under natural disease. Cases of the last description are generally very embarrassing; for if, instead of medicine, a poison be administered, whose symptoms resemble the natural disease, suspicion may not arise till it is too late to collect evidence.

It must be apparent from the preceding observations, that the characters common to the symptoms of general poisoning are by no means universally applicable. Yet on reviewing them attentively it will also appear, that, considering the little knowledge possessed by the vulgar of the action of poisons, and consequently the rude nature of their attempts to commit murder by poisoning, the exceptions to the general statements made above will not be numerous.

It now remains to be seen how far these characters distinguish the symptoms of poisoning from those of natural disease ; and

1. As to *the suddenness of their invasion and rapidity of their progress*, it is almost needless to observe, that many natural diseases commences with a suddenness and prove fatal with a rapidity, which few or no poisons can surpass. The plague may prove instantaneously fatal ; and even the continued fever of this country may be fully

* See subsequently the Chapter on Arsenic, Section ii.

formed in an hour, and may terminate fatally, as I have once witnessed, at the beginning of the second day. Inflammation of the
stomach also begins suddenly and terminates soon. Cholera likewise
answers this description : I have known the characters of ordinary
cholera fully developed within an hour after the first warning symptom, and frequently in hot climates, nay, in some rare instances even
in Britain, it proves fatal in a few hours. Malignant cholera frequently proves fatal in a few hours. Inflammation of the intestines,
too, may begin, or at least seem to begin, suddenly and end fatally
in a day : One variety of it, now well known to affect the mucous
membrane, may remain quite latent till the gut is perforated by ulceration, and then the patient is attacked with acute pain, vomiting,
and mortal faintness, and frequently perishes within twenty-four
hours.* But in particular many organic diseases of the heart prove
suddenly fatal, without any previous warning ; and this is also true
to a certain extent even of apoplexy ; for, as will afterwards be seen,
it is an error to suppose that apoplexy is always, or even generally,
preceded by warning symptoms. The first characteristic, therefore,
as applied to the symptoms of poisoning generally, contrasted with
those of general disease, must appear by no means distinctive. But
opportunities will occur afterwards for showing, that it is sometimes
a good diagnostic in the case of particular poisons.†

2. As to the uniformity or *uninterrupted increase of the symptoms*,
it is equally the attribute of many common diseases. I am not aware,
that in speedily fatal cases of the internal *phlegmasiæ* a considerable
remission is often observed. Apoplexy, too, very frequently continues its course without interruption ; and the same may be said of
cholera, and indeed of most acute diseases, when they prove rapidly
fatal.

3. It was stated above, that the third character, *uniformity in kind*
throughout their progress, is by no means an invariable circumstance.
Still less is it distinctive ; for many diseases are marked by great uniformity of symptoms. It has been enumerated nevertheless among
the general characters of poisoning, because, although its presence
can hardly ever add any weight to the evidence in favour of death
by poison, its absence may sometimes afford even positive proof in
favour of natural death. That is, changes of a certain kind occurring
in the symptoms during their progress may be incompatible with the
known effects of a particular poison or of all poisons, and capable
of being accounted for only on the supposition of natural disease
having been at least the ultimate cause of death. This statement,
which is one of some importance, is illustrated by a pointed case,
that of Charles Munn, mentioned at the close of the present section.

4. In the next place, it was observed that some reliance may be
placed on the fact, that the symptoms of poisoning *appear very soon
after a meal.* But we also know this to be the most frequent occa-

* Archives Générales de Médecine, i. 17 ; also Abercrombie on Diseases of the Stomach, &c. 273.
† See Oxalic Acid and Nux Vomica.

sion on which some natural disorders begin. An attack of apoplexy after a hearty meal is a common occurrence. That kind of cholera which follows the immoderate use of acid fruit likewise comes on soon after eating. Sometimes mere excessive distension of the stomach after a meal proves suddenly or instantaneously fatal. Drinking cold water when the body is overheated likewise causes at times immediate death. It appears that perforation of the stomach, the result of an insidious ulcer of its coats, and likewise rupture of the stomach from mechanical causes, are most apt to occur during the digestion, and therefore soon after the taking of a meal.

These few observations will make it evident that the appearing of violent symptoms soon after eating may arise from other causes besides the administration of poison. At the same time, as the diseases which are apt to commence suddenly at that particular time are few in number, and none of them by any means frequent, it is always justly reckoned a very suspicious circumstance; and when combined with certain points of moral proof, such as that several people, who have eaten together, were seized about the same time with the same kind of symptoms, the evidence of general poisoning becomes very strong indeed. Sometimes the evidence from the date of their commencement after a meal may singly supply strong evidence, as in the case of the mineral acids and alkalis, or corrosive sublimate, which begin to act in a few seconds or minutes.

On the other hand, if the symptoms do not begin soon after food, drink, or medicine has been taken (the circumstances being such as to exclude the possibility of poison being introduced by a wound, by the lungs, or by any other channel but the stomach), the presumption on the whole is against poisoning; and sometimes the evidence to this effect may be decisive. The principle now propounded may be often a very important one in the practice of medical jurisprudence; for when united with a little knowledge of the symptoms antecedent to death, it may be sufficient to decide the nature of the case. Thus it is sufficient, in my opinion, to decide the celebrated case of the Crown Prince of Sweden. The prince, while in the act of reviewing a body of troops on the 28th May, 1810, was observed suddenly to waver on his horse; and soon afterwards he fell off while at the gallop, was immediately found insensible by his staff, and expired in half an hour. As he was much beloved by the whole nation, a rumour arose that he had been poisoned; and the report took such firm root in the minds of all ranks, that a party of military, while escorting the body to Stockholm, were attacked near the city by the populace, and their commander, Marshal Fersen, murdered; and Dr. Rossi, the prince's physician, after narrowly escaping the same fate, was in the end obliged to quit his native country. Now, no other poison but one of the most active narcotics could have caused such symptoms, and none of them could have proved so quickly fatal unless given in a large dose. It was proved, however, that on the day of his death the prince had not taken any thing after he breakfasted; and an interval of nearly four hours elapsed after that till he fell from his horse. This fact alone, independently of the marks of apoplexy found in the head after death, and the warning symptoms he repeatedly had, was quite enough to show that he could not have died of poison, as it was incompatible with the known action of the only poisons which could cause the symptoms. This is very properly one of the arguments used by the Medical Faculty of Stockholm, which was consulted on the occasion.*

The same circumstances will often enable us to decide at once a set of cases of frequent occurrence, particularly in towns, — where the sudden death of a person in a family, the members of which are on bad terms with one another, is rashly and ignorantly imputed to poison, without any particular poison being pointed at ; and where, consequently, unless the morbid appearances clearly indicate the cause of death, a very troublesome analysis might be necessary. In several cases of this kind, which have been submitted to me, I have been induced to dispense with an analysis by resting on the criterion now under consideration. The following is a good example.

A middle-aged man, who had long enjoyed excellent health, one afternoon about two o'clock returned home tired, and after having been severely beaten by his wife went to bed. At a quarter past two one of his workmen found him gasping, rolling his eyes, and quite insensible ; and he died in a few minutes. As his wife had often maltreated and threatened him, a suspicion arose that he had died of poison, and the body was in consequence examined judiciously by Sir W. Newbigging and myself. The only appearance of disease we could detect was a considerable tuberculation of the septum cordis and anterior parietes of both ventricles. This disease might have been the cause of death ; for there is no disease of the heart which may not remain long latent, and prove fatal suddenly. But, as the man never had a symptom referrible to disease of the heart, it was impossible to infer, in face of a suspicion of poisoning, that it must have been the cause of death ; since the man might very well have died of poison, the disease of the heart continuing latent. Poisoning, however, was out of the question. The man had taken nothing whatever after breakfasting about nine. Now no poison but one of the most active narcotics in a large dose could cause death so rapidly as in this case ; and the operation of such a poison in such a dose could not be suspended so long as from nine till two. An analysis was therefore unnecessary.

5. Little need be said with regard to *the symptoms beginning, while the body is in a state of perfect health ;* because in truth almost all acute diseases begin under the same circumstances. Connected with this subject, however, a point of difference should be noticed which may be of use for distinguishing poisoning by the irritants from acute diseases of the inflammatory kind : — the latter rarely begin without some adequate and obvious natural cause.

On considering all that has now been said regarding the cha-

* Rossi. Ueber die Art und Ursache des Todes des hochseligen Kronprinzen von Schweden. Berlin, 1812.

racteristics of the symptoms of general poisoning, as contrasted with those of natural disease, no one can hesitate to allow, that from them alone a medical jurist can never be entitled to pronounce that poisoning is certain. At the same time he must not on that account neglect them. For, in the first place, they are of great value as generally giving him the first hints of the cause of mischief, and so leading him to search in time for better evidence. Next, they will often enable him to say that poisoning was possible, probable, or highly probable ; which, when the moral evidence is very strong, may be quite enough to decide the case. Thirdly, although they can never entitle him to say that poisoning was certain, they will sometimes enable him to say, on the contrary, that it was impossible. And to conclude, when the chemical or moral evidence proves that poison was given, the characters of the symptoms may be necessary to determine whether it was the cause of death.

As the last statement is one of consequence, and yet has been overlooked by some authors on medical jurisprudence in this country, it may be illustrated by one or two comments. It does not follow, because a poison has been given, that it is the cause of death ; and therefore in every medico-legal inquiry the cause of the first symptoms and the cause of death should be made two distinct questions. The question, whether a poison, proved to have been administered, was the cause of death, is to be answered by attending to the second and third characteristics mentioned above, and considering whether the symptoms went on progressively increasing, or altered their nature during the course of the patient's illness, and whether the alteration, if any, was such as may occur in the case of poisoning generally, or of the special poison given. These remarks are very well exemplified by a case, of which I have related the particulars elsewhere,* that, namely, of Charles Munn, tried at the Inverary Spring Circuit of 1824 for the double crime of procuring abortion, and of murder by poisoning. The moral evidence and symptoms together left no doubt that arsenic had been given, and that the deceased, a girl with whom the prisoner cohabited, laboured under the effects of that poison in a very aggravated and complex form for twelve days. After that she began to recover rapidly, and in the course of a fortnight more was free of every symptom except weakness and pains in the hands and feet : In short, all things considered, she was thought to be out of danger. But she then became affected with headache and sleeplessness, and died in nineteen days more under symptoms of obscure general fever, without any local inflammation. Dr. Duncan, junior, and I, who were consulted by the Crown in this case, were of opinion, — that granting the girl's first illness, as appeared from moral and medical evidence, was owing to arsenic, her death could not be ascribed to it with any certainty. It is true that in a few instances the primary irritant symptoms caused by arsenic have been

* Edinburgh Medico-Chirurgical Transactions, ii. 309.

known to pass into an obscure general fever, which has ended fatally ; and that this mode of termination coincides with the effects ascribed to arsenic as the chief ingredient in the celebrated *Aqua Toffana*. But the latter phenomena, at best of doubtful authenticity, are not represented to have been preceded by the ordinary symptoms of violent irritation, or to have been developed except under the use of continuous small doses ; and as for the more recent and less ambiguous cases of fever succeeding the usual primary effects of a large dose, in no instance yet recorded was there an intermission between the two stages.

So much, then, for the force of the evidence drawn from the characters of the symptoms of general poisoning. According to the example of others, I might consider in the present place the force of evidence derived from the symptoms themselves, which distinguish the three classes of poisons. But this subject, together with the special natural diseases which imitate the symptoms of poisoning, will be treated of more conveniently as an introduction to each of the classes.

Section II. — *Of the Evidence from Morbid Appearances.*

The appearances left in the dead body after death by poison used formerly to be relied on as strongly as the symptoms during life ; and with even less reason. Except in the instance of a very few poisons, the morbid appearances alone can never distinguish death by poison from the effects of natural disease, or from some other kinds of violent death. There is not much room, therefore, for general remarks under the present head.

It was at one time thought by the profession, and is still very generally imagined by the vulgar, that unusual blackness or lividity of the skin, indicates death by poison generally. But every experienced physician is now well aware, that excessive lividity is by no means universally produced by poison, and that it is likewise produced by so many natural diseases as not even to form, in any circumstances whatever, the slightest ground of suspicion. Neither is there any difference in kind, as some imagine, between the lividity which succeeds death by poison, and that which follows natural death. Yet it is right for the medical jurist to be aware that lividity as a supposed consequence of poison ought to be strictly attended to by medical inspectors and law officers while investigating charges of poisoning, because the vulgar belief on the subject sometimes leads to such conduct or language on the part of the poisoner as betrays his secret at the time, and constitutes evidence of his guilt afterwards.

Another appearance equally unimportant is early putrefaction of the body. Early putrefaction, at one time much insisted on as a criterion of poisoning,* cannot even justify suspicion. It is by no means invariably, or even generally caused by poisons ; nay, some-

* Alberti, Systema Jurispr. Medic. i. c. 13. § 4.

times a state precisely the reverse appears to be induced;* and it is seen quite as frequently after natural death.

Some other appearances, not more conclusive, might also be mentioned here ; but they belong properly to the effects of individual poisons, or of classes of poisons, not to those of poisoning generally. It may merely be remarked at present, therefore, that the appearances after death, which are really morbid, and which may be produced by poisons, are, in one great class, the signs of inflammation of the alimentary canal in its progressive stages, — in another class, the signs of congestion within the head, — and in a third, a combination of the effects of the two preceding classes ; that neither set of appearances is invariably caused by the poisons which usually cause them ; that congestion within the head is really seldom produced by those which are currently imagined to produce it ; and that most of the appearances of both kinds are exactly similar to those left by many natural diseases.

But although, on the whole, the appearances after death, when considered singly, can seldom supply evidence of poisoning even to the amount of probability, they may nevertheless prove very important under other points of view. Thus, in connection with the symptoms and the general evidence, the appearances after death may furnish decisive proof; and even should the history of the symptoms be unknown, or have been unskilfully collected, the appearances after death, by pointing out the nature of the previous illness, may furnish evidence enough to decide the case, when the moral proof is strong. Again, in cases of alleged *imputation of poisoning* they are necessary to determine whether a poison actually found in the body was introduced during life or after death. Besides, the very absence of morbid appearances may afford presumptive proof in some circumstances, — when, for example, the question is, whether a person has died of apoplexy or of poisoning with narcotics ? Farther, a few poisons, as was formerly stated, occasionally produce appearances so characteristic, as not to be capable of being confounded with the effects of any other agent whatsoever: It will be found hereafter, for example, that the mineral acids have at times left behind them in the dead body unequivocal evidence of their operation. And finally, in cases where no doubt can be entertained that poison was taken, the evidence from morbid appearances may be useful or necessary for settling whether or not it was the cause of death. Two pointed examples of this kind will be noticed under the next section.

When signs of the action of poison are not found in the dead body, and on the contrary marks are found of the operation of natural disease, the presumption of course is that the person died a natural death. But here a few words of caution must be added with regard to the drawing of that inference in cases where the history of the symptoms is not known. It does not follow merely because certain appearances of natural disease are found, that their cause was the

* See Arsenic — Morbid appearances.

cause of death. For death may have arisen from a totally different cause, such as poisoning. This remark is not, as some may imagine, the offspring of hypothetical refinement, but a necessary caution, drawn from actual and not unfrequent occurrences. Thus, for example, the following cases will show, that there may be found in the dead body diseased appearances, arising from pleurisy, hydrothorax, or peripneumony, sufficient to cause death, or to account for death in ordinary circumstances; and that nevertheless the disease may have been completely latent, and death have arisen from poison. In Rust's Magazin is related the case of a German apothecary, who poisoned himself with prussic acid, and in whose body the lower lobe of the left lung was found consolidated and partly cartilaginous.* In Corvisart's Journal an army-surgeon has described the case of a soldier, who died of a few hours' illness, and whose right lung was found after death forming one entire abscess; yet to the very last day of his existence he daily underwent all the fatigues of a military life; and in fact he died of poisoning with hemlock.† In Pyl's Memoirs and Observations, there is a similar account of a woman who enjoyed tolerable health, and died during a fit of excessive drinking, and in whose body the whole left lung was found one mass of suppuration.‡ Under the next section will be mentioned other equally pointed cases of death by poison, where the apparent cause of death was external violence.

The conclusions to be drawn from these facts are that, at all events, the medical inspector in a question of poisoning, must take care not to be hurried away by the first striking appearances of natural disease which he may observe, and so be induced to conduct the rest of the inspection superficially; and likewise, that he should not so frame his opinion on the case, as to exclude the possibility of a different cause from the apparent one, unless the appearances are such as must necessarily have been the cause of death. It may be said, that in requiring this condition for an unqualified opinion, a rigour of demonstration is exacted, which can rarely be attained in practice. But, on the one hand, it must not be forgotten, that an unqualified opinion is not always necessary; and on the other hand, although it were, I think it might be shown, if the subject did not lead to disproportionate details, that we may often approach very near the rigour of demonstration required. At present no more need be said, than that the inspector should be particularly on his guard in those cases, in which the appearances, though belonging to the effects of a deadly disease, are trifling; and still more in those in which the appearances, though great, belong to the effects of a disease, whose whole course may be latent. And I may add, that, from what I have observed of medico-legal opinions, the caution now given is strongly called for.

It may be right to allude here also to another purpose which may

* Magazin für die gesammte Heilkunde, xiv. 104.
† Journal de Médecine, xxix. 107.
‡ Aufsätze und Beobachtungen aus der gerichtlichen Arzneiwissenchaft, v. 103.

8

be served by a careful consideration of the morbid appearances. In cases in which the history of the symptoms is unknown or imperfect the extent and state of progress of the appearances will sometimes supply strong presumptive evidence of the duration of the poisoning. This is an obvious and important application of the knowledge of the pathology of poisoning ; but the simple mention of it is all which can be here attempted, as special rules can hardly be laid down on the subject.

SECTION III. — *Evidence from Chemical Analysis.*

The chemical evidence in charges of poisoning is generally, and with justice, considered the most decisive of all the branches of proof. It is accounted most valid, when it detects the poison in the general textures of the body, or in the blood, or in the stomach, intestines or gullet, then in the matter vomited, next in articles of food, drink or medicine of which the sufferer has partaken, and lastly, in any articles found in the prisoner's possession, and for which he cannot account satisfactorily.

When poison is detected in any of these quarters, more especially in the stomach or intestines, it is seldom that any farther proof is needed to establish the fact of poisoning. In two circumstances, however, some corroboration is necessary.

In the first place, in cases where a defence is attempted by a charge of imputation of poisoning it may be necessary to determine by an accurate account of the symptoms, or by the morbid appearances, or by both together, whether the poison was introduced into the body before or after death. For it is said, that attempts have been made to impute crime by introducing poison into the stomach or anus of a dead body ; and although I have not been able to find any authentic instance of so horrible an act of ingenuity having been perpetrated, it must nevertheless be allowed to be quite possible.

Secondly, an account of the symptoms and morbid appearances is still more necessary, when the question at issue is, not so much whether poison has been given, as whether it was the cause of death, granting it had been taken. Some remarks have been already made on this question in the two former sections. In the present place some farther illustrations will be added from two very striking cases. They are interesting in many respects, and particularly as showing the importance of strict medico-legal investigation : I am almost certain that but a few years ago their real nature would not have been discovered in this country. The first to be noticed occurred to Dr. Wildberg of Rostock. Wildberg was required to examine the body of a girl, who died while her father was in the act of chastising her severely for stealing, and who was believed by all the bye-standers, and by the father himself, to have died of the beating. Accordingly, Wildberg found the marks of many stripes on the arms, shoulders and back, and under some of the marks blood was extravasated in considerable quantity. But these injuries, though severe, did not appear to him adequate to account for death. He therefore proceeded to examine the cavities; and on opening the stomach, he found it very much inflamed, and lined with a white powder which proved on analysis to be arsenic. It turned out, that on the theft being detected the girl had taken arsenic for fear of her father's anger, that she vomited during the flogging, and died in slight convulsions. Consequently, Wildberg very properly imputed death to the arsenic. In this case the chemical evidence proved that poison had been taken; but an account of the symptoms and appearances was necessary to prove that she died of it.* The other case occurred to Pyl in 1783. A woman at Berlin, who lived on bad terms with her husband, went to bed in perfect health; but soon afterwards her mother found her breathing very hard, and on inquiring into the cause discovered a wound in the left side of the breast. A surgeon being immediately sent for, the hemorrhage which had never been great, was checked without difficulty; but she died nevertheless towards morning. On opening the chest it appeared that the wound pierced into it, and penetrated the pericardium, but did not wound the heart; and although the fifth intercostal artery had been divided, hardly any blood was effused into the cavity of the chest. Coupling these circumstances with the trifling hemorrhage during life, and the fact that she had much vomiting, and some convulsions immediately before death, Pyl satisfied himself that she had not died of the wound: and accordingly the signs of corrosion in the mouth and throat, and of irritation in the stomach, with the subsequent discovery of the remains of some nitric acid in a glass in her room, proved that she had died of poison.†

Causes of the disappearance of poison from the body. — Chemical evidence is not always attainable in cases of poisoning. Various causes may remove the poison beyond reach. Hence although poison be not detected in the body, — the experimenter being supposed skilful and the poison of a kind which is easily discovered, — still it must not be concluded from that fact alone that poison has not been the cause of death. For that which was taken into the stomach may have been all discharged by vomiting and purging, or may have been all absorbed, or decomposed; and that which has been absorbed into the system may have been all discharged by the excretions.

1. It may have been discharged by vomiting and purging. Thus on the trial of George Thom for poisoning the Mitchells, held at Aberdeen at the Autumn Circuit of 1821, it was clearly proved, that the deceased had died of poisoning by arsenic; yet by a careful analysis none could be detected in the stomach or its contents; for the man lived seven days, and during all that time laboured under frequent vomiting.‡ In a remarkable case related by Dr. Roget, arsenic could not be found in the matter vomited twenty-four hours after it had been swallowed;§ in another related by Professor Wagner

* Wildberg, Praktisches Hanbuch für Physiker, iii. 227.
† Aufsätze und Beobachtungen, &c. ii. 122.
‡ Edinburgh Medical and Surgical Journal, xviii. 171.
§ London Medico-Chirurgical Transactions, ii. 158.

of Berlin, that of an infant who died in twelve hours under incessant
vomiting after receiving a small quantity of arsenic, none could be
detected in the stomach ;[*] in another which I have described in a
paper on arsenic, although the person lived only five hours, the
whole arsenic which could be detected in the tissues and contents of
the stomach did not exceed a fifteenth part of a grain ;[†] in an American Journal there is a striking case of a grocer, who died eight
hours after swallowing an ounce of arsenic, and in whose body none
could be found chemically, — at a period however antecedent to the
late improvements in analysis ;[‡] and in a case communicated to me
not long ago by Mr. Hewson of Lincoln, where arsenic was given in
solution, and death ensued in five hours, none of the poison could
be detected either in the contents or tissues of the stomach by a
careful analysis conducted according to the most modern principles.

Nevertheless, it is singular how ineffectual vomiting proves in expelling some poisons from the stomach. Those which are not easily
soluble, and have been taken in a state of minute division, may remain adhering to the villous coat, notwithstanding repeated and violent efforts to dislodge them by vomiting. Many instances to this
effect have occurred in the instance of arsenic. Metzger has related
a case, where, after six hours of incessant vomiting, three drachms
were found in the stomach.[§] Mr. Sidey, a surgeon of this city, has
mentioned to me an instance of poisoning with king's yellow, in
which he found the stomach lined with the poison, although the patient had vomited for thirty hours. In three cases which I have investigated arsenic was detected, although the people lived and vomited much for nearly two days ;[‖] and Professor Orfila has noticed
a similar instance in which that poison was found in the contents of
the stomach, although the person had vomited incessantly for two entire days.[**]

It is not easy to specify the period after which a poison that has
excited vomiting need not be looked for in the stomach. It must
vary with a variety of circumstances whose combined effect it is almost impossible to appreciate, such as the solubility and state of division of the poison, the frequency of vomiting, the substances taken
as remedies, and the like. When the poison is in solution and the
patient vomits much, an analysis may be expected to prove frequently
abortive, even though the individual survive but a few hours, as in
Mr. Hewson's case already noticed. In other circumstances, however, as various facts quoted above will show, poisons may frequently
be found after two days incessant vomiting; and on the whole it may
be stated, that the recent improvements in analysis render the period
much longer than it has generally been, and would naturally be
imagined. Metzger has related the case of a woman poisoned with

* Archiv für Medizinische Erfahrung, 1834, p. 754.
† Edinburgh Medico-Chirurgical Transactions, ii. 303.
‡ New York Medical and Philosophical Journal, iii. No. 1.
§ De Veneficio caute dijudicando in Schlegel's Collectio opusculorum, &c. iv. 22.
‖ Edinburgh Medico-Chirurgical Transactions, ii. 291, Edinburgh Medical and Sur-
gical Journal, xxvii. 457, and xxix. 26.
** Archives Générales de Médecine, ii. 58.

arsenic mixed with currants, in whose body, after eight days of frequent vomiting, he found ten or twelve currants, which gave out an odour of garlic when burnt ;* but here the dose, if there was really arsenic, must have been repeated recently before death, for it is not possible to conceive how currants could remain in the stomach so long, whatever may be thought of the possibility of arsenic remaining. It is farther proper to add, that Professor Henke of Erlangen, one of the highest living authorities in Germany, once found grains of arsenic in the gullet, although he found none in any other part of the body, of a person who survived the taking of the poison four days.† Allowing to this fact all the weight derived from the high name of its author, I must neverthelesss express great doubt whether the arsenic was not repeated more recently before death.

2. The poison may have disappeared, because it has been all absorbed. It has several times happened that in the bodies of those poisoned with laudanum, or even with solid opium, none of the drug could be detected after death. Sometimes indeed it is found, even though the individual survived the taking of the poison many hours. Thus a case related by Meyer of Berlin, in which the person lived ten hours after taking the saffron-tincture of opium ; and nevertheless it was detected in the stomach by a mixed smell of saffron and opium.‡ But more commonly it all disappears, unless the dose has been very large. In a case of poisoning with laudanum, which I examined here along with Sir W. Newbigging in 1823, none could be detected, although strong moral circumstances left no doubt that laudanum had been swallowed seven or eight hours before death. An instance of the same kind has been minutely related by Pyl. It was that of an infant who was poisoned with a mixture of opium and hyoscyamus, and in whose stomach and intestines none could be detected by the smell.§ Similar observations have been often made on animals ; and several additional cases of the same purport, occurring in man, will be related under the head of opium.

It might be of use to quote some of the numerous errors committed by medical witnesses, in consequence of having overlooked the effect of absorption in removing poisons beyond the reach of chemical analysis. But not to be too prolix, I shall be content with mentioning a single very distinct case in point, which happened at a Coroner's Inquest in London, in 1823. A young man one evening called his fellow-lodger to his bedside ; assured him he had taken laudanum, and should be dead by the morrow ; and desired him to carry his last farewell to his mother and his mistress. His companion thought he was shamming ; but next morning the unfortunate youth was found in the agonies of death. The moral evidence was not very satisfactory ; but that is of little consequence to my present ob-

* Materialien für die Staatsarzneikunde, 130.
† Ueber die gerichtlich-medizinische Beurtheilung der Vergiftungen.   Kopp's Jahrbuch, vii. 159.
‡ Rust's Magazin für die gesammte Heilkunde, iii. 24.
§ Aufsätze und Beobachtungen, viii. 92.

8*

ject.   The point in the case I would particularly refer to is the declaration of the medical inspector, that laudanum could not have
been taken, because he did not find any by the smell or by chemical analysis in the contents of the stomach.*

3. Poisons may not be found, because the excess has been decomposed.

Vegetable and animal poisons may be altogether destroyed by the
process of digestion.   This observation will explain why sometimes
no poison could be found in cases of poisoning with crude opium or
other vegetable solids. A French physician, M. Desruelles, has related
the case of a soldier, who died six hours and a half after swallowing
two drachms of solid opium, and in whose stomach nothing was
found but a yellowish fluid, quite destitute of the smell of the drug.†

Some mineral poisons, such as corrosive sublimate, lunar caustic,
and hydrochlorate of tin, are also decomposed in the stomach.   But
they are not removed beyond the reach of chemical analysis.   The
decomposition is the result of a chemical, not of a vital process ;
and the basis of the poison may be found in the solid contents of the
stomach under some other compound form.   Other poisons again may
be apt to elude detection by altering their form, by combining with
other substances, without themselves undergoing decomposition.
Thus it appears from a case related by Mertzdorff of Berlin, that, in
poisoning with sulphuric acid, after the greater part of the poison is
discharged by vomiting, the remainder may escape discovery by being neutralized : For, although he could not find any free acid in the
contents of the stomach, he discovered $4\frac{1}{2}$ grains in union with ammonia by precipitation with muriate of baryta.‡

It may be also right to mention another kind of decomposition
which may render it impossible to detect a poison that has been really
swallowed — namely, that arising from decay of the body.   In several recent cases bodies have been disinterred and examined for
poison months or even years after death.   In these and similar cases
it would be unreasonable to expect always to find the poison, even
though it existed in the stomach immediately after death.   Some
poisons, such as oxalic acid, might be dissolved and then exude ;
others, such as the vegetable narcotics, will undergo putrefaction ;
and others, such as prussic acid, are partly votalized, partly decomposed, so as to be undistinguishable in the course of a few days only.
The mineral poisons, those at least which are solid, are not liable to
be so dissipated or destroyed.   Some authors, indeed, have said that
arsenic may disappear in consequence of its uniting with hydrogen disengaged during the progress of putrefaction, and so escaping in the form
ot arseniuretted hydrogen gas ; and they have endeavoured to account
in this way for the non-discovery of it in the bodies of the people
who had been killed by arsenic, and disinterred for examination many
months afterwards.§   But the supposition is by no means probable :

* Morning Chronicle, Jan. 8, 1823.
† Journal Universel des Sciences Médicales, xix. 340.
‡ Horn's Archiv für Medizinische Erfahrung. 1823, i. 451.
§ Bachmann.   Einige auserlesene gerichtlich-medizinische Abhandlungen, von
Schmitt, Bachmann, &c. p. 21.

at least arsenic has been detected in the body fourteen months, nay, even seven years, after interment. For farther details, on this curious topic, the reader may turn to the article Arsenic.

On the whole, the result of the most recent researches is that the effect of the spontaneous decay of dead animal matter in involving poisons in the general decomposition appears to be much less considerable than might be anticipated. For this most important medico-legal fact, the toxicologist is indebted to the experimental inquiries of MM. Orfila and Lesueur.* The poisons tried by them were — sulphuric and nitric acids, arsenic, corrosive sublimate, tartar-emetic, sugar of lead, protomuriate of tin, blue vitriol, verdigris, lunar caustic, muriate of gold, acetate of morphia, muriate of brucia, acetate of strychnia, hydrocyanic acid, opium, and cantharides. They found that after a time the acids become neutralized by the ammonia disengaged during the decay of animal matter ; — that by the action of the animal matter the salts of mercury, antimony, copper, tin, gold, silver, and likewise the salts of the vegetable alkaloids, undergo chemical decomposition, in consequence of which the bases become less soluble in water, or altogether insoluble ; — that acids may be detected after several years' interment, not always, however, in the free state ; — that the bases of the decomposed metallic salts may also be found after interment for several years ; — that arsenic, opium, and cantharides undergo little change after a long interval of time, and are scarcely more difficult to discover in decayed, than in recent animal mixtures ; — but that hydrocyanic acid disappears very soon, so as to be undistinguishable in the course of a few days.

4. Lastly, the poison which has been absorbed into the system, and may consequently be detected in certain circumstances in the textures of the body at a distance from the alimentary canal, may also be removed beyond the reach of analysis, by being gradually discharged along with the excretions. It has been fully proved in recent times, that in poisoning with arsenic the poison may be found in ordinary cases, for some days after being swallowed, in the liver especially, but also in the other textures, in the blood, and in the urine ; but that if a flow of urine be established and kept up, in nine or ten days, and sometimes much sooner, it can no longer be discovered anywhere by the nicest analysis.†

Is the discovery of poison in the body or the evacuations essential to establish a charge of poisoning? It was mentioned at the commencement of the present section, that the chemical evidence is generally, and correctly, considered the most decisive of all the branches of proof in cases of poisoning. But some toxicologists have even gone so far as to maintain that without chemical evidence, or rather, in more general terms, without the discovery of poison either in the body itself or in the evacuations, — no charge of poisoning ought to be held as proved. This, however, is a doctrine to which I cannot assent. In the preceding observations on the evidence of general

* Revue Médicale, 1828, ii. 469.
† Orfila, in Journ. de Chim. Med. 1842, p. 77.

poisoning it has been several times alluded to as unsound ; and repeated opportunities of establishing exceptions will occur in the
course of this work, under the head of individual poisons.   At present
it may be well to illustrate its unsoundness in reference to those
charges of poisoning, where no particular poison is pointed at by
the medical evidence, but where a whole class of poisons must be
kept more or less in view.   Even here I apprehend there may be
sufficient evidence in the symptoms and morbid appearances, without
any chemical facts, — to render poisoning so highly probable, that in
conjunction with strong moral evidence, no sensible man can entertain any doubt on the subject.   Several illustrations might be here
given ; and some will be found scattered throughout the work.   In
the present place a few instances will be mentioned which cannot be
conveniently arranged any where else, and which are well worthy of
notice, as being striking examples of the decision of questions of
poisoning without chemical evidence.

   A man of doubtful character and morals, well acquainted with
chemistry and medical jurisprudence, and of disordered finances, was
known to harbour a design on a friend's wife, who possessed a considerable fortune.   At last he one morning invited the husband to
breakfast with him at a tavern ; and they breakfasted, in a private
apartment, on beef-steaks, fried potatoes, eels, claret, and rum.
They had scarcely commenced the meal when his guest complained
of feeling unwell ; and soon afterwards he vomited violently.   This
symptom continued, along with excruciating pain in the belly, for a
long time before the prisoner sent for medical aid ; indeed he did not
procure a physician till the sufferer had been also attacked with
very frequent and involuntary purging.   The physician, who, before
seeing his patient, had received the prisoner's explanation of the apparent cause of the illness, was led at first to impute the whole to
cholera caught by exposure to cold ; but on returning at seven in
the evening, and finding the gentleman had been dead for an hour,
he at once exclaimed that he had been poisoned.   On the body being
inspected much external lividity was found, contraction of the fingers, and great inflammation of the stomach and intestines, presenting an appearance like that of gangrene.*   On analyzing some fluid
left in the stomach, no arsenic or other poison could be detected.   The
attention of the inspectors was turned specially to arsenic, because the
prisoner was proved to have bought that poison, and to have made
a solution of some white powder in his kitchen not long before the
deceased died.   The prisoner in his defence stated, that the deceased had been for some time much weakened by the use of mercury, and while in this state was seized with cholera ; and he likewise attempted to make it probable that the man, in despair at his
not recovering from a venereal disease, might have committed suicide.   The council of physicians who were required to give their
opinion on the case state on the contrary, that the diseased was a
healthy man, without any apparent disposition to disease ; that there

* Probably black extravasation.

was no pretext whatever for supposing suicide ; that the inflammatory state of the stomach and bowels supplied strong probability of poisoning with arsenic, but not certain evidence ; that acute gastritis from natural causes is always attended with constipation ; that the deceased presented symptoms of stupor and other signs of derangement of the nervous system remarked in rapid cases of poisoning with arsenic ; that cholera is very rare at the end of November, the season when this incident occurred ; and that the poison might well be discharged by vomiting.   Although all the prisoner's statements in defence were contradicted by satisfactory proof, and the medical evidence of poisoning was supported by a chain of the strongest general circumstances, the crime was considered by the court as not fully proved, because the prisoner could not be induced to confess, and because poison was not actually detected in the body.   But on account of the very strong probability of his guilt, he was, in conformity with the strange practice of German courts in the like cases, condemned to fifteen years' imprisonment.*   In this instance — considering the kind of symptoms, their commencement during a meal, the rapidity of death, the signs of violent inflammation in the stomach after so short an illness, and the facility with which the absence of poison in the contents of the stomach may be accounted for, more especially if it be supposed that the poison was administered in solution, — I consider the medical evidence of death by poisoning so very strong, that, the general evidence being also extremely strong, the prisoner's guilt was fully demonstrated.

A case of the same kind, but of still greater interest, is that of Mary Anne M'Conkey, who was tried at the Monaghan Assizes in 1841 for the murder of her husband.   I am indebted for the particulars to Dr. Geoghegan, one of the principal Crown witnesses. The prisoner who had been too intimate with another man, and had been heard to express her intention of getting rid of her husband, was observed one day before dinner to separate some greens for him from the plateful intended for the rest of the family.   None of the latter suffered at all.   But her husband was taken violently ill immediately after dinner, and died ; and a neighbour accidentally present, who partook, though sparingly, of the same dish with him, was also similarly and violently affected but recovered.   The deceased before finishing the greens said they had a disagreeable sharp taste, and was seized soon after with burning at the heart, tenderness at the pit of the stomach, vomiting, coldness, a sense of biting in the tongue and tingling through the whole flesh, excessive restlessness, occasional incoherence, locked-jaw, clenching of the hands, and frothing at the mouth; and he expired three hours after the meal.   His neighbour, two minutes after finishing his greens, experienced a sense of pricking in the mouth and burning in the throat, gullet, and stomach ; then salivation, a feeling of swelling in the face without actual fulness, general numbness and creeping in the skin ; next excessive

* Marx, die Lehre von den Giften, i. ii, 429, from Hitzig's Zeitschrift für die Criminal-Rechts-Pflege, I. i. l.

restlessness, coldness of the integuments, dimness of sight, and stupor; about an hour after the meal he became speechless, repeatedly fainted, frothed at the mouth, and clenched his hands ; vomiting ensued, with considerable relief, and subsequently he had frequent attacks of it, with purging, tenderness of the epigastrium, cramps, and tingling in the flesh ; and from these symptoms he recovered so slowly as to be unable to work for five weeks. The only morbid appearance of any note in the body of the deceased was a number of irregular brownish-black patches on the inside of the stomach. No poison could be detected in the contents or tissues of the stomach ; none could be discovered in the house except a corrosive-sublimate solution which the prisoner used for a gargle ; and none could be traced into her possession. A variety of circumstances of a general nature, which are passed over here for brevity, as not strictly appertaining to the present view of the case, threw very great suspicion over the prisoner. The medical witnesses deposed, that poisoning could alone explain the medical circumstances ; and Dr. Geoghegan was of opinion that death was owing to some vegetable poison, although he could not specify the particular substance. He suspected, however, that it was monkshood. In these views, when consulted by him before the trial, I entirely concurred. Considering the taste observed by the deceased at the time he ate the greens, the rapidity with which he was taken ill afterwards, and the very peculiar symptoms, unlike those of any natural disease with which physicians are acquainted, and agreeing with those which are produced by monkshood, —considering also that another individual, who partook of the same dish with him, was similarly and simultaneously attacked, and with a severity proportioned to the quantity he took, while other persons who ate the same food from a different dish, did not suffer at all, — it appears to me that poisoning was clearly established ; and I also think that the general evidence brought home the charge of administering the poison to the prisoner. She was condemned and executed, and confessed before execution, that she did poison her husband, and that the substance she used was the powdered root of monkshood, which is well known as a poison to the peasantry of Monaghan under the name of Blue Rocket.

It is scarcely necessary to add, that great caution must be observed in applying the general principle here inculcated. But the opposite doctrine, that no charge of poisoning can be established without the discovery of poison in the body or in the evacuations, appears to me a great error, though upheld by no mean authority. Under that doctrine few criminals would be brought to justice, were they to resort to a variety of vegetable poisons, which in certain seasons are within the reach of every one.

SECTION IV. — *Evidence from Experiments on Animals.*

Evidence from experiments on animals with articles supposed to contain poison is more equivocal than was once imagined. But it may be doubted whether some medical jurists have not overstepped the proper limits, when they hold it to constitute little or no proof at all.

Evidence from express experiments should rarely form part of a regular medical inquiry into a charge of poisoning. For in the first place, to make sure of performing an experiment well requires more experimental skill than the generality of practitioners can be expected to possess ; then, as will seen in the sequel, evidence procured from this source can very rarely be more than presumptive ; and lastly, if the quantity of poison in the suspected substance is great enough to affect one of the perfect animals, it may generally be recognized to a certainty by its physical or chemical properties.

For these reasons it is not likely, that, in an inquiry undertaken by a skilful toxicologist, he will put himself in the way of delivering an opinion on the force of such evidence. But it is nevertheless necessary for me to consider it in detail, because he may have to give his opinion regarding experiments made inconsiderately by others, or accidents caused by domestic animals eating the remains of substances suspected to be poisoned.

The matter subjected to trial may be either suspected food, drink, or medicine ; or it may be the stuff vomited during life, or found in the stomach after death ; or it may be the flesh of poisoned animals.

1. The evidence derived from *the effects of suspected food, drink, or medicine* is better than that drawn from the effects of the vomited matter or contents of the stomach. But an important objection has been made to both, namely, that what is poison to man is not always poison to the lower animals, and that, on the other hand, some of the lower animals are poisoned by substances not hurtful to man.

A good deal of obscurity still hangs over the relative effects of poisons on man and the lower animals. There are two species, however, whose mode of life in respect to food closely resembles our own, and which, according to innumerable experiments by Orfila, are affected by almost all poisons exactly in the same way as ourselves, namely, the cat and dog, but particularly the latter.

In general poisons act less violently on these animals ; thus two drachms of opium are required to kill a middle-sized dog,[*] while twenty grains have killed a man, and undoubtedly less would be sufficient. It appears that one poison, alcohol, acts more powerfully on them than on man. There are also some poisons, such as opium, which, although deleterious to them as well as to man, nevertheless produce in general different symptoms. Yet the differences alluded to are probably not greater than exist between man and man in regard to the same substances ; and therefore it may be assumed, that, on the whole, the effects of poisons on man differ little from those produced on the dog and cat.

* Charret, in Revue Médicale, 1827, i. 514.

The present objection is generally and perhaps justly considered a stronger one, when it is applied to other species of animals. But it must be confessed after all, that our knowledge of the diversities in the action of poisons on different animals is exceedingly vague, and founded on inaccurate research ; and there is much reason to suspect, that, if the subject is studied more deeply, the greater number of the alleged diversities will prove rather apparent than real. Both reasoning and experiment, indeed, render it probable, that some orders, even of the perfect animals, such as the *Ruminantia*, are much less sensible than man to many poisons, and especially to poisons of the vegetable kingdom. But so far as may be inferred from the only accurate inquires on the subject, their effects differ in degree more than in kind. Some exceptions will without doubt be found to this statement. For example, oxalic acid, besides inflaming the stomach, causes violent convulsions in animals, but in man it for the most part excites merely excessive prostration ; and opium most generally excites in man pure sopor, in animals convulsions also. Other exceptions, too, exist by reason of functional peculiarities in certain animals. Thus irritant poisons do not cause vomiting in rabbits or horses, because these animals cannot vomit ; neither do they appear to cause much pain to rabbits, because rabbits have not the power of expressing pain with energy. But exceptions like these, and particularly such as are unconnected with functional peculiarities, will probably prove fewer in number, and less striking than is currently imagined. For it is, on the other hand, well ascertained, that many, indeed most of the active poisons whose effects have been examined by a connected train of experiments, produce nearly the same effects on all animals whatever from the highest to the lowest in the scale of perfection. It has been fully proved, that arsenic, copper, mercury, the mineral acids, opium, strychnia, conia, white hellebore, hydrocyanic acid, cyanogen gas, sulphuretted hydrogen, and many others, produce nearly the same effects on man, quadrupeds, birds, amphibious animals, and even on fishes and insects.*

* As a specimen of the vague, desultory, and erroneous nature of the investigations which have been made by authors on this subject, I may quote some remarks published by Virey in the Journal Universel (vi. 26), and drawn, he says, from a comparison of statements in various works. He states that arsenic, which is so fatal to animals in general, merely purges dogs and wolves more or less; that nux vomica is less fatal to man than to dogs; that pepper is fatal to hogs, parsley to parrots, the agrostis arundinacea to goats, elder-berries to poultry, chenopodium vulvaria to swine; that on the contrary the goat eats with impunity hemlock, daphne gnidium, and some species of euphorbia; that the camel eats all species of euphorbia, the hedgehog cantharides, the horse monkshood, ranunculus flammula, and buckthorn ; asses and mules white hellebore, swine yew-berries ; all which are poisonous to animals in general. He does not state special authorities for these facts ; but they are taken from authors not of the most modern times, and must be received, in my opinion, with great reserve, notwithstanding the respect which he claims for the older writers. Some of the statements are plainly false.

In a more recent paper Virey lays it down as a general principle, that poisons from the inorganic kingdom act more or less on the whole animated creation, but that vegetable and animal poisons are such only in respect to particular animals; that carnivorous animals are more sensible to the action of vegetable poisons, but less so

Accordingly there are cases, in which the evidence from experiments on animals with suspected articles of food is unequivocal.   For

to that of animal poisons, than herbivorous or graminivorous animals; and that the activity of poisons on different animals bears a ratio in the first place to their relative sensibility, and secondly, to the digestive power of their stomach.   I question whether these views will be generally admitted by toxicologists, without much more extensive and more careful inquiries than any hitherto made. [Journ. de Chim. Méd. vii. 214.]

Another singular illustration of the facility with which facts are admitted in proof of the varying effects of poisons on different animals, is a statement by a German naturalist, Dr. Lenz, to the effect that the hedgehog altogether resists the most powerful poisons.   He states that he has seen one receive ten or twelve wounds from a viper on the ears, muzzle, and tongue, without sustaining any harm; and that ultimately it kills and devours the snake.   He quotes Palas for the fact that it has taken 100 cantharides flies without injury, and says a medical friend who wished to dissect a hedgehog, gave it successively hydrocyanic acid, arsenic, opium, and corrosive sublimate, without being able to kill it [L'Institut. ii. 84].   His countryman Reich, however, contradicts these statements, observing that he has poisoned the hedgehog with hydrocyanic acid, arsenic, and corrosive sublimate, but that doses considerably larger are required for a dog or cat.   Ninety grains of medicinal hydrocyanic acid, thirty of arsenic, and twenty of corrosive sublimate, occasioned death.   [Annalen der Pharmacie, i. 358.]   One of my colleagues having lately quoted Lenz's assertion in his lectures, some of his pupils brought me two hedgehogs to be subjected to experiment. A drop of the pure acid put upon the tongue killed each within a minute.

The following experiments by Professor Gohier of the veterinary school of Lyons are worth mentioning; but in order to be satisfactory would require to be performed in a more consecutive train.   Muriate of soda in the dose of two or three pounds causes in the horse great disorder and even death.   Calomel has no effect.   The juice of rhus toxicodendron has no effect on the *solipedes* either internally or applied to the skin.   Ten drachms of opium cause in the horse tympanitis and stupor, not somnolency.   Thirty-six grains of opium had no effect on a dog.   Cantharides does not injure the horse in the dose of a drachm, or the dog in that of nine grains.   When the sheep swallows yew-leaves it is soon seized with locked-jaw and convulsive movements of the lips and flanks: in the horse they cause dilated pupil, convulsive movements of the eyes, and restlessness: the goat and dog eat them with impunity [Corvisart's Journal de Médecine, xix. 156]: man is severely affected by them.   Hyoscyamus, stramonium, hemlock, and other narcotic vegetables, though powerfully narcotic to man, will not affect the domestic animals unless given in doses 100 times as great as those given to man.   [Ibid. 154.]

The most important researches I have yet seen in this line of inquiry are those of Professor Viborg of Copenhagen, read in the Royal Danish Society of Sciences in 1792.   He instituted a connected series of experiments, expressly to determine how far the effects of poisons on man correspond with those on the lower animals.   The results were, that mineral poisons appeared to act nearly in the same manner on all orders of animals, antimonial and barytic salts alone excepted, the former of which acted powerfully on man, the carnivorous animals, and swine, but scarcely at all on ruminating and herbivorous animals, while the latter in doses of a drachm had no effect on horses: That animal poisons resemble mineral poisons in their leading effects on most animals: That the vegetable acrids also act pretty uniformly on most animals: and that of the vegetable narcotics there are few which possess poisonous properties in regard to certain animals only.   Yew-leaves kill all ruminating animals, and, notwithstanding Virey's statement, swine, mules, and horses, also chickens; and they produce violent symptoms in geese, ducks, cats and dogs, although Gohier says dogs eat them with impunity.   An ape ate a large quantity of the Æthusa cynapium without injury.   Dogs took from an ounce and a half to three ounces of belladonna without dangerous symptoms. [Marx, die Lehre von den Giften, — from Viborg's Sammlung von Abhandlungen für Thier. rate. i. 277.]

Professor Mayer of Bonn, in an inquiry into the effects of the Coriaria myrtifolia, found that rabbits are not affected at all by a drachm of the extract of the juice given internally, or applied to a wound; while half a drachm swallowed by a cat kills it in a few hours, and three grains will have the same effect when introduced

9

example ; — a sexton and his wife, who had got a bad name in their village in consequence of informing against the bailiff for smuggling, and who were on that account shunned by all the neighbours, accused the bailiff and his wife of having tried to poison them by mixing poison with their bread. Immediately after eating they were attacked, they said, with sickness, griping, swelling, and dizziness ; and they added, that a cat was seized with convulsions after eating a part of it, had sprung away, and never returned. A large portion of the loaf was therefore sent to the Medical Inspector of the district ; who reported, that it seemed exactly similar to another unsuspected loaf ; — that, although he was not able to detect any poison, it might after all contain one, — vegetable poison particularly ; — but that he could hardly believe it did, for he fed a dog, a cat, and a fowl several days with it, and they not only did not suffer any harm, but even appeared very fond of it.* In this case it was clear that poisoning was out of the question. On the other hand, the effects of some poisons on man may be developed so characteristically in animals as to supply pointed evidence. Thus, in the case of Mary Bateman, an infamous fortune-teller and charm-worker, who after cheating a poor family for a series of years, at last tried to avoid detection by poisoning them, it was justly accounted good evidence, that a portion of the pudding and the honey, supposed to have been poisoned, caused violent vomiting in a cat, killed three fowls, and proved fatal to a dog in four days, under symptoms of irritation of the stomach such as were observed in the people who died.†

into a wound. He likewise found that it is a deadly poison to the dog, the hawk, and the frog. [Journal der Praktischen Heilkunde, lxviii. 4, 43.]

Professor Giacomini of Padua says, that " in many experiments performed by him on dogs and rabbits, he has constantly observed, that the former, as being carnivorous by nature, sustain stimulating substances tolerably well; while rabbits, being herbivorous, stand stimulants ill, but sedatives well." " Hence many herbivorous animals eat with impunity large quantities of vegetable poisons of the sedative kind which prove fatal to carnivorous animals." [Annali Univ. di Med. 1841, i. 372.] This may be true as a general rule. But it is not universally applicable ; for alcoholic fluids kill dogs with great swiftness in no great dose.

An extraordinary statement was lately brought before the French Institute, to the effect that 120 sheep, affected with an epidemic pleurisy, got each about 500 grains of arsenic without sustaining the slightest harm ; and that it was also ascertained to have no poisonous action upon sheep even in a state of health. A commission of the Institute, however, which was appointed to test this assertion, found that healthy sheep were killed by a dose of 155 grains, if they had fasted for some time before [Annales d'Hyg. Publ. &c. 1843, xxix. 468.] It is reasonable to suppose, that ruminating animals, whose alimentary canal is scarcely ever empty should suffer less than carnivorous animals from such poisons as arsenic.

Lassaigne, in some experiments with arsenic, incidentally remarked, that 246 grains of solid arsenic given daily for four days had no effect whatever on a horse ; but that this result seemed to depend on the difficulty which the stomach must experience in appropriating it among the bulky materials of its food ; for 154 grains in solution killed the same animal in six hours [Journ. de Chim. Méd. 1841, 82].—Gianelli of Lucca found that a horse was killed in eight hours by 185 grains of powder of arsenic given in the form of bolus [Annales d'Hyg. Publ. &c. 1842, xxviii. 88].

I might easily extend these extracts. But the result would be merely a mass of contradiction, from which no sound conclusion could be drawn, otherwise the subject would have been discussed in the text.

* Pyl's Aufsätze und Beobachtungen, i. 29.   † Celebrated Trials, vi. 55.

It has been farther objected to experiments on animals with suspected articles of food, drink, or medicine, that it is difficult to administer poison to them in a state of concentration, and to prevent it from being discharged by vomiting. This objection, however, may be obviated by performing the experiment in the way recommended by Professor Orfila. A small opening is made into the gullet, previously detached from its surrounding connexions, the liquid part is introduced by a funnel thrust into the opening, and the solid portion previously made into little pellets is then squeezed down. Lastly, the gullet is tied under the aperture. The immediate effect of the operation is merely an appearance of languor ; and no very serious symptom is observable till four or five days at soonest after the tying of the gullet. Hence if signs of poisoning commence within twenty-four hours, they are independent of the injury done by the operation.* This process requires some adroitness to execute it well. It cannot be tried successfully but by a practised operator, who, for reasons already given, would hardly ever try experiments of the kind with suspected articles. Mention is here made of it, therefore, chiefly because it is the best mode of experimenting in those cases in which it is necessary, as will presently be seen, to determine disputed points in the physiology of poisons.

I may here shortly notice a method which has been lately proposed for detecting poisons that enter the blood, and which is founded on their effects on animals. M. Vernière suggests that advantage may be taken of the extreme sensibility of the medicinal leech to procure at least presumptive evidence, when no evidence can be procured in any other manner. He has related some experiments to prove that the leech, when placed in the blood of dogs killed by nux-vomica, is affected even when the quantity of the poison is exceedingly small.† It is extremely doubtful whether any importance can be attached to this criterion, as every one knows that the leech is apt to suffer from a variety of obscure causes, and among the rest from some diseased states of the body.

2. In the case of *the vomited matter* or *contents of the stomach* there are other and weightier objections to experiments on animals. — In the first place, the poison which has caused death may have been either in part or wholly vomited before-hand, or absorbed, or transmitted into the intestines, or decomposed by the process of digestion. Secondly, though abounding in the matter vomited or which remains in the stomach, it may be so much diluted, as not to have any effect on an animal. And, thirdly, the animal fluids secreted during disease are believed to act occasionally as poisons.

The first two objections are so plainly conclusive as scarcely to require any illustration. It may be well, however, to mention as a pointed practical lesson, that Professor Orfila once detected a considerable quantity of arsenic in the contents of the stomach, where

* Toxicologie Générale, ii. 676.

† Journal des Progrès des Sciences Médicales, 1827, iv. 124. See subsequently the articles Oxalic Acid and Narcotine.

a prior investigation had shown that the same article produced no effect on two animals, and where the reporters from this and other circumstances declared, that in their opinion death was not owing to poison.*

The last objection is a very important one; but there is reason for suspecting that it has been a good deal exaggerated by medical jurists. — Animal fluids are certainly poisonous when putrid. The repeated and fatal experience of anatomists, together with the precise experiments of M. Gaspard and M. Magendie,† leave no doubt that putrid animal fluids, when introduced into an external wound, cause spreading inflammation of the cellular tissue ; and although Magendie says he has found such fluids harmless when introduced into the stomach of dogs,‡ it is probable, from their effects on man, that they will act as irritants on animals not habituated to their use. I believe, too, that independently of putrefaction, vomited matter or the contents of the stomach may be apt to make dogs vomit on account of their nauseous taste ; and perhaps we may infer, that they will also cause some of the other symptoms of poisoning with the irritants, particularly if not vomited soon after being administered. — As to the influence of disease in rendering the contents of the stomach deleterious, it is to be observed that the effects just mentioned are probably owing to the influence of disease on the secretions, but that beyond this we know very little of the subject. In authors I have hitherto found only one fact to prove that disease can render the contents of the stomach decidedly poisonous; and on the negative side of the question there exists no facts at all. Morgagni describes the case of a child who died of tertian ague, amidst convulsions, and in whose stomach a greenish bile was found, which proved so deleterious, that a little of it given with bread to a cock caused convulsions and death in a few minutes, and a scalpel stained with it, when thrust into the flesh of two pigeons, killed them in the same manner.§ It is not easy to say what to think of this experiment; which, if admitted to the full extent of the conclusions deducible from it, would lead to the admission, that disease may impart to the secretions the properties of the most active narcotics. Farther researches are certainly required before this admission can be made unreservedly.

On the whole, it appears that in the present state of our knowledge, experiments or accidental observations on the effects of the contents of the stomach, or of vomited matter, on animals are equivocal in their import. At the same time it may be observed, as with regard to articles of food, drink, or medicine, that the effects of some poisons on man may be developed so characteristically on animals by the contents of the stomach, as to supply very pointed evidence indeed. Of the force of this statement the following example is a striking illustration. In the case of a girl, who was proved to have died of accidental poisoning with laudanum, the inspector evaporated

* Journal de Chimie Méd. vii. 131.
† Journal de Physiologie, ii. 1, and iii. 81.   ‡ Ibidem, iii. 84.
§ De Sedibus et Causis Morborum, T. ii. Ep. lix. 18.

the contents of the stomach to dryness, made an alcoholic extract from the residue, and giving this to several dogs, chickens, and frogs, found that they were all made lethargic by it, some of them oftener than once, and that a few died comatose.* Facts such as these, agreeing so pointedly with the known effects of the poison suspected, appear to me to yield evidence almost unimpeachable.

3. The effects of *the flesh of poisoned animals*, eaten by other animals, constitute the least conclusive of all the varieties of the present branch of evidence. For the flesh of animals that have died of poisoning is not always deleterious; while on the other hand flesh is sometimes rendered so by natural causes, as will be seen in the Chapter on Diseased and Decayed Animal Matter.

This subject stands much in need of careful and methodic investigation. And it is of more practical importance than might be imagined at first sight. For the question has actually occurred in a legal inquiry in this country,—Whether poisoning in the human subject may be caused by the flesh of a poisoned animal?

In regard to some poisons it is well established, that animals killed by them may be eaten with impunity, such as game killed with the wourali poison, or fish by cocculis-indicus. This seems the general rule. But it is not clear that all poisons are similarly circumstanced.

The only systematic researches hitherto undertaken on this question are some recently made at Lucca by Professor Gianelli; of which however I have only seen an abstract. He found that the blood, urine, and lungs of animals poisoned with arsenic acted as a poison on small birds, such as sparrows, whether the parts were taken from the body while the animal was alive, or after death; but that alcohol, cherry-laurel water, corrosive sublimate, sulphate of copper, tartar-emetic, acetate of lead, nitrate of silver, tris-nitrate of bismuth, chloride of tin, sulphate of zinc, laudanum, acetate of morphia, strychnia, and cantharides, had no such effect.† Orfila has since shown some reason for doubting the conclusiveness of Gianelli's investigations; and on repeating them, obtained such results as render it doubtful whether any reliance can be put upon experiments made upon small birds.‡ Guérard however has ascertained, that dogs, fed on the flesh and entrails of sheep which had taken arsenic, were attacked with vomiting and purging, became reduced in flesh, and at length would not eat what was put before them; but none of them perished, or seem to have been seriously ill. Arsenic was detected in their urine.§

The importance of the inquiry, which the preceding experiments are intended to elucidate, will appear from the following singular case, for the particulars of which I am indebted to the kindness of Mr. Jamieson of Aberdeen, who was employed by the authorities to inves-

* Knape und Hecker's Kritische Jahrbucher der Staatsarzneikunde, ii. 100.
† L'Examinateur Médical, 1 Juin, 1842, from Bulletino delle Scien. Med, Jan. 1842.
‡ Annales d'Hyg. Publ. et de Méd. Lég: 1842, xxviii. 84.
§ Ibid. 1843, xxix. 471.

9*

tigate it. An elderly woman, who kept fowls which occasionally trespassed on a neighbour's fields, one morning observed four of them very sickly; and in the course of the day they became so ill that she killed them. She cleaned and prepared two of them for cooking, buried another, and gave away the fourth to a beggar, who was afterwards lost sight of. Next day soup made with the half of one of the fowls was given to a little girl, who suffered severely from sickness and vomiting, and also to a cat, which was similarly affected for the whole evening. On the day afterwards the woman herself and a female lodger, took broth made with what remained of the fowls, and also eat the gizzards; but the remainder was thrown with the offal upon the dunghill. In the course of five or six hours both women were attacked with severe illness. One had sickness, vomiting and great coldness; but after encouraging the vomiting with hot water and then taking some spirits, she got better in the night-time, and next morning was pretty well. The other, who was the owner of the fowls, was seized somewhat later than her friend with great thirst and shivering, and next day with pains in the stomach, severe sickness, and fruitless efforts to vomit. On the sixth day, when a medical man first saw her, she had great pain throughout the abdomen, much thirst, difficult breathing, a red, dry tongue, and a very frequent, small pulse. Next day the pain and difficult breathing became worse; and in the evening, after an attack of sneezing, she became gradually insensible and motionless, in which state she remained till the tenth day, when she expired. The stomach and intestines did not present any distinct morbid appearance; but the vessels of the brain were turgid, there were about two ounces of serosity in the lateral ventricles, both corpora striata were softened anteriorly, and a clot of blood as big as an almond was contained in the right anterior lobe of the brain. — A judicial investigation being ordered, it was ascertained that the fowl which the woman buried as well as the remains of the other fowls which were thrown upon the dunghill, had been carried off. But on searching the dunghill more carefully afterwards, the contents of one of the crops, which had been taken out and examined by the lodger, were discovered in the rubbish; and in the mass Mr. Jamieson detected a considerable quantity of arsenic.

This incident happened in 1836. More lately the same gentleman met with another extraordinary attempt of the same kind. A farmer, about to be married, gave directions for killing in the evening some fowls which were to be sent to the house of his bride where the ceremony was to take place. The killing of them however was accidentally delayed; and next morning, on the hen-house door being opened, the fowls ran furiously to the well, drank water incessantly, and died in an hour. On examining the bodies, Mr. Jamieson found arsenic in large quantity in their crops and gizzards.

On each of these occasions a particular-individual came under suspicion; but the evidence against them was too slight to justify the authorities in bringing a formal charge; and consequently the proceedings did not go farther. In the former instance the evidence in favour of the flesh of poisoned animals being sometimes poisonous is strong ; and the history of the woman's case, although death seems to have been caused directly by apoplexy, renders it probable that even dangerous results might accrue.

The preceding remarks will enable the medical witness to know under what circumstances accidental observations or intentional experiments on animals furnish satisfactory proof.

Before quitting the subject, however, I have to add, that there is another purpose, besides procuring direct evidence, to which experiments with animals may be applied with great propriety ; — namely, the settling disputed questions regarding the physiological and pathological properties of a particular poison. The science of toxicology is not yet by any means so perfect, but in particular cases topics may arise, which have not hitherto been investigated, and which it may be necessary to determine by experiment. Experiments on animals instituted for such purposes by a skilful toxicologist are not liable to any important objection. On the trial of Charles Angus at Liverpool in 1808, for procuring abortion and murder by poison, a trial of great interest, which will be referred to more particularly afterwards, it appeared from the evidence of the crown witnesses, that the poison suspected, corrosive sublimate, could not be discovered in the stomach by certain methods of analysis; and that, although corrosive sublimate is a powerful irritant, the villous coat of the stomach was not inflamed. But then it was proved by experiments made by one of their number, Dr. Bostock, that animals might be killed with corrosive sublimate without the stomach being inflamed, and without the poison being discoverable after death by the tests he used in the case.* An attempt was made on the side of the prisoner to throw out this line of evidence as incompetent, on the ground of the discrepant effects of poisons on man and on the lower animals. But it was admitted by the judge, on the plea that it was only to illustrate a general physiological fact, and not to infer proof of poisoning. The importance of experiments on animals to settle incidental physiological questions has lately been again acknowledged in a very pointed manner in an English court of law : for a set of experiments, to settle the question of the rapidity with which hydrocyanic acid acts, was instituted before the trial by the medical witnesses, at the request of the judge who was to try the case.†

SECTION V. — *Of the Moral Evidence.*

It is not my object to treat under this head of the moral evidence generally, which is required to establish a charge of poisoning. But as it is well known that in criminal trials medical witnesses have for

---

* Trial. — This is a good illustration. Nevertheless, it will be seen under the head of morbid appearances caused by the irritant class of poisons, that Dr. Bostock's experiments, though conclusive as to the statement in the text, did not affect the real questions in the case.

† See trial of Freeman — *article* Hydrocyanic Acid.

the most part nothing to do with the moral proof, while at the same time in cases of poisoning the medical and moral circumstances are always intimately interwoven and apt to be confounded together, it is necessary for me to specify those particulars of the moral evidence, which either require some medical skill to appreciate them, or fall naturally under the cognizance of the physician in his quality of practitioner. I shall enter into greater details under this section than may perhaps appear to the medical reader necessary, chiefly that I may redeem the pledge given in the introduction to the lawyer and general reader, and endeavour to show how powerful an instrument a medico-legal investigation may become in skilful hands, for throwing light on almost every branch of the evidence.

The moral or general proof in charges of poisoning is almost always circumstantial only. The circumstances of which it usually consists relate, 1. To suspicious conduct on the part of the prisoner before the event, such as dabbling with poisons when he has nothing to do with them in the way of his profession, or conversing about them, or otherwise showing a knowledge of their properties not usual in his sphere of life : — 2. To the purchase or possession of poison recently before the date of the alleged crime, and the procuring it in a secret manner, or under false pretences, such as for poisoning rats when there are none on his premises, or for purposes to which it is never applied : — 3. To the administration of poison either in food, drink, medicine, or otherwise : — 4. To the intent of the prisoner, such as the impossibility of his having administered the poison ignorantly, or by accident, or for beneficial purposes, alleged or not alleged : — 5. To the fact of other members of the family besides the deceased having been similarly and simultaneously affected : — 6. To suspicious conduct on the part of the prisoner during the illness of the person poisoned, — such as directly or indirectly preventing medical advice being obtained, or the relations of the dying man being sent for, or showing an over-anxiety not to leave him alone with any other person, or attempting to remove or destroy articles of food or drink, or vomiting matter which may have contained the poison, or expressing a foreknowledge of the probability of speedy death : — 7. To suspicious conduct after the person's death, such as hastening the funeral, preventing or impeding the inspection of the body, giving a false account of the previous illness, showing an acquaintance with the real or supposed effects of poison on the dead body : — 8. To the personal circumstances and state of mind of the deceased, his death-bed declaration, and other particulars, especially such as tend to prove the impossibility or improbability of suicide : — 9. To the existence of a motive or inducement on the part of the prisoner, such as his having a personal quarrel with the deceased, or a hatred of him, — his succeeding to property by his death, or being relieved of a burthen by it, — his knowing that the deceased was with child by him.

Upon many of the particulars now enumerated, important evidence may be derived from the medical part of the investigation ; and not unfrequently such evidence can be collected or appreciated only by means of a medico-legal inquiry.

1 and 2. On the first two articles, suspicious conduct or conversation on the part of the prisoner before the crime, and the possession or purchase of poison by him, little or nothing need be said. The medical witness may of course be asked whether the conduct or conversation proved betokens an unusual acquaintance with poisons and their effects. And his opinion may be referred to regarding the nature of suspected articles found in the prisoner's possession. As to the purchase of arsenic under the false pretence of poisoning rats, it may be observed, that a great deal more stress is usually laid on such evidence than it seems to deserve ; for there are few houses, in the country particularly, which are not more or less infected by them. On the other hand, too little weight is attached to the circumstance of the purchaser not having warned his household of poison being laid. Such conduct ought in my opinion to be accounted extremely suspicious ; for so far as I have remarked, the fear with which unprofessional persons regard the common poisons is such, that I can hardly believe any master of a house would actually lay poison without warning the servants and other inmates of his having done so.

3. The next article, which relates to the proof of the administration of poison, will require some details.

Direct proof of the administration of poison by the actual giver is very rarely attainable, that part of the transaction being for the most part easily concealed. The proof of this point is justly accounted, however, a very important part of the evidence ; nay, on some recent trials in this country the prosecution has failed apparently for want of such evidence, although the case was complete in every other particular. It is generally constituted by a chain of circumstances, and these are often strictly medical, as will now be shown by a few examples.

In the first place, pointed evidence as to the individual who gave the poison may be derived from the chemical investigation, — for example, from the comparative results of the analysis of the poisoned dish, and of the articles of which it consisted. I am indebted to my colleague, Dr. Alison, for the following excellent illustration from the case of William Muir, who was condemned at Glasgow in 1812 for poisoning his wife. In the course of the day on which she took ill she was visited by a farmer of the neighbourhood, who had studied physic a little in his youth. He learned from her that she had breakfasted on porridge a short time before she felt herself ill, and that she suspected the porridge to have been poisoned. He immediately procured the wooden bowl or *cap* in which the cottagers of Scotland keep the portion of meal used each time for making the porridge ; and finding in it some meal, with shining particles interspersed, he wrapped a sample in paper, and took the proper measures for preserving its identity. He then secured also a sample from the family store in a barrel.

The two particles were produced by him on the trial; and from experiments made in court the late Dr. Cleghorn was enabled to declare, that the meal from the bowl contained arsenic, and that the meal from the barrel did not. These facts, besides proving that the woman had next to a certainty taken arsenic in the porridge, likewise, in conjunction with other slight moral circumstances, established that the poison had been mixed with the meal in the house, and on the morning when the deceased took ill, before any stranger entered the house. The procedure of this farmer was precisely that which ought to be followed by the medical practitioner in a similar conjuncture.

Au instance of an opposite description related by M. Barruel also deserves notice, as showing how evidence of this kind may afford, in otherwise suspicious circumstances, a strong presumption of accidental poisoning. Sixteen people near Bressières in France having been severely affected with vomiting and colic immediately after dinner, the bread, which was suspected, was examined by Barruel, and found to contain a little arsenic. The flour of which the bread was made had been taken from a large store of it, which, on being examined, was also found to be similarly impregnated. As it was extremely improbable that any one either could or would poison so large a mass of flour, to attain any malicious object, it was inferred that the arsenic had been mixed with it accidentally, and that the accident might have arisen from grain having been taken by mistake to the flour-mill to be ground, which had been intended originally for seed, and sprinkled with arsenic to destroy insects.[*]

It may be worth while observing, in the present place, that in the instance of poisoned wine very important evidence may be obtained by examining whether the wine with which the cork is impregnated contains any traces of the poison. This method of investigation occurred to me in a very singular case of poisoning with arsenic in champaign, which happened in a baronet's family in Scotland. In this instance, however, such analysis was proved to be unnecessary; for the gentleman himself brought the bottle from his cellar, broke the wires and drew the cork, immediately before the wine was drunk.[†]

All evidence of the like nature, though it is at present often procured from other sources, should, for obvious reasons, be invariably collected, if possible, with the aid of a medical person. If again a medical man is called to a patient evidently affected with suspicious symptoms, and finds himself obliged to declare such to be his opinion, his thoughts, as soon as he has given directions for the treatment, should be turned towards that part of the evidence, for the securing of which he is naturally looked to as the person best qualified by previous education and his opportunities at the mo-

---

[*] I have unfortunately mislaid the reference to this interesting fact, which was taken, I think, from a French periodical. In this country arsenic is never employed for the purpose mentioned in the text.

[†] Edinburgh Med. and Surg. Journal, xxxiii. 67.

ment. With this view, therefore, having ascertained in what articles it is possible for poison to have been administered, he should at once endeavour to secure the remains of the particular portion partaken of by his patient, as well of the general dish, if it is an article of food, and of the ingredients of which the dish was ostensibly made, not forgetting the salt with which it was seasoned. A case occurred some years ago in the north of Scotland, in which arsenic was administered in porridge by mixing it with the salt.

It is of great consequence, before proceeding to analyze such articles, for example suspected dishes, — to be particular in investigating every thing connected with the cooking, serving, and eating of them. By doing so, not only will the chemical analysis be facilitated, but likewise facts in it will be accounted for, which might otherwise prove embarrassing, and even lead to the drawing of false conclusions from the result of the analysis. This statement is very well exemplified by the following incident which occurred to myself. In 1827 a family in Portobello were poisoned by the maid-servant; and it was believed, that, for the sake of a trick, she had, while carrying to the oven the beef subsequently used at dinner, maliciously mixed with it tartar-emetic or some other poison. One-half of the beef having been preserved, and two persons of the family having been very severely affected, Dr. Turner and I, to whom the case was remitted, made little doubt that we should discover the poison by chemical analysis: but we did not. Being subsequently employed by the sheriff to inquire into the particulars, I found that the poison had been mixed with the gravy, which had been consumed almost to the last drop, — that the gravy had been poured over the beef, — that the upper half of the beef had been eaten, — and that the remainder which we analysed had been transferred upon a different plate from that on which it was served for dinner. These particulars accounted sufficiently for the poison not having been discovered.

Another mode in which the chemical part of the inquiry may contribute to discover the individual who administered the poison is by a comparative examination of the persons of the deceased and the accused. The following very pointed illustration has been published by MM. Ollivier and Chevallier of Paris. — A woman who lived on bad terms with her husband was found dead on a roadside the morning after having been seen drunk in his company in the neighbourhood. The mouth, throat, and gullet were proved by a careful analysis to be corroded with nitric acid, the stains and traces of which were also found on various parts of her dress, and on the hair, neck, and arms, but not on her hands, and not lower down the alimentary canal than the upper fourth of the gullet. Ollivier, suspecting from these appearances, that she had not taken the acid voluntarily, requested to see the husband; whereupon there were found on his coat, trousers, and hands, a great number of stains, which, like those on the deceased, were proved by chemical analysis to have been produced by nitric acid. Here it was scarcely possible to avoid inferring, that the man got these stains while endeavouring to force his intoxicated wife to take the posion. Marks of nail scratches were also observed round the mouth and on the throat; whence it was reasonably inferred, that, having failed in his original plan, he had suffocated her with his hands.*

While these illustrations are given of the conclusiveness of the chemical evidence in fixing the administration of poison on a particular individual, it is essential likewise to observe that the same kind of evidence may be at times equally conclusive of the innocence of a person unjustly suspected. This obvious and important application of a chemical inquiry is forcibly suggested by the following particulars of an incident related by M. Chevallier : — An individual was accused by a woman of having tried to poison her ; and she represented that he had put the poison into her soup, while it stood from one day to another in an iron pot. On making a careful analysis of some of the soup which remained, Chevallier found it so strongly impregnated with copper, that, supposing the sulphate was the salt mixed with the soup, ten ounces must have contained twenty-two grains. It then occurred to him, that it was important to examine the iron pot, in which the poisoned soup was represented to have been kept; for the probability was that a large quantity of the copper, if any salt of that metal had really been contained in the soup, would have been thrown down by the superior affinity of the iron, and consequently that a coppery lining would be found on the inside. He was led, however, to anticipate that no copper would be found there, because there was no iron dissolved in the soup, as would have been the case if copper had been precipitated from it by the iron of the pot. And accordingly he not only found no copper lining the inside of the pot ; but likewise, on following the process described by the accuser as the one pursued in cooking the soup and in subsequently poisoning it, he satisfied himself by express trial that there was nothing in the circumstances of the case which could have prevented the iron from exerting its usual action on the salts of copper. These conclusions, coupled with certain facts of general evidence, proved substantially that the suspected person had nothing to do with the crime charged against him ; and he was therefore discharged.† A case somewhat similar will be related under the head of Imputed Poisoning.

In the second place, evidence as to the person who administered the poison may be procured by considering the commencement of the symptoms, in relation to the time at which particular articles have been given in a suspicious manner by a particular individual. The import of facts of this nature can be properly appreciated only by the medical witness ; for he alone can be acknowledged as conversant with the symptoms which poisons produce, the intervals within which they begin to operate, and the circumstances in which their operation may be put off or accelerated.

Few cases will occur in which it is not possible to procure evidence of the kind, when diligently sought for. It is often too very decisive in its operation on judicial proceedings. In the case of Margaret Wishart tried at the Perth Spring Circuit in 1827 for poisoning her blind sister, a man who lodged with the prisoner and cohabited both with her and with the deceased, appeared at first from general circumstances to be implicated in the crime. He had left the house, however, on the morning of the day before that on the evening of which the deceased took ill; and he did not return till after her death. Now her illness commenced suddenly and violently; and arsenic was the poison which caused it.* It was quite clear, therefore, that the poison could not have been administered, at least in a dangerous dose, so early as the day before she was taken ill; and such I stated to be my opinion, on a reference from the Lord Advocate. The evidence being also otherwise insufficient, the man was set at liberty. In the case of Mrs. Smith tried here in February of the same year, this branch of the evidence was made the subject of question under more doubtful circumstances. The deceased certainly died of poisoning with arsenic, and the prisoner was strongly suspected of being the poisoner for many reasons, and among others because, on the evening before the morning on which the deceased took ill, the prisoner gave her in a suspicious manner a white-coloured draught. Here the possibility of the draught having been the cause of the symptoms must be admitted. But as they did not appear for eight hours after the draught was taken, I stated in my evidence that it was improbable the dose, if it contained arsenic at all, contained a quantity sufficient to cause the violent symptoms and death which followed.†

The correspondence in point of time between the appearance of symptoms of poisoning, and the administration of suspicious articles by an individual, constitutes still more decisive proof in a set of cases, in which it is of great value, as the chemical evidence is generally defective, — namely, where poisoning is attempted with repeated moderate doses. If the several renewals or exacerbations of illness correspond with the periods when suspicious articles have been given by the same individual, the circumstantial evidence of the administration may be even tantamount to direct proof. Thus, on the trial of Miss Blandy for the murder of her father, it was proved, that Mr. Blandy on several occasions, after the prisoner received certain suspicious powders from her lover, was taken ill with vomiting and purging; and that on two occasions recently before his death, when he got from his daughter a bowl of gruel which contained a gritty sediment, he was attacked after a very short interval with pricking and heat in the throat, mouth, stomach, and bowels, —

* Edin. Med. and Surg. Journal, xxix. 23.

† Ibid., xxvii. 441. On considering, however, this and other instances of the kind which have since come under my notice, I suspect the case is rendered intelligible by the effect of sleep in suspending or delaying for a time the action of arsenic and other simply irritating poisons. See above — *evidence from symptoms beginning soon after a meal,* p. 46. — also *article* Arsenic.

10

with sickness, vomiting, gripes, and bloody diarrhœa.* Here the proof of administration by the prisoner was complete.

These examples will show how the evidence of a particular person's criminality may be affected by the relation subsisting in point of time between the commencement of the symptoms and the suspicious administration of particular articles. But farther, the special period at which the symptoms begin may even at times supply strong evidence of his instrumentality, although there may be no direct proof from general evidence of his having been concerned in administering anything whatever in a suspicious manner. This statement is well exemplified by the case of Mrs. Humphreys, who was convicted at the Aberdeen Autumn Circuit in 1830 for poisoning her husband, by pouring sulphuric acid down his throat while he was asleep. It was clearly proved, as will be seen under the head of sulphuric acid, that the deceased died of this poison; and the administration was brought home to the prisoner in the following singular manner. The only inmates of the house were the deceased, the prisoner, and a maid-servant. The deceased got a little intoxicated one evening at a drinking party in his own house; and after his friends all left the house, and the street-door was barred inside, he went to bed in perfect health, and soon fell fast asleep. But he had slept scarcely twenty minutes, when he suddenly awoke with violent burning in his throat and stomach; and he expired in great agony towards the close of the second day. Now sulphuric acid, when it occasions the violent symptoms observed in this instance, invariably excites them in a few seconds, or in the very act of swallowing. It was, therefore, impossible that the man could have received the poison at the time he was drinking with his friends; and as he knew he had not taken any thing else afterwards, and it was fully proved that he had been asleep before his illness suddenly began, — it followed that the acid must have been administered after he fell asleep, the accomplishment of which was rendered easy by a practice he had of sleeping on his back with his mouth wide open. But, after he gave the alarm, the door was found barred as when he went to bed. Consequently no one could have administered the poison except his wife or servant; and it was satisfactorily proved, that no suspicion could attach to the latter. Such was one of the principal train of circumstances, which, as it were by a process of elimination, led to the inference that the wife was undoubtedly the person who administered the poison. Other circumstances of a similar tendency were also derived from the medical evidence; but these it is unnecessary to detail at present. I have related the particulars of the whole case fully elsewhere.† The prisoner strenuously denied her guilt after being sentenced, but confessed before her execution.

4. The next article in the moral evidence relates to the intent of the person who is proved to have administered poison. When the

* Howell's State Trials, xviii.
† Edinburgh Med. and Surg. Journal, xxxv. 298.

administration is proved, little evidence is in general required to establish the intent. It is sufficient that the giver knew the substance administered was of a deadly nature ; and in regard to any of the common poisons this knowledge is sufficiently constituted by his simply knowing its name.

In some cases, however, the exact nature of the poison is not established with certainty ; and then something else may be required to prove the prisoner's knowledge, and through that knowledge his intent.   In the case of Charles Munn, formerly alluded to [p. 50], arsenic was the poison presumed to have been taken by the deceased.   But the purchase or possession of it by the prisoner was not for some time satisfactorily established ; neither was there any chemical evidence, the deceased having lived forty days and upwards after taking the poison.   It was proved, however, that whatever it was which had been administered, the prisoner knew very well that what he gave was deleterious ; because he persuaded the deceased, who was pregnant by him, to take it by assigning to it properties which no drug either possesses, or is so much as thought by the vulgar to possess. On one occasion he persuaded her that it would show whether she was with child, and on another that it would prevent people from knowing she was with child. In such cases, then, good evidence may be derived from the arguments used by the giver to persuade his victim to take the poison ; and sometimes, as in the instance now mentioned, it will lie with the medical witness to inform the court whether or not the reasons assigned are false.

Sometimes it has been pleaded by the prisoner that he gave the poison by mistake.   In all such cases, if he descends to particulars, which he cannot help doing, there is every likelihood that the falsehood of the defence will be made evident by the particulars of the story not agreeing with other particulars of the moral or medical evidence.   At present it is only necessary to allude to inconsistencies in his story with the medical facts.   No general rules can be laid down on the method of investigating a case with a view to evidence of this kind : I must be satisfied with an illustration from an actual occurrence. On the trial of Mr. Hodgson, a surgeon, at the Durham Autumn Assizes in 1824, for attempting to poison his wife, it was clearly proved, that pills containing corrosive sublimate, and compounded by the prisoner, were given by him to her in place of pills of calomel and opium, which had been ordered by her physician. But it was pleaded by him, that, being at the time intoxicated, he had mistaken, for the shop-bottle which contained opium, the corrosive-sublimate bottle which stood next it.   This was certainly an improbable error, considering the opium was in powder, and the sublimate in crystals. But it was not the only one which he alleged he had committed. Not long after his wife took ill, the physician sent the prisoner to the shop to prepare for her a laudanum draught, with water for the menstruum.   When the prisoner returned with it, the physician, in consequence of observing it to be muddy, was led to taste it, before he gave it to the sick lady : and finding it had the taste of corrosive sublimate, he preserved it, analyzed it, and discovered that it did contain that poison. The prisoner stated in defence, that he had a second time committed a mistake, and instead of water had accidentally used for the menstruum a corrosive-sublimate injection, which he had previously prepared for a sailor. This was proved to have been impossible ; for the injection contained only five grains to the ounce, while the draught, which did not exceed one ounce, contained fourteen grains.*

I believe it must be allowed, that, as the medical inquiries preparatory to trial are commonly conducted without the inspector being made acquainted with the moral circumstances in detail, it is rarely possible for him to foresee what points should be attended to, with the view of illustrating the intent. But the case now related will show that it is impossible for him to render his inquiries too minute or comprehensive ; and more particularly, it shows the propriety of ascertaining, whenever it is possible, not only the nature but likewise the quantity of the poison.

5. The next article among the moral circumstances, — the simultaneous illness of other members of the family besides the person chiefly affected, — depends for its conclusiveness almost entirely upon the researches and opinion of the medical witnesses.

The fact, that several persons, who partook of the same dish or other article, have been seized about the same time with the same symptoms, will furnish very strong evidence of general poisoning. A few diseases, such as those which arise from infection or from atmospheric miasmata, may affect several persons of a family about the same time ; and hysteria, and epilepsy, have been communicated to several people in rapid succession.† But I am not aware, that, among the diseases which resemble well marked cases of poisoning either with irritants or with narcotics, any one ever originates in such a way as to render it possible for several persons in a family to be attacked simultaneously, except through the merest and therefore most improbable accident. Cholera perhaps is an exception. But when cholera attacks at one time several people living together, it arises from bad food, and is properly a variety of poisoning. In such cases, too, the fallacy may in general be easily got the better of, by finding that the store or stock, from which the various articles composing the injurious meal have been taken was of wholesome quality.

Hence it may be laid down as a general rule, that, perhaps if two, but certainly if three or more persons, after taking a suspected article of food or drink, are each affected with symptoms, furnishing of themselves presumptive evidence of poisoning, and have been seized nearly about the same time, and within the interval after eating within which poisons usually begin to act, — the proof of poisoning is decisive. Several late cases might, in my opinion, have been

* Edinburgh Medical and Surgical Journal, xxii. 438.

† For a very striking example of the latter description see Hufeland's Journal der Praktischen Heilkunde, xii. i. 110. Fourteen people were seized about the same time in a charity workhouse.

decided by this rule. Thus it might have decided the important case of George Thom tried at Aberdeen in 1821 for poisoning the Mitchells, and likewise that of Eliza Fenning, about whose condemnation some clamour was made in London in 1815. In both instances, as will be mentioned under the head of arsenic, the symptoms were developed so characteristically, that from them alone poisoning with arsenic might have been inferred almost to a certainty. But even if the symptoms had been somewhat less characteristic, all doubt of general poisoning was set aside by the fact, that four persons in the former case, and five in the latter, were similarly and simultaneously affected, and all of them at an interval after eating, which corresponded with the interval within which arsenic usually begins to act.

Sometimes it happens, that while one or more of a party at a certain meal suffer, others escape. Such an occurrence must not be hastily assumed as inconsistent with poison having been administered at that meal. For the guilty person may have slipped the poison into the portion taken by the individual or individuals affected.

If it be proved that all who ate of a particular dish have suffered, and all who did not have escaped, the kind of moral evidence now under review becomes strongest of all. It is well for the medical jurist to remember also, that such evidence is very useful in directing him where chiefly he should look for poison.

At other times it happens that the several people affected, suffer in proportion to the quantity taken by each of a particular dish. Too much importance ought not to be attached to the absence of that relation; for it has been already mentioned that habit, idiosyncrasy, and the state of fulness of the stomach at the time, will modify materially the action of poisons. But when present, it will often form strong evidence. — A good illustration of what is now said may be found in the case of Thomas Lenargan, tried in Ireland for the murder of his master, Mr. O'Flaherty. He had for some time carried on an amour with O'Flaherty's wife ; and afterwards, to get rid of the troublesome surveillance of the husband, contrived to despatch him by poison. The crime was not suspected for two years. Among the facts brought out on the trial the most pointed were, that O'Flaherty's daughter and two servants were affected at the same time with the very same symptoms as himself; that they had partaken of the same dish with him ; that the severity of their several complaints was in proportion to the quantity each had taken ; and that others of the family, who did not eat it, were not affected.*

Another remarkable instance of this kind has been recorded by Morgagni. A clergyman, while travelling in company with another gentleman and two ladies, was setting out one afternoon to resume his journey after dining at an inn, when he was suddenly taken ill with violent pain in the stomach and bowels, and soon after with

* Having mislaid the copy I possessed of this trial, I am unable to give here the reference.

10*

vomiting and purging.   One of the ladies was similarly affected, but
in a less degree; and likewise the other gentleman, though in a
degree still less: but the other lady did not suffer at all.   Morgagni
found, that this lady was the only one of the party who had not tasted
a dish of soup at the commencement of dinner.   But he was puzzled
on finding that the gentleman who suffered least had taken the largest share of the soup, while the clergyman had taken less than
either of the two that were seized along with him.   He then remembered, however, that in the district where the accident happened, it
was the custom to use scraped cheese with the soup in question;
and on inquiry he was informed that they had each added to the soup
a quantity of cheese proportioned to the severity of their illness.
Here, therefore, Morgagni was led to suspect the presence of poison;
and accordingly, after the whole party had fortunately recovered, the
innkeeper acknowledged, that in the hurry of preparation, he had
served up to his guests cheese seasoned with arsenic to poison rats.[*]
This interesting anecdote shows, that the truth in such cases is not
always to be discovered without minute inquiry and considerable
adroitness.   In the case of poisoning with arsenic in wine formerly
alluded to, — where all the individuals at table, to the amount of
six, were severely affected during dinner, — the soup was the article
suspected, because all had partaken of it; and, accordingly, the soup
and vomited matter were sent to me for analysis.   On detecting a
trace of arsenic in the vomited matter, but none in the soup, I suggested that some other article might have been used in common by
the party, and mentioned the wine as a probable article of the kind.
It turned out that all had drunk a single glass of champaign from a
particular bottle; and in the wine remaining in this bottle arsenic
was found in the proportion of half a grain per ounce.[†]

Cases of this nature are so instructive that no apology need be
made for mentioning one example more which lately came under my
own notice.   In the case of Mary Anne Alcorn, convicted here in
the summer of 1827, of having administered poison to her master
and mistress (a case already referred to for another purpose, p. 75),
it was proved that a white powder was introduced in a suspicious
manner into the gravy of baked beef, which gravy was subsequently
poured over the beef.   Now the master of the family dined heartily
on beef, potatoes and rice-pudding, and mixed the greater part of the
beef gravy with his pudding; the mistress ate moderately of the first
slices of the beef, took very little gravy, even to the beef, and none
at all to the pudding; a little girl, their niece, dined on pudding
alone, without gravy; and the prisoner dined after the family on the
beef and potatoes.   Accordingly the master suffered so severely as for
two or three days to be in danger of his life, the mistress was also
severely, but by no means so violently affected, the little girl did not
suffer at all, and the servant had merely slight pain and sickness at
stomach.   The evidence thus procured was exceedingly strong, more

* De Sedibus et Causis Morborum, T. ii. Ep. lix. 7.
† Edin. Med. and Surg. Journal, xxxiii. 67.

particularly when coupled with the fact, that the beef used was half of a piece, the other half of which had been used by the family two days before, without any ill consequences.

6. The next article of the moral evidence relates to suspicious conduct on the part of the prisoner during the illness of the person poisoned. Under this head it is necessary merely to state what I conceive to be, with reference to the present branch of the proof, the duty of the medical practitioner who happens to attend a case of poisoning.

In such a conjuncture he is undoubtedly placed in a situation of some delicacy. But on considering the matter attentively, good reasons will appear why he should adopt the course, which, I believe, our courts of justice will expect of him, and keep some watch over the actions of any individual who is suspected of having committed the crime. On the one hand, no one else is by education and opportunities so capable of remarking the motions of the different members of the family dispassionately, without officiousness, and without being observed. And on the other hand, it is undoubtedly a part of his private duty as practitioner, to protect his patient against any farther criminal attempts, as well as part of his public duty to prevent the vomited matter and other subjects of analysis from being secretly put away or destroyed. No one can be so occupied without many accessary particulars coming under his notice. And certain it is, that on several trials the practitioner has contributed, with great credit to himself, a considerable part of the pure moral proof. For an example of discreet and able conduct under these trying circumstances, the reader will do well to refer to that of Dr. Addington, the' chief crown witness, both as to medical and moral facts, in the case of Miss Blandy.* It is almost unnecessary to add, that in acting as now recommended, the physician must conduct himself with circumspection, in order to avoid giving unnecessary offence, or alarming the guilty person.

7, and 9. On the seventh article, which respects the conduct of the prisoner after the death of the deceased, and on the ninth, which relates to the existence of a motive or inducement to the crime, nothing need be said here. But on the

8th article of the moral evidence, — comprehending the death-bed declaration of the deceased, his state of mind, his personal circumstances and other points which prove the possibility or impossibility of voluntary poisoning — a few remarks are required, because an important and little understood part of the practitioner's duty is connected with this branch of the proof.

The question as to the possibility of the poisoning being voluntary is one upon which the medical attendant will be expected to throw some light, and into which he will also naturally inquire for his own satisfaction. In doing so his attention will be turned to circumstances purely moral, which may not only decide that question, but may also criminate a particular individual. His inquiries must there-

* Howell's State Trials, xviii.

fore be conducted with discretion, and for obvious reasons should be confined as much as possible to the patient himself. They are to be conducted not so much by putting questions, as by leading him to disburden his mind of his own accord ; and it is well to be aware, that there is no one of whom a patient is so ready to make a confident on such an occasion as his medical attendant.

If disclosures of consequence are made, and the attendant should feel it his duty to look forward to the future judicial proceedings and to the probability of his appearing as a witness, he ought to remember the general rule is, that his account of what the patient told him is not evidence in the eye of the law, unless it was told under the consciousness of the approach of death. Of late, however, the rigour of this principle in law has been occasionally departed from in Scottish practice ; and in regard to medical facts ascertained in the way here mentioned, many strong reasons might be assigned for such relaxation. Evidence of the kind is technically called the death-bed declaration of the deceased, and is justly accounted very important.

Here it is right to take notice of a part of the death-bed evidence, although it does not properly belong to the question of suicide, because it should always be collected if possible by the medical attendant, and with much greater care than is generally bestowed on it even by him — I mean the history of the symptoms previously to his being called in. On this part of the history, including particularly the time and manner in which the illness began, medical conclusions of extreme consequence are often subsequently founded : On a single fact or two may depend the fate of the prisoner. It is not enough, therefore, in my opinion, that such evidence formed a part of the death-bed declaration. If a fact derived at second hand from the deceased, and stated too by him from memory, is a material element of any of the medical opinions on the trial, it is of much importance that the information be procured by a medical man ; and that the person who procured it, whether professional or not, was aware at the time of the probability of its becoming important. Such evidence, although not collected with these precautions, is admissible ; but I have so often had occasion to witness the carelessness with which the previous history of cases is inquired into both in medical and medico-legal practice, that I do not see how it is possible to put trust in evidence of the kind, unless it bear marks of having been collected with care, and under an impression of its probable consequence. These statements are well illustrated by the following example : — On the trial of Mrs. Smith for poisoning her maid-servant with arsenic, it was proved that some drug was administered by the prisoner in a suspicious manner on a Tuesday evening. Now it appeared at the trial improbable that this drug contained a fatal dose of arsenic, because to her fellow-servants, of whom one slept with her, and others frequently visited her, the deceased did not appear to be ill at all for eight hours after, or seriously ill for nearly a day. On the contrary, however, a surgeon, who was called to see her on the following Saturday, a few hours before her death, deposed that, according to information communicated by herself, she had been ill with sickness, vomiting, purging, and pain in the stomach and bowels since the Tuesday evening. This evidence, if it could have been relied on, would have altered materially the features of the case, as it would have gone far to supply what all the medical witnesses considered defective, namely, proof of the administration. But at the time the surgeon made his inquiries, he did not even suspect that the girl laboured under the effects of poison. Neither he therefore nor his patient could have been impressed with that conviction of the importance of the information communicated, which was necessary to insure its accuracy, particularly as it related to a matter usually of so little consequence in ordinary medical practice as the precise date of the commencement of an illness ; and it would consequently have been rash to adopt it in face of more direct and contrary evidence. Any one who examines the details of this trial as I have reported them, will at once see how much the case turned on the point now alluded to.*

CHAPTER III.

OF IMAGINARY PRETENDED, AND IMPUTED POISONING.

The present seems the most convenient place for noticing the general mode of procedure by which the medical jurist may detect cases of imaginary, feigned, and imputed poisoning. It is by no means easy to lay down rules for the investigation of cases suspected to be of such a kind. But an attempt will be made to state the leading points to be attended to, and to illustrate them by the circumstances of a few examples of each variety.

Imaginary poisoning should rarely be the occasion of deception or embarrassment. The same wandering of the imagination which has led to a belief of injury from poison, will commonly also lead to such extravagant notions relative to the mode of administration and the symptoms, as will infallibly point out the true nature of the case to one who is well acquainted with the real effects of poisons. It is easy, nevertheless, to conceive cases which may be embarrassing ; and certainly, in every instance, the physician should proceed in his inquiries with caution.

It appears to me that in the first place, without seeming to take up at once the conviction of his patient, he should scrupulously abstain from treating it lightly, and should on the whole act rather as if he suspected poison had been given. Allowing his patient therefore apparently credit for the truth of his suspicions, the medical attendant should request him to give a full history of existing symptoms, of

* Edin. Med. and Surg. Journal, xxvii. 441. The reader will remember that what was considered defective in the proof in this trial, the connection between the administration of a suspicious article and the first invasion of the symptoms, would now appear less so, for the reason assigned in note † p. 77.

their origin and progress, of their relation in point of time to various meals, and of the mode and vehicle in which the supposed poison was administered. No unprofessional person can possibly go through such a narrative, without stating many circumstances which are wholly irreconcilable with the idea of poisoning generally, and still more of the administration of a particular poison.

I have met with two instances of imaginary poisoning, the nature of which was thus at once made obvious by a host of impossibilities in the narrative of the patient. One of these may be here given as an example. An elderly lady, who had certain expectancies of the death of a relation, conceived that the family of her relative had re-solved to defraud her of her supposed rights. She afterwards ima-gined that an attempt was made to poison her, and camphor was the poison she fixed on as the article which had been administered. In its general or moral particulars the narrative was all plausible and suspicious enough ; but unluckily for its consistency, she stated that the poison could only have been given in wine, — that she did not remark any particular taste in the wine, — that her illness did not begin till the day after she took it ; and although she alleged, without any leading question on my part, that camphorous perspiration was exhaled on the subsequent day, the whole train of symptoms differed entirely in every other respect from a case of poisoning, and resembled closely in their origin and progress a case of slight general fever. The incompatibility of her story with the idea of poisoning with camphor will be readily understood by referring to what is afterwards said of the effects of that substance.

Feigned or *pretended poisoning* is more apt to escape suspicion, and when suspected is commonly more difficult to develope satisfac-torily ; for the actor has it in his power to lay his plans with care, and even to become acquainted with the properties of the poisons whose effects he intends to feign. Still he can rarely enact his part so well as to deceive a skilful physician both by existing symptoms and by his history of their origin and progress ; much less can he contrive his scheme so adroitly that it shall not be unfolded by the refinements of chemical analysis.

The investigation of such a case will be directed of course in the first instance to the state and progress of the symptoms. Here, as in imaginary poisoning, it is of moment to conceal from the individual the suspicion entertained of his falsehood. For even if a person who has actually taken poison knows he is unjustly suspected of feigning, it is not improbable that he might try to mend his story with impos-sibilities, and so lead the physician into error. In a case of feigned poisoning an excellent mode of investigation is, after hearing out the individual's own story, to put a number of questions involving an al-ternative answer, one alternative being compatible and the other in-compatible with the alleged nature of his illness. No unprofessional person can stand such a system of interrogation, if skilfully pursued. Not only will his answers be often wrong ; but likewise his manifest perplexity how to answer will of itself supply evidence of falsehood.

In the next place, great attention must be paid to the chemical analysis. A person who feigns poisoning will commonly produce the poisoned remains of a dish, or some other article, which he represents himself to have swallowed. Sometimes the substance contained in it will prove on analysis not to be poison at all, as in an instance I remember reading some years ago in a London newspaper of pretended poisoning with arsenic, where the dregs of a bowl of gruel contained, not arsenic, but finely pounded glass. Sometimes the quantity of a real poison contained in the remains of a dish may indicate, in what is said to have been swallowed, a portion wholly incompatible with the mildness or severity of the symptoms. Sometimes the vomited matter, even the matter first vomited, may not contain any of the alleged poison. Sometimes poison found in matter alleged to have been vomited may yield compounds during analysis which are not animalized, showing that it never was in the stomach. Sometimes the quantity of poison contained in such matter may be greater than that alleged to have been taken. Sometimes the quantity contained in the first matter vomited may be less than that contained in what is vomited or said to be vomited subsequently. By these and many other such inconsistencies the falsehood of the story may be unequivocally unfolded.

The following example will illustrate some of the rules now laid down. A young married female, in the seventh month of pregnancy, having been discovered by her friends to be secretly addicted to dram-drinking, appeared to be much annoyed in consequence of the discovery; and one evening was found apparently very ill by her husband on his return from work. She represented that she had taken arsenic with a view to self-destruction, that she was in great torture, and that she was sure she must soon die. It was accordingly found, on reference to a neighbouring apothecary, that she had the same forenoon purchased about a drachm and a half of arsenic for the pretended purpose of poisoning rats; and in the bottom of a teacup, in which she said she mixed it, there was left a small quantity of white powder, that proved on analysis to be pure oxide of arsenic. Notwithstanding these strong facts, the mildness of the symptoms and the composure with which she complained of her tortures led her friends to suspect she was feigning. On investigating her case I first ascertained, in farther corroboration of her story, that the powder was nowhere to be found. But she then stated in reply to questions involving an alternative answer, that the arsenic had a sour taste, and that the pain began in the lower part of the belly, and spread upwards. She likewise said that she vomited a mouthful or two into a chamber-pot twenty minutes after taking the poison; that she vomited no more till the apothecary was sent for, who gave her emetics of sulphate of zinc, carefully preserving the discharges; and that she only vomited when emetics were given. When I first saw her, five hours after the alleged date of the taking of the arsenic, the skin was warm and moist, the face full and flushed, the pulse frequent and firm, the muscular strength natural. The chamber-pot contained only a small quantity of the faeces of a child and apparently a little water, but no vomited matters, and no white powder. The fluid discharged in presence of the apothecary was found on careful analysis to contain a large quantity of zinc, but not an atom of arsenic. She gradually recovered from the illness under which she laboured at the time I saw her, and in two days she admitted she was quite well, but continued to insist that she had taken the poison. — M. Tartra has related a singular case of the same kind, where a young woman feigned poisoning with nitric acid, and was not detected for several days.*

Imputed poisoning differs in general from feigned poisoning only in so far as the symptoms which are feigned are imputed to the agency of another.

The imputation of the crime of poisoning by feigning or actually producing the symptoms, and contriving that poison shall be detected in the quarters where in actual cases it is usually sought for, has been not unfrequently attempted. Two important continental cases have already been referred to for other purposes [pp. 66, 76]; and I may here relate the heads of two English cases, which are of great interest, and will serve to illustrate the mode of procedure in such circumstances.

The first of these, which I have related elsewhere in detail,† is a striking example of the power of science in eliciting the truth, and redounds highly to the credit of Mr. Thackrah, the medical gentleman who conducted the investigation.

Samuel Whalley was indicted at York Spring Assizes in 1821, for maliciously administering arsenic to Martha King, who was pregnant by him. The woman King swore, that the prisoner, after twice trying, but in vain, to prevail on her to take drugs for the purpose of procuring abortion, sent her a present of tarts, of which she ate one and a half, — that in half an hour she was seized with symptoms of poisoning with some irritant poison, — and that she continued ill for a long time after. Mr. Thackrah found arsenic in the tarts that remained untouched, and likewise in some matter that was vomited in his presence after the administration of an emetic, as well as in other vomited matters which were preserved for him between his first and second visits. Her appearance, however, did not correspond with the complaint she made of her sufferings, her pulse and tongue were natural, and on careful investigation the following inconsistencies were farther detected. 1. She said she felt a coppery taste in the act of eating the tarts, a taste which arsenic certainly does not possess. 2. From the quantity of arsenic in the tarts which remained she could not have taken above ten grains, while even after repeated attacks of vomiting, the alleged matter subsequently preserved contained nearly fifteen grains. 3. The matter first vomited contained only one grain, while the matter alleged to have been vomited subsequently contained fifteen grains. 4. The time at which these fifteen grains were alleged to have been vomited was not till between two and three hours after

* Sur l'Empoisonnement par l'acide nitrique, p. 243.
† Edinburgh Medical and Surgical Journal, xxix. 19.

the symptoms began ; in which case the symptoms would before that time have been in all probability violent. The prisoner was acquitted, and the prosecutor and another woman who corroborated her deposition afterwards confessed that they had entered into a conspiracy to impute the crime to him, because he had deserted her on finding she was too intimate with other men.

Another case not less interesting in its details was communicated to me by my colleague Dr. Traill, who was consulted by the medical attendant, Mr. Parr of Liverpool. A man accused his sister-in-law of administering poison in his tea. He stated that he was seized with pain in the stomach and uneasiness in the head half an hour after taking the tea ; and when visited soon after, the countenance was anxious, the skin pallid, the pulse frequent, the throat red ; and while Mr. Parr was examining the throat, a quantity of matter was vomited, containing a white, gritty, crystalline substance, which was afterwards ascertained to be oxalic acid. The following circumstances, however, proved that the poison could not have been given in the tea. The man alleged that he remarked in the very first mouthful an acrid taste, followed by sweetness, which is not the taste of oxalic acid. Notwithstanding this warning, he drank the greater part of the tea. He stated that the poison was dissolved in the tea, yet he vomited some oxalic acid in the solid form. Granting he was mistaken in supposing the whole poison dissolved, the quantity swallowed must in that case have been large ; and nevertheless the symptoms were mild, though no vomiting took place for about an hour, and next day he was almost well. Four other individuals had tea at the same time from the same tea-pot, without sustaining any harm ; and what remained of the infusion did not contain any oxalic acid. Finally, his niece took what he left of his tea in the cup, without remarking any unusual taste ; and in the unwashed cup not a trace of oxalic acid could be detected. It was quite plain, therefore, that the man's accusation was false ; and certain points of general evidence, coupled with the medical facts, afterwards proved that he must have taken the oxalic acid himself.

It has been alleged, that attempts have been made to impute the crime of poisoning by introducing poisonous substances into the body after death; and although I have not been able to find any actual instance of such ingenious atrocity mentioned by authors, it must be acknowledged to be quite possible ; and the medical jurist should therefore be prepared for the requisite investigations. Every case may be clearly made out by attending to the relative effects of poisons on the dead and on the living tissues ; — a subject which will receive some notice under the head of the principal poisons in common use.

11

PART SECOND.

OF INDIVIDUAL POISONS.

CHAPTER I.

OF THE CLASSIFICATION OF POISONS.

AFTER the preliminary observations on General Poisoning, I proceed next to treat of Poisons Individually. The subsequent remarks will be confined in a great measure to the most common poisons, which will be examined minutely. The rest being mere objects of curiosity, and hardly ever taken by man either intentionally or by accident, it will be sufficient to point out their leading properties.

It may be well to point out in the first instance the poisons in most general use. These will appear from the following Tables. The first is compiled from a Parliamentary Return of the cases of fatal poisoning brought before the coroners of England in two years ending with 1838.

1. *Arsenical* . White arsenic . 185
Yellow arsenic . . . 1
———186

2. *Acids* . . . . Sulphuric acid . . 32
Nitric acid 3
Oxalic acid 19
— 54

3. *Mercurials.* Corrosive sublimate 12
White mercury . . . 1
Turbith-mineral . . . 1
Mercury (?) 1
— 15

4. *Other mine-* Tartar-emetic 2
ral irritants Sulphate of iron . . 1
Chloride of tin 1
Subacetate of lead . . 1
Bichrom. of potash . 1
Percussion powder . 1
Carbonate of potash . 1
Black-ash 1
— 9

5. *Veget. irri-* Colchicum 3
tants Hellebore 1
Savin 1
Cayenne 1
Castor seeds 1
Morison pills 1
— 8

6. *Anim. irrits.* Cantharides 3
7. *Opium* . Opium or Laudan. . 180
Opium & nitric acid . 1
Poppy-syrup 4
Godfrey's Cordial . . 6
Morphia 1
Acetate of morphia . 1
———193

8. *Hydrocya-* Med. Hydroc. acid . 27
nic acid Do. and Laudanum . 1
Ess. oil of Almonds . 5
Bay-leaves 1
— 34

9. *Other veget.* Nux-vomica 3
Narcotics Strychnia 2
Belladonna 2
Hemlock 1
Monkshood 2
Spirits 4
Fungi 4
— 18

10. *Narcot. gases.* Coal-gas 3
11. Unascertained 22

Total 543

In France, in seven years, from 1825 to 1831, inclusive, there were 216 trials for poisoning, at which 273 persons were charged with the crime, and only 102 condemned. In 94 cases occurring between November 1825 and October 1832, the substances employed were as follows.*

Arsenic	54	Tartar-emetic	1	Cantharide	
Orpiment	1	Sulphate of zinc	1	Nux-vomica	4
Verdigris	7	Acetate of lead	1	Opium	1
Corrosive sublimate	5	Cerusse	1	Sulphuric acid	1
Fly-powder	3	Mercurial ointment	1	Nitric acid	1
		Unascertained	5		

In the subsequent seven years there were 218 trials, and 153 prisoners condemned. Among 194 of these the following were the poisons used.†

Metallic arsenic	5	Tartar-emetic	1	Belladonna	1
Arsenious acid	132	Cerusse	1	Opium	3
Arsenite of copper	1	Sulphuric acid	5	Morphia	1
Compounds of copper	13	Nitric acid	2	Nux-vomica	1
Corrosive sublimate	10	Muriatic acid	1	Cantharides	10
Artificial orpiment	3	Hydrocyanic acid	1		
Sulphate of zinc	1	Ammonia	1		

In Denmark, in five years ending with 1835, there were 99 cases of poisoning of all sorts, 16 by arsenic, 74 by sulphuric or nitric acid, 4 by potash, 1 by an unascertained caustic substance, 2 by opium, 1 by litharge, and 1 by copper. Only 5 cases, namely, 3 by arsenic and 2 by sulphuric acid, were cases of murder, or attempt to murder.‡

The classification of poisons has hitherto defied the ingenuity of toxicologists. Formerly it was thought sufficient to arrange them in three great classes, according as they are derived from the mineral, the vegetable, or the animal kingdom. It is evident, however, that the only sound basis of arrangement is their action on the animal economy; for such a classification is the only one which can be useful in practice. Now, when we consider what has been said on their mode of action, or the symptoms produced in consequence of that action, it must at once be perceived, that no system founded on either of these circumstances can be logically correct. It would be very desirable, if their mode of action could be adopted as the basis of arrangement; but both reasoning and experience have proved this to be impracticable. One very distinct class indeed might be formed of purely local poisons, comprehending the mineral acids, the fixed alkalies, and one or two of their chemical compounds. But a vast proportion of the other poisons which act locally have also a general or remote action; and on the other hand there are few of the latter description which do not likewise act locally. Hence if all which possess this double action were arranged in one class, that class would include nine-tenths at least of known poisons; so that, in truth, the labour of classification would still remain to be overcome.

* MM. Chevallier et Boys de Loury, in Annales d'Hyg. Publ. et Méd. Lég. xivv. 400.

† MM. Lecanu and Chevallier in Annales d'Hyg.Publ. 1840, xxiv. 282.

‡ London Medical Gazette, 1839-40, i. 575.

It would be even more fruitless to attempt an arrangement of poisons according to their medium of action; for no sure criterion is known, by which a poison acting through direct transmission of an impulse along the nerves can be distinguished from one that acts by entering the blood.

Neither is the embarrassment of the toxicologist materially less, if he attempts to classify poisons according to the symptoms they induce in man.   This is the principle now generally followed, and which in common with others I shall pursue.   But the reader will be at no loss to discover that the partitions which separate the classes are exceedingly slight, and that very many poisons might be arranged without impropriety in either of two classes.

The preceding statements show the impossibility of founding a good system of arrangement on the only basis which can be acknowledged philosophical and practical; and consequently, that, as the science of toxicology now stands, we must altogether despair of forming one that shall be even moderately satisfactory.

On the whole I see no reason for deviating from the classification adopted in the first edition of the present work, being a modification of that previously followed by Professor Orfila.   In this classification poisons are divided into irritants, narcotics, and narcotic-acrids.

The class of irritants includes all poisons whose sole or predominating symptoms are those of irritation or inflammation; the narcotics those which produce stupor, delirium, spasms, paralysis, and other affections of the brain and nervous system; and the narcotico-acrids those which cause sometimes irritation, sometimes narcotism, sometimes both together.   Some writers still adopt a fourth class, called septics, because they give rise to putrefaction in the living body. But modern physiology will scarcely sanction the continuance of such a class of poisons.   For assuredly no substance can cause putrefaction in the living body.

CHAPTER II.

CLASS FIRST.

ON IRRITANT POISONS GENERALLY.

THE class of irritant poisons comprehends all whose sole or predominant action consists in exciting irritation or inflammation.   That is, it comprises both those which have a purely local, irritating action, and likewise many which also act remotely, but whose most prominent feature of action still is the inflammation they excite wherever they are applied.

This subject will be introduced with an account of the general symptoms and morbid appearances caused by the irritants, and a comparison of these with the symptoms and morbid appearances of the natural diseases which are chiefly liable to be confounded with irritant poisoning, or mistaken for it.

SECTION I. — *Of the Symptoms of the Irritant Poisons, compared with those of natural diseases.*

The symptoms caused by the irritating poisons, taken internally, are chiefly those of violent irritation and inflammation of one or more divisions of the alimentary canal.

The mouth is frequently affected, especially when the poison is easily soluble, and possesses a corrosive as well as irritating power. The symptoms referrible to the mouth are pricking or burning of the tongue, and redness, swelling and ulceration of the tongue, palate, and inside of the cheeks.

The throat and gullet are still more frequently affected; and the affection is commonly burning pain, sometimes accompanied with constriction and difficulty in swallowing, and always with redness of the visible part of the throat and gullet.

The affection of the throat and mouth precedes every other symptom when the poison is an active corrosive, and more particularly when it is either a fluid poison or is easily dissolved. Nay, sometimes burning pain of the mouth, throat, and gullet occurs during the very act of swallowing. — On the contrary if the poison is soluble with difficulty, and is only an irritant, not a corrosive, and still more if it is only one of the feebler irritants, the throat is frequently not affected sooner than the stomach, occasionally not at all.

The stomach is the organ which suffers most invariably from the operation of irritant poisons. The symptoms referrible to their operation on it are acute and general burning pain, sometimes lancinating or pricking pain, — sickness, vomiting, tenderness on pressure, tension in the upper part of the belly, and occasionally swelling. Of these symptoms the sickness is generally the first to develope itself. In the instance of corrosive irritants pain commonly commences along with it. The matter vomited is at first the contents of the stomach, afterwards tough mucus, streaked often with blood and mingled with bile, frequently clots of purer blood. The powerful corrosives affect the stomach the moment they are swallowed; irritants which are either liquid or very soluble also affect it very soon; but the more insoluble irritants, such as arsenic, generally do not begin to act till half an hour or even more than a whole hour has elapsed. — The stomach may be affected without any other part of the alimentary canal participating in the injury; but much more frequently other parts suffer also, and in particular the intestines.

The action of irritant poisons on the intestines is marked by pain extending over the whole belly, sometimes even to the anus. This pain, like that of the stomach, is often a sense of burning; but it is also frequently a pricking or tearing pain, and still more frequently a twisting, intermitting pain like that of colic. It is seldom attended with much swelling, but often with tension, and tenderness of the whole belly; and at times the inflammatory state of the mucous coat of the intestines is clearly indicated by excoriation of the anus and prolapsus of the rectum, which is of a bright red colour. The pain

11*

of the bowels is most generally attended by purging, rarely with constipation, frequently with tenesmus. The matter discharged, after the alimentary and feculent contents have passed, is chiefly a mucous fluid, often abundant, often also streaked with blood or mixed with considerable quantities of blood. In some cases the intestines are affected when no other part of the alimentary canal suffers, not even the stomach. But much more generally the stomach and intestines are affected together.

In a few very aggravated cases of poisoning with the irritants the whole course of the alimentary canal, from the throat to the anus, is affected at one and the same time.

The symptoms now briefly enumerated are accompanied in almost every instance with great disturbance of the circulation—quick, feeble pulse—excessive prostration of strength,—coldness, and clammy moisture of the skin.

The other symptoms, which are often united with the preceding, do not belong to the irritants as a class. Perhaps, however, among the symptoms of the class may be mentioned those of irritation and inflammation of the windpipe and lungs, and those of irritation in the urinary organs. A great number of the irritant poisons cause hoarseness, wheezing respiration, and other signs which indicate the spreading of the inflammation of the throat to the windpipe: some likewise cause darting pains throughout the chest: and not a few are very apt to cause strangury and other signs of inflammation of the urinary passages.

Of the effects of the irritants when applied externally little need be said at present. Their most striking external symptoms will be noticed under the head of one of the orders of this class, the vegetable acrids. In the chapter on the local action of poisons some account was given of the several effects which are produced by the application of poisons to the skin. It is there stated that some produce merely redness, that others cause blistering, that others bring out a crop of deep-seated pustules, that others corrode the tissues chemically, and so give origin to a deep slough, and that others excite spreading inflammation of the cellular tissue under the skin and between the muscles.

Such is a general view of the symptoms caused by the irritant poisons. This topic will be afterwards taken up in detail under the head of the several species. At present an important subject remains for consideration, namely, the natural diseases whose effects are apt to be mistaken for the effects of poison. The remarks now to be made might be extended to many diseases. In fact, they might be extended to all which prove fatal suddenly, for all such diseases are apt in peculiar circumstances to give rise to a suspicion of poisoning. But those only will be here noticed which occasion the greatest embarrassment to the medical jurist, and which are most likely to come under his review in courts of law. They are the following:—Distension and rupture of the stomach; rupture of the duodenum, biliary ducts, uterus, or other organs in the belly; the effects of drinking cold water; bilious vomiting and common cholera; malignant cholera; inflammation of the stomach; inflammation and perforation of the intestines; inflammation of the peritonæum; spontaneous perforation of the stomach; melæna and hæmatemesis: colic, iliac passion and obstructed intestine.

1. *Distension of the Stomach.* — Mere distension of the stomach from excessive gluttony may cause sudden death. Generally indeed the symptoms and appearances in the dead body show that death is the consequence of apoplexy; but sometimes not. In order to preserve the continuity of the succeeding remarks on the diseases of the stomach which imitate poisoning, it may be useful to consider in the present place all the varieties of the effects of distension.

Excessive distension of the stomach, then, sometimes causes sudden death by inducing apoplexy, which is commonly of the congestive kind, — that is, without rupture of vessels. Mérat has related an instructive case of this kind. A man in good health, while greedily devouring an excellent dinner, became suddenly blue and bloated in the face; a clammy sweat broke out over his body; and he died almost immediately. On dissection the stomach was found enormously distended with food, and the vessels of the brain were so gorged, that the brain appeared too large to be contained within the skull.*

There is reason, however, to suppose that death from distension is the consequence not always of apoplexy, — but sometimes of an impression on the stomach itself. Sir Everard Home relates the case of a child, who, being left by its nurse beside an apple-pie, was found dead a few minutes afterwards, and in whose body no appearance of note could be discovered, except enormous distension of the stomach with the pie. — A still more distinct case in point forms the subject of a medico-legal report by Wildberg. A corpulent gentleman died suddenly fifteen minutes after dinner; and as he lived on bad terms with his wife, a suspicion arose that he had been poisoned. His wife said that he fell asleep immediately after dinner; but had not slept many seconds, when he suddenly awoke in great anguish, called out for fresh air, exclaimed he was dying, and actually expired before his physician, who was instantly sent for, could arrive. Wildberg found the stomach so enormously distended with ham, pickles, and cabbage-soup, that, when the belly was laid open, nothing could be seen at first but the stomach and colon. Some white powder, found on the villous coat of the stomach, was at first suspected to be arsenic; but it proved on analysis to be merely magnesia, which the gentleman had been in the habit of taking frequently. The diaphragm was pushed high into the chest by the distended stomach. There was not any particular congestion in the brain. Wildberg very properly ascribed death to simple over-distension of the stomach.† — In all such cases the symptoms may be suspicious; but when carefully considered they can scarce be said to re-

* Dictionnaire des Sciences Médicales, Art. Indigestion, xxiv. p. 374.
† Praktisches Handbuch für Physiker, iii. 292.

semble closely the effects of irritant poisoning; and at all events the
appearances in the dead body will at once distinguish them.

2. *Rupture of the Stomach* is not a common occurrence; but it
sometimes imitates in its symptoms the effects of the irritant poisons.
It is generally the consequence of over-distension, combined with
efforts to vomit. The cause of it seems to be, that the abrupt turn
which the gullet makes in entering an excessively distended stomach
acts as a valve, so that the contents cannot be discharged by vomiting. A case of this kind is related by M. Lallemand in his Inaugural Dissertation at Paris in 1818.* A woman convalescent from a
tedious attack of dyspepsia, being desirous to make amends for her
long privations as to diet, ate one day to satiety. Ere long she was
seized with a sense of weight in the stomach, nausea, and fruitless
efforts to vomit. Then she all at once uttered a piercing shriek, and
exclaimed that she felt her stomach tearing open; afterwards she
ceased to make efforts to vomit, soon became insensible, and in the
course of the night she expired. In the fore part of the stomach there
was a laceration five inches long; and a great deal of half-digested
food had escaped into the cavity of the abdomen. The coats of the
body of the stomach were healthy; but the pylorus or opening into
the intestines was indurated; which had been the cause of her dyspepsia.

In other cases of death from rupture the laceration is caused not
by the accumulation of food, but by the accumulation of gases arising
from depraved digestion, constituting a disease almost the same as
that which attacks cattle that have fed on wet clover. A singular
example of this rare affection, in which death was preceded by the
symptoms of irritant poisoning, has been noticed by Professor
Barzelotii.† — Another case, which appears to have been of the
same kind, is mentioned in a late French journal. A child, a twelvemonth old, after eating cabbage-soup, died during the night unper-
ceived by its mother. On the body being examined, a great quantity
of fetid gas escaped from the abdomen, and a smooth laceration like
an incised wound, three inches in length, was found in the lesser
arch of the stomach.‡

In other cases, however, it is not easy to say what occasions the
injury. An instance, for example, has been related, where the accident followed the drinking of a little shrub and water. The individual, a man of middle age, who had been long liable to fits of
severe pain in the stomach, going off with vomiting, was suddenly
seized the day after one of his fits with violent pain in the epigastrium, extreme tenderness and tension of the muscles, and for a short
time with violent vomiting. In seventeen hours he expired. On
dissection a dark-brown fluid was found in the cavity of the belly,
and the fore part of the stomach presented a laceration four inches
long. There were likewise several lacerations, one of them three
inches long, which intersected the peritonæal coat alone.§ A case

* See also Dictionnaire des Sciences Médicales, *Art.* Rupture, xlix. 225.
† Médicina Legale, ii. 22.   ‡ Archives Générales de Médecine, **xx. 433.**
§ Mr. Weekes, in London Medico-Chirurgical Transactions, xiv. 447.

probably similar in nature has been described by Dr. Roberts of London, that of a man who died of convulsions in five hours, and presented after death a long rent in the stomach, with escape of its contents into the general cavity of the belly.*

Another rare variety of rupture of the stomach must also be particularly noticed, because the course of the symptoms imitates very closely a case of poisoning with the irritants. It is *partial rupture,* — or laceration of the inner coat only. A very interesting case of that description has been related by Mr. Chevalier. A youth of fourteen, on the evening after a Christmas feast, at which he ate and drank heartily, was attacked with violent and frequent vomiting. Next morning he said he felt as if the blood in his heart was boiling, he was unable to swallow, the pulse became irregular, and pressure on the heart or stomach gave him excruciating agony. These symptoms continued till the following day, when he vomited two pounds of blood at successive intervals, and soon afterwards expired. The inner coat of the stomach was torn in many places, and that of the duodenum was lacerated almost completely round. No other disease existed in the bowels or elsewhere.†

Some of the cases now mentioned could hardly be distinguished from the effects of certain irritant poisons by the symptoms only. But the morbid appearances in the stomach will at once determine their real nature.

Rupture of the stomach, it may be observed, does not always occasion the symptoms hitherto related. Sometimes it causes instant death. Thus a healthy coal-heaver in London, while attempting to raise a heavy weight, suddenly cried out, clapped his hand over his stomach, drew two deep sighs, and died on the spot. On dissection a lacerated hole was found in the stomach, big enough to admit the thumb; and the stomach did not contain any food.‡ This case, along with those of Dr. Roberts and Mr. Weekes, will show that rupture may take place without previous distension.

3. *Rupture of the Duodenum* is a very rare accident from internal causes. The following instance resembles considerably the symptoms of irritant poisoning. A gentleman, 48 years old, quarrelled violently with another while playing billiards immediately after dinner. Soon afterwards he was seized suddenly with violent pain in the stomach, vomiting, cold extremities, and a failing pulse; and he died very soon. The mucous coat of the duodenum was found much inflamed, and four inches and a half from the pylorus there was a lacerated hole involving a third of the circumference of the gut.‡

4. Under the next head may be classed rupture of the other organs of the belly. *Rupture of the Biliary Ducts* for example, an extremely rare accident, has been known to imitate the symptoms of irritant poisoning, as the following case will show. — An elderly lady, after a slight attack of jaundice, was seized with violent pain in the stomach,

* London Medical and Physical Journal, June, 1831, vol. lxvi.
† London Medico-Chirurgical Transactions, v. 93.
‡ London Medical Repository, xvii. 108.
§ Bulletins des Sciences Médicales, x. 64.

and vomiting recurring in frequent fits, and in seventeen hours with extreme tenderness, tension of the muscles, coldness of the skin, and failure of the pulse.   She expired in twenty-four hours ; and after death the hepatic duct was found torn across, a gall-stone lay at the opening of the cystic duct, the peritonæum was here and there inflamed, and three pounds of blood and bile were effused into the cavity of the abdomen.*— The nature of such cases will be always apparent on dissection, but by no means always from the symptoms.

In like manner *rupture of the uterus or its appendages* may in certain circumstances occasion similar symptoms, and so be mistaken for the operation of poison.   A striking example of the kind once came under my notice.   A middle-aged woman much addicted to drinking, and on that account living on indifferent terms with her husband, was suddenly seized at two in the afternoon with pain in the belly, afterwards with vomiting and purging, then with extreme exhaustion and coldness of the extremities ; and at ten in the evening she expired.   A suspicion of poisoning having arisen in the neighbourhood, a judicial inspection was ordered by the sheriff of Linlithgowshire, where the case happened ; and the examination was entrusted to her medical attendant, Mr. Robertson, and myself.   On inquiry, it was found that she had taken nothing whatever after breakfasting at eight in the morning, six hours before ; and farther, that the pain had begun violently in the lower part of the belly.   These two circumstances alone were almost, if not altogether, incompatible with the idea of irritant poisoning having been the occasion of death. But all doubt was completely removed by the inspection of the body ; for the lower part of the belly was filled with a great quantity of clotted blood, which had proceeded from the rupture of a Fallopian conception.

5. The next accident which may be noticed on account of its being liable to be mistaken for the effects of poison is *sudden death from drinking cold water*.

In Britain the most common form of death from this cause appears to have been instant death, arising from the impression on the stomach. It is not an uncommon thing for people to drop down instantaneously and die on the spot, in consequence of drinking freely of cold water or other fluids while over-heated.†   There is an interesting report on a case of this kind by Pyl in his Memoirs and Observations.   The individual had been quarrelling with a companion, and in the height of a fit of violent passion swallowed a glass of beer ; when he dropped down senseless and motionless, and died immediately.   His wife suspecting the administration of poison, demanded a judicial inquiry ; but nothing was found in the body to account for death.   Pyl therefore came to the conclusion that the man died from the sudden impression caused by the cold beer.‡   Dr. Currie, after quoting several instances of the like kind, relates the following remarkable case which

* Journal des Progrès des Sciences Médicales, xiv.
† For an instance, see Bulletins des Sciences Médicales, ix. 249.
‡ Aufsätze und Beobachtungen aus der gerichtlichen Arzneiwissenschaft, v. 89.

occurred to himself. A young man, having just sat down, panting and bathed in sweat, after a severe match at tennis, drank greedily from a pitcher of water fresh drawn from a neighbouring pump. Suddenly he laid his hand on his stomach, bent forward, became pale, breathed laboriously, and in a few minutes expired.[*]

But when combined with exposure to a burning sun, as in hot climates, drinking cold water when the body is over-heated seems often to excite along with irritation in the stomach congestive apoplexy. Dr. Watts has given a good account of these effects as they occurred in the neighbourhood of New York during the hot season of 1818. During the summer of that year the thermometer often stood in the shade so high as 92° ; and the labourers in consequence could not be restrained from drinking frequently and excessively of cold water. Many were attacked with pain in the stomach, sickness, giddiness, and fainting ; next with difficult breathing, and rattling in the throat ; then with apoplexy ; and not a few perished.[†] These symptoms are very like the effects of some narcotico-acrid poisons.

Lastly, drinking cold water sometimes causes symptoms more nearly allied to those of the pure irritants. Thus some persons, on eating ices, or drinking iced-water, or cold ginger-beer in the hot days of summer, are attacked with violent colic. Others in the like circumstances are attacked with violent fits of vomiting.[‡] Haller has even mentioned an instance of a man, who after swallowing a large draught of cold water while over-heated, was seized with symptoms of acute gastritis, and died in fifteen days : and in the dead body the stomach was found gangrenous and ulcerated at its fundus.[§] M. Guérard relates a similar case, that of a quarter-master who, swallowing iced-beer after a hurried journey in a hot day, was attacked in six hours with shivering, then with heat and tightness in the pit of the stomach, vomiting of every thing he took, anxiety, thirst and frequency of the pulse ; next with extreme prostration, cessation of pain, hiccup, and lividity of the face ; and he expired in five days. Signs of inflammation were found in the stomach, such as great redness internally, with spots of extravasation, and a blackish matter like what he vomited.[||] Cholera has also been sometimes referred to the same cause. In the hot summer of 1825 it was remarked that a great number of persons who used to frequent a particular coffee-house in the Palais-Royal at Paris, and the owner among the rest, were severely affected with cholera. Poison being suspected to be the cause, a judicial inquiry was instituted. It was proved, however, that similar accidents had been observed at other coffee-houses, in other cities, and likewise in former hot seasons ; and when the whole medical evidence was referred to a commission of physicians and chemists, they gave their opinion, that the disease was owing to the incautious use of ices and iced-water in an unusually hot summer.[¶]

[*] Med. Rep. on the Effects of Cold Water, 1798, p. 96.
[†] New York Medical Register.
[‡] Ann. d'Hyg. Publ. et de Méd. Lég. xxvii. 57.
[§] Abercrombie on Diseases of the Stomach, &c. 14.
[||] Ann. d'Hyg. Publ. xxvii. 60.   [¶] Bulletins des Sciences Médicales, vi. 34.

Perhaps cholera arising thus may prove fatal. The following extraordinary case, which appears to have been of this nature, was communicated to me by the late Dr. Duncan, junior. A bookbinder in this city, previously in excellent health, rose one morning at six to kindle his fire, and took a large draught of cold water from a pitcher used in common by the whole family. He went immediately to bed again, complaining of pain in the pit of the stomach, and extreme anxiety, and affected with incessant vomiting. In twelve hours he died without any material change in the symptoms, and no disease whatever could be detected in the dead body. Dr. Duncan satisfied himself from general circumstances, that poisoning was quite out of the question; so that, however extraordinary it may appear, his death could be accounted for in no other way than by ascribing it to the cold water. — Hoffmann says he was acquainted with instances where fatal inflammatory fever was induced by drinking too freely of cold water, and a suspicion of poisoning in consequence excited.[*]

6. *Of Bilious Vomiting and Simple Cholera.* — Of all the diseases which are apt to be confounded with the effects of the irritant poisons, there is none which it is of so much importance that the medical jurist should be able to distinguish as cholera. A trial for poisoning with the common poisons hardly ever occurs, but an attempt is made to ascribe death to that disease; for it is very frequent, and its symptoms bear a close resemblance to those of the principal poisons of the class we are now considering.

It is unnecessary to give here a detailed account of the symptoms of simple cholera. There is the same burning pain in the stomach and bowels as in irritant poisoning, the same incessant vomiting and frequent purging, the same tension and tenderness of the belly, the same sense of acridity in the throat, and irritation in the anus, the same depression and anxiety, the same state of the pulse.

It would be wrong, however, to infer from these resemblances that the two affections are always undistinguishable. Some cases of irritant poisoning certainly cannot be distinguished by their symptoms from cholera. Many other cases are similarly circumstanced, because their particulars cannot be accurately collected. But there is no doubt that in others the distinction between poisoning and cholera may be drawn by the physician who has been able to ascertain the symptoms in detail. At present those points of difference only will be noticed which relate to the irritants as a class; others will be mentioned under the head of poisons individually.

The first difference is, that in cholera the sense of acridity in the throat does not precede the vomiting, as it sometimes does in poisoning. In cholera this sensation is caused by the vomited matter irritating the throat, or perhaps by the irritation in the stomach being propagated upwards by continuity of surface. But, whatever may be its cause, it is certain that the sense of acridity or burning sometimes remarked in cholera never begins before the vomiting. In many cases of poisoning, though certainly not in all, it is the first

[*] De cauta et circumspecta veneni dati accusatione, § 12.

symptom. — The next difference is, that in cholera the vomiting is never bloody. I have been at some pains to investigate this point: and I have been unable to find any instance of the cholera of this country, which has been accompanied with sanguinolent vomiting; neither is such a symptom mentioned in any accounts I have read of malignant cholera. This article of diagnosis will, of course, be open to correction from the experience of other practitioners. Lastly, a material difference is, that the simple cholera of this country very seldom proves fatal so rapidly as poisoning with the irritants usually does. Death from irritant poisoning is on the whole seldom delayed beyond two days and a half, and frequently happens within thirty-six hours, sometimes within six hours, or even less. Malignant cholera frequently proves fatal in as short a time; but with regard to the cholera of this country, I believe it may be laid down as a rule hitherto unshaken by all the controversy to which the subject has given rise, — that death is not often caused by it at all, and that death within three days is 'very rare indeed. A few cases of death within that period, nay, even within twelve hours, have certainly occurred; but their great rarity is obvious from the fact, that many practitioners of experience have not met with a single instance, and others with only one case in the course of a long practice. Dr. Duncan, senior, mentioned to me a case, the only one of the kind he had met with, which commenced soon after the individual eat a sour orange in the Edinburgh theatre, and which proved fatal in twelve hours. Dr. Duncan, junior, also met with a single case, which was the instance already noticed of cholera produced by drinking cold water. Dr. Abercrombie also once, and once only, met with a case fatal within two days.* Mr. Tatham, a late writer on this subject, met with an instance which proved fatal in twelve hours.† Dr. Burne of London has likewise related an instance of death within fifteen hours occurring in a child.‡ And I was informed in 1831 of a case at Leith which ended fatally in twenty-six hours, and was at first supposed by the unprofessional inhabitants of the place to be an instance of epidemic or malignant cholera. My colleagues, Drs. Home, Alison, and Graham, never met with an instance fatal in so short a time as two or three days; at a meeting of the Medico-Chirurgical Society of this city, none of the members present could remember to have seen such a case;§ and of the witnesses who were brought to swear to this point on a well-known trial, all of them physicians of extensive practice, not one could depose that such a case had ever come within his personal observation.‖ It has been stated however in a controversial publication written by the late Dr. Mackintosh of this place, that the author had seen many cases fatal within the

* Edinburgh Medical and Surgical Journal, xxviii. 88.
† Ibid. xxix. 70.
‡ London Medical Gazette, viii. 496.
§ Edinburgh Medical and Surgical Journal, xxviii. 99.
‖ Trial of Donnal. — See Paris and Fonblanque's Medical Jurisprudence, iii. Appendix, 277, et seq.

12

period now mentioned.* This is incomprehensible. For my own part, I cannot help repeating, as the result of the whole inquiry, that simple cholera rarely causes death in this country, in the period within which irritant poisoning commonly proves fatal,— that, consequently, every case of the kind will naturally be apt to lead, in peculiar circumstances, to suspicion of poisoning, — and that in charges of poisoning, rapid death under symptoms of violent irritation in the alimentary canal, like those of cholera, must always be considered an important article of a chain of circumstantial or presumptive evidence.

7. *Of Malignant Cholera.*— The history of this disease affords a fair promise that, in so far as British practitioners are concerned, it may ere long be excluded from the list of those which imitate irritant poisoning. Meanwhile, however, malignant cholera must be allowed to bear, in its essential symptoms and their course, a marked resemblance to poisoning with the irritants. So much indeed is this the case that some authors have actually compared its phenomena to the effects of arsenic, tartar-emetic, and other powerful acrids. In many cases the two affections are undoubtedly not so distinguishable by symptoms as to warrant a physician to rely on the diagnosis in a medico-legal inquiry. But in many other instances the distinction may be drawn satisfactorily. Thus the uneasiness in the throat which sometimes attends cholera never precedes the vomiting. The vomiting in cholera is never bloody. The colour and expression of the countenance and whole body are peculiar. In frequent instances the early signs which resemble poisoning are followed by a secondary stage, sometimes of simple coma, sometimes of typhoid fever, which a practised person may easily distinguish from the secondary phenomena produced by some irritants. Lastly, no mistake can arise where the patient, before presenting the symptoms common to both affections, experiences violent burning pain or certain tastes, during or immediately after the swallowing of food, drink, or some other article.

8. *Of Inflammation of the Stomach.* — Chronic inflammation of the stomach is a common disease ; which, however, on account of the slowness of its course, is not liable to be confounded with the ordinary effects of irritant poisons. Acute inflammation, on the contrary, follows precisely the same course as that of irritant poisoning. But great doubts may be entertained whether true acute gastritis ever exists in this country as a natural disease. Several of my acquaintances, long in extensive practice, have stated to me, that their experience coincides entirely with that of Dr. Abercrombie, who observes he has " never seen a case which he could consider as being of that nature."† An important observation of the same purport has been made by M. Louis, one of the most experienced and accurate pathologists of the present time. He says, that during six years' service at the hospital of La Charité, during

* Edinburgh Medical and Surgical Journal, xxviii. 87.
† On Diseases of the Stomach and other Abdominal Viscera, p. 15.

which he noticed the particulars of 3000 cases and 500 dissections, he did not meet with a single instance of fatal primary gastritis. The disease only occurred as a secondary affection or complicating some other disease which was the canse of death.* So far as I have hitherto been able to inquire among systematic authors, the descriptions of idiopathic acute gastritis appear to have been taken from the varieties caused by poison.

The following are the only specific accounts I have hitherto met with of an affection of the nature of idiopathic acute gastritis; and the reader will be at no loss to perceive that in each of them it admits of being viewed differently. The first two are the cases of inflammation referred by Haller and Guérard to drinking cold water incautiously [p. 100]. The next is a remarkable incident related by Lecat, and occurring in 1763. A girl, nineteen years old, was attacked while in good health with shivering, faintness, acute pain in the belly, cold extremities and imperceptible pulse; and she died in sixteen hours. The stomach was found red, and checkered with brownish patches and gangrenous pustules (probably warty black extravasation): yet it was supposed to have been ascertained that she had not taken any thing deleterious.† This narrative is certainly to appearance pointed. But when it is added, that the girl's mother was attacked about the same time with precisely the same symptoms and died in four hours, I think the reader, when he also considers the imperfect mode in which chemical inquiries were then conducted, will by no means rest satisfied with Lecat's assurance that nothing deleterious was swallowed. The last is an equally singular case given by Dr. Hastings, of Worcester, where poisoning with cantharides was suspected. A young lady, liable to indigestion, but at the moment in better health than usual, was attacked with sickness before breakfast and after it with vomiting. Three days elapsed before she was seen by her medical attendant, who found her sinking under incessant vomiting, severe pain in the loins, strangury, bloody urine, and swelling of the clitoris, attended with red extravasation of the eyes, and a red efflorescence on the skin. Death followed next day amidst convulsions; and there was found in the dead body extravasation of blood between the kidneys and their outer membrane, into the pelvis of each kidney, and into the bladder, — redness of the bronchial membrane, and gorging of the air-cells with blood, — and general redness of the inside of the stomach, with numerous extravasated spots in the submucous coat.‡ It seems to have been clearly proved at the coroner's inquest that poisoning was here out of the question. But the case appears rather to have been one of renal irritation or inflammation than of gastritis, and the affection of the stomach secondarily merely.

* Recherches sur la Gastro-entérite, ii. 51.

† Laisné sur les Perforations Spontanées, p. 206, from Recueil des observations des Hopitaux Militaires, i. 375. — This case is also given by MM. Petit and Serres in their treatise entitled " de la Fièvre Entéro-Mésenterique," p. 197, and is considered by them an instance of that particular disease.

‡ Trans. of Provinc. Med. and Surg. Association, vol. i.

The question as to the possibility of acute gastritis being produced by natural causes is one of very great interest to the medical jurist. For its possible occurrence is the only obstacle in the way of a decision in favour of poisoning, from symptoms and morbid appearances only, in certain cases by no means uncommon, which are characterised by signs of violent irritation during life, early death, and unequivocal marks of great irritation in the dead body, namely, bright redness, ulcers, and black, granular, warty extravasation. In regard to these effects, it may with perfect safety be said, that they can very rarely indeed all arise from natural causes ; and for my own part, the more the subject is investigated, the more am I led to doubt whether they ever arise in this country from any other cause than poison. The possible occurrence of a case of the kind from natural causes must be granted. But this concession ought not to take away from the importance of the contrary fact as one of the particulars of a chain of circumstantial proof.

In whatever way the fact as to the existence of idiopathic acute gastritis may eventually be proved to stand, an important criterion of this disease, as of cholera, will be that the sense of burning in the throat, if present at all, does not precede the vomiting.

9. *Inflammation of the Intestines* in its acute form is more common than inflammation of the stomach, as a natural disease. It is generally accompanied, however, with constipation of the bowels. Acute enteritis, unless we choose with some pathologists to consider cholera as of that nature, is very rarely attended with purging.

There is a variety of intestinal inflammation, observed only of late by pathologists,* but now well known, which bears a close resemblance to the effects of the irritants. It is a particular variety of ulceration commonly situated near the end of the small intestines, accompanied at first with trifling or insidious symptoms, and terminating suddenly in perforation of the gut. It begins with tubercular deposition under the mucous membrane in roundish patches. Then an ulcer appears on the middle of one or more of these patches, gradually spreads over them, and at the same time penetrates the other coats. At last when the peritoneal coat alone is left, some trifling accident ruptures it, the fæcal matters escape into the sac of the peritonæum, and the patient dies in great agony in the course of one or two days, or in a few hours. Such cases, if not distinguished by the symptoms, will be at once recognized by the morbid appearances. Perforation of the intestines, with similar symptoms, also takes place without the previous tubercular deposit, by simple ulceration of the coats.†

Another form of intestinal inflammation may also be here particularized, because it imitates the effects of the irritants in the cases in which they prove slowly fatal. It is a form of aphthous ulceration

---

* Louis in Archives Générales de Médecine, i. 17, or Edin. Med. and Surg. Journal, xxi. 239, also Abercrombie on Diseases of the Stomach, &c. 273, and Louis Recherches sur la Gastro-entérite, *passim*.

† Abercrombie on Diseases of the Stomach, &c. pp. 156 and 243.

of the mucous membrane of the alimentary canal, which appears to affect almost every part of it from the throat downwards, and begins commonly in the throat. I once met with a remarkable case in which it appeared in the form of little white ulcers in the back of the throat, and gradually travelled downwards to the stomach and from that to the intestines, — being characterized by burning pain in every one of its seats, and successively by difficulty of swallowing, by sickness, vomiting, and tenderness of the stomach, and finally by purging. Such cases resemble the slow forms of poisoning with arsenic. But they differ in attacking the several divisions of the alimentary canal in turn, while in the examples of poisoning with arsenic now alluded to, the whole canal from the mouth to the anus is affected simultaneously. Dr. Abercrombie has described a similar disorder, which he appears to have occasionally seen affecting both the stomach and intestines at the same time ; but he seems to doubt whether it ever occurs as an idiopathic disease, or independently of some co-existing or preceding fever or local inflammation.*

10. *Inflammation of the Peritonæum*, or lining membrane of the belly, will not require many remarks. When acute, it is rarely attended in its early stage by vomiting ; rarely also by irregular action of the intestines, and never by diarrhœa ; and it is at once distinguished in the dead body by unequivocal marks of peritonæal inflammation, which are very seldom caused by irritant poisons.†

11. The subject of *Spontaneous Perforation of the Stomach* is an important topic for the medical jurist, because both the symptoms before death and the appearances in the dead body are occasionally very like the effects of some of the most active irritant poisons. The following is a statement of the most material facts hitherto ascertained on this subject; but it must be premised that a good deal of obscurity still hangs over some parts of it.

Spontaneous perforation of the stomach is of three kinds. One is the last stage of some varieties of scirrhus. The indurated membrane ulcerates, the ulcer penetrates first the villous, then the muscular, and at last the outer or peritoneal coat, so that the contents of the stomach escape into the belly. The symptoms of the perforation are a sense of something giving way in the pit of the stomach, acute pain gradually extending over the whole abdomen, great tenderness and tension, excessive prostration, and death commonly within twenty-four hours. The symptoms which precede the perforation in general clearly indicate organic derangement of the stomach, namely, aggravated dyspepsia of long standing. Several cases of this description may be seen in a thesis by M. Laisné,‡ a pupil of Professor Chaussier. Two characteristic cases have been published by Dr.

* Abercrombie on Diseases of the Stomach, &c., p. 52.

† For cases of this disease, see Abercrombie on Diseases of the Stomach, &c. p. 156 and 181.

‡ Considérations Medico-légales sur les perforations spontanées de l'estomac, 1819. This thesis, published with three others on medico-legal subjects, is understood to have been in a great measure the work of the late Professor Chaussier.

12*

Crampton ;* and Mr. Alfred Taylor has referred to several others, the stomachs of which are preserved in Guy's Hospital Museum, and gives the particulars of some which had occurred in the practice of that institution or to his friends.† Occasionally no symptom exists prior to the perforation, as in an instance related by Dr. Kelly of a stout healthy servant, who was suddenly seized with excruciating pain in the stomach and expired in eighteen hours, and in whose body the stomach was found perforated in the middle of an extensive thickening and induration of the villous coat.‡

The second variety of perforation takes place by simple ulceration without previous scirrhus. In one of Dr. Crampton's papers will be found some remarks by Mr. Travers, along with a case of this kind. The subject of it was a man of a strumous habit, who enjoyed good health, till one day at dinner he was suddenly attacked with acute pain in the pit of the stomach, and died in thirteen hours. The stomach was found perforated in the centre of a superficial ulcer of the mucous coat, occupying two-thirds of the ring of the pylorus.§ This case shows that the present variety of perforation may take place without the preliminary organic disease being indicated by any symptom. The circumstances under which it commenced are peculiarly important in relation to the medical jurisprudence of poisoning. Another case which has been lately described with great exactness by M. Duparcque, was preceded only by very trivial dyspeptic symptoms. Here the whole mischief arose from a small ulcer eight lines long and five in breadth on the inside of the stomach, and not more than a line and a half in diameter at the perforation through the peritonæum.‖ Several excellent examples of the same disease have been related by Dr. Abercrombie.¶ In one of these the ulcer in the centre of which the perforation had been formed, was not bigger than a shilling, and the rest of the stomach quite healthy. A very instructive case of a similar nature, but of unusual duration, has been related by Mr. Alfred Taylor. A young woman, after suffering for some time from nausea and constant craving for food, but inability to indulge it, and occasionally from pain in the stomach, was attacked suddenly with the usual symptoms of perforation, and died forty-two hours afterwards. The villous coat of the stomach, though generally healthy, presented at the lesser curvature several small elevated points, and in the middle of two of these a sharply-defined ulcer, one affecting the mucous coat only, while the other, which was half an inch in diameter where it affected the mucous coat, perforated the muscular and peritonæal coats by a hole no bigger than a crow-quill.** A case still more remarkable has

* Trans. of the Dublin College of Physicians, i. 2, and London Medico-Chirurgical Transactions, viii. 228.
† Guy's Hospital Reports, 1839, iv. 20.
‡ Abercrombie on Diseases of the Stomach, 41.
§ London Medico-Chirurg. Transactions, viii. 233.
‖ Archives Générales de Médecine, xxvi. 123.
¶ On Diseases of the Stomach, pp. 35, 37.
** Guy's Hospital Reports, 1839, iv. 16.

been also related by the same author, where the circumstances naturally gave rise to a strong suspicion of poisoning. A young female in a noble family, subject to slight dyspepsia, was suddenly attacked, three hours after a meal, with violent vomiting and pain in the belly. Collapse soon ensued, and in fifteen hours she died, under so strong suspicions of poisoning that various antidotes were administered. This suspicion was in some measure borne out by proofs of an intrigue having been carried on between her and a male person in the house, and by the discovery after death of the signs of recent sexual intercourse. On examining the cavity of the abdomen, however, there was found, at the upper and back part of the stomach near the pylorus, an oval perforation, half an inch wide, surrounded by a firm, smooth, almost cartilaginous margin, without any inflammation near it. Mr. Taylor properly points out, that the sudden occurrence of such violent symptoms so long after a meal is incompatible with the action of any poison which could cause perforation in fifteen hours ; and that the characters of the perforation were those of a natural disease long latent. He could not detect a trace of any poison in the stomach.[*] — In some cases, as in that of M. Duparcque, the pain at the moment the perforation is completed is not at first violent, because the close proximity of some adjoining organ, such as the liver, prevents the contents of the stomach from escaping for a time, so that inflammation of the peritonæum is but gradually developed.

The third variety of spontaneous perforation is of a much more singular kind. It is produced not by ordinary ulceration, but by a jelly-like softening of the coats. The gelatinization sometimes extends over a great extent of surface, affecting chiefly the villous coat, so that the aperture through the other membranes is surrounded by extensive pulpiness of the internal membrane. It is seldom accompanied by vascularity. Its symptoms are exceedingly obscure. In adults there is very rarely any symptom at all till the perforation is complete ;[†] in children, as appears from a paper by Dr. J. Gairdner of this city, and another by Dr. Pitschaft, a German author,[‡] the early symptoms indicate an obscure chronic gastritis. The nature of this singular disease will be discussed in the section on the morbid appearances. At present it may merely be observed, that the injury caused to the coats of the stomach seems to be precisely the same with the gelatinization, which is sometimes found after death in persons who had no symptoms of an affection of the stomach, and which is ascribed by John Hunter,[§] and most British pathologists, to the solvent action of the gastric juice in the dead body. This disease is well described by Laisné in his thesis formerly quoted. The following is a good example : a young lady, previously in good health, was awakened at three one morning with excruciating pain in the stomach, which nothing could alleviate. She expired seven hours

* Guy's Hosp. Rep. 1839, 52.　　† Edinb. Med-Chirurgical Transactions, i. 311.
‡ Rust's Magazin für die gesammte Heilkunde, xxi. 199. This paper is analysed in Edinburgh Med. and Surg. Journal, xxvi. 451.
§ Philosophical Transactions, lxii. 447.

after ; and on dissection two holes were found in the back part of the stomach, surrounded with much softening of the villous coat.* Another case will be mentioned in page 118. — The appearances produced by this disease have been mistaken for the effects of corrosive poisons.

12. The *gullet* may be perforated in a similar manner either with or without symptoms. Under the head of the morbid appearances [119] two instances will be mentioned in which there were no corresponding symptoms. In the following case symptoms did pre-exist. A man, six weeks after being bit by a dog, which was killed without its state of health having been ascertained, was attacked with a sense of strangling, impossibility of swallowing, delirium, excessive irritability, glairy vomiting ; and he died within twenty-four hours. The gullet, a little above the diaphragm, was perforated by a hole two-thirds of an inch in diameter, with thin edges ; and effusion had taken place into the posterior mediastinum.†

13. *Perforation of the alimentary canal by worms* may here also be noticed shortly as a disease liable in careless hands to be confounded with irritant poisoning. This is far from being a common accident, and very rarely takes place during life. In most of the cases in which it has been witnessed the symptoms antecedent to death were those not of irritant, but of narcotic poisoning, and were then owing simply to the great accumulation of worms in the alimentary canal. On this subject the reader is referred to the article Epilepsy in the introductory remarks on the effects of the narcotic class of poisons. But at times the symptoms have been like those of irritant poisoning. Thus the following is a case of perforation by worms during life giving rise to all the phenomena and symptoms of peritonæal inflammation. A soldier at Mauritius was seized with slight general fever and severe pain, at first in the pit of the stomach, and afterwards over the whole belly, which on the third day began to enlarge. A tendency to suppression of urine and costiveness ensued, then bilious vomiting ; and he died on the fourth day, the belly having continued to increase to the end. On dissection, several quarts of muddy fluid were found in the sac of the peritonæum, the viscera were agglutinated by lymph, a round worm was discovered among the intestines between the navel and pubes, and the ileum was perforated six inches from the colon by a hole corresponding in size with the worm.‡ — A singular case, not however fatal, but which confirms the fact, that worms may make their way through the intestines and other textures during life, is mentioned in Rust's journal. A woman after a tedious illness first vomited several lumbrici, and was then seized with a painful swelling in the left side, which in the process of time suppurated, and discharged along with the purulent matter three other worms of the same species.§ Another

* Gastellier in Leroux's Journal de Médecine, xxxiii. 24.
† Archives Générales de Médecine, xi. 463.
‡ Mr. Kell in London Medical Gazette, ii. 649.
§ Magazin für die gesammte Heilkunde, xviii. 107.

instance of the same kind, where the perforation of the gut succeeded strangulated hernia, and was followed by the discharge of two lumbrici and ultimate recovery, is detailed in the Revue Médicale.*

Symptoms like those of narcotico-acrid poisoning may be caused by worms without perforation. A girl, eight years old and in excellent health, was suddenly seized with violent colic pains, vomiting, bloody stools, tenderness and swelling of the belly, followed by convulsions and coma, and proving fatal in seven hours. No other explanation of the case could be discovered on dissection except the presence of several hundred ascarides in the intestines and thirteen in the stomach.†

14. The next diseases to be mentioned are melæna and hæmatemesis, or purging and vomiting of pure or of altered blood. It is hardly possible to mistake them for poisoning, as the pain which accompanies them is seldom acute, and the discharge of blood generally profuse.

15. The last are *colic, iliac passion,* and *obstructed intestine.* As the symptoms of some poisons are the same with those of colic, it is of course sometimes impossible to distinguish the natural disease from the effects of poison by attending to the abdominal symptoms only. But the distinction in severe cases of poisoning may almost always be drawn from collateral symptoms and extraneous circumstances. — The iliac passion is distinguished by a complete reversion of the vermicular motion of the intestines in consequence of which the fæces are often discharged by vomiting. I am not aware that stercoraceous vomiting is ever caused by poisoning. — A case has been recorded in Corvisart's journal, in which iliac passion, originating in obstruction of the ileum by hardened fæces, and proving fatal in twenty-six hours, gave rise to a judicial inquiry into the possibility of poisoning.‡ Another instance, that led to a strong suspicion of poisoning, has been lately published by M. Rostan, in which there was continued vomiting and pain of abdomen, proving fatal in two days, and arising from the small intestines being obstructed by an adventitious band.§ In this case the first inspectors failed to observe the true cause of the symptoms; but Rostan and Orfila, who were appointed to examine the body a second time, discovered the constriction, and were unable to find any poison in the stomach by analysis. Stercoraceous vomiting occurred during life; which might have been held sufficient to settle the real nature of the case. — Obstruction of the intestines arising from twisting of the gut, intussusception, foreign bodies, or strangulated hernia, is easily known by the seat where the pain begins, by the obstinate constipation, and also by the excessive enlargement of the belly, — which last, however, is rather an equivocal symptom.

The preceding observations will enable the medical jurist to de-

* Revue Médicale, 1826, i. 100.
† Jahrbuch des Oesterreiches Staates, xxii. 54, or Arch. Gén. de Méd. xlvi. 480.
‡ Journal de Médecine. xxxiv. 25.
§ Affaire Hullin. Archives Générales de Médecine, xix. 332.

termine, how far a diagnosis may be drawn from the symptoms between poisoning with the irritant and the diseases which resemble it. It will be remarked that the most embarrassing disease, on account of its frequency, and peculiar symptoms, is cholera. Cholera, however, may be recognised in some instances even considered in regard to the irritants as a class; and we shall presently find that it may be distinguished still better from the effects of some individual poisons.

SECTION II. — *Of the Morbid Appearances caused by Irritant Poisons, compared with those of certain natural diseases.*

The next subject for consideration is the morbid appearances produced by the irritants as a class, together with those of a similar nature, which arise from natural causes.

The powerful irritants, which are not corrosives, produce simply the appearances characteristic of inflammation of the alimentary canal in its various stages, — in the mouth, throat, and gullet vascularity, and also, if the case has lasted long enough, ulceration ; — in the stomach, vascularity, extravasation of blood under and in the substance of the villous coat and likewise into the cavity of the organ, abundant secretion of tough mucus, deposition of coagulable lymph in a fine network, ulceration of the membranes, occasionally perforation, preternatural softness of the whole or of part of the villous coat, and on the other hand sometimes uncommon hardness and shrivelling of that coat ; in the intestines vascularity, extravasation, and ulceration. — Sometimes several of these appearances are to be seen in the whole alimentary canal at once. In poisoning with arsenic or corrosive sublimate it is no unusual thing to meet with redness or ulceration of the throat, great disease in the stomach, vascularity of the small intestines, ulcers in the great intestines, and excoriation of the anus. — When the poison is an active corrosive much more extensive ravages are sometimes caused, particularly in the stomach. After poisoning by the mineral acids, for example, the whole mucous membrane of the stomach is at times found wanting; nay, large patches of the whole coats may be wanting, and the deficiency supplied by the adhesion of the margin of the aperture to the adjoining viscera, and the conversion of the outer membrane of these viscera into an inner membrane for the stomach.

Of the appearances here briefly enumerated the particulars will be related partly under what is now to be said of the appearances arising from natural causes, which are liable to be confounded with the effects of poisons, partly under the head of individual poisons.

Of redness of the stomach and intestines from natural causes, and its distinction from the redness caused by poisons.

Simple redness of the alimentary mucous membrane in all its forms, whether of mere vascularity, or actual extravasation, not only does not distinguish poisoning from inflammatory disorders of natural origin, but will even seldom distinguish the effects of poison from those of processes that occur independently of disease, and subsequent to death. On the subject of real inflammation, as distinguished from redness originating after death, or pseudo-morbid redness, as it is commonly termed, — a subject of great consequence to the medical jurist, — the reader may consult with advantage a paper by Dr. Yelloly,[*] an essay by MM. Rigot and Trousseau,[†] or that of M. Billard.[‡] The former authors proved by experiment, that various kinds of pseudo-morbid redness may be formed, which cannot be distinguished from the parallel varieties caused by inflammation ; that these appearances are formed after death, and not till three, five, or eight hours after it ; that they are to be found chiefly in the most depending turns of intestines, and in the most depending parts of each turn, or of the stomach ; and that after they have been formed, they may be made to shift their place, and appear where the membrane was previously healthy, by simply altering the position of the gut. M. Billard, on the other hand, has laid down their characters, and made a minute arrangement of the several kinds. He has divided them into ramiform, capilliform, punctated, striated, laminated, and diffuse redness, — terms which need hardly be explained. I must be content with merely referring to these sources of information for a particular account of the appearances in question. But it may be right at the same time to quote an instance of the most aggravated form of pseudo-morbid redness, in order to convince the reader that all forms may equally arise from the same causes. Among other exsample, then, which have been related of laminated redness, or redness in patches from extravasation, M. Billard mentions the case of a man who hanged himself, and in whose body was found, on the mucous membrane of the small intestine where it lay in the right flank, " a large, amaranth-red patch, six finger-breadths wide, covered with bloody exudation, and not removable by washing:" and in the lower pelvis there was a similar patch of even larger dimensions.[§]

Although morbid and pseudo-morbid redness of the inner coat of the alimentary canal cannot be distinguished from one another by any intrinsic character, M. Billard thinks this may be done by attending to collateral circumstances. According to his researches, redness is to be accounted inflammatory only when it occurs in parts not depending in position, or is not limited to such parts : when the mesenteric veins supplying the parts are not distended, nor the great abdominal veins obstructed at the time of death ; when the reddened membrane is covered with much mucus, particularly if thick, tenacious, and adhering ; when the mucous membrane itself is opaque, so that when dissected off and stretched over the finger, the finger is not visible ; when the cellular tissue which connects that membrane

[*] London Medico-Chirurgical Transactions, iv. 371.
[†] Archives Générales de Médecine, Oct. and Nov. 1826; also Edin. Medical and Surgical Journal, xxviii. 149.
[‡] De la Membranes Muqueuse Gastro-intestinale, 1825.
[§] Ibid. p. 220.

with the subjacent coat is brittle, so that the former is easily scratched off with the nail.

Some observations may be here also made on another appearance, allied to the present group, but which there is strong reason to believe always indicates some violent irritation at least, if not even irritation from poison only, in the organ where it is found. It is an effusion under the villous coat of the stomach, and incorporation with its substance, of dark brownish-black, or as it were charred, blood; which is thus altered either by the chemical action of the poison, or by a vital process. In many cases of poisoning with the mineral acids, oxalic acid, arsenic, corrosive sublimate, and the like, there are found on the villous coat of the stomach little knots and larger irregular patches and streaks, not of a reddish-brown, reddish-black, or violaceous hue, like pseudo-morbid redness, but dark-grayish-black, or brownish-black, like the colour of coal or melanosis, — accompanied too with elevation of the membrane, frequently with abrasion on the middle of the patches, and surrounded by vascularity. This conjunction of appearances I have never seen in the stomach, unless it had been violently irritated; and several experienced pathologists of my acquaintance agree with me in this statement. It bears a pretty close resemblance to melanosis of the stomach;[*] but is distinguished by melanotic blackness being arranged in regular abruptly-defined spots, and still better by melanosis not being preceded by symptoms of irritation in the stomach.

Referring to what was already said under the head of the symptoms of gastritis [p. 102], I must again express my doubts whether the appearances now described ever arise in this country from natural disease. In the intestines they are sufficiently familiar to the physician, as arising from idiopathic enteritis, and from dysentery. But in the stomach their existence as the effect of natural disease is very doubtful.

Another kind of coloration of the inner membrane of the stomach, which may be shortly alluded to, because it has actually been mistaken for the effect of irritation from poison, although by no means like it, — is staining of the membrane with a reddish, brownish, yellowish, or greenish tint, observed in bodies that have been kept some time, and produced by the proximity of the liver, spleen, or colon if it contains fæces. No unprejudiced and skilful inspector could possibly mistake this appearance for inflammation. But under the impulse of prejudice it has been considered such, and imputed to poison. On the occurrence of such stains an attempt was made by the French to ascribe to poison the death of the republican general Hoche. He died rather suddenly on his way from Frankfort to join his troops; and as poisoning was suspected, the body was opened in the presence of three French army-surgeons, and a French and two German physicians. The only appearance of note in the alimentary canal was two darkish spots on the villous coat of the stomach. The surgeons drew up a report which imputed his death to poison; but

* For a case of this rare and singular disease, see Edin. Medical and Surgical Journal, xxvi. 214.

the physicians refused to sign it; and other medical people who were subsequently added to the commission decided with the latter.* The surgeons probably would not have been so hasty, if they had not known that the result of their complaisance would have been the levying of a heavy fine on the inhabitants.

The last kind of discoloration of the inner coat which requires mention is dyeing from the presence of coloured fluids in the contents. A remarkable instance has been recorded where redness of this nature was mistaken for inflammation, and the death of the individual in consequence ascribed at first to poison. A person long in delicate health died suddenly after taking a laxative draught; and the sto-mach, as well as the gullet, being found on dissection red and livid in various places, it was hastily inferred by his medical attendants, that these appearances were the effect of poison, and that the apothe-cary had committed some fatal error in compounding the draught. But another physician, who was acquainted with the deceased, al-though he did not attend him professionally, strongly suspected he had died a natural death; and happening to know he was in the practice of taking a strong infusion of corn-poppy, inferred that the supposed signs of inflammation were merely stains arising from the habitual use of this substance. Accordingly, on making the experi-ment, he found that in dogs to which a similar infusion was given, appearances were produced identically the same.†

Of the effusion of mucus and lymph from natural causes. — The abundant secretion of tough mucus in the stomach is a sign of that organ having been irritated. But the effusion of lymph is more cha-racteristic. This may be produced by natural inflammation as well as by irritating poisons. As arising from either cause, however, it is rare; and certainly by no means so common as would be supposed from what is said in systematic works; for tough mucus has been often mistaken for it. Reticulated lymph adhering to the villous coat, and accompanied with corresponding reticulated redness of that coat, such as I have seen in animals poisoned with arsenic or oxalic acid, is an unequivocal sign of inflammation.

Of idiopathic ulcers and perforation of the stomach and intestines, and their distinction from those caused by poison. — Both ulceration and perforation may be produced by natural disease. In the ulcera-tion produced by poisons there is generally speaking nothing to distin-guish it from natural ulcers; but that caused by some poisons, such as iodine, is said to differ by the surrounding coloration of the mem-brane; and when the ulcer is caused by a sparingly soluble poison in a state of powder, such as arsenic, the cavity of the ulcer is some-times filled with the powder. Perforation is a rare effect of the sim-ple irritant poisons; but it is often caused by corrosives. It is imi-tated by two of the varieties of perforation from natural disease.

The form of natural perforation caused by a common ulcer is pre-cisely the same as that caused by the simple irritants, and is inca-

* Kopp's Jahrbuch der Staatsarzneikunde, ii. 169.
† Journal de Médecine, vii. 333. Also Foderé, Traité de Médecine-Legale, iv. 282.

pable of being distinguished, except when it is attended with scirrhus.

By far the most remarkable variety, however, of spontaneous perforation is that which takes place, without proper inflammatory action, from simple gelatinizing of the coats. It is very apt to be mistaken, and in a celebrated trial, which will be immediately noticed, was actually mistaken for the effect of corrosive poison.

It may be situated on any part of the stomach, but is oftenest seen on the posterior surface. It is sometimes small, more often as big as a half-crown, frequently of the size of the palm, and occasionally so great as to involve an entire half of the stomach. Sometimes there is more than one aperture. The margin is of all shapes, commonly fringed, and almost always formed of the peritoneum, the other coats being more extensively dissolved. In one instance, however, the peritonæal surface was on the contrary the most extensively destroyed;[*] and in a case which occurred in the infirmary here, and was pointed out to me by the late Dr. W. Cullen, the peritonæum alone was extensively softened, and partly dissolved, so as to lay the muscular coat bare on its outer surface. The gelatinization therefore sometimes, though very rarely, begins on the outside of the stomach. Internally the whole is surrounded by pulpiness of the mucous coat, generally white, occasionally bluish or blackish, never granulated like an ulcer, very rarely vascular; and when vascular, the blood may be squeezed out of the loaded and open vessels. The organs in contact with the hole are also frequently softened. Thus an excavation is sometimes found in the liver or spleen; or the diaphragm is pierced through and through. The margins of the latter holes are without any sign of vascular action, but are generally besmeared with a dark pulpy mass, the remains of the softened tissue. The pulp never smells of gangrene; with which, indeed, this species of softening is wholly unconnected. The edge of the hole in the stomach never adheres to the adjoining organ; yet, even when the hole is very large, the contents of the stomach have not always made their escape. Often the dissolution of the coats is incomplete. John Hunter and others, indeed, have said that a stomach is rarely seen without more or less solution of the mucous coat.[†] The best account of the appearances in this state is given by Jaeger of Stuttgardt.[‡]

The circumstances under which this extraordinary appearance occurs are singularly various. Professor Chaussier and the French pathologists conceive it to be always a morbid process constituting a peculiar disease; and doubtless cases have occurred in which death appears to have arisen from the stomach being perforated during life by gelatinization.[§] But it has been found much more frequently, when death was clearly the consequence of a different disease, and when there did not exist during life a single sign of disorder in the

* Nouvelle Bibliothéque Médicale, 1828, iii. 141.
† Philos. Trans. lxii. 459.
‡ See Analysis of his Essay by Dr. Gumprecht, Lond. Med. Repos. x. 416.
§ Laisné, Sur les Perforations Spontanées, 149.

stomach. Thus it has been found in women who died of convulsions after delivery, — in children who died convulsed or of hydrocephalus, — after death from suppuration of the brain, both natural and the result of violence, — from coma following an old ulcer of the back, which communicated with the spinal canal, — from diseased mesenteric glands, — from phthisis, — from nervous fever, — and after sudden death from fracture of the skull or hanging :* and in all of these circumstances it has occurred without any previous symptom referrible to a disorder in the stomach.

The opinions of pathologists are divided as to its nature. The French conceive it arises from a morbid corrosive action, which, however, may extend after death, in consequence of the fluids acquiring a solvent power. Hunter ascribed it entirely to the solvent power of the gastric juice after death. There are difficulties in the way of both doctrines. A full examination of the whole inquiry, which is one of much interest and considerable complexity, would be misplaced in this work; but some remarks are called for, by reason of the important medico-legal relations of the subject, and the uncertainty in which it is at present involved.

In the first place, then, it appears difficult, if not impossible, to comprehend how a vital erosive action can account for the perforations observed after death from diseases wholly unconnected with the stomach, and unattended during life by any symptom of disorder in that organ. For, not to dwell on other less weighty arguments, — on the one hand, there is during life no symptom of perforation, an accident which if deep stupor be not present at the same time is always attended with violent symptoms when it arises from any cause but gelatinization, — and on the other hand, there is frequently no escape of the contents of the stomach into the cavity of the abdomen, though the hole is of enormous size, and its edge not adherent to the adjoining organs. — All such perforations, however, are perfectly well accounted for, on the other theory, by what is now known of the properties of the gastric juice. This will appear from the following exposition.

The power of the gastric juice to dissolve the stomach and other soft animal textures was long thought to be fully proved by the well-known researches of Spallanzani,† Stevens,‡ and Gosse.§ In later times doubts were entertained on the subject in consequence of negative results having been obtained by other experimentalists, more especially by Montégre.‖ But these apparently discrepant facts and opinions have been reconciled by the ulterior experiments of Tiedemann and Gmelin on digestion;¶ who found that the nature and

---

* The last cases were observed by Hunter. See Philos. Transactions, lxii. 452.

† Fisica Animale e Vegetabile. Dissertazione quinta, § ccxxiii.-ccxxxi. T. ii. 86-89, Edit. Venezia, 1782.

‡ De Alimentorum Concoctione. Diss. Inaug. Edinburgi, 1777.

§ Experiments on Digestion. Appendix to Spallanzani's Dissertations relative to the Natural History of Animals and Vegetables. London Edition, 1784, i. 317.

‖ Expériences sur la Digestion dans l'homme. Paris, 1814, pp. 20, et seq.

¶ Die Verdauung nach Versuchen, &c. Heidelberg, 1825, or the French Edition, Recherches Expérimentales Physiologiques et Chimiques sur la Digestion, 1826, passim.

quality of the fluid secreted by the stomach vary much in different circumstances, — that, when its villous coat is not subjected to some stimulus, the fluid which lines it is not acid, and does not possess any particular solvent action, — but that when the membrane is stimulated by the presence of food or other sources of excitement, the quality of the secretion is materially changed, for it becomes strongly acid and is capable of dissolving alimentary substances both in and out of the body. And still more lately the solvent power of the proper gastric juice over the stomach, and its capability of producing perforation in animals after death, have been established in the most satisfactory manner by Dr. Carswell,[*] who has shown by a series of incontrovertible facts, — that in the rabbit when killed during the digestion of a meal, and left for some hours afterwards in particular positions, all the phenomena of spontaneous gelatinized perforations observed at times in man, may be easily produced at will, — that acidity of the gastric juice is an invariable circumstance when such perforations are remarked, — and that the appearances in question as they occur in the rabbit are the result of chemical action alone, and occur only after death. Thus, then, the physiological experiments of Tiedemann and Gmelin, together with the investigations of Carswell, not merely establish positively the fact, that the stomach may be perforated after death by the gastric juice, but likewise account clearly for the negative results obtained by other experimentalists. For example, passing over earlier experiments, they explain sufficiently the negative results obtained by Dr. Pommer of Heilbronn,[†] an experimentalist of some reputation in Germany ; for, falling into the error of some of the less recent experimentalists on this subject, he made his observations on animals killed slowly by starving, — in which circumstance there is no proper gastric juice in the stomach, and consequently no solvent action can exist.

These statements relative to the causes and phenomena of gelatinized perforation in the stomach supply the strongest possible presumption which analogy can furnish, that a great proportion of spontaneous gelatinized perforations in the human subject are owing to the action of the gastric juice after death. And this presumption is increased to something not far removed from demonstration by the circumstance, that in man the process of softening has actually been traced extending in the dead body. This interesting fact was first noticed by Mr. Allan Burns.[‡] In the body of a girl who died of diseased mesenteric glands he found an aperture in the fore part of the stomach with the usual pulpy margin, and the liver in contact with the hole uninjured. In two days more the liver opposite the hole had become pulpy, and its peritonæal coat quite dissolved ; and the back part of the stomach opposite the hole was also dissolved, so that only its peritonæal coat remained. Dr. Sharpey has communicated to me a similar observation. On finding in the body of a child the stomach

---

* Inquiry into the Chemical Solution of the stomach after death. Edinburgh Med. and Surg. Journal, xxxiv. 282.

† Medizinisch chirurgische Zeitung, 1828, ii. 57, 77, 93, and 107.

‡ Edinb. Med. and Surg. Journal, vi. 135.

perforated and gelatinized, but the adjoining organs uninjured, he sewed up the body, to show the appearances to some of his friends next day. By that time the peritonæal surfaces of the spleen and left kidney were found much softened and pulpy where they lay in contact with the hole in the stomach. I have since met with a similar occurrence where the perforation affected the duodenum (p. 120).

It must be admitted, then, that the action of the gastric juice after death is quite sufficient to account for the greater number of gelatiniform perforations in the human stomach.

But in the second place, it seems scarcely possible to explain every perforation of the kind in this way. The solvent action of the gastric juice for example, affords no explanation of a singular case related by M. Récamier,[*] where, after death in the secondary stage of small-pox, the stomach was transparent and brittle, and perforated in the splenic region by a gelatinized hole large enough to admit the fist, — although the fluid in the stomach was subsequently found incapable of dissolving another stomach, and almost destitute of free acid. And still less will the solvent action of the gastric juice account for such cases as those of Laisné and Gastellier, quoted in pp. 107-8, or the French medico-legal case to be mentioned in p. 118, — where death is preceded by a short illness, indicating a violent disorder of the stomach, and sometimes even characterized by all the marked symptoms of perforation. In the last description of cases, which are comparatively very rare, it seems necessary to admit that the gelatinization takes place during life; unless, indeed, it be supposed that the stomach is first perforated during life by ordinary ulcerative absorption, and then gelatinized after death, in consequence of the irritation existing before death having given rise to an unusual secretion of gastric juice.

Passing now to the differences between these gelatinized perforations, and the perforations caused by corrosive poisons, it may in the first instance be observed, that the margin of a corroded aperture is sometimes of a peculiar colour, — for example, yellow with nitric acid, brown with sulphuric acid or the alkalis, orange with iodine. But a much better, perhaps indeed an infallible criterion, and one of universal application, is the following. Either the person dies very soon after the poison is introduced, in which case vital action may not be excited in the stomach: or he lives long enough for the ordinary consequences of violent irritation to ensue. In the former case, as a large quantity of poison must have been taken, and much vomiting cannot have occurred, part of the poison will be found in the stomach: In the latter case, the poison may have been all ejected ; but in consequence of the longer duration of life, deep vascularity, or black extravasation must be produced round the hole, and sometimes too in other parts of the stomach ; changes which will at once distinguish the appearance from a gelatinized aperture. There is no doubt that the stomach may be perforated by the strong corrosives,

* Journal Complémentaire du Dict. des Scien. Med. xxxvii. 194.

13*

and yet hardly any of the poison be found in the stomach after death. Thus in a case related by Mertzdorff of poisoning with sulphuric acid, where life was prolonged for twelve hours, he could detect by minute analysis only $4\frac{1}{2}$ grains of the acid in the contents and tissue of the stomach. But then the hole was surrounded by signs of vital reaction, and so was the spleen upon which the aperture opened.[*] Judging from what I have often seen in animals killed with oxalic acid, which is the most rapidly fatal of all corrosives, so that little time is allowed for vital action, and also several times in persons who had died quickly from the action of sulphuric acid, I believe no poison can dissolve the stomach, without such unequivocal signs of violent irritation of the undissolved parts of the villous coat, as will secure an attentive observer from the mistake of confounding with these appearances the effects of spontaneous erosion. Spontaneous erosion is very generally united with unusual whiteness of the stomach, and there is never any material vascularity.

Resting on the description now given of the spontaneous and poisonous varieties of corrosion, it is an easy matter to decide a controversy, which at the time it occurred made a great deal of noise, and upon which the opinions of toxicologists have been unnecessarily divided. It is the question regarding death by poison which occurred in the trial of Mr. Angus at Liverpool in 1808 for the murder of his housekeeper Miss Burns. The poison suspected was corrosive sublimate. The symptoms were those of irritation in the alimentary canal, — vomiting, purging, and pain. In the dead body there was not any particular redness either of the intestines or of the stomach. But on the fore part of the stomach an aperture was found between the size of a crown piece and the palm of the hand; it had a ragged, pulpy margin; and the dissolution of the inner coat extended two inches from it all round the hole. No mention is made of adhesion or coloration of the margin. This description, it will be remarked, answers exactly that given above of spontaneous gelatinized perforation; and the absence of the signs of vital action around the hole and in the rest of the stomach is incompatible with the effects of a strong corrosive poison, unless death had occurred very soon after it was swallowed. This, however, was out of the question; for then the poison would have been found in the stomach, — which it was not.[†]

The case of Angus is not the only instance in recent times of spontaneous perforation having given rise to an opinion by medical men in favour of poisoning, and consequently to a criminal trial. Six years afterwards a similar incident occurred in France. A young woman near Montargis having died of a short illness, and a large erosion having been found in the stomach after death, six practitioners, on a view of the parts, and without referring to the antecedent symptoms or attempting an analysis of the contents of the stomach, declared that she died of the effects of some corrosive poison. The husband and mother-in-law, against whom there does not appear to

[*] Horn's Archiv für Medizinische Erfahrung, 1823, i. 45.
[†] Trial of Angus for the murder of Margaret Burns, 1808.

have been a shadow of general evidence, were therefore imprisoned and subsequently tried for their lives. Luckily, however, an intelligent physician of the town saw the error of the reporters, and after vainly endeavouring to persuade them to revise their opinion, was the means of the case being remitted to the medical faculty of Paris. That distinguished body, with Professor Chaussier at its head, gave a unanimous and decided opinion, not only that there was not any proof of poisoning, but likewise that the woman could have died of nothing else than spontaneous perforation. The leading features of the medical evidence will at once show how indefensible the conduct and opinion of the original reporters were. The last meal taken by the woman before she became ill, and the only one at which poison could have been administered by the prisoners, was her supper; her illness did not begin till past six next morning; the symptoms were mortal coldness, fainting, general pains, headache, pain in the stomach, purging and colic, without vomiting, and she died after twenty-four hours' illness; the morbid appearances were general redness of the stomach, softening and pulpy destruction of a third part of its posterior parietes, and nevertheless the presence in the stomach of a pint and a half of fluid matter, containing evidently the remains of soup taken by the woman after she felt unwell. On the decision of the Parisian faculty the prisoners were discharged; and the original reporters were deservedly handled with great severity in several publications that appeared not long after.*

Of perforations of the Gullet and Intestines from natural causes, and their distinctions from those produced by poisons. — The intestines, and sometimes even the gullet, may be perforated by the same erosive or solvent process as the stomach. Thus Mr. Allan Burns observes, that in four plump children, whose previous history he could not learn, he found every part of the alimentary canal, from the termination of the gullet down to the beginning of the rectum, reduced to a gluey, transparent pulp, like thick starch. The bodies were quite free from putrefaction ; but the abdomen exhaled a very sour smell when opened. No other organic derangement could be detected.†
The particulars of a similar case, with an account of the symptoms, have been lately published by Mr. Smith, a London surgeon. In the body of a child who died of protracted diarrhœa subsequent to weaning, the whole intestines, from the duodenum to the sigmoid flexure of the colon, were found fourteen hours after death gelatinous, semi-transparent, and so soft and brittle that they could not bear their own weight, but tore when lifted between the fingers. The stomach and rectum were healthy.‡ I lately met with the following instance, where the erosion clearly took place after death. In the body of a girl who died within twelve hours of poisoning with red-precipitate, the stomach and duodenum were found much inflamed, but quite

* Laisné sur les Perforations de l'Estomac, p. 190, and Billiard, Considérations sur l'Empoisonnement par les Irritans, *passim.*
† Edin. Med. and Surg. Journal, vi. 137.
‡ London Medical Gazette, ii. 619.

entire and firm three days after death. Eighteen days afterwards, when I had an opportunity of examining these organs, their textures remained firm everywhere, except a few inches below the pylorus, where I found two apertures in the duodenum, each as big as a crown, and surrounded by extensive jelly-like softening.

The following case from Laisné's treatise shows that the gullet may be also dissolved in the same way. A woman three days after delivery was attacked with puerperal peritonitis, and died in four days. In the belly were found the usual morbid appearances of peritonitis : but in addition there was in the lower part of the gullet a large oval aperture two inches long, which penetrated through the posterior mediastinum into the lungs.* Another singular instance of the same kind has already been mentioned under the head of the symp- toms (see p. 107). Another has been described by Dr. Marshall Hall. In a child who died of bronchitis, an opening was found in the gullet about the size of a pea, so that the canal of the gullet communicated with the sac of the pleura ; and several veins appeared also to have been opened.† The stomach was likewise perforated.

It is not difficult to draw the distinction between these perforations and the effects of poison. The throat and gullet may be partially disorganized or corroded by the strong corrosives ; but they are very rarely penetrated, since the greater part of the poison must pass into the stomach or be rejected by vomiting. Destruction of the mucous coat is a common consequence, and stricture occasionally follows ; but I have hitherto met with only one instance among the innumerable published cases of poisoning with the mineral acids, alkalis, and other corrosives, where the gullet was perforated. In that case the perfora- tion was the result of slow ulceration from poisoning with sulphuric acid, where life was prolonged for two months.‡ Perforation from simple corrosion never occurs. The intestines are never perforated by chemical corrosion from within, for either the poison is in a great measure expelled from the stomach by vomiting, or the pylorus con- tracts and prevents the passage of every poison that is sufficiently concentrated to corrode. Both the small and great intestines might be corroded from without, in consequence of the poison escaping through a hole in the stomach. I am not acquainted, however, with any case of the kind where intestinal perforation has oc- curred.

When the intestines are pierced by true ulceration, it is im- possible to tell whether it arose from natural disease or an irritant poison.

The mode of forming a diagnosis between the symptoms and appearances of irritant poisoning and those of natural disease being thus explained, the different species of poisons which have been arranged in the class of irritants will now be considered in their order.

* Laisné. &c. p. 564.
† Edin. Med. and Surg. Journal, xxxii 38.   ‡ London Med. Gazette, xiv. 30.

The irritant class of poisons may be divided into five orders: the acids and their bases; the alkalies and their salts; the metallic compounds; the vegetable and animal irritants; the mechanical irritants. In a short appendix some substances will be mentioned which are not usually considered poisonous, but are capable of causing violent symptoms when taken in large doses.

The greater number of poisons included in the first order have a very powerful local action. Most of them possess true corrosive properties when they are sufficiently concentrated. Most of them likewise act remotely. One of them, oxalic acid, is evidently not so much an irritant as a narcotico-acrid; but since its most frequent action as seen in man is irritation, it seems inexpedient to break the natural arrangement for the sake of logical accuracy. This is far from being the only instance where the toxicologist is compelled to violate the principles of philosophical classification.

In the present Order are included four of the mineral acids, the sulphuric, nitric, muriatic and phosphoric, with their bases, phosphorus, sulphur, and chlorine: To these may be added iodine and bromine, with their compounds, and also oxalic and acetic acid, two of the vegetable acids.

CHAPTER III.

OF POISONING WITH THE MINERAL ACIDS.

Of the mineral acids, the most important, because the most common, are *sulphuric*, *hydrochloric*, and *nitric* acids. They are remarkably similar in their effects on the animal economy. Phosphoric acid is of much less consequence, and will be noticed cursorily.

Sulphuric acid (*vitriolic acid, vitriol — oil of vitriol*), hydrochloric acid (*muriatic acid, — spirit of salt*) and nitric acid (*aqua-fortis*), have been long known to be possessed of very energetic properties; and consequently cases of poisoning with them have often been observed. The instances of the kind hitherto published have been chiefly the result of suicide; a considerable number have originated in accident; and, however extraordinary it may appear, a few have been cases of murder. Tartra, in an excellent memoir on the subject of poisoning with nitric acid, quotes an instance of a woman having been poisoned while in a state of intoxication by that acid being mixed with wine and poured down her throat.[*] Valentini has related the case of a woman who was killed by frequent doses of sulphuric acid given under the pretence of administering medicines.[†] In 1829 an hospital servant was condemned at Strasbourg for trying to murder his wife in like manner, by first making her ill with tartar-

* Traité de l'Empoisonnement par l'acide Nitrique, 1802, p. 87.
† Novellæ Medico-legales, Cas. xxix. p. 211.

emetic and then giving her sulphuric acid in syrup, under the pretence of curing her.* At the Aberdeen autumn circuit in 1830 a woman Humphrey was convicted of murdering her husband by pouring the same acid down his throat while he lay asleep with his mouth open.† On the whole, considering the powerful taste and excessively acrid properties of these poisons, it is probable that they will seldom be resorted to for the purpose of making away with another person, who is an adult, and in a state of consciousness. Of late, however, there have been several instances in our country of murder committed on infants in this barbarous manner. A woman Malcolm was executed here in 1808 for murdering her own child, an infant of eighteen months, by pouring sulphuric acid down its throat ;‡ another woman Clark was tried for the same crime at Exeter in 1822 ; a man was executed lately at Manchester for murdering in the same way his son, a child four years and a half old ;§ and the particulars of an interesting trial will be presently noticed, that of Overfield, who was executed at Shrewsbury in 1824, for poisoning his child in the like manner.‖

In a medico-legal point of view, the mineral acids are interesting on another account. Of late a new crime has arisen in Britain, the disfiguring of the countenance by squirting oil of vitriol on it. It originated in Glasgow, during the quarrels in 1820, between masters and workmen regarding the rate of wages,¶ and became at last so frequent, that the Lord Advocate, in applying for an act of Parliament to extend the English Stabbing and Maiming act to Scotland, added a clause which renders the offence now alluded to capital. In 1828 a woman Macmillan was tried here and condemned under that act.** The crime afterwards became common in England. Three cases were noticed in the newspapers as having occurred in London, in November, 1828 ; and two others near Manchester in the spring of 1829. It is now much less frequent.

The mineral acids are also very interesting on scientific grounds. They afford the purest examples of true corrosive poisons, their poisonous effects depending entirely on the organic injury they occasion in the textures to which they are applied. It is of use to set out, in investigating the effects of poisons, by determining the phenomena presented under such circumstances. When made aware of the rapidity with which other irritating poisons prove fatal, and the slight signs they commonly leave of their operation, one cannot fail to be struck with discovering what the animal frame will sometimes endure from these the most violent of all irritants, and nevertheless recover.

In laying down the mode of determining by chemical evidence a

* Bulletins des Sciences Médicales, Janvier, 1830.
† Edinburgh Medical and Surgical Journal, xxxv. 298.
‡ Burnett on Criminal Law, 544. *Note.*
§ Edinburgh Med. and Surg. Journal, xxxvi. 102.   ‖ Ibidem, xxii. 222.
¶ Report of the Committee of the House of Commons on the Combination Laws, June, 1825, pp. 323-328. Evidence of Mr. Campbell and Mr. Robinson.
** Cases and Observations in Medical Jurisprudence, Case iii. Edin. Med. and Surg. Journal, xxxi. 229.

case of supposed poisoning with any of the three mineral acids mentioned above, it will be unnecessary to notice any of their chemical properties, except those from which their medico-legal tests are derived.

The only common properties that require notice are, their power of reddening the vegetable blue colours, for showing which litmus-paper is commonly used, and is most convenient : and their power of staining and corroding all articles of dress, especially such as are made of wool, hair, and leather. This last property is specified, though a familiar one, because it always forms important evidence in criminal cases. In order to give precision to such evidence, it is necessary to remember, that if the article of dress is a coloured one, it is generally rendered red by the mineral acids ; but that the vegetable acids also will redden most articles of dress, although they do not corrode them.

I. — OF POISONING WITH SULPHURIC ACID.

Sulphuric acid is extensively employed in very many trades, is used even for some domestic purposes, and is consequently familiar to every one. Hence it is the mineral acid which has been most commonly used as a poison, especially for committing suicide. Of 35 cases of poisoning with the mineral acids which occurred in England in the years 1837 and 1838, 32 were caused by this acid (p. 90).

SECTION I. — Of the Tests for Sulphuric Acid.

Sulphuric acid is known as a poison chiefly in the form of the concentrated commercial acid. But a few cases of poisoning have also been produced by blue-liquor or the solution of indigo in strong sulphuric acid ; and one instance* has been recorded of poisoning with the aromatic sulphuric acid of the Pharmacopœias, which is an infusion of aromatics in a mixture of sulphuric acid, ether and alcohol. In the following remarks on its tests, it will be sufficient to consider it *first* in the concentrated form, — *secondly*, in a state of simple dilution, — and *thirdly*, when mixed with various impurities, more especially with vegetable and animal matter. The acid solution of indigo may be known by the tests for the concentrated acid, and its blue colour, removable by a solution of chlorine ; and the aromatic sulphuric acid may be distinguished by its odour and the tests for the diluted acid.

1. *When concentrated* it is oily-looking, colourless, or brownish from having acted on organic particles, without odour, much heavier than water, and capable of quickly corroding animal substances. If from these properties, and its effect in reddening litmus, its exact nature be not considered obvious, it may be heated with a few chips of copper ; when sulphurous acid is disengaged and may be readily recognised by its odour.

* London Med. Gazette, 1839-40, i. 944.

2. *When diluted*, it may be distinguished from all ordinary acids by solution of nitrate of baryta occasioning a heavy white precipitate of sulphate of baryta, which is insoluble in nitric acid. Selenic and sulphurous acids, however, and also, as Mr. Alfred Taylor informs me he has lately found, the fluo-silicic acid, are similarly acted on in all respects. But selenic and fluo-silicic acids in all forms, and sulphurous acid in a state of solution, are so seldom met with, being known only in the laboratory of the scientific chemist, that they can scarcely be considered sources of fallacy. Sulphuric acid may at once be distinguished from sulphurous acid, by the latter possessing a peculiar pungent odour. From the two other acids it may be distinguished by collecting and drying the barytic precipitate, mixing this with charcoal, converting it into sulphuret of barium by heating it in a platinum spoon before the blowpipe, and then adding diluted muriatic acid to the sulphuret, so as to disengage sulphuretted-hydrogen-gas, — which again is easily known by its odour, or its property of blackening paper dipped in solution of acetate of lead. A much more important source of fallacy than these is the possible presence of a bisulphate in solution, or a neutral sulphate along with any other free acid ; for these substances will present the same reactions with litmus and barytic salts as free sulphuric acid itself. Much has been published lately upon this point ; but the difficulty has not yet been satisfactorily overcome. It may be got rid of indeed by proving, that no bisulphate or neutral sulphate is present. Their absence may be shown by no solid residuum being left on evaporating the suspected fluid, or at least no more than a mere haziness, owing to the sulphate of lead which commercial sulphuric acid always contains in small quantity. Or as Orfila suggests, we may establish their absence still better by concentrating the fluid, and finding that neither carbonate of soda, which would cause a precipitate with earthy or metallic bases, nor chloride of platinum, which would do so with potash or ammonia in combination, nor fluo-silicic acid, which precipitates soda salts, has any effect when applied to separate portions of the subject of inquiry. But suppose it appear in the course of these trials that one or more bases are actually present, how is it to be settled whether the sulphuric acid, indicated by litmus and a salt of baryta, is really free or not? To this question I must reply, that no method has yet been proposed, which is at once satisfactory and easily available. Mr. Alfred Taylor proposes to concentrate the fluid, and agitate it with alcohol, in the hope that the alcohol will remove sulphuric acid, and not a sulphate, from the water.* But it removes sulphuric acid from a bisulphate even when dry, and still more when a little water is present. Orfila† proposes, in the case of sulphuric acid in vinegar, — where there is both a vegetable acid and a neutral sulphate of lime, — to concentrate to a sixth, and agitate the residuum with four times its volume of sulphuric ether, in the expectation that this fluid will remove the free acid alone, and separate it from sulphates. But notwithstanding the authority of his

* A Manual of Medical Jurisprudence, 1844, p. 94.
† Toxicologie Générale, 1843, i.

name for the fact, pure ether will not remove sulphuric acid from a watery fluid; and etherized alcohol, which does remove it, takes it away also, like alcohol itself, from bisulphates. These results I have observed in some careful trials made along with Dr. Douglas Maclagan. I suspect, therefore, that where sulphates or bisulphates do exist, there is no absolutely satisfactory way of determining whether free sulphuric acid also coexists, except by a quantitative analysis, for ascertaining whether the amount of acid and of bases corresponds with this supposition or not. And it is scarcely necessary to add, that so operose a method is scarcely applicable to ordinary medico-legal investigations.

3. It is seldom that the medical jurist is called on to search for sulphuric acid in either of the states already mentioned. Much more generally it has mingled with and acted on various organic substances. The circumstances in which it has usually to be sought for in the practice of medical jurisprudence are twofold, — on the one hand, in stains on clothes, — and on the other, in vomited matter, the contents of the stomach, or organic mixtures generally.

Process for analyzing stains on clothes. — When sulphuric acid is thrown upon your clothes, it produces a permanent red, reddish-brown, or yellowish stain, destroys the cloth entirely or renders it brittle, and in consequence of its strong attraction for water keeps the stain long in a moist state. In the course of the decomposition of the cloth a part of the acid is itself decomposed, sulphurous acid being disengaged. But it is an important medico-legal fact, that after a time the change either goes on very slowly, or is arrested altogether, possibly by the dilution of the acid with moisture from the atmosphere; and that consequently it may be discovered in a free state in stains after a much longer interval than would à *priori* be expected. In the case of Macmillan formerly alluded to, Dr. Turner and I, who were employed by the crown to examine the different injured articles of dress, found on a man's hat, stock, shirt-collar and coat many discoloured and corroded spots, which were sour to the taste fourteen days after the crime was committed; in the subsequent case of Mrs. Humphrey I discovered six-tenths of a grain of free sulphuric acid in two small spots on a blanket seven weeks after the crime; and from an express experiment on the same blanket with two drops of acid of known strength, it appeared that only one-half of the acid disappeared in seven weeks. It may therefore be inferred, that, in every instance where stains have been produced by concentrated sulphuric acid on clothes, at least on woollen clothes, and no attempt has been made to remove the remaining acid by washing or neutralization, a sufficient quantity will be present even after several weeks to admit of being satisfactorily detected by chemical analysis.

The following are the steps of the process which appear to me the most delicate and equivocal. Cut away the stained spots; boil them for a minute or two in several successive small portions of distilled water; and filter if necessary. Next prove the acidity of the fluid by litmus, and likewise by the taste if the quantity of solution is large

14

enough to allow of so coarse a test being used ; and with a few drops
ascertain the existence of sulphuric acid in one form or another by
nitrate of baryta and nitric acid, as mentioned in the process for the
pure diluted acid.   If no precipitate appears, the search for sulphuric
acid is at an end.   But if a precipitate is produced, ascertain the absence of bisulphates and sulphates by proving the absence of bases,
according to the method described in the process for the simple diluted acid.   If, however, bases be found in material proportion to
the acid, the analysis is subject to all the difficulties mentioned above
in speaking of the detection of the diluted acid in similar circumstances.

Process for the contents of the stomach and other complex mixtures. —
When sulphuric acid has been mixed with various mineral and organic substances, it may in no long time cease to exist in the free
state.   Part may be decomposed by organic matter in the way formerly mentioned.   Or the whole may be neutralized at once by earthy
or alkaline carbonates, administered purposely as antidotes.   Or it
may also be neutralized more slowly by the gradual development of
ammonia in consequence of the decay of the animal matter co-existing in the mixture.   Thus in a case mentioned by Mertzdorff of a
child killed in twelve hours with sulphuric acid, the contents of the
stomach did not redden litmus, but on the contrary had an ammoniacal odour ; and they contained a considerable quantity of a soluble
sulphate, probably the sulphate of ammonia.*   In like manner MM.
Orfila and Lesueur found that when this acid was left some months in
a mixture which contained putrefying azotized matter, it was gradually neutralized by ammonia.†   It appears from Orfila's latest researches,‡ that in most cases of acute poisoning with this substance
some free acid will be found in the contents or tissues of the
stomach, provided alkalis or earths were not given as antidotes, and
the examination of the body be made before decay sets in.

The detection of sulphuric acid in complex organic mixtures, simple
though it appears at first sight, is one of the most difficult problems
in medico-legal chemistry.   The difficulty arises from a variety of
sources, — from the probable presence of neutral sulphates along
with free hydrochloric, acetic, or some other acid, — the possible
presence of a bisulphate, — the occasional neutralization of the sulphuric acid by antidotes given during life, or ammonia evolved during
decay after death, — or its neutralization, together with the development of a different free acid, by its having displaced this acid from a
salt existing in the mixture.

The subject was investigated in most of its relations in the last
edition of the present work, and a process proposed which overcame
some difficulties, but left others untouched.   The inquiry has been
since undertaken also by M. Devergie and Professor Orfila, but with
most success in Germany by Dr. Simon.§   The result of all these

* Archiv für Medizinische Erfahrung, 1823, i. 456.
† Revue Médicale, 1824, ii. 469.
‡ Toxicologie Gén. 4ème edition, 1843, i. 112.
§ Poggendort's Annalen der Physik und Chemie, xli. 643.   Buchner's Repertorium,
1838, lxiv. 20.

researches is, that a satisfactory process for detecting sulphuric acid in organic mixtures still remains to be discovered. Meanwhile the most eligible method appears to me to be the following.

a. *If the mixture be acid,* add distilled water, if necessary, boil, filter, and test a few drops of the fluid with nitrate of baryta, followed by nitric acid. If there be no precipitate, the search for sulphuric acid is at an end. If a precipitate form, distil the fluid from a muriate of lime or oil bath, at a temperature not above 240°, till the residuum acquire a thick syrupy consistence ; and preserve apart the last sixth of the distilled liquor. In this liquor test for hydrochloric acid by litmus-paper and nitrate of silver, and for acetic acid by litmus-paper, and the odour and taste of the liquid. If these acids be not in the distilled fluid, they are not in the residuum. In a portion of this residuum search for nitric acid, and in another portion for oxalic acid, by the processes for these poisons in complex mixtures. If all these acids be thus proved to be absent, it is most unlikely that the acidity of the mixture is owing to any other but sulphuric acid, especially in the case of the contents or textures of the stomach.

Dilute now what remains of the syrupy extract, and add nitrate of baryta with nitric acid. If a precipitate arise, there is a strong presumption that the acidity of the mixture was owing either to a bisulphate or to free sulphuric acid. And between these the question may be almost settled, first by the probability or improbability of a bisulphate having come in the way, and secondly, by the symptoms and morbid appearances. The result however cannot justify more than a presumptive opinion. — But if hydrochloric, acetic or nitric acid be indicated in the subject of analysis, or an acid sulphate, the whole process is vitiated, and it is scarcely possible to arrive at any trustworthy conclusion.

The difficulties adverted to above have been made the groundwork of various processes ; which however seem to me all imperfect. — It has been proposed to divide the mixture into two equal parts, to precipitate one directly by a barytic salt, to do the same with the other after drying and incinerating it, to compare the weight of the precipitates, and to infer the presence of free sulphuric acid if the former is more than double the latter. Various objections however may be brought against this check, not the least serious being its difficulty in ordinary hands, whenever the precipitates are none of them considerable. — Simon proposes to exhaust the residuum of evaporation with absolute alcohol, in the hope that free sulphuric acid will alone be taken up ;* but he himself found that neutral sulphates are dissolved partially ; and besides, alcohol removes sulphuric acid from bisulphates. — Orfila proposes to remove free sulphuric acid by agitating the concentrated liquor with sulphuric ether, and separating and evaporating off the ether ; for he holds that all neutral and acid salts of sulphuric acid are insoluble in ether.† This proposal is unaccountable. Simon stated in his paper three years before, that ether does not remove sulphuric acid from watery fluids containing it. And Dr. Douglas Maclagan and I, on inquiring into the matter, found

* Buchner's Repertorium, lxiv. 32.　　† Journal de Chimie Médicale, 1841, 474.

that we could not, by means of ether, separate a particle of sulphuric acid from an ounce of rice soup and mucilage to which ten drops of the acid had been added.   The process of Orfila for establishing the absence of bases in a simple watery solution is applicable to organic mixtures also, after incineration.   But if bases be present in material quantity, all the difficulties now in question remain in full force.

b. *When the mixture is neutral,* sulphuric acid may be detected in it by the first steps of the preceding process.   But the inference, that it once existed free can only be drawn when the subject of examination is not in a state of decay, when the quantity of sulphate of baryta obtained is considerable, when the administration of an antidote is proved, and when the ashes after incineration contain the antacid base which is said to have been administered.   Even then the inference is only presumptive.

SECTION II.— *Of the Mode of Action of Sulphuric Acid, and the Symptoms caused by it in Man.*

It was formerly observed that the action of the strong mineral acids is independent of the function of absorption.   They act by the conveyance along the nerves of an impression produced by the irritation or destruction of the part to which they are applied.   There is very little difference between the three acids in the symptoms they excite or the action they exert.

When sulphuric acid is introduced directly into a vein it causes death by coagulating the blood.   Thus, when Professor Orfila injected in the jugular vein of a dog half a drachm diluted with an equal weight of water, he observed that the animal at once struggled violently, stretched out its limbs, and expired ; and on opening the chest immediately, he found the heart and great vessels filled with coagulated blood.* — Nitric acid and hydrochloric acid act in the same way.

If, on the other hand, they are introduced into the stomach, the blood as usual remains fluid for some time after death ; the symptoms are referrible almost solely to the abdomen ; and in the dead body the stomach is found extensively disorganised, and the other abdominal viscera sometimes inflamed.   If the dose be large, and the animal fasting, death may take place in so short a time as three hours : but in general it lives much longer.†

When the strong mineral acids are applied outwardly, they irritate, inflame, or corrode the skin.   The most rapid in producing these effects is the nitric, or rather the nitrous acid.   The strong, fuming nitrous acid even causes effervescence when dropped on the skin.

Orfila has proved that sulphuric acid, as well as the two other mineral acids, is absorbed ; for they may be detected in the urine, when they are introduced either into the stomach or through a

* Toxicologie Gén. i. 77.   † Ibidem, 78.

wound.* He could not succeed, however, in detecting any of them in the liver or spleen; in which organs it will be seen, hereafter, that various other poisons may be discovered by chemical analysis. But Mr. Scoffern seems to have found sulphuric acid in the kidney, even although the individual survived the taking of the poison nearly two days.† It is also worthy of remark, that, as will be proved presently, these acids may pass through the coats of the stomach by transudation, and so be found on the surface of the other organs in the belly.

Toxicology is indebted to M. Tartra for the first methodic information published respecting the symptoms caused in man by sulphuric acid and the other mineral acids:‡ but many important additional facts have been made known by numberless cases of poisoning which have since appeared, chiefly in the periodic journals.

The symptoms caused by all the three acids are so nearly the same, that after a detailed account of those occasioned by sulphuric acid, it will not be necessary to add much on the subject under the head of nitric and muriatic acid.

M. Tartra considers that four varieties may be observed in the effects of the mineral acids. 1. Speedy death from violent corrosion and inflammation; 2. Slow death from a peculiar organic disease of the stomach and intestines; 3. Imperfect recovery, the person remaining liable ever after to irritability of the stomach; 4. Perfect recovery.

1. The most ordinary symptoms are those of the first variety, — namely, all the symptoms that characterise the most violent gastritis, accompanied likewise with burning in the throat, which is increased by pressure, swallowing, or coughing;§ — eructations proceeding from the gases evolved in the stomach by its chemical decomposition; — and an excruciating pain in the stomach, such as no natural inflammation can excite. The lips are commonly shrivelled, at first whitish, but afterwards brownish in the case of sulphuric acid. Occasionally there are also excoriations, more rarely little blisters. Similar marks appear on other parts of the skin with which the acid may have come in contact, such as the cheeks, neck, breast, or fingers; and these marks undergo the same change of colour as the marks on the lips. I had an opportunity of witnessing this in the case of the man who was disfigured by the Macmillans (p. 122) with sulphuric acid. He was cruelly burnt on the face as well as on the hands, which he had raised to protect his face; and the marks were at first white, but in sixteen hours became brownish. The inside of the mouth is also generally shrivelled, white, and often more or less corroded; and as the poisoning advances, the teeth become loose and yellowish-brown about the coronæ. The teeth sometimes become brown in so short a time as three hours.‖ Occasionally the tongue, gums, and inside

* Journal de Chimie Médicale, 1842, 266.
† London Medical Gazette, 1841-42, ii. 254.
‡ Traité de l'Empoisonnement par l'acide nitrique, 1802.
§ Lebidois, Arch. Gén. de Med. xiii. 367.
‖ Martini in Rust's Magazin für die gesammte Heilkunde, xviii. 159.

14*

of the cheeks are white, and as it were polished, like ivory.* There
is almost always great difficulty, and sometimes complete impossibility, of swallowing. In the case of a child related by Dr. Sinclair, of Manchester, fluids taken by the mouth were returned by
the nose ; and the reason was obvious after death ; for even then
the pharynx was so much contracted as to admit a probe with difficulty.† On the same account substances taken by the mouth have
been discharged by an opening in the larynx which had been made
to relieve impending suffocation. The matter vomited, if no fluids
be swallowed, is generally brownish or black, and at first causes
effervescence, if it falls on a pavement containing any lime. Afterwards this matter is mixed with shreds of membrane, which resemble the coats of the stomach, and sometimes actually consists of
the disorganised coats, but are generally nothing more than coagulated mucus. The bowels are obstinately costive, the urine scanty
or suppressed ; and the patient is frequently harassed by distressing
tenesmus and desire to pass water. The pulse all along is very
weak, sometimes intermitting, and towards the close imperceptible.
It is not always frequent ; on the contrary, it has been observed
of natural frequency, small and feeble in a patient who survived
fifteen days.‡ The countenance becomes at an early period glazed
and ghastly, and the extremities cold and clammy. The breathing
is often laborious, owing to the movements of the chest increasing
the pain in the stomach, — or because pulmonary inflammation is
also at times present, — or because the admission of air into the
lungs is impeded by the injury done to the epiglottis and entrance
of the larynx. To these symptoms are added occasional fits of
suffocation from shreds of thick mucus sticking in the throat, and
sometimes croupy respiration, with sense of impending choking.

Such is the ordinary train of symptoms in cases of the first
variety. But sometimes, especially when a large dose has been
swallowed, instead of these excruciating tortures, there is a deceit-
ful tranquillity and absence of all uneasiness. Thus, in the case of
a woman who was poisoned by her companions making her swallow
while intoxicated aqua fortis mixed with wine, although she had
at first a good deal of pain and vomiting, there were subsequently
none of the usual violent symptoms ; and she died within twenty
hours, complaining chiefly of tenesmus and excessive debility.§
Occasionally eruptions break out over the body :‖ but their nature
has not been described.

Death is seldom owing to the mere local mischief, more generally to sympathy of the circulation and nervous system with that
injury. According to Bouchardat death arises from the acid entering the blood in sufficient quantity to cause coagulation.¶ But

* Correa de Serra in Journal de Chimie Médicale, ii. 209, on the third day.
† Edinburgh Med. and Surg. Journal, xxxvi. 103.
‡ Archives Générales de Médecine, xiii. 367.   § Tartra, iii. 87.
‖ Desgranges, Recueil Périodique de la Société de Médecine, vi. 22. Tulpius, Ob-
servationes Medicinales, iii. 43.
¶ Annales d'Hygiène Publique, xvii. 362.

although this certainly happens sometimes to the blood in the vessels of the stomach and adjacent organs, as will be proved under the head of the morbid appearances, there is no evidence that the same takes place throughout the bloodvessels generally, or in the great veins and heart in particular. Bouchardat's proofs of the detection of sulphuric acid in the blood are not satisfactory.

The duration of this variety of poisoning with the acids is commonly between twelve hours and three days. But sometimes life is prolonged for a week* or a fortnight;† and sometimes too death takes place in a very few hours. The shortest duration among the numerous cases of adults mentioned by Tartra is six hours;‡ but Dr. Sinclair, of Manchester, has related a case which lasted only four hours and a half;§ a man lately died in the Edinburgh Infirmary within four hours; and Professor Remer of Breslau once met with a case fatal in two hours.‖

The quantity required to produce these effects has not been ascertained, and must be liable to the same uncertainty here as in other kinds of poisoning. The smallest fatal dose of sulphuric acid I have hitherto found recorded was one drachm. It was taken with sugar by mistake for stomachic drops by a stout young man, and killed him in seven days.¶ An infant of twelve months has been killed in twenty-four hours by half a tea-spoonful, or about thirty minims.** A man has recovered after taking six drachms.††

2. The second variety of symptoms belong to a peculiar modification of disease, which is described by Tartra in rather strong language. It begins with the symptoms already noticed; but these gradually abate. The patient then becomes affected with general fever, dry skin, spasms and pains of the limbs, difficult breathing, tension of the belly, salivation, and occasional vomiting, particularly of food and drink. Afterwards membranous flakes are discharged by vomiting, and the salivation is accompanied with fœtor. These flakes are often very like the mucous membrane of the stomach and intestines; and such they have often been described to be. More probably, however, they are of adventitious formation; for the mere mucous coat of the alimentary canal cannot supply the vast quantity that is evacuated. There is no doubt, however, that the lining membrane of the alimentary canal is occasionally discharged. Dr. Wilson has mentioned an instance of the ejection by coughing of about nine inches of the cylindrical lining of the pharynx and gullet six days after sulphuric acid was taken.‡‡ Sometimes worms are discharged dead, and evidently corroded by the poison.§§ Digestion is at the same time deranged, the whole functions of the body are languid, and the patient falls into a state of marasmus, which reduces

* Journal der Praktischen Heilkunde, vii. ii. 18.
† Archives Générales, xiii. 367.   ‡ Tartra, p. 160.
§ Edinburgh Med. and Surg. Journal, xxxvi. 102.
‖ Journal der Praktischen Heilkunde, xlix. iii. 60.
¶ Journal der Praktischen Heilkunde, vii. ii. 18.
** Mr J. B. Thomson in London Med. Gazette, 1841-42, i. 146.
†† Martini's case.   ‡‡ London Med. Gazette, 1834, xiv. 489.
§§ Tendering in Horn's Archiv für Medizinische Erfahrung, 1825, i. 458.

him to a mere skeleton, and in the end brings him to the grave. Death may take place in a fortnight, or not for months. In one of Tartra's cases the patient lived eight months. The vomiting of membranous flakes continues to the last.

3. The third variety includes cases of imperfect recovery. These are characterized by nothing but the greater mildness of the primary symptoms, and by the patient continuing for life liable to attacks of pain in the stomach, vomiting of food and general disorder of the digestive function.

4. The last variety comprehends cases of perfect recovery, which are sufficiently numerous even under unpromising appearances. From the average of 55 cases recorded by Tartra it appears that the chances of death and recovery are nearly equal. Twenty-six died, 19 of the primary, 7 of the secondary disorder. Twenty-nine recovered, and of these twenty-one perfectly. Suicidal are for obvious reasons more frequently fatal than accidental cases.

Tartra has not taken notice in his treatise of another form of poisoning with the strong acids, — in which the injury is confined to the gullet and neighbouring parts. In Corvisart's Journal there is the case of a man, who began to drink sulphuric acid for water while intoxicated, but suddenly found out his error before he had swallowed above a few drops; and consequently the chief symptoms were confined to the throat. After his physician saw him he was able to take one dose of a chalk mixture; but from that time he was unable to swallow at all for a fortnight.* Martini likewise met with a similar instance of complete dysphagia from stricture in the gullet caused by sulphuric acid.† His patient recovered.

It also appears exceedingly probable, that the strong acids may cause death, without reaching the stomach or even the gullet, by exciting inflammation and spasm of the glottis and larynx. Such an effect may very well be anticipated from an attempt to commit murder with these poisons; as the person, if he retains consciousness at the time, may become aware of their nature before he has swallowed enough to injure the stomach.

Thus, Dr. A. T. Thomson says in 1837, that he once met with the case of a child, who, while attempting to swallow strong sulphuric acid by mistake for water, died almost immediately, to all appearance from suffocation caused by contraction of the glottis; and it was ascertained after death that none of the poison had reached the stomach.‡ Professor Quain describes a similar case, occurring also in a child, where impending death was prevented by artificial respiration, and acute bronchitis ensued, which proved fatal in three days. In this instance thickening of the epiglottis and great contraction of the upper opening of the larynx showed the violent local injury inflicted there, inflammation could be traced down the trachea into the bronchial tubes, but no trace of injury could be detected in the gullet and stomach.§ In a very interesting and carefully detailed

* Journal de Médecine par Corvisart, xix. 263.
† Rust's Magazin für die gesammte Heilkunde, xxiii. 156.
‡ Lancet, 1836-37, ii. 835.   § Lancet, 1836-37, i. 195.

case by Mr. Arnott, where the poison taken was the nitric acid, the injury was confined in a great measure to the gullet and larynx, — the stomach, which was distended with food at the time, being very little affected. The chief symptoms at first, besides great general depression, were croupy respiration and much dyspnœa, which became so urgent, that laryngotomy was performed, and with complete relief to the breathing. But the patient nevertheless rapidly sunk under the symptoms of general exhaustion, and died in thirty-six hours without presenting any particular signs of the operation of the poison on the stomach; and the traces of action found there after death were trifling.*

The importance of the fact established by these cases will appear from the following medico-legal inquiries. A Prussian medical college was consulted in the case of a new-born child, in which the stomach and intestines were healthy, and did not contain poison, but in which the cuticle of the lips was easily scraped off, the gums, tongue, and mouth yellowish-green, as if burnt, the velum and uvula in the same state, the rima glottidis contracted, and the epiglottis, larynx, and fauces violently inflamed. The College declared, that a concentrated acid had been given, and that death had been occasioned by suffocation. Sulphuric acid was found in the house; and the mother subsequently confessed the crime.† A case was formerly quoted (p. 75), where MM. Ollivier and Chevallier found traces of the action of nitric acid on the lips, mouth, throat and upper fourth of the gullet, but not lower. In this instance the reporters came to the opinion from the absence of injury in the more important parts of the alimentary canal, as well as from the marks of nail-scratches on the neck, and the gorged state of the lungs, that death had been produced by strangling, after an unsuccessful attempt by the forcible administration of nitric acid. It is quite possible, however, that death might quickly ensue from the effects of the poison on the throat and gullet. In the course of the judicial inquiries M. Alibert stated that he had known repeated instances of death from swallowing nitric acid, although none of it reached lower down than the pharynx. Ollivier in his paper doubts the accuracy of this statement; but the cases quoted above show clearly that such injury may be done to the glottis as will be adequate of itself to occasion death.‡

It seems farther not improbable that, among the terminations of poisoning with the strong mineral acids, scirrhous pylorus must also be enumerated. This is a very rare effect of the action of corrosive poisons. But M. Bouillaud has related an instance of death from scirrhous pylorus in its most aggravated shape, which supervened on the chronic form of the effects of nitric acid, and which proved fatal in three months.§

In some circumstances the stomach seems to acquire a degree of insensibility to the action of the strong acids. Tartra, in alluding to what is said of certain whisky-drinkers acquiring the power of swal-

* London Medical Gazette, xii. 219.   † Augustin's Repertorium, i. ii. 15.
‡ Archives Gén de Méd., xxi. 372, *note.*   § Journal Hebdomadaire.

lowing with impunity small quantities of the concentrated acids, has related the case of a woman at Paris, who, after passing successively from wine to brandy and from that to alcohol, at last found nothing could titillate her stomach except aqua-fortis, of which she was seen to partake by several druggists of veracity.*   The fire-eating mountebanks too are said to acquire the same power of endurance ; but much of their apparent capability is really legerdemain.   On the other hand, a very extraordinary sensibility to the action of the diluted mineral acids has been supposed to exist in the case of infants at the breast, — so great a sensibility, that serious symptoms and even death itself have been ascribed to the nurse's milk becoming impregnated with sulphuric acid, in consequence of her having taken it in medicinal doses.   By two writers in the London Medical Repository griping pains, tremors and spasms have been imputed to this cause ;† and a writer in the Medical Gazette says he has seen continued griping, green diarrhœa and fatal marasmus ensue, — apparently, he thinks, from ulceration of the gastro-intestinal mucous membrane.‡   Without questioning the great delicacy and tenderness of that membrane in infants, I must nevertheless express my doubts whether so small a quantity taken by a nurse, amounting in the cases in question only to four or six drops a day, could really produce fatal or even severe effects on her child.

Sulphuric acid is not less deadly when admitted into the body through other channels besides the mouth.   Thus, it may prove fatal when introduced into the rectum.   A woman at Bruges in Belgium had an injection administered, in which, being prepared hastily in the middle of the night, sulphuric acid had been substituted by mistake for linseed-oil.   The patient immediately uttered piercing cries, and passed the remainder of the night in excessive torture.   In the morning the bed-clothes were found corroded, and a portion of intestine had apparently come away ; and she expired not long afterwards.§

Death may also be occasioned by the introduction of this acid into the ear.   Dr. Morrison relates a case of the kind, where nitric acid, which is analogous in action, was poured by a man into his wife's ear, while she lay insensible from intoxication.   She awoke in great pain, which continued for two or three days.   In six days an eschar detached itself from the external passage of the ear ; and this was followed by profuse hemorrhage, which recurred daily more or less for a month.   On the day after the eschar came away, and without any precursory symptom referrible to the head, she was attacked with complete palsy of the right arm, and in eight days more with tremors and incomplete palsy of the rest of that side of the body. These symptoms subsequently abated ; but they again increased after an imprudent exertion, and she died in a state of exhaustion seven weeks after the injury.   The whole petrous portion of the temporal

* Tartra, p 124.   † Dr. Bartley, iv. 289, and Mr. Diamond, v. 110.
‡ Mr. Bevan, i. 756.   § Journal de Chimie Médicale, 1835, 426.

bone was found carious, but without any distinct disease of the brain or its membranes.*

Sulphuric acid and the other mineral acids are equally poisonous when inhaled in the form of gas or vapour; and they then act chiefly by irritating or inflaming the mucous membrane of the air-passages and lungs. For some observations on their effects in this form both on plants and animals the reader may refer to the Chapter on Poisonous Gases.

Sulphuric acid belongs to the poisons alluded to under the head of General Poisoning, — of whose operation satisfactory evidence may be occasionally drawn from symptoms only. If immediately after swallowing a liquid which causes a sense of burning in the throat, gullet, and stomach, violent vomiting ensues, particularly if the vomited matter is mixed with blood; if the mouth becomes white, and stripped of its lining membrane, and the cheeks, neck, or neighbouring parts show vesications, or white, and subsequently brown excoriated spots; — if the clothes show red spots and are moist and disintegrated there, — I cannot see any objection to the inference, that either sulphuric or muriatic acid has been taken. In this opinion I am supported by a good authority, Dr. Mertzdorff, late medical inspector at Berlin.†

SECTION III. — *Of the Morbid Appearances caused by Sulphuric Acid.*

The outward appearance of the body in cases of Tartra's first variety in the action of the acids is remarkably healthy; every limb is round, firm, and fresh-looking.

On the lips, fingers, or other parts of the skin, spots and streaks are found where sulphuric acid has disorganized the cuticle. These marks are brownish or yellowish-brown, and present after death the appearance of old parchment or of a burn; sometimes there are little blisters.‡

The lining membrane of the mouth is more or less disorganized, generally hardened, and whitish or slightly yellowish. The pharynx is either in the same state, or very red or even swelled. The rima glottidis, as in the case described by Dr. Sinclair and in that of Mr. Arnott, is sometimes contracted, the epiglottis swelled, or on the contrary shrivelled, and the commencement of the larynx inflamed.§ The gullet is often lined with a dense membrane, adhering firmly, resembling the inner coat, but probably in general a morbid formation; and the subjacent tissue is brown or red. Sometimes, however, the inner coat or epithelion of the gullet loses its vitality, and is detached in part or altogether. In Mr. Arnott's case the pharynx and upper gullet were lined by a pale lemon-coloured membrane, which in the lower two-thirds of the canal was completely detached and was plainly the œsophageal membrane; in the case related by

* Dublin Journal of Med. and Chem. Science, No. 25.
† Horn's Archiv für Medizinische Erfahrung, 1823, i. 465.
‡ Ibid. 452.
§ Edin. Med. and Surg. Journal, xxxvi. 101. Lond. Med. Gazette, xii. 221.

Mertzdorff, the whole inner coat of the gullet, as well as that of the throat, epiglottis, and mouth, was stripped from the muscular coat ;* and in Dr. Wilson's case (p. 131), which proved fatal in ten months, the upper third of the gullet shone like an old cicatrix, and the lower two-thirds were narrowed, vascular, and softened on the surface.† In a few rare cases of chronic poisoning with the mineral acids the gullet is found perforated by an ulcerative process ;‡ but it is never perforated by their corrosive action in quickly fatal cases. Occasionally the gullet is not affected at all, though both the mouth and the stomach are severely injured ; and an instance has even been published where the acid, in this instance the nitric, left no trace of its passage downwards till near the pylorus.§

The outer surface of the abdominal viscera is commonly either very vascular or livid, or bears even more unequivocal signs of inflammation, namely, effusion of fibrin and adhesions among the different turns of intestine ; and these appearances may take place although the stomach is not perforated.|| The cause of this appearance, which is seldom observed in poisoning with other irritants, more especially with the metallic irritants, is that the acid passes through the membranes of the stomach by transudation during life, — as will be proved immediately. It must be observed, that the peritonæum is sometimes quite natural after death from sulphuric acid, even although the stomach was perforated. I have seen this in a case which proved fatal in twelve hours. An important appearance in the abdomen, to which less attention has been hitherto paid than it deserves, is gorging of the vessels beneath the peritonæal membrane of the stomach and adjoining organs with dark, firmly coagulated blood, arising from the acid having transuded through the membranes and acted on the blood chemically. My attention was first turned to this appearance by an interesting case, which I saw in 1840 in the Royal Infirmary of this city, and of which an able account has been published by Dr. Craigie.¶ The whole vessels of the stomach were seen externally to be most minutely injected and gorged, and the blood in them was coagulated into firmly-cohering cylindrical masses, as if the vessels had been successfully filled with the matter of an anatomical injection. This appearance was also observed in the superior mesenteric arteries, in the omental vessels, and over the greater part of the mesentery. It was occasioned by the chemical action of the acid coagulating the colouring matter and albumen ; for the clotted blood was strongly acid to litmus-paper. So too was the peritoneal surface of the stomach, omentum and intestines. And the acid had transuded through the stomach and into the omentum and tissues of the intestines during life ; for in the first place, there was no perforation of the stomach, and secondly, I ascertained that

* Horn's Archiv, &c. 453.
† London Medical Gazette, xiv. 489, and 1837-8, ii. 76.
‡ Louis, ibidem, xiv. 30.
§ Philadelphia Journal of Med. and Phys. Sciences, iv. 410.
|| London Medical Gazette, viii. 76.
¶ Edinburgh Med. and Surg. Journal, liii. 406.

there was no free acid either in the matter discharged from the stomach before death after the free administration of antacids, or in the contents of the stomach obtained at the examination of the dead body.

The stomach, if not perforated, is commonly distended with gases. It contains a quantity of yellowish-brown or black matter, and is sometimes lined with a thick paste composed of disorganized tissue, blood and mucus. The pylorus is contracted.

The mucous membrane is not always corroded. If the acid was taken diluted, the coats may escape corrosion ; but there is excessive injection, gorging, and blackness of the vessels, general blackness of the membrane, sometimes even without softening, as in a case related by Pyl of a woman who first took aqua-fortis and then stabbed herself.* More commonly, however, along with the blackness there is softening of the rugæ or actual removal of the villous coat, and occasionally regular granulated ulceration with puriform matter on it.† The stomach is not always perforated. But if it is, the holes are commonly roundish, and the coats thin at the margin, coloured, disintegrated, and surrounded by vascularity and black extravasation. In some rare cases there is no mark of vital re-action except in the neighbourhood of the aperture. A case of this kind is related by Mertzdorff: The margin of the hole was surrounded to the distance of half an inch with apparent charring of the coats, and this areola was surrounded by redness ; but the rest of the stomach was grayish-white.‡ I examined with the late Dr. Latta of Leith a similar case, where the limitation of the injury was evidently owing to the stomach having been at the time filled with porridge. The patient, a child two years old, died in twelve hours ; and on the posterior surface of the fundus of the stomach, towards the pylorus, there was a hole as big as a half-crown, which was surrounded to the distance of an inch with a black mass formed of the disorganized coats, and of incorporated charred blood. But the rest of the stomach was quite healthy. The most remarkable instance of chemical destruction of the coats yet known to me is a case mentioned by Mr. Watson of this city, where suicide was effected by cutting the throat about half an hour after two ounces of sulphuric acid had been swallowed. The individual was at first thought to have died simply of the wound of the throat. But on dissection the usual signs of acid poisoning were found ; and among other effects, it was observed that nearly three-fourths of the stomach had been entirely destroyed.§ The perforation, if the patient lives long enough, is generally accompanied with a copious effusion into the belly of the usual muddy liquor of peritonitis ; and the outer surface of the viscera feels unctuous, as if from a slight chemical action of the acid on them. The acid has

* Aufsätze und Beobachtungen, ii. 122.
† Archives Générales de Médecine, xiii. 368.
‡ Horn's Archiv, &c. 1823, i. 456.
§ Edin. Med. and Surg. Journal, liii. 401.

15

actually been found in the contents poured out from the stomach into
the sac of the peritonæum.*

One would expect to find the acid always in the stomach when it
is perforated. Nevertheless it is sometimes almost all discharged.
In Mertzdorff's case, that of an infant who was killed in twelve
hours, a hole was found in the stomach ¾ths of an inch in diameter,
and the contents of the stomach were effused into the belly : yet by
a careful analysis the whole acid he could procure from the contents
and tissues together was only 4½ grains. Sometimes of course the
disappearance of the acid may be owing, as in Dr. Craigie's case, to
the effectual administration of antacids during life.

The inner coat of the duodenum often presents appearances closely
resembling those of the stomach. Sometimes, however, as in the
case just related from Mertzdorff, and in the infant I examined, the
inner coat of the small intestines is not affected at all, probably because in such rapid cases the pylorus retains a state of spasmodic
contraction till death or even after it.

The urinary bladder is commonly empty. The thoracic surface of
the diaphragm is sometimes lined with lymph, indicating inflammation of the chest. In the case which was fatal in two hours [p.
131], Professor Remer found the surface of the lungs, as well as that
of the liver and spleen, brown and of a leathern consistence, and the
tissue beneath scarlet ; — appearances which he thinks arose from
the acid penetrating in vapour and acting chemically. I have not
found this appearance mentioned by any other writer ; but I have
seen it in animals poisoned with oxalic acid. The blood in the
heart and great vessels has been several times seen forming a firm
black clot. Kerkring† relates an instance of the kind ; in Dr. Latta's
case the appearance was very distinct; and it is dwelt on strongly in
a recent paper by M. Bouchardat.‡ Bouchardat thinks this state of
the blood is simply the effect of the absorbed acid ; but coagulation of
the blood in the heart and great vessels, — a striking appearance in
contradiction to what is observed after death from most other poisons,
— is more probably the healthy state of the blood, and not the effect
of the particular poison.

The general appearance of the body of those who have died of the
second or chronic variety of poisoning with the acids, is that of
extreme emaciation. The stomach and intestines are excessively
contracted : The former has been found so small as to measure only
two inches and a half from the cardia to the pylorus, and two inches
from the lesser to the greater curvature.§ Tartra says the intestines
are sometimes no thicker than a writing quill. They are in other
respects sound outwardly, except that they sometimes adhere together.

Internally the pylorus is contracted. In a case of slow poisoning,
fatal in three months, which has been described by Dr. Braun of

* Edin. Med and Surg. Journ. xxii. 222, and xxxvi. 103.
† Kerkringii opera omnia, p. 146.
‡ Annales d'Hygiène Publique, &c. xvii. 362.
§ Robert in Nouvelle Bibliothéqeu Médicale, 1827, iv. 415.

Fürth, the chief appearance besides excessive emaciation was a thickening of the coats round and behind the pylorus to such a degree that the opening of the pylorus was formed of an almost cartilaginous ring several lines broad, and only wide enough to pass a quill.* There are spots over the stomach apparently of regenerated villous tissue, smoother and redder than the natural membrane. At the points where the stomach adheres to the neighbouring organs, its coats are sometimes wanting altogether, so that when its connections are torn away, perforations are produced. The other parts of the body are natural.

It may in some circumstances be necessary to determine from the appearances in the dead body whether sulphuric acid has been the occasion of death or has been introduced into the body after death. This may always be easily done. If a few drachms of sulphuric acid be injected into the anus immediately after death, and the parts be examined in twenty-four hours, it will be found, that wherever the acid touches the gut, its mucous coat is yellowish and brittle, its muscular and peritonæal coats white, as if blanched, and the blood in the vessels charred ; the injury is confined strictly to the parts actually touched, is surrounded by an abrupt line of demarcation, and shows no sign of inflammatory redness. Nitric acid produces nearly the same effects. The whole tunics are yellow, and the disorganization is greater. For these facts we are indebted to Orfila.†

In closing this account of the morbid appearances, some observations will be required on the force of evidence derived from them ; because circumstances may exclude all other branches of medical proof. In many instances both of acute and of chronic poisoning with the strong acids, I conceive, contrary to the general statements of most systematic writers on modern medical jurisprudence, that distinct evidence might be derived from morbid appearances only. Thus, what fallacy can intervene to render the following opinion doubtful? In a case several times alluded to as described by Mertzdorff, there were vesicles and brown streaks on the lips, neck, and shoulders, similar to the effects of burning, — almost total separation of the lining membrane of the mouth, throat, epiglottis, and gullet, — perforation of the stomach, with a margin half an inch wide, which was extensively charred, and surrounded by a red areola. From the appearances alone Mertzdorff declared that the child must have been poisoned with sulphuric acid. Perhaps he should have said sulphuric or muriatic acid.

Or take the case of Richard Overfield, who was condemned at Shrewsbury Assizes in 1824 for murdering his own child, a babe three months old, by pouring sulphuric acid down its throat. In the dead body the following appearances were found : The lips were blistered internally and of a dark colour externally ; the gullet was contracted and its inner coat corroded ; the lining membrane of the mouth and tongue of a dull white colour ; the great curvature of the stomach corroded and converted into a substance like wet brown paper ; the

* Henke's Zeitschrift für die Staatsarzneikunde, xxxii. 161.
† Toxicologie Générale, ii. 689.

stomach perforated and a bloody-coloured fluid in the sac of the peritonæum.* If to these appearances be added the fact that the child's dress was reddened, what is there to prevent the medical jurist from declaring, without reference to chemical evidence, that this case must have been one of poisoning by sulphuric acid or some other mineral acids?

In like manner in the case of Mrs. Humphrey, who was condemned at Aberdeen in 1830 for murdering her husband by pouring sulphuric acid down his throat while he was asleep, there was found, on examining the dead body, two brown spots on the outside of the lips,— whiteness of the inside of the lips and of the gums, — glazing of the palate,— redness, with here and there ash-coloured discoloration, of the uvula, posterior part of the throat, pharynx and epiglottis,—abrasion of most of the inner coat of the gullet,— erosion and dark-red ulceration of the inner coat of the stomach in winding furrows.   When to these appearances it is added, that the man was in good health only forty-seven hours before death, and was taken ill instantaneously and violently with burning pain in the throat and stomach,† it is not easy to see what other opinion could be formed of the case, unless that he died of poisoning with a mineral acid, and probably with sulphuric acid.

Among the appearances justifying an opinion where chemical evidence happens to be wanting, not the least important seems to me to be the peculiar turgescence and induration of vessels under the peritonæum of the stomach and neighbouring organs, occasioned by the chemical coagulation of blood in them.   It is an appearance, which, when once seen, cannot be confounded with any natural morbid phenomenon I have ever witnessed.

I am far from desiring to encourage rashness of decision, or to revive the loose criterions of poisoning relied on in former times. But there cannot, in my opinion, be a rational doubt that in the instance of sulphuric acid there may often be distinct exceptions to the general law regarding the feebleness of the evidence from morbid appearances ; and that a witness would certainly be guilty of thwarting the administration of justice, if, relying on general rules, he refused to admit such exceptions.   What natural disease could produce appearances like those described above ?   Assuredly no form of spontaneous perforation bears any resemblance to that caused in most cases of death from sulphuric acid ; nor is it easy to mention any combination of natural diseases which could produce the peculiar conjunction of appearances remarked in the case of the man Humphrey.

Section IV. — *Of the Treatment of Poisoning with Sulphuric Acid.*

Since this acid and the other mineral acids act entirely as local irritants, it may be inferred that their poisonous action will be prevented by neutralizing them.   But in applying that principle to the

---

* Edinburgh Med. and Surg. Journal, xxii. 222.   † Ibidem, xxxv. 302.

treatment it is necessary to bear in mind their extremely rapid operation ; for if much time is lost in seeking for an antidote, irreparable mischief may be caused before the remedy is taken. Should it be possible then to administer chalk or magnesia without delay, these are the antidotes which ought to be preferred ; but it may be well for the physician to remember, that in the absence of both he may at once procure a substitute in the plaster of the apartment beat down and made into thin paste with water. M. Chevallier, in a paper on the antidotes for the mineral acids, quotes five cases of poisoning with sulphuric acid and two with nitric acid, where life seems to have been saved by the speedy and free administration of magnesia, although in some cases so large a quantity as two ounces of the poison had been swallowed.[*] — A solution of soap is another antidote of no small value. While the antidote is in preparation, the acid should be diluted by the free use of any mild fluid, such as milk or oleaginous matters. — The alkaline bicarbonates are also excellent antidotes ; but their carbonates are ineligible, being themselves possessed of corrosive properties. In a paper on poisoning with the mineral acids by Dr. Lunding of Copenhagen, the author is disposed to ascribe the large proportion of deaths in his practice to the system pursued in the Copenhagen hospital of administering carbonate of potass as an antidote daily for weeks together.[†] On the other hand however it may be mentioned, that in a late memoir, on this description of poisoning Dr. Ebers of Breslau endeavours to show, that there is no reason to dread the administration of the alkaline carbonates, even the carbonate of potash, provided they be given with mucilaginous fluids and syrup in a rather concentrated form ; and he gives three cases illustrative of the good effects of this mode of treatment, which he maintains to be free of all danger, and preferable to every other antidotal method, because the remedy may be administered in small volume, — an advantage possessed by it especially over chalk or magnesia.[‡]

After the proper antidote has been given to a sufficient extent, the use of diluents ought to be continued, as they render the vomiting more easy. — Some have recommended the stomach-pump for administering antidotes and diluents ; but this is unnecessary. When it is wished to evacuate the stomach, there is an advantage in allowing it to do so by its own efforts, if possible ; because the evacuation is accomplished in this way more completely than by the stomach-pump. Besides, if the patient cannot swallow fluids, still less can he suffer the tube of the stomach-pump to be introduced. On several occasions, indeed, it has been found impracticable to introduce it.[§]

The treatment of the surpervening inflammation does not differ from that of inflammation of the stomach. Where there is great diffi-

[*] Journal de Chimie Médicale, 1840, 30.
[†] Medizinisch-Chirurgische Zeitung, 1824, iv. 276.
[‡] Rust's Magazin für die gesammte Heilkunde, 1837, 1. 501.
[§] Dr. Sinclair. Edin. Med. and Surg. Journal, xxxvi. 99 ; and case of Humphrey. Ibidem, xxxv. 301.

culty of breathing, evidently from obstruction of the larynx, and where
the absence of abdominal pain, tension or vomiting affords a presumption that little injury has been done to the stomach, laryngotomy appears an advisable remedy, and has been known to give very great
relief.*   But the patient may nevertheless die soon of the sympathetic disorder of the circulation.

II. — Of Poisoning with Nitric Acid.

Nitric acid is more frequently used as a poison abroad than in this
country.   But even in Britain it is not an uncommon cause of severe
accidents and death.

Of the Tests for Nitric Acid.

1. *When concentrated,* nitric acid is easily known by the odour of
its vapour, which is peculiar.   When pure, the acid as well as its
vapour is colourless ; when mixed with nitrous acid it is of various
tints, and generally yellow.   The acid of commerce is at times rendered impure by sulphuric acid, a circumstance which must be attended to in applying the subsequent tests. — The simplest test for nitric
or nitrous acid is the action of copper, lead, or tin.   If any of these
metals in small fragments, or powder, be thrown into either
acid previously diluted with an equal volume of water, an effervescence takes place, which in the case of lead or copper is much accelerated by heat ; nitric oxide gas is disengaged ; and ruddy fumes
of nitrous acid gas are formed when the gas comes in contact with
the oxygen of the air.   Another characteristic test, which has the advantage of being applicable on an extremely small scale, is morphia,
the alkaloid of opium.   This substance is turned in a few seconds to
a beautiful orange-red colour by nitric acid, and after longer contact
forms with it a bright yellow solution.   No other acid has this effect.
Muriatic acid, as Dr. O'Shaughnessey has remarked,[†] does not act
at all on morphia, and sulphuric acid chars and blackens it.   When
nitric acid is added to a solution of narcotin in sulphuric acid, the
colour of the solution is changed from yellow to blood-red.[‡]   When
it is added to a solution of proto-sulphate of iron, the solution becomes brown, and the addition of sulphuric acid then alters the colour
to violet.[§]   When it is added even in the most minute proportion
to sulphuric acid, the addition of a few particles of the alkaloid brucia will render the whole fluid red, passing gradually to yellow.[§] —
Many other characteristic tests might be mentioned ; but those now
specified are more than enough.

2. *In a diluted state* this acid is not so easily recognised as the other
mineral acids, for it does not form any insoluble salt or precipitate
with bases.

* London Medical Gazette, xii. 219.   Mr. Arnott's Case.
† Lancet, 1829-30, ii. 330 and 432.
‡ Orfila. Journal de Chimie Médicale 1842, p. 5.
§ Peligot. Journal de Pharmacie, 1833, p. 644.
‖ Barthemot. Journal de Pharmacie, 1841, 560.

The most convenient process consists in first ascertaining the acidity of the fluid, then neutralizing it with potass, evaporating to dryness, and heating the residue in a tube with sulphuric acid. The vapour disengaged, if abundant, may be known by its orange colour in the tube and its odour. But if small in quantity it is best to distil over the vapour in a proper apparatus, and to subject the condensed product to the tests of morphia, narcotin dissolved in sulphuric acid, and protosulphate of iron dissolved in water. A convenient tube for the purpose is that represented in Fig. 3; into which the materials are introduced by the funnel, Fig. 4. The wide part of the tube may then be drawn out in the spirit-lamp flame to any length or fineness that may be necessary, so as to conduct the vapour into another tube as a condenser, or directly into the substances to be used as tests.

3. *When in a state of compound mixture*, nitric acid, like sulphuric acid in similar circumstances, may be after a time partly decomposed and partly neutralized ; and when the matter with which it is mixed belongs to either of the organic kingdoms, more particularly to the animal world, its decomposition is more rapid than that of sulphuric acid. Still it is an important fact, that some of the acid may be discovered after a considerable interval. M. Ollivier detected it in various stains on the skin at least a day after it had been applied ;* Dr. O'Shaughnessey detected it in a stain on cloth sent to him from Ireland to Edinburgh ;† and I have found it in stains made on broad-cloth with detached drops seven weeks before.

Process for Stains. Nitric acid produces on the skin a yellow stain, which gradually becomes dirty orange, and finally of a dirty yellowish-brown ; but in all of these states it is at once rendered for a time lively yellow by the action of ammonia. I am not aware that any other yellow stain is similarly affected. Stains on cloth are generally yellow, reddish-yellow, or brownish-yellow, and are attended with more or less disintegration of the texture of the cloth. The method of analyzing all these stains is as follows : — The stained parts is to be boiled in a few drachms of pure water several times in succession ; and the liquid is then filtered, and may be subjected to litmus-paper for the purpose of ascertaining its acidity. It is then to be rendered neutral, or for the sake of greater facility, feebly alkaline, by adding a few drops of a diluted solution of caustic potass, after which the whole is evaporated to dryness, and in a vapour-bath, if practicable. The residuum is then to be decomposed by sulphuric acid in the same way as recommended above for the simple diluted acid. — Orfila thinks it advantageous to let the stains macerate for some hours in a solution of bicarbonate of soda rather than to boil them in water. In that case, however, it is necessary to ascertain the acidity of the stains with litmus-paper before proceeding to macerate them.

Process for Mixtures. The detection of nitric acid in compound mixtures, such as the contents of the stomach, is not so easy a matter

* Archives Générales de Médecine, xxi. 365. † Lancet, 1829-30, ii. 840.

as its detection in stains ; and indeed a sure and delicate process is still a desideratum in medico-legal chemistry.   The process varies, as in the case of sulphuric acid, according as the subject of analysis is acid or neutral.

a. *If the mixture be acid*, and the proportion of the acid considerable, it may be detected without difficulty.   It is merely necessary to ascertain the acidity of the mixture by litmus-paper, to neutralize with potass, water being added if necessary, and then to filter and evaporate to a convenient degree of concentration.   Crystals will form on cooling, which may be decomposed by sulphuric acid in the usual way.   But the medical jurist ought not to flatter himself with the expectation of meeting often with a proportion large enough to admit of being discovered by so coarse a method of analysis.   In general the crystallization of the nitrate of potass is prevented by co-existing animal or vegetable matter.   When the proportion appears inconsiderable, therefore, a different process must be pursued. In preparing the former edition of this work, the present topic was investigated with some care, and a method suggested which appeared to me at that time more effectual, delicate, and conclusive than any previously made public.   Since then Professor Orfila has also investigated the subject attentively, and after trying various methods, has ended in adopting one which is substantially the same as that now referred to, but without a precaution, which seems to me essential for success in certain probable enough circumstances.*   I am therefore disposed to retain my former process, with some variations and additions in the details.

Macerate the subject of analysis for a few hours in distilled water, if it be not already liquid enough ; and then boil for a few minutes, and filter it.   Ascertain now whether the fluid be acid to litmus ; and if it be so, neutralize it with solution of potash, or as Orfila suggests, with a solution of the purer salt, the bicarbonate of soda. Evaporate gently, to obtain crystals if possible ; and if these do not tend to the cubical form, distil them with sulphuric acid, and proceed as directed for nitric acid simply diluted.   If crystals do not appear, or their form tend to the cube, — in which case chloride of sodium is present, — re-dissolve the whole residue of evaporation in distilled water ; add a slight excess of a warm solution of acetate of silver, to throw down organic matter and the chlorine of any chlorides that may be present; filter and evaporate to dryness, and distil the residuum with sulphuric acid, applying as usual to the vapour the tests of litmus-paper and morphia, — also, as Orfila proposes, the solution of narcotin in sulphuric acid, and proto-sulphate of iron in water, — and if the quantity of vapour be great enough, the sense of smell and the action of copper with the condensed vapour.

b. *If the mixture be neutral*, proceed exactly as above, except that it becomes unnecessary to neutralize the liquid with potash or bicarbonate of soda.   This variety in the process will be principally required, where earths or alkalis have been administered as antidotes.

* Annales d'Hygiène Publique, &c. xxviii. 200.   Also Toxicologie Générale. 1843, i. 142.

The process now detailed requires a word or two of commentary. — Organic matter is inconvenient because it prevents the nitrate of potash or soda in the mixture from crystallizing. But it will not prevent the evolution of nitric acid vapour by distillation with sulphuric acid, even although the material be a simple extract without crystals. At the same time it is better to get rid of as much organic matter as possible, if distinct crystals be not obtained by evaporation. A more serious difficulty, however, to which Orfila does not advert, arises from the co-existence of a chloride. For, in that case, distillation with sulphuric acid may disengage not nitric acid, but chlorine, in consequence of the reaction which takes place between the nitric and hydrochloric acids in the act of being liberated. This is a more important reason for purifying the liquid by acetate of silver before subjecting it to concentration ; but in addition, by removing organic matter, this precaution increases the chance of crystals of nitrate of potash or soda being obtained. Its necessity, where a chloride co-exists, will appear from the following experiment. Four drops of nitric acid neutralized with potass were mixed with six ounces of strong barley-broth ; from which half an ounce of limpid fluid was procured by filtration. One-half of this evaporated to dryness gave a crystalline residue, which, heated with sulphuric acid in a tube, emitted a strong odour of chlorine; and the moisture which bedewed the tube scarcely affected morphia. The residuum of the other half of the filtered fluid was re-dissolved, treated with acetate of silver, again filtered, and evaporated to dryness; and the residue was gently heated in a tube with sulphuric acid. An odour of nitric acid was now disengaged, and the moisture on the tube close to the mixture turned a fragment of morphia to bright orange-red.

Acetate of silver is prepared by mixing strong solutions of acetate of potass and nitrate of silver, draining and compressing between folds of bibulous paper the crystalline precipitate which forms, dissolving this precipitate by agitating it in boiling water, and finally crystallizing the salt again by refrigeration. The crystals, which are sparingly soluble in cold water, should be then separated, slightly washed with a little water, and again dried by compression. When put to use, a solution should be made by agitating the salt in boiling water, because at low temperatures water retains very little of the salt; but actual ebullition should be avoided, because acetate of silver is thus quickly decomposed.

In all medico-legal analyses for nitric acid, care must be taken that the different reagents used are free of this acid, and also of nitrates. Sulphuric acid often contains a little nitric, or rather nitrous acid; which may be discovered by the sulphuric acid becoming brown or dark-red when a solution of proto-sulphate of iron is gently poured over it in a test-tube ; and which may be removed either by boiling the acid with a few grains of sugar, according to the formula of the Edinburgh Pharmacopœia, or, as Orfila directs, by boiling it with sulphate of ammonia.

SECTIONS II. III. IV.— *Of the Action, Symptoms, Morbid Appearances, and Treatment of Poisoning with Nitric Acid.*

All the observations made on these topics under the head of sulphuric acid apply, with few exceptions, to the nitric acid also. A few statements therefore on the peculiarities ascertained to exist in the latter case are all that will be required in the present sections.

Nitric acid is not less powerful as a corrosive and irritant than sulphuric acid. It will act with energy as an irritant even when considerably diluted, for example with six or eight parts of water or even more. — The lips which are rendered at first whitish by all the acids, and eventually brownish by sulphuric acid, becomes soon yellow with nitric acid. The tongue too sometimes acquires a yellow colour instead of a white glazed appearance ; but this character is not invariable. — All spots caused by it on the skin become speedily yellow, and long retain this hue ; or if the tint become dull, which generally happens in a few days, it is enlivened and the yellow colour restored for a time, by ammonia, potash, soda, or soap. — An important fact, for which toxicology is indebted to Professor Orfila, is that the acid may be often found in the urine, both when it had been swallowed, and when it had been introduced through the medium of the cellular tissue.* It is to be discovered by the process for compound mixtures. Orfila adds that he has hitherto been unable to find it in the liver or spleen.

A difference of tint in the lining membrane of the mouth and gullet is the only difference observed in the morbid appearances caused by nitric and sulphuric acid. The former sometimes renders these parts yellow; but this appearance is far from being invariable.

The treatment in both instances is the same in every respect.

III. — OF POISONING WITH HYDROCHLORIC ACID.

This acid occurs more rarely than any of the other mineral acids in medico-legal cases ; a fact which appears singular enough on considering, that it is a powerful corrosive, and more perhaps in the hands of the working-classes than any other.

SECTION I.— *Of the Tests for Hydrochloric Acid.*

Like the other acids, hydrochloric acid occurs in the concentrated shape, in a state of simple dilution, and mixed with various matters, especially from organic kingdoms.

1. Hydrochloric acid, *in its concentrated state,* is colourless, if pure, but yellowish as usually sold ; and it is easily known by the peculiar appearance and odour of its fumes. A convenient additional test, which, however, is not absolutely distinctive, is the formation of white vapour when a rod dipped in it is brought near another dipped in ammonia. If any farther evidence be desired, the strong acid must be diluted with water, and examined by the tests for it in a diluted state.

* Journal de Chim. Médicale, 1842, 266.

2. *When diluted*, it is recognised with facility, first by litmus-paper, and then by the nitrate of silver, which forms with it a dense, white precipitate, the chloride of silver. This is soluble in ammonia, re-appears on neutralizing the ammonia by nitric acid, and is not re-dissolved by a large excess of nitric acid, even aided by heat. Its permanence under an excess of nitric acid distinguishes it from every other silver salt, but the cyanide ; which again is known by disap-pearing when boiled with a large excess of the acid.

3. In the last edition of this work I proposed for the detection of hydrochloric acid in *compound organic mixtures* a process, to which Professor Orfila has since made an important addition,* and which the investigations of that toxicologist, as well as my own, lead me to suppose superior to any other yet suggested, although it is not en-tirely free from objection. This process divides itself into two, ac-cording as the subject of analysis is acid or neutral ; but in the latter case its indications are of dubious import.

a. If the matter to be examined be acid, boil it with water if ne-cessary, filter, and distil it with a gentle heat till the residue acquire the consistence of a very thin syrup. Subject the distilled liquor to the tests for diluted hydrochloric acid. It will seldom be found there, however, because it is apt to be retained by the co-existence of or-ganic matter. If it be not found, add to the thin extract in the retort a slight excess of a strong solution of tannin, filter, and distil the fil-tered liquid by means of a hot bath of solution of hydrochlorate of lime (consisting of two parts of crystallized salt and one of water,) — taking care that the temperature of the bath never exceeds 240° ; and stop the distillation just before the residuum becomes dry. Ex-amine now the distilled liquor with the tests for diluted hydrochlo-ric acid.

Hydrochloric acid has a tendency to adhere with obstinacy to or-ganic matters, especially when these are abundant; and therefore Orfila properly proposes to remove organic principles as far as pos-sible by precipitating them with solution of tannin. I have found, as he did, that the acid may be obtained by distillation after this measure, when it could not be obtained previously. — Orfila objects to the process however that hydrochlorate of ammonia will pass over in the distillation. But I have not found this to be the fact, when the temperature did not rise above 240° ; which in his experiments seem to have been considerably exceeded. — A more important fal-lacy is, that hydrochloric acid will be indicated by the process in a mixture which contains both a neutral chloride, such as common salt, and sulphuric acid. This fallacy can only be obviated by as-certaining that sulphuric acid is not present. — But the most import-ant fallacy of all is, that free hydrochloric acid constitutes an essen-tial part of the gastric juice, and an ingredient of the secretions of the stomach in various states of disordered digestion.† It is not

* Annales d'Hygiène Publique, 1842, xxviii. 317.

† Prout, Philosophical Transactions, 1824, p. 45.— Tiedemann and Gmelin, Die Ver-dauung nach Versuchen, *passim*. — *Children*, Annals of Philosophy, 1824, viii. 68.

easy to see how this fallacy can be obviated, unless the acid be obtained in large quantity ; nor am I prepared to say what quantity
would justify the conclusion, that the acid had been derived from an
external source.   Dr. Prout once found between four and five grains
of pure acid in sixteen ounces of the fluid of water-brash.*   The
quantity of hydrochloric acid is to be known by drying, heating and
weighing the chloride of silver thrown down in the distilled fluid by
nitrate of silver, and allowing 100 parts of concentrated commercial
acid for 145 of chloride.

b. When the mixture is neutral, hydrochloric acid can be no longer
detected in it without the aid of sulphuric acid to decompose the
chloride that has been formed.   This should be added to the filtered
fluid obtained after organic matter has been separated by solution of
tannin.   Hydrochloric acid will then distil over. — It is seldom
however that the discovery of the acid in this way will warrant the
conclusion, that it had ever existed free in the mixture whence it is
obtained.   For it may have proceeded from chlorides contained in
the subject of analysis from the first, more especially chloride of sodium, which exists in small quantity in all animal fluids and solids,
and more largely in many articles of food and drink.   The only circumstance indeed in which the detection of hydrochloric acid by decomposition with sulphuric acid will yield any evidence, — and even
then the evidence will only be presumptive, — is when it is known
that an earth or alkali was given as an antidote, and when the alkali
or earth which was used is found in the suspected substance.

SECTION II. — *Of the Action and Symptoms produced by Hydrochloric
Acid.*

Hydrochloric acid has been found by Professor Orfila to exert the
same action as sulphuric and nitric acids ; but it is a less powerful
corrosive and irritant. — In the gaseous state, it is a most destructive
poison to vegetables, as will be shown in the article on the Poisonous
Gases.

The symptoms it occasions in man are very like those produced
by sulphuric acid.   As few cases however of poisoning with this
substance have yet been published, its effects are not so well known
as those of the other powerful acids ; and it may therefore be right to
mention the leading particulars of some of the cases which are met
with in authors. — Mr. Quekett has related the case of a man, who,
on arriving at home one day, told the woman he lodged with that he
had poisoned himself with spirit of salt, but presented at the moment
so little sign of uneasiness, that she at first scarcely believed him.   In
a short time however he suddenly became faint and fell down.   On
being removed to the London Hospital, magnesia and milk were
given, about three hours after the acid had been taken ; but no relief
was experienced.   He suffered intense thirst, complained of excessive pain in the stomach and throat, and expired in about fifteen

* Philosophical Transactions, 1824, p. 49.

hours.* — Mr. J. F. Crawfurd of Newcastle has related a still more
rapid case which was occasioned by two ounces of an equal mixture
of hydrochloric acid and "tincture of steel," probably the tincture of
chloride of iron. Vomiting occurred soon afterwards, but subsequently ceased; there was no complaint made either of pain or heat
anywhere, or of thirst; and questions were answered intelligently.
But the pulse was imperceptible, and the muscles of the extremities
contracted; and death took place in five hours and a half.† — Orfila
mentions that an hospital patient, affected with inflammation of the
brain after a fall on the head, having got by mistake from his nurse
45 grammes, or two fluidounces, of hydrochloric acid, was attacked
with acute pain in the stomach, efforts to vomit, hiccup, extreme
restlessness, a small pulse, a fiery red tongue, blackness of the lips,
and a burning skin; and next day he died in a state of constant delirium, and covered with a cold clammy sweat.‡

These cases present nearly the same violence and variety of action
with that which results from the two other acids.

Section III. — *Of the Morbid Appearances caused by Hydrochloric
Acid.*

The morbid appearances are on the whole similar to what are
caused by sulphuric acid. In Mr. Quekett's case the stomach outwardly was leaden-coloured and its vessels gorged with black blood;
the intestinal peritonæum injected and speckled with fibrinous effusion; the villous coat of the stomach lined with yellow, curdled milk,
and itself irregularly black here and there, as if charred, and in some
places softened and corroded, so that a rent was made in handling
it; the inner membrane of the duodenum similarly affected, and also
even the jejunum, though more irregularly. The contents of the
stomach were not acid, and did not contain any chloride. — In Mr.
Crawfurd's case the villous coat presented black elevated ridges, as
if charred, and the furrows between were scarlet-red; black granular
extravasation had taken place at many points into the submucous
tissue; similar appearances were seen in the duodenum and jejunum;
and the lower part of the gullet looked as if it had been cauterized.
— In the case related by Orfila the gullet and pharynx were red, and
at one or two places excoriated; the stomach inflamed externally,
and its inner membrane spotted with gangrenous (?) patches, and very
brittle; the duodenum thickened, and the jejunum perforated by a
round-worm.

CHAPTER IV.

ON POISONING WITH PHOSPHORUS AND THE OTHER BASES OF THE MINERAL ACIDS.

Of *Poisoning with Phosphorus.* — The only other mineral acid that

* London Medical Gazette, 1839-40, i. 285.
† Lancet, 1839-40, i. 899.   ‡ Toxicologie Générale, i. 155.

deserves mention is the phosphoric. It possesses properties nearly analogous, and hardly inferior to those of the three acids already mentioned. On its own account, however, it does not merit any notice here, since it is much too rare to be within reach of a person who intends to give or take poison. But it must be attended to, because it is formed in the course of the action of a more common poison, phosphorus. An attempt has actually been made to perpe-trate murder by means of this substance. A woman at Mengshausen tried to poison her husband by putting into his soup a mixture of phosphorus, flour, and sugar, used for poisoning rats. But the soup having been kept warm on the stove, the man's suspicions were excited by its phosphorescence, and phosphorus was detected in it.[*]

Orfila found that two drachms of phosphorus given to dogs in frag-ments caused death in twenty-one hours, that the whole stomach and intestines were more or less inflamed, and that the phosphorus had lost much of its weight, though vomiting had been prevented by a ligature on the gullet; in fact the poison was partly oxidated. In a state of minute division, as when dissolved in oil, twenty-four grains caused death in less than five hours with all the symptoms of the most acute irritant poisoning; and after death the stomach was found extensively corroded, and perforated by two holes.[†] Other experi-mentalists have found that half a grain melted in hot water could kill a dog;[‡] and that water, in which phosphorus had been simply re-ceived in the process for preparing it, proved in small quantities fatal to poultry.[§]

There is no doubt, therefore, that phosphorus is a dangerous poison to animals. Its effects on man have not been often witnessed; but the observations hitherto made will show that it is not less injurious to him than to the lower animals. A grain and a half have actually proved fatal to man, as appears from a case mentioned by M. Worbe.[‖] The subject of the case was a stout young man who took a grain and a half in hot water, after having previously taken half a grain with-out sustaining injury. In seven hours, and not till then, he was at-tacked with pain in the stomach and bowels, then with incessant vomiting and diarrhœa, excessive tenderness and tension of the belly, — all the symptoms in short of irritant poisoning; and he died ex-hausted in twelve days. Another fatal case somewhat similar in its circumstances has been related by M. Julia-Fontenelle.[¶] An apothe-cary, after taking in one day first a single grain and then two grains of phosphorus without experiencing any particular effects, swallowed next day three grains at once in syrup. In the evening he felt gene-rally uneasy, from a sense of pressure in the belly, which continued for three days; and then he was also seized with violent, continual vomiting of a matter which had an alliaceous odour. On the seventh day he had also spasms, delirium, and palsy of the left hand; and

* Lins in Buchner's Repertorium, lxviii. 389.   † Toxicologie Générale, i. 56.
‡ Worbe in Mémoires de la Société Médicale d'Emulation, ix. 507.
§ Annales de Chimie, xxvii. 87.
‖ Worbe, &c. and Edin. Med. and Surg. Journal, xxviii. 228.
¶ Revue Médicale, 1829, iii. 429.

death speedily ensued. — Dr. Maier of Ulm relates a singular case occasioned by a portion of lucifer-match composition having been swallowed intentionally. Vomiting and pain in the belly ensued, then anxiety, restlessness, and excessive thirst, and death in about fifteen hours.* — M. Martin-Solon relates the case of a patient, affected with lead-palsy, who having taken considerably less than a grain in the form of emulsion, was attacked with burning along the gullet and in the stomach, mucous vomiting, tenderness of the belly, general coldness and feebleness of the pulse. Afterwards the pulse became imperceptible, the limbs neuralgic, the intellect clouded, and the breathing stertorous; and he died in little more than two days.† — In the only other case I have hitherto found recorded death took place in forty hours, and the symptoms were violent pain in the stomach and continual vomiting, together with the discharge by clysters of small fragments of phosphorus, which were discovered by their shining in the dark, and subsequently by the appearance of burnt spots on the bed-linen. In this case, which is described by Dr. Flachsland of Carlsruhe,‡ the quantity of the poison taken was not ascertained. The patient, a young man, took it on bread and butter at the recommendation of a quack, to cure constipation, general debility, and impotence.

At one time it was the custom to give small doses of phosphorus in medical practice; but the uncertainty and occasional severity of its operation have perhaps properly expelled it from most modern pharmacopœias. Among other properties ascribed to it in medicinal doses, it is said to be a powerful aphrodisiac: No such symptom occurred in the first of the fatal cases just related, or is mentioned in any of the others; but there is no doubt that medicinal doses sometimes produce it.

As to the morbid appearances, the same changes of structure may be expected as in the instance of the mineral acids generally. In Worbe's case quoted above, the skin was generally yellow, and here and there livid; the lungs gorged with blood; the muscular coat of the stomach inflamed, but the other coats not, except near the two extremities of the organ, where they were black. In Flachsland's case much fluid blood was discharged from the first incisions through the skin of the belly; the omentum and outside of the stomach and intestines were red; the villous coat of the stomach presented an appearance of gangrenous inflammation (probably black extravasation only); the inner membrane of the duodenum was similarly affected; the great intestines were contracted to the size of the little finger; the mesenteric glands enlarged; and the kidneys and spleen inflamed. In Maier's case the peritonæum and omentum were dry and vascular, the stomach and small intestines pale, the great intestines contracted, almost empty, brownish-red, and here and there inflamed, the liver large, and the blood everywhere liquid. The contents of

* Buchner's Repertorium für die Pharmacie, lxxi. 341.
† Diction. de Méd. et de Chir. Pratiques, xii. 707.
‡ Medizinisch-Chirurgische Zeitung, 1826, iv. 183.

the caput cœcum had an odour of phosphorus, and here were found two yellowish lumps weighing eight grains, which shone when rubbed, exhaled a phosphoric odour, and contained 0·6 of a grain of phosphorus. In Martin-Solon's case the gullet was cherry-red and its epithelion brittle, the villous coat of the stomach grayish and brittle, the solid viscera in the abdomen soft, and the cerebral membranes congested.

Phosphorous acid, the effects of which have been examined experimentally by Professor Hünefeld of Greifswalde, differs in its operation from phosphoric acid. Twenty-five grains had no effect on a rabbit; but a drachm caused difficult breathing, restlessness, bloody vomiting, slight convulsions, and death in twelve hours; and the stomach was found not much injured. The urine contained phosphoric acid.*

Of Poisoning with Sulphur.—It does not appear that sulphur, which resembles phosphorus in many particulars, bears any resemblance to it in physiological properties;—which may be ascribed to its not being susceptible of spontaneous acidification. It certainly possesses, however, slight irritating properties. It is often given as a purgative, which is sufficient to prove that it is not altogether inert; and the veterinary school at Lyons found that a pound killed horses by producing violent inflammation, recognizable during life by the symptoms, and after death by the morbid appearances.†

Of Poisoning with Chlorine. — Chlorine in its gaseous state acts powerfully as an irritant on the windpipe and lungs, and on that account will be noticed under the head of the poisonous gases. But even in solution it retains to a certain degree its poisonous qualities. Orfila says that five ounces of a strong solution of chlorine will kill a dog in twenty-four hours, if it is kept in the stomach by a ligature, and that two ounces diluted with twice its volume of water will prove fatal in four days;—that the symptoms are those of irritation of the stomach;—and that in the former case he found general redness and blackness—in the latter ulceration of its villous coat.‡

Of Poisoning with Iodine.

Iodine is a poison of more consequence than chlorine, both because it is becoming a more common article, and because it is more violent in its effects on the animal economy.

Tests of Iodine.—Iodine when pure is a solid substance easily known by its scaly form, its resemblance in colour and resplendence to polished iron, its peculiar odour, the violet fumes it forms when heated, and the fine blue colour it produces with a solution of starch. It is very sparingly soluble in water, but readily so in rectified spirit and in aqueous solutions of certain salts, more especially the iodide of potassium. Its ordinary forms in the shops are iodine itself, the

* Horn's Archiv für Medizinische Erfahrung, 1830, ii. 861.
† Corvisart's Journal de Médecine, xxi. 70.
‡ Toxicologie Genéralé, i. 141.

tincture, and the compound solution, where the solvent is a solution of iodide of potassium in water. It stains the skin brownish-yellow; but the stain is not permanent. Its fumes are intensely irritating to the nostrils, throat, and lungs.

When dissolved in water or in solutions of neutral salts, it communicates to the fluid a yellowish-brown or reddish-brown colour, which is destroyed by sulphuretted hydrogen, because the iodine is converted into hydriodic acid. In the colourless fluid thus formed, if treated with chlorine, — or in the original brown fluid without chlorine, — a solution of starch, obtained by ebullition and subsequently cooled, produces a fine blue colour and precipitate ; and these, if the solution be sufficiently diluted, disappear on boiling, reappear on sudden cooling, and are removed permanently by a stream of sulphuretted hydrogen. This is a very delicate and characteristic system of tests. The best mode of using chlorine for decomposing hydriodic acid is to let it descend in the gaseous form from the mouth of a bottle of nitro-hydrochloric acid upon the fluid to be examined ; In this way an excess is easily avoided, which bleaches out the blue colour. Sulphuric acid, though often recommended for the purpose, does not act unless it contains nitrous acid, — from which however the sulphuric acid of commerce is seldom quite free.

When mingled with organic substances, the discovery of it is a matter of some nicety ; because many substances of this nature, especially in the living body, quickly convert it into hydriodic acid.* Hence few cases can occur in medico-legal practice, where iodine will be discoverable in its free state. The following method of analysis will meet all possible cases.

Process for Compound Mixtures. — Add water if necessary, and filter. If either the fluid or solid part is little or not at all coloured, test it with cold solution of starch, assisting the action of the test on the solid part by trituration in a mortar. If a blue colour be struck, which disappears under ebullition, and reappears under refrigeration alone, or on subsequently allowing chlorine gas to descend on the surface of the fluid, there can be no doubt of the existence of iodine. — If the colour of the suspected mixture after filtration is so deep that the action of the starch cannot be expected to yield characteristic appearances, then both the solid and fluid parts should be agitated with a third of their volume of ether ; and after the ethereal solution has arisen to the surface, it is to be removed and tested with solution of starch. The blue colour will be now perhaps struck, because the ether, in carrying off the iodine from the mixture, leaves many coloured organic principles behind.

Should free iodine not be thus detected, strong presumptive evidence may still be procured of its actual presence, or of its having been at one time present, by continuing the examination with the view to detect hydriodic acid. This is described in p. 159.

By following this method of analysis, I have found that one grain of iodine of potassium, which is equivalent to three-quarters of a grain

* Dr. O'Shaughnessey, in Lancet, 1829-30, ii. 632.

16*

of iodine, may be easily discovered in six ounces of urine,— a flui d
as complicated as can well be conceived.

The process adopted by Professor Orfila is so nearly the same with
this, as scarcely to require being detailed. He uses nitric acid instead of chlorine for decomposing the hydriodic acid. Chlorine,
however, is the most delicate reagent for the purpose, if it be used
in the way described above.

Action of Iodine and Symptoms in Man. — Iodide has a twofold
action, one local and irritating, the other general, and produced only
when it has been administered long in frequent small doses.

Orfila remarked that in doses of two drachms it excited in dogs
symptoms of irritation in the stomach ; that death slowly ensued in
seven days, without the symptoms having ever become very violent ;
and that the villous coat of the stomach was here and there yellow,
had also patches of yellow mucus lining it, and exhibited numerous
little ulcers of a yellow colour. He could not observe much injury
from iodine introduced into the cellular tissue ; and more lately, Dr.
Cogswell remarked that in this way it merely induces phlegmonous
inflammation and the usual consequences.[*]

An important circumstance in regard to the physiology and medical jurisprudence of this poison and its compounds is, that it may undoubtedly be detected in the blood, both when a single large dose
has been taken, and in those persons who have used it for some time
medicinally. Cantu, an Italian experimentalist, discovered iodine in
such circumstances in the blood, sweat, urine, saliva and milk ;[†] and
Bennerscheidt, a German chemist, also found it in the blood, when
it had been employed outwardly.[‡] In the latter instance it could not
be detected in the serum, but it was detected in the crassamentum
by means of starch. Some interesting facts of the same nature have
also been ascertained by Dr. O'Shaughnessey, from which it appears
that even in acute poisoning with this substance, satisfactory proof
of its administration may be procured several days afterwards by ana-
lysing certain secretions. In a dog poisoned with iodine, he detected the poison in forty minutes in the urine, and occasionally in
the same secretion so late as the fifth day, when it died. It is singular, however, that he could not find it in the same quarter on the
third day, although it existed at that time abundantly in the saliva.[§]
In these experiments the iodine was always found in the form of hydriodic acid, having been converted into that compound in the alimentary canal. This change takes place with such rapidity, that on
one occasion, in the vomited matter discharged by a dog fifteen minutes only after the administration of iodine, Dr. O'Shaughnessey
could find no iodine, but a large quantity of hydriodic acid.[‖]
Orfila has found it not only in the urine, but likewise in the liver of
animals.[¶]

* Experimental Essay on Iodine, &c. 1837, p 21.
† Journal de Chimie Médicale, ii. 291.   ‡ Ibid. iv. 388.
§ Lancet, 1830-31, vol. i. 613.   ‖ Ibidem, 612.
¶ Annales d'Hygiène Publique, xxviii. 431.

Considerable uncertainty prevails as to the circumstances in which we may expect iodine to be detected in the organs or secretions of persons who have taken it. Thus it has been stated by an Italian physician, Dr. Cristin, that in many individuals affected with dropsy, struma, epilepsy, and other diseases, he had sought for iodine to no purpose in the urine, bronchial mucus, and other excretory fluids.*

With regard to its operation on man, Orfila says, he has tried the effects of four or six grains on himself, and that he found this dose produce a sense of constriction in the throat, sickness, pain in the stomach, and at length vomiting and colic. There is no doubt, therefore, that in larger doses it will prove a dangerous irritant to man as well as to dogs. Accordingly, Dr. Gairdner has noticed the case of a child four years old, who died in a few hours after taking about a scruple in the form of tincture;† but he has not mentioned the symptoms. Dr. Jahn of Meiningen mentions a case where an over-dose produced violent pain in the belly, vomiting, profuse bloody diarrhœa, coldness and blanching of the skin, rigors, quivering of the sight and rapid pulse.‡ Two similar cases are related in a recent French journal; in one, which was produced by a drachm and a half of the ioduretted solution of hydriodate of potass, nausea, with acute pain and sense of burning in the pit of the stomach, followed immediately; in an hour there was vomiting of a yellowish matter which had the taste of iodine; excessive restlessness ensued, with headache, giddiness and paleness of the countenance; and these symptoms were not entirely dissipated for five days.§ In the other case two drachms and a half of iodine were swallowed for the purpose of self-destruction. A sense of dryness and burning from the throat down to the stomach was immediately produced; lacerating pain in the stomach and fruitless efforts to vomit succeeded; and in an hour, when the relater of the case first saw the patient, there was suffusion of the eyes, excessive pain and tenderness of the epigastrium, and sinking of the pulse. Vomiting, however, was then brought on by warm water; copious yellow discharges, possessing the smell and taste of iodine, took place; and in nine hours the patient was well.‖

There is a singular uncertainty, however, in the action of one or more large doses. Magendie says he has taken two drachms of the tincture, containing about ten grains of iodine, without injury;¶ Dr. Gully, that he has given three times as much daily for some time; Dr. Kennedy, that he gave an average of twelve grains daily in the form of tincture for eighty days without observing any effect at all; and Mr. Delisser, that he has given a patient thirty grains in a day without injury.** Dr. Samuel Wright met with the case of an infant, not more than three years old, who took three drachms of the tinc-

* Annali Universali di Med. 1833.
† Essay on the Effects of Iodine, 1824, p. 20.
‡ Horn's Archiv für Medizinische Erfahrung, 1829, i. 340.
§ Dessaigne in Journal de Chim. Médicale, iv. 65.
‖ Moncourrier, Ibidem, iv. 216.
¶ Formulaire pour les Nouveaux Médicamens, 1825, p. 161.
** Quoted in Dr. Cogswell's Experimental Essay, p. 23.

ture at once, and suffered only from attempts to cough, some retching and much thirst.*

It further appears that in medicinal doses, such as a quarter of a grain, frequently repeated, it is a dangerous poison, unless its effects are carefully watched. For in consequence of accumulation in the system, or gradually increasing action, it produces when long used some very singular and hazardous symptoms; and like mercury, foxglove, and some other poisons, it may be taken long without effect, and at length begin to operate suddenly. The symptoms which it then occasions are sometimes those of irritation; namely, incessant vomiting and purging, acute pain in the stomach, loaded tongue, rapid and extreme emaciation, violent cramps and small frequent pulse. These symptoms may continue many days, and even when subdued to a certain extent, vomiting and cramps are apt to recur for months after.† A fatal case of this form of affection has been related by M. Zink, a Swiss physician. His patient, after taking too large doses of iodine for about a month, was seized with restlessness, burning heat of skin, tremors, palpitation, syncope, excessive thirst, a sense of burning along the gullet, frequent purging of bilious and black stools, priapism, and tremulous pulse. The symptoms of local inflammation went off in a few days; but those of general fever continued; and he died after six weeks' illness.‡ Another fatal case has been described in Rust's Journal. The leading symptoms were pain in the region of the liver, loss of appetite, emaciation, quartan fever, diarrhœa, excessive weakness; and after the emaciation was far advanced a hardened liver could be felt. The patient appears to have died of exhaustion.§ From this case, and another of which the appearances after death will be presently noticed, it is not improbable that iodine possesses the power of inflaming the liver.

In another and more common affection, the patient is attacked with tremors, at first slight and confined to the fingers, afterwards violent and extending to the whole muscles of the arms and even of the trunk. At the same time there is excessive and rapidly increasing weakness, a sense of anxiety and sinking, a total suspension of the function of digestion, rapid and extreme muscular emaciation, tendency to fainting, and violent continued palpitation,‖ accompanied sometimes with absorption of the testicles in man, and of the mammæ in females. In the midst of these phenomena the curative powers of the poison over the disease for which it has chiefly been used, namely, goître, are developed. It has been remarked in particular, that the diminution of the goître keeps pace with the diminution of the breasts, though at times either effect has been developed without the other. An instance is related in Rust's Journal of a female, whose breasts began to sink after she had used iodine for four months; and in four weeks hardly a vestige of them remained;

* Quoted in Dr. Cogswell's Experimental Essay, p. 27.
† Gairdner on the Effects of Iodine, p. 9.
‡ Journal Complémentaire, xviii. 126.
§ Magazin für die gesammte Heilkunde, xvi. 111.
‖ Gairdner, &c. p. 12.

but her goître was not affected.* An American physician, Dr. Rivers, has twice noticed barrenness apparently induced by the prolonged use of iodine ; and as in these instances the females were young and previously very prolific, but ceased to bear children from the time the iodine was used, his observations seem worthy of attention.† Dr. Jahn‡ specifies among the leading effects of the poison when slowly accumulated in the body, — absorption of the fat, — increase of all the excretions, — dinginess of the skin, with frequent clammy sweat, — hurried anxious breathing, — diuresis and an appearance of oil floating in the urine, — increased discharge of fæces, which are unusually bilious, but free of mucus, — increased secretion of semen, — increased menstrual discharge, — swelling of the subcutaneous veins and lividity of the lips, — feebleness of the pulse, with superabundance of serosity in the blood, — impaired digestion and diminished secretion of saliva and mucus. This affection, which, in conformity with the name he has given it, may be termed Iodism [*Iodkrankheit*], he contrasts with mercurialism, the constitutional effect of the accumulation of mercury in the body ; and he considers the former not more unmanageable than the latter. The dose required to produce these effects are very various. Some people appear almost insensible to its action ; in one instance, nine hundred and fifty-three grains were taken in daily portions varying from two to eighteen grains, without any bad effect ;§ and I have known an average of four grains daily taken for fifteen months, with the effect only of increasing the appetite. On the other hand, Dr. Gairdner has seen severe symptoms commence when half a grain was taken three times a day for a single week ;‖ and Coindet has seen bad effects from thirty drops of the solution of ioduretted hydriodate taken daily for five days.¶

Iodine and iodide of potassium in medicinal doses have been supposed by Dr. Lawrie to be capable of exciting in certain constitutions an affection resembling *cynanche laryngea* in its symptoms, consisting of inflammation of the salivary glands, glottis, and other adjacent parts, and proving sometimes fatal.** This property is doubtful ; but several instances have been published of profuse salivation and soreness of the mouth during a course of iodine ; it is apt to cause chronic irritation of the Schneiderian membrane ; and some think that it may affect in like manner the bronchial membrane in the lungs.††

Morbid Appearances from Iodine. — The only account I have seen of the appearances left in the body after death from slow poisoning with iodine is contained in the essay of Dr. Zink. In a second fatal case which came under his notice he found enlarged abdomen from

* Magazin für die gesammte Heilkunde, xxii. 291.
† American Journal of Medical Science, viii. 546.
‡ Archiv für Medizinische Erfahrung, 1829, i. 342.
§ Johnson's Preface to his Translation of Coindet on Iodine, p. ix.
‖ Gairdner, p. 20.   ¶ Coindet on Iodine, p. 17.
** London Medical Gazette, 1839-40, ii. 588.
†† Cogswell's Essay, p. 42.

distension of the intestines with gases, enlargement of the other viscera and serous effusion into the peritonæum ; adhesion of the viscera to one another; redness of the intestines, in some places approaching to gangrenous discoloration ; redness and excoriation of
the peritonæal coat of the stomach, and also of its villous coat; enlargement and pale rose-red coloration of the liver. In the chest
serum was found in the sac of the pleura. The gullet was contracted
in diameter, and red internally.

On Poisoning with Iodide of Potassium.

To these remarks on iodine a few observations may be added on
the iodide of potassium, one of its compounds, which is now generally substituted in medicine for the simple substance. The tests
and actions of this poison have been examined by M. Devergie ; and
more lately its medico-legal chemistry has been investigated by Dr.
O'Shaughnessey and Professor Orfila.

It is sold in the shops of various degrees of purity. Pure iodide
of potassium is in white crystals, tending to the cubical form, permanent in the air, possessing a faint peculiar odour, and easily
soluble in both water and rectified spirit. Another variety has the
same form, but possesses an odour of iodine, is often yellowish in
colour, and deliquesces slightly in moist air. This contains an excess of iodine, but may be otherwise pure. A third variety is impure. It presents less tendency to assume a crystalline form, is more
or less deliquescent, dissolves but partially in alcohol, and when dissolved effervesces with acids. The principal ingredient in this
article is carbonate of potass ; and sometimes the proportion of iodide
is inconsiderable. In one specimen I procured 74·5 per cent. of
carbonate of potass, 16 of water, and only 9·5 of iodide of potassium.

In the solid state the iodide of potassium may be known by the
effect of strong sulphuric or nitric acid, which turns it brown with
effervescence, and when aided by heat disengages violet fumes of
iodine.

In solution many tests will detect it, such as chlorine, nitric acid,
corrosive sublimate, acetate of lead, protonitrate of mercury, muriate
of platinum, and starch with chlorine or nitric acid. Chlorine or
nitric acid forms a brown or orange-coloured solution by disengaging
iodine. Corrosive sublimate forms a fine carmine-red precipitate,
the biniodide of mercury ; acetate of lead a fine yellow precipitate,
the iodide of lead ; protonitrate of mercury a yellow protiodide of
mercury, which gradually fades into a dirty-brown. Solution of
starch, followed by chlorine in solution or in vapour, strikes a deep
blue colour, which, if the fluid is sufficiently diluted, disappears on
boiling, reappears on sudden cooling, and is permanently removed
by a stream of sulphuretted hydrogen gases. Of these tests the most
characteristic is starch with chlorine; and it is also extremely delicate. Too much chlorine however bleaches the blue colour away.

In compound mixtures most and sometimes all of these tests are useless. If the mixture is deeply coloured, none will act characteristically. If carbonate of potass be present in such proportion as is often met with in the shops, the tests cannot be trusted to.

Process for Compound Mixtures.—The following method of analysis is applicable to all mixtures, organic and inorganic. Add water, if necessary, and filter ; and if the fluid which passes through is tolerably free from colour, test a little of it with solution of starch and chlorine. If the colour is too deep to admit of this trial, or the test on trial does not act, unite the fluid and solid parts and transmit sulphuretted hydrogen to convert any free iodine into hydriodic acid. Drive off the excess of gas, supersaturate with a considerable excess of potass, filter, and evaporate to dryness. Char the residue at a low red heat in a covered crucible ; pulverize the charcoaly mass, and exhaust with water. This solution will probably act characteristically with starch and chlorine; but on the whole it is better in the first instance to remove some of the salts by evaporating to dryness, and exhausting the residuum with alcohol. The alcoholic solution contains the hydriodate of potass, with some other salts ; and on being evaporated to dryness, a residuum is left, on which, when dissolved in water, the starch and chlorine will act characteristically. No other test is necessary ; and frequently no other test will act, on account of coexisting salts.

I have found that a grain of iodide of potassium may thus be easily detected in six ounces of urine, which must be considered a very complicated fluid. In the solution ultimately procured nitrous acid struck a pale brown tint, and on the addition of solution of starch a dark-blue precipitate was formed ; which, after being sufficiently diluted, disappeared under ebullition, leaving a colourless fluid. On cooling, no change took place ; but on the subsequent addition of a drop of sulphuric acid, the blue colour and precipitation were immediately restored. No other reagent acted characteristically, although there was a sufficient quantity of solution to try the starch test ten times at least.

Dr. O'Shaughnessey has proposed a more complex method by precipitation with chloride of platinum.* Professor Orfila says it is sufficient to boil and filter the suspected matter, and to heat first the liquid and then the solid part with solution of chloride, when violet vapours of iodine are disengaged, which may be condensed and subjected to various tests.† I have not compared this method with the one I have been in the practice of using ; but, notwithstanding the strong assurances of its proposer, its superiority in point of delicacy seems dubious, although no one can deny its simplicity.‡

Action and Symptoms in Man. — From the experiments of Devergie on animals, iodide of potassium seems to be in large doses an irritant, though not a powerful one. Two drachms in an ounce of water killed a dog in three days with violent vomiting, and signs of

* Lancet, 1829-30, ii. 635.
† Toxicologie Générale, 1843, i. 74.   ‡ Lancet, 1829-30, ii. 638.

irritation were found in the stomach, namely, black extravasated spots and ulcers in the middle of them. A solution injected into the cellular tissue caused only local inflammation. Injected into the jugular vein in the dose of four grains, it produced tetanus and death in a minute and a half.*   The latter investigations of Dr. Cogswell confirm essentially these results.

Discrepant accounts have been given of the effects of iodide of potassium on man.   When first introduced into medicine, it was conceived to be an active poison, not much inferior to iodine itself. Many however have since had an opportunity of observing that it is in general by no means so energetic.   Its medicinal doses were gradually raised from one grain to five, ten, twenty grains ; and at last Dr. Elliotson gave to not a few patients so much as two, four, or even six drachms daily in divided doses, without observing any remarkable effect.†   These and other similar observations however were made at a period when the salt used in British practice was much adulterated, often indeed containing eighty or ninety per cent. of impurity ; at the same time it does appear that large doses of a pure salt have been occasionally taken with impunity.   On the other hand it has evidently in some instances acted with great force.   Mr. Alfred Taylor mentions a case, on the authority of Mr. Ericksen, where five grains produced alarming dyspnœa, attended with inflammation of the nostrils and conjunctiva of the eyes.‡   An instance has been published where twelve grains in four doses occasioned shivering, vomiting, purging, general fever, and extreme prostration ; and the purging continued for some days.§   Dr. Moore Neligan informs me he met with the case of an elderly lady in 1841, who, on taking three five-grain doses for two days, while labouring under irregular gout, was seized with severe headache, thirst, and swelling of the face ; which symptoms were succeeded in two days by swelling of the tongue, ulceration of the gums, and profuse salivation for a week. Dr. Lawrie says he has known two grains and a half given thrice in one day, followed by great dyspnœa and irritation in the throat ; and is even inclined to think that death resulted on two occasions from repeated medicinal doses.‖   It would farther appear from some important researches made in France, that the protracted use of iodide of potassium in small doses with the food may produce serious derangement of the health, — swelling of the face, headache, urgent thirst, inflammation of the throat, violent colic pains, and frequently bloody diarrhœa.   A disease characterized by the symptoms now described appeared repeatedly as an epidemic a few years ago in various parts of France, and spread so widely in one parish, that not less than a sixth of the whole population were attacked.   After several careful investigations, it seems to have been fully proved that the affection was owing to the use of salt fraudulently adulterated with an impure salt, obtained from kelp after the separation of car-

* Archives Générales de Médecine, x. 255.   † Lancet, 1831-32.
‡ Manual of Medical Jurisprudence, 128.
§ London Medical Gazette, 1841.   ‖ Ibidem, 1839-40, i. 588.

bonate of soda, and consequently impregnated with an appreciable proportion of hydriodate of potass.*

It is difficult to arrive at any satisfactory conclusions from these statements as to the nature and energy of the action of this salt as a poison. But on the whole it appears to be not in general very active ; and the few instances of unusual activity which have occurred may probably be put to the account of idiosyncrasy. The most remarkable of its idiosyncratic effects from medicinal doses are salivation, and a series of symptoms which imitate sometimes catarrh, and sometimes a cold in the head. I do not know any facts to warrant the general statement of M. Devergie that 18 or 30 grains may constitute a fatal dose.† The present question is far from being unimportant in a medico-legal point of view. Mr. A. Taylor mentions the heads of a case, very dubious however in its nature, where it was suspected that a single dose of six grains of iodide of potassium had been the occasion of death.‡

It is important to remember in medico-legal researches, that iodide of potassium may be detected in the blood, liver, spleen, muscles, urine, and other textures and secretions ; and especially that it may be found in the urine, when it may no longer exist in the alimentary canal or in vomited matters. These interesting facts have been clearly proved by the researches of Wöhler,§ Stehberger,‖ O'Shaughnessey,¶ and Dr. Cogswell.**

Of Poisoning with Bromine. — This singular substance is not an object of much interest in relation to medical jurisprudence, because it is rare, and only to be met with in the laboratory of the chemist. Hence, although it appears to be a poison of some activity, it scarcely requires to be dwelt on particularly.

It is easily known from all other substances by its fluidity, its great density, which is thrice as great as that of water, its reddish-brown colour by reflected, and blood-red colour by transmitted light, the orange fumes which occupy the upper part of a bottle partly filled with it, and its intensely acrid suffocating vapour, which is so irritating that an incautious inhalation is followed by all the phenomena of severe coryza and catarrh. Its odour, however, apart from its acridity, is very far from being so disagreeable as its discoverer in naming it seems to have imagined. In its properties it bears a close resemblance to chlorine and iodine.

The toxicological effects and medico-legal relations of bromine have

---

* This adulteration and its effects have been indicated by various chemists. For the best account, see Chevallier, sur les falsifications qu'on fait subir au sel marin, Annales d'Hyg. Publ. et de Méd. Lég. viii. 250. At one time he found about a third of the salt in Paris thus sophisticated.

† Cours de Médecine-Légale, 1840, iii. 183.

‡ Manual of Medical Jurisprudence, p. 38.

§ Zeitschrift für Physiologie, ii.

‖ Ibidem.

¶ Lancet, 1830-31, i. 613.

** Experimental Essay on Iodine, &c. 1837, p. 91.

17

been examined by M. Barthez,* Dr. Butske,† Dr. Dieffenbach,‡ and Dr. M. Glover.§

M. Barthez has given the following process for detecting bromine in compound mixtures, such as the contents of the stomach or vomited matter. First separate the fluid matter by filtration, and subject it to the action of chlorine, which will produce a fine orange-colour. Should this effect not result, or the change of colour be observed by the deep tint of the fluid, treat the solid matter with solution of caustic potass; filter and add what passes through to the former fluid; evaporate to dryness and char by a red heat; act on the residue with distilled water. The solution contains the bromide of potassium, and is therefore turned orange-red by chlorine. The orange tint, whether struck at once in the fluid part of the mixture, or after carbonization and solution of the residue, is removed by agitation with ether; and the etherial solution of bromine in its turn loses colour when treated with solution of caustic potass, hydro-bromate of potass being again formed.

M. Barthez found, that a solution of twelve grains injected into the jugular vein of a dog, sometimes occasioned immediate tetanus and death; and that the heart was gorged with clotted blood. Sometimes however even seventeen drops did not prove fatal, but produced merely restlessness, difficult breathing, dilated pupil, frequency of the pulse, and sneezing. Dieffenbach remarked similar effects in the rabbit: The animal either died immediately, or soon recovered altogether. In a cat, after the injection of twelve drops of a concentrated solution into its jugular vein, death took place in fifteen minutes; but in another from which a little blood was drawn after the symptoms were fully formed, complete recovery gradually ensued. Butske found a horse suffer so much from mortal prostration immediately after five grains dissolved in two ounces of water were injected into its jugular vein, that he supposed it was about to die; but it quickly revived, and ultimately got quite well. Dr. Glover obtained similar results. When recovery took place, the leading symptoms were panting, sneezing, discharge from the nostrils, rigors and debility.

When introduced into the stomach of dogs, M. Barthez found that twenty drops on a full stomach had no particular effect; that thirty drops occasioned vomiting, and temporary acceleration of the pulse and breathing; and that from forty to sixty drops on an empty stomach brought on violent vomiting, sneezing, cough, dilated pupil and prostration, succeeded in a few hours by languor without any other symptom, and by death in four or five days. In the dead body he remarked numerous little ulcers of the villous coat, some of which had an ash-gray appearance at the bottom, while others were covered

---

* De l'Action du Brôme et de ses combinaisons sur l'économie animale. Thèse Inaug. à Paris, 1828.

† Hufeland's Bibliothek der Praktischen Heilkunde, Sept. 1829; or Archives Gén. de Méd. xxiv. 289.

‡ Meckel's Archiv für Anatomie und Physiologie, xiv. 222.

§ Edin. Med. and Surg. Journal, lviii. 120.

with a black slough, easily removed by friction. When the gullet was tied to prevent vomiting, less doses proved more quickly fatal. He likewise observed that the matter vomited in these experiments, even a few minutes after the administration of the poison, had no appearance or odour of bromine; whence it is reasonable to conclude, that, as in the instance of iodine, a chemical change takes place with the aid of certain vital operations, so that the bromine becomes hydrobromic acid. — The experiments of Dr. Butske assign to it more activity as a poison than those now related. For he found that a dog died in a day from taking only five grains dissolved in two ounces of water; and the symptoms were laborious breathing, loud cries, and convulsions. In the dead body he found the stomach internally chequered with bloody extravasation, and filled with bloody mucus, the duodenal mucous membrane universally injected, but the rest of the alimentary canal in a healthy state. — Dr. Glover remarked in such cases, besides the usual symptoms of an irritant action on the stomach, coryza, sneezing, salivation and difficult breathing. Sixty minims killed a cat in seventeen minutes, two fluidrachms a dog in five hours and a half, ten grains a rabbit in five minutes. A dog twice got twenty grains in solution and recovered, but died after a third dose of the same amount. Another got twenty grains in solution every two or three days for a month without injury. In some of these experiments hydrobromic acid was detected in the blood and urine.

Little is yet known of the effects of bromine on man. Butske found that a drop and a half in half an ounce of water produced a sense of heat in the mouth, gullet, and stomach, and subsequently colic pains; and that two drops and a half in an ounce of mucilage excited, in addition to the preceding symptoms, great nausea, hiccup, and increased secretion of mucus. On the other hand M. Fournet, who gave doses gradually increasing from two to sixty drops daily for many weeks, observed that the lowest doses exited itching in the hands and feet, and sometimes colic; that an increase in the quantity caused heat in the chest and nausea; and that forty-five drops occasioned also severe burning and sense of acidity in the stomach, which however were temporary. The appetite was in general rather improved, and the body became more plump.* — Bromine appears on the whole to be a pure local irritant. It acts mot energetically when most thoroughly dissolved in water.

Hydrobromic acid seems from the experiments of Dr. Glover to be a pure irritant and corrosive, allied in action and energy to hydrochloric acid. The same experimentalist found that *bromine of potassium* in the dose of forty grains had sometimes little or no effect on dogs when injected into the blood-vessels, while in other instances less doses cause speedy death by paralysing the heart. Barthez observed that half a drachm in solution produced dulness and depression in dogs, but no other bad effect; and that two drachms retained in the stomach by tying the gullet occasioned death in three days with symptoms of irritant poisoning. M. Maillet observed that two

* Bulletins de Thérapeutique, Fevrier, 1830.

ounces of this salt in the form of ointment, administered to a dog by rubbing it over his nose, and letting him lick it off and swallow it, had no effect whatever.*

CHAPTER V.

OF POISONING WITH ACETIC ACID.

ACETIC acid, although in its ordinary state undoubtedly possessed of little activity as a poison, has nevertheless proved in some circumstances deleterious, and capable of occasioning death even in the human subject. It exists in various forms. The most common is ordinary vinegar, in which it is much diluted. Another common form is the pyroligneous vinegar, pyroligneous acid, or pyroligneous acetic acid, as it is variously called, which when impure has a reddish-brown colour, but when pure is almost or altogether colourless, and the strength of which is much greater than that of common vinegar. What is called proof vinegar has a density about 1005, and contains about four per cent. of concentrated acid. The pyroligneous acid sold in the shops of this town has a density about 1035, and contains about 25 per cent. ; but the pyroligneous acid of the London Pharmacopœia is stronger, for its density is 1050, and 100 parts contain about 50 of the strong acid. A third form is the concentrated or pure acetic acid of the apothecary, which is familiarly known as the chief ingredient and menstruum of a common perfume, aromatic vinegar.

SECTION I. — *Of the Tests for Acetic Acid.*

In all its forms acetic acid is easily known by its very peculiar odour, together with its acid reaction on litmus. But if farther evidence of its nature be required, it will be requisite to neutralise the fluid suspected to contain it with carbonate of potass, and then to procure the acetate of potass by evaporation. This salt is known by its extreme tendency to deliquesce, and by a concentrated solution in water, yielding, when distilled with sulphuric acid, a fluid possessing the peculiar odour and pungency of concentrated acetic acid.

When in a state of compound admixture with organic substances, such as the contents of the stomach, it has been proved by late researches of Orfila,† that this acid may be present in considerable proportion without distinctly reddening litmus. For such mixtures the following process of analysis, devised by the Parisian professor, will be found convenient and effectual. The fluid being put into a retort with a receiver attached, the retort is to be heated in a muriate of lime bath till the residuum be dry. The distilled fluid may then be tested tentatively for sulphuric and muriatic acids; and these being

---

* Journal de Chimie Médicale, 1837, 227.
† Annales d'Hygiène Publ. et de Méd Lég. vi. 169.

proved to be absent, the acidity and peculiar smell of the liquid will supply strong presumption of the presence of acetic acid. This presumption may be turned to certainty by forming acetate of potass, as already directed for the pure diluted acetic acid.

Orfila has omitted in his paper a serious fallacy to which this, as well as every process for the detection of acetic acid in the contents of the stomach is exposed, — namely, that the natural secretions of the stomach, according to the researches of many physiologists, but more especially in recent times those of Tiedemann and Gmelin in Germany, and those of Leuret and Lassaigne in Paris, frequently contain a small proportion of acetic acid. Hence, the inference in favour of the introduction of acetic acid into the stomach from without, founded on the process related above, is only legitimate when the quantity discovered is considerable. — The medical jurist ought also to keep in mind that vinegar is a common remedy with the vulgar for many diseases, and especially for poisoning.

SECTION II. — *Of the Effects of Acetic Acid on Man and Animals.*

In the first edition of this work, it was stated that acetic acid could scarcely be considered a poison. And in illustration, a case was mentioned which fell under my own notice, — that of a gentleman, who during dinner swallowed at a draught about eight ounces of vinegar by mistake for beer, and who nevertheless sustained no harm although he retained it all, and as the only measure of precaution, swallowed after it an equal quantity of port wine. In farther confirmation of what is here mentioned, it may be added, that an ounce of acid equal in strength to the pyroligneous vinegar, has been found by Schubarth of Berlin to produce very little effect when administered to a dog. The animal merely frothed a little at the mouth; cried and became restless for a time; then had one or two attacks of vomiting; and in an hour appeared quite well again.[*] Nay, it has even been found by Pommer of Heilbronn, that a considerable quantity of diluted acetic acid may be injected into the blood without causing any mischief. He injected six drachms of distilled vinegar into the femoral vein of one dog, and an ounce into the jugular vein of another, but observed no effect whatever, except a slight labour of respiration for a short time afterwards.[†]

It appears, however, from some experiments performed by Professor Orfila on occasion of a judicial case to be mentioned presently, that all the forms of acetic acid will prove injurious and even fatal to dogs, if given in sufficient quantity and prevented from being discharged by vomiting. An ounce of pyroligneous vinegar, administered to dogs of middle size, and retained in the stomach by a ligature on the gullet, produces efforts to vomit, evident suffering, prostration of strength, and death in five, seven, or nine hours. An

[*] Beiträge zur Kentniss der Wirkungen der Arzneimittel und Gifte. Horn's Archiv. 1824, i. 59.
[†] Medizinische Zeitung, 1828, ii. 256.

17*

ounce of concentrated acetic acid occasioned death in one hour and a quarter ; and four or five ounces of common vinegar proved fatal in ten or fifteen hours.   These experiments would make it appear that acetic acid is scarcely less active as an irritant poison than even the mineral acids.*   They are in some measure confirmed by the prior experiments of Schubarth ; who operated, however, with an impure reddish-brown pyroligneous acid, and was led to ascribe its energy to the presence of some empyreumatic oil, because he found, as was already remarked, that a pure acid of equal strength appeared almost inert.   From half an ounce to an ounce of the impure acid given to dogs, caused fruitless efforts to vomit, sometimes free vomiting, occasionally great flow of tears, always weakness in the hind-legs, and feeble, irregular pulse, and death either in two days without any new symptom of consequence, or more rapid death in four or five hours, with previous convulsions, and sometimes insensibility.† These experiments were made with an acid which neutralized 50 grains of carbonate of lime per ounce, consequently contained at least 50 grains of concentrated acid, or about a tenth of its weight.

To these observations it may be added, that according to the experiments of Hébréart, a small quantity of acetic acid dropped into the windpipe, produces hissing respiration, rattling in the throat, and death in three days from true croup.‡

In all the preceding experiments distinct evidence was obtained in the dead body of the irritant action of the poison.   The stomach contained brownish-black blood, the villous coat was blackish, and the subjacent cellular tissue injected with black blood ; sometimes there was an appearance of erosion on the surface of the villous coat ; and in the instance of the concentrated acid perforations were found. In the experiments of Hébréart the lining membrane of the windpipe was covered with a fibrinous pseudo-membrane, exactly as after croup.

Although acetic acid in its various forms is daily in the hands of every body, one case only of poisoning with it in the human subject has hitherto been made public.   It is described by MM. Orfila and Barruel.§   A girl was seen in a village near Paris at eleven at night apparently intoxicated.   Five hours afterwards she was found lying on the ground in great agony; and after complaining of pain in the stomach and experiencing several attacks of convulsions, she expired.   On the subsequent examination of the body considerable lividity was observed on the skin of the depending parts.   The back of the tongue was brownish and leathery, and the inner membrane of the gullet blackish-brown, intersected by a fine network of vessels. The stomach presented internally several large, black, firm elevations, owing to the injection of coagulated blood into the sub-mucous cellular tissue ; and elsewhere it had a grayish-white tint, with here

* Ann. d'Hyg. Publ. et de Méd. Lég. vi. 160.
† Beiträge, &c.   Horn's Archiv, 1824, i. 56.
‡ Corvisart's Journal de Médecine, xxiv. 215.
§ Annales d'Hyg. Publ. et de Méd. Lég. vi. 159.

and there a reddish colour ; but the mucous membrane was perfectly entire. The cavity contained above eight ounces of a thick, blackish fluid ; and a thicker pulpy matter of the same colour adhered firmly to the villous coat. The intestines were healthy, and so also were the other organs in the belly and chest. The uterus contained a fœtus two months and a half old. The contents of the stomach were subjected to a careful analysis by MM. Orfila and Barruel, who found that they did not contain any appreciable quantity of free sulphuric or muriatic acid, or of any of the common metallic poisons ; and by the process of analysis formerly described, they succeeded in separating from the impure mass three drachms of a pure, and tolerably concentrated acetic acid, besides two drachms more from the contents of the intestines. As the residue of the distillation left behind in the retort did not yield any bitter principle to boiling alcohol, so as to countenance the idea of a vegetable alkaloid having been given along with the acetic acid, they inferred that this acid had been swallowed alone ; and the experiments of Orfila on dogs, performed for the occasion, induced them to conclude that it was the cause of death.

To these observations it is only farther necessary to add, that the concentrated acid is a powerful irritant and even corrosive when applied externally; which properties are owing to its power of dissolving many of the soft animal solids.*

CHAPTER VI.

OF POISONING WITH OXALIC ACID.

The last poison of this order is oxalic acid. It is a substance of very great interest; for it is a poison of great energy, and in this country is in common use for committing suicide, and has been often taken by accident for Epsom salt.

It is certainly ill adapted for the purposes of the murderer ; for although it might be easily given to a sick person instead of a laxative salt, yet its real nature would betray itself too soon and too unequivocally for the chief object of the prisoner, — secrecy. Nevertheless, attempts of the kind have been made. At the trial of James Brown for assaulting his wife, held at the Middlesex Autumn Assizes 1827, it was brought out in evidence that he had previously tried to posion her by giving her oxalic acid in gin ;† and Mr. Alfred Taylor says he is acquainted with two similar cases, where an attempt was made to administer it in tea.‡

It was first made known as a poison by Mr. Royston in 1814.§ Its properties have been examined by Dr. A. T. Thomson of Lon-

* See Trousseau and Blanc, Arch. Gén. de Med. Sept. 1830.
† London Courier, September 22, 1827.
‡ Manual of Medical Jurisprudence, 116.
§ London Medical Repository, i. 382.

don,* and Dr. Perey of Lausanne;† in 1823, the whole subject of poisoning with oxalic acid in its medico-legal relations was examined by Dr. Coindet of Geneva and myself;‡ and in 1828, another experimental inquiry, which confirms most of the results we obtained, was published by Dr. Pommer of Heilbronn.§

Section I. — *Of the Tests for Oxalic Acid.*

Oxalic acid is commonly in small crystals of the form of flattened six-sided striated prisms, transparent, colourless, free of odour, very acid to the taste, and permanent in the air. Two other common vegetable acids, the citric and tartaric acids, present a totally different crystalline form. In general appearance it greatly resembles the sulphate of magnesia, for which it has been so often and so fatally mistaken. So close, indeed, is the resemblance, that repeatedly, on desiring several persons to point out which was the poison and which the laxative, I have found as many fix on the wrong as on the right parcel. The sulphate of magnesia has of course a very different taste, being strongly bitter. Various plans have been devised for preventing the accident to which this unlucky resemblance has given rise. The best of them imply the use of a safeguard by the patient before he takes his laxative draught. It seems to have escaped the notice of those who have proposed the plans in question, that, if accidents are to be prevented in this manner, by far the simplest and most effectual security will be to let the public know, that a laxative salt ought always to be tasted before being swallowed. Its solubility has been much overrated by some chemists. It does not appear to me soluble in less than eleven parts of water.

In determining the medico-legal tests for oxalic acid, it will be sufficient to consider it in two states, — dissolved in water, — and mixed with the contents of the stomach and intestines or vomited matter. If the substance submitted to examination is in the solid state, the first step is to convert it into a solution.

1. In the form of a pure solution, its nature may be satisfactorily determined by the following process.

The acidity of the fluid is first to be established by its effect on litmus paper. — A small portion is next to be tested with ammonia, which, if the solution of the acid be sufficiently concentrated, will produce a radiated crystallization, as the oxalate of ammonia formed is much less soluble than oxalic acid itself. This property, according to Dr. O'Shaughnessey, distinguishes it from every other acid.‖ The remainder of the fluid is next to be subjected to the following reagents.

Hydrochlorate of lime causes a white precipitate, the oxalate of lime ; which is dissolved on the addition of a drop or two of nitric

* Lond. Med. Rep. iii. 382.
† Dissertatio Inauguralis de Acidi Oxalici vi venenata, Edin. 1821.
‡ Edinburgh Med. and Surg. Journal, xix. 163.
§ Medizinisch-Chirurgische Zeitung, 1828, ii. 203, *et seq.*
‖ Lancet, 1830-31, i. 96

acid, — and is not dissolved when similarly treated with hydrochloric acid, unless the acid is added in very large proportion.

The easy solubility of the oxalate of lime in nitric acid distinguishes the precipitate from the sulphate of lime, which the present test might throw down from solutions of the sulphates, and which is not soluble in a moderate quantity of nitric acid without the aid of heat. The insolubility of the oxalate of lime in hydrochloric acid on the other hand distinguishes the precipitate from the tartrate, citrate, carbonate and phosphate of lime, which the test might throw down from any solution containing a salt of these acids. The last four precipitates are redissolved by a drop or two of hydrochloric acid ; but the oxalate is not taken up till a large quantity of that acid is added.

Sulphate of lime in solution causes a white precipitate with oxalic acid, and not with any other.*

Sulphate of copper causes a faint bluish-white, or greenish-white precipitate, which is not re-dissolved on the addition of a few drops of hydrochloric acid. The precipitate is the oxalate of copper. It is re-dissolved by a large proportion of hydrochloric acid.

This test does not precipitate the sulphates, hydrochlorates, nitrates, tartrates, citrates. But with the carbonates and phosphates it forms precipitates resembling the oxalate of copper. The oxalate, however, is distinguished from the carbonate and phosphate of copper by not being re-dissolved on the addition of a few drops of hydrochloric acid.

Nitrate of silver causes a dense, white precipitate, the oxalate of silver ; which, when collected on a filter, dried and heated, becomes brown on the edge, then fulminates faintly and is dispersed.

The object of the supplementary test of fulmination is to distinguish the oxalate of silver from the numberless other white precipitates which are thrown down by the nitrate of silver from solutions of other salts. The property of fulmination, which is very characteristic, requires, for security's sake, a word or two of explanation, in consequence of the effect of heat on the tartrate and citrate of silver. The citrate when heated becomes altogether brown, froths up, and then deflagrates, discharging white fumes and leaving an abundant, ash-gray, coarsely fibrous, crumbly residue, which on the farther application of heat becomes pure white, being then pure silver. The tartrate also becomes brown and froths up, but does not even deflagrate, white fumes are discharged, and there is left behind a botryoidal mass, which, like the residue from the citrate, becomes pure silver when heated to redness. Another distinction between the oxalate and tartrate is that the former continues permanent at the temperature of ebullition, while the latter becomes brown. The preceding process or combination of tests will be amply sufficient for proving the presence of oxalic acid, free or combined, in any fluid, which does not contain animal or vegetable principles.

2. The only important modifications in the analysis rendered ne-

* Mr. A. Taylor. Manual of Medical Jurisprudence, p. 120.

cessary by the admixture of organic principles, occur in the case of the contents of the alimentary canal or vomited matters.

Dr. Coindet and I proved, that oxalic acid has not any chemical action with any of the common animal principles except gelatin, which it rapidly dissolves; — and that this solution is of a peculiar kind, not being accompanied with any decomposition, either of the acid or of the gelatin.* Consequently oxalic acid, so far as concerns the tissues of the stomach or its ordinary contents, is not altered in chemical form, and remains soluble in water.

In such a solution, however, a variety of soluble principles are contained, which would cause abundant precipitates with two of the tests of the process, — sulphate of copper and nitrate of silver ; so that the oxalates of these metals could not possibly be detached in their characteristic forms. The process for a pure solution, therefore, is inapplicable to the mixtures under consideration.

But changes of still greater consequence are effected on the poison by exhibiting antidotes during life. It is now generally known, that the proper antidotes for oxalic acid are magnesia and chalk. Each of these forms an insoluble oxalate ; so that if either had been given in sufficient quantity, no oxalic acid will remain in solution, and the proofs of the presence of the poison must be sought for in the solid contents of the stomach or solid matter vomited.

The following process for detecting the poison will apply to all the alterations which it may thus have undergone.

Process for Compound Mixtures.—If chalk or magnesia has not been given as an antidote, the suspected mixture is to be macerated if necessary for a few hours in a little distilled water, then filtered, and the filtered fluid neutralized with carbonate of potass. If on the other hand chalk or magnesia has been given, the mixture is to be left at rest for some time, and the supernatant fluid then removed. This fluid, if not acid, may be thrown away; but if acid, it may be treated as already directed for a suspected mixture, where chalk or magnesia has not obtained entrance. After the removal of the supernatant liquid, pick out as many solid fragments of animal or vegetable matter as possible ; and add as much pure water to the insoluble residue as will give the mass a sufficiently thin consistence. Add now to the mixture about a twentieth of its weight of carbonate of potass, and boil gently for two hours, or till the organic matter is all dissolved. While dissolution thus takes place, a double interchange is effected between the elements of the carbonate of potass on the one hand, and those of the earthy oxalate on the other, so that an oxalate of potass will at length exist in solution. The fluid when cold is next to be filtered, then rendered very faintly acidulous with nitric acid, then filtered and rendered very faintly alkaline with carbonate of potass, and filtered a third time. At each of these steps some animal matter will be thrown down.

From this point onwards the process proceeds in the same way, whatever may have been the original form in which the acid existed

* Edin. Med. and Surg. Journal, xix. 168.

in the mixture; for the oxalate of lime or magnesia in the second case is converted into oxalate of potass.

Add now the solution of acetate of lead to the fluid as long as any precipitate is formed. Collect the precipitate on a filter, wash it well, and dry it by compression between folds of bibulous paper. Remove this precipitate, which consists of oxalate of lead and organic matter in union with oxide of lead, and rub it up very carefully while damp with a little water in a mortar. Transmit sulphuretted hydrogen gas briskly for an hour, so that the whole white precipitate shall be thoroughly blackened; filter and boil. In this manner is formed a sulphuret of lead, which retains a great deal of animal matter; and the oxalic acid being set free, is found in the solution tolerably pure. Filtration before boiling is an essential point in this step, to prevent animal matter being dissolved by the water from the sulphuret of lead. More animal matter may still be separated by evaporating the liquid to dryness at 212°, keeping it at that temperature for a few minutes, and re-dissolving and filtering. The solution will now exhibit the properties of oxalic acid.

I have found that when this process was applied to a decoction of an ounce of beef in six ounces of water, with which one grain of anhydrous oxalic acid had been mixed, all the tests acted characteristically on the solution ultimately procured. I have farther found, that when two grains of oxalate of lime, which correspond with one grain of oxalic acid, were mixed with a similar decoction in which some fragments of beef were purposely left to complicate the process, a solution was eventually obtained, which gave with muriate of lime a white precipitate insoluble in a little muriatic acid, with sulphate of copper a greenish-white precipitate also insoluble in a little muriatic acid, and with nitrate of silver a white precipitate which fulminated and was almost all dispersed, but left a little charcoal, owing to its containing a small proportion of animal matter. In a case which lately happened in London, every test acted as here described, except that the oxalate of lime did not fulminate, owing to the presence of organic impurities.* In order to try the test of fulmination in such circumstances, it is essential to dry the precipitated oxalate of silver thoroughly before raising the temperature to the point at which fulmination usually occurs.

The process now recommended is both delicate and accurate. An objection has been advanced against it, — that acetate of lead will throw down chloride of lead as well as the oxalate of lead; that both will subsequently be decomposed by the sulphuretted-hydrogen? and that the hydrochloric acid thus brought into the solution with the oxalic acid will be precipitated by the nitrate of silver, and form a mixture of salts which will not fulminate characteristically.† This objection is not well founded. Chloride of lead being soluble in thirty parts of temperate water, it will seldom be thrown down from such fluids as occur in medico-legal inquiries; and besides it is easily removed, as I have ascertained, by washing the precipitate with moderate care on the filter.

* Mr. Davies in Lancet, 1838-39, i. 30.   † Lancet, 1830-31, i. 197.

Professor Orfila has advanced another objection, — that the process will yield all the indications mentioned above, if binoxalate of potash be present, or sorrel-soup, which contains a little of that salt.* The objection is valid, were these substances apt to come in the way. But the binoxalate of potash is not put to any medicinal use in Britain, and English cookery does not acknowledge the " soupe à l'oseille." The process he recommends to meet the difficulty, an important one in France, is the following : 1. Having made a watery solution as above, evaporate nearly to dryness, agitate the residue with cold pure alcohol, repeatedly during a period of several hours ; decant the tincture, and repeat this step with more alcohol ; evaporate to obtain crystals, if possible ; dissolve these again in cold pure alcohol, and crystallize a second time by evaporation. If crystals do not form on first concentrating the alcoholic solution, evaporate it till a pellicle begins to form, agitate the residue with cold pure alcohol, and concentrate again to obtain crystals. Lastly, examine the crystals by the tests for pure oxalic acid. The object of these steps in the process is to separate binoxalate of potass, oxalate of magnesia and oxalate of lime, which, he says, are all either not soluble, or very sparingly so, in absolute alcohol. 2. More oxalic acid may be got by acting with distilled water on the matter left by the action of alcohol, evaporating this watery solution nearly to dryness, agitating the residuum with cold alcohol as before, and so on. 3. The preceding operations may have left oxalate of magnesia and oxalate of lime unacted on by the water among the solids remaining on the filter. The former compound may be dissolved out by cold hydrochloric acid diluted with four times its volume of water ; and by an excess of pure carbonate of potass, the oxalate of magnesia in the solution is converted into insoluble carbonate of magnesia and soluble oxalate of potass, from which oxalic acid is to be obtained by a salt of lead and sulphuretted-hydrogen, as explained in my own process. 4. Oxalate of lime, which may still remain, is to be sought for by boiling the residuum of the action of hydrochloric acid with solution of bicarbonate of potass, so as to obtain here also an oxalate of potass in solution. I have not had an opportunity of trying this method. But I find, that, contrary to Orfila's statement, binoxolate of potass, though sparingly soluble in cold alcohol of the density of 800, is sufficiently so to vitiate the principle on which the process is founded.

Caustic potash must not be used for decomposing oxalate of lime or magnesia, because the pure alkali, as Gay-Lussac has shown, produces oxalic acid in acting on animal substances at a boiling temperature. Carbonate of potass has no such effect.

The discovery of oxalic acid in the form of oxalate of lime in the stomach or vomited matter is exposed to a singular fallacy, if a material quantity of rhubarb has been taken recently before death, or before the discharge of the vomited matter. For according to the researches of M. Henry of Paris, rhubarb root always contains some

---

* Toxicologie Gén. 1843, i. 190.

oxalate of lime, and some samples yield so much as 30 and even 33 per cent.*

SECTION II. — *On the Action of Oxalic Acid and the Symptoms it causes in Man.*

The action of oxalic acid on the animal economy is very peculiar. When injected in a state of concentration into the stomach of a dog or cat, it causes exquisite pain, expressed by cries and struggling. In a few minutes this is succeeded by violent efforts to vomit; then by sudden dulness, languor, and great debility; and death soon takes place without a struggle. The period which elapses before death varies from two to twenty minutes, when the dose is considerable, — half an ounce, for example. After death the stomach is found to contain black extravasated blood, exactly like blood acted on by oxalic acid out of the body; the inner coat of the stomach is of a cherry-red colour, with streaks of black granular warty extravasation; and in some places the surface of the coat is very brittle and the subjacent stratum gelatinized, evidently by the chemical action of the poison.† If the stomach is examined immediately after death, little corrosion will be found, compared with what is seen if the inspection be delayed a day or two.‡

Such are the effects of the concentrated acid. When considerably diluted, the phenomena are totally different. When dissolved in twenty parts of water, oxalic acid, like the mineral acids in the same circumstances, cease to corrode; nay it hardly even irritates. But, unlike them, it continues a deadly poison; for it causes death by acting indirectly on the brain, spine, and heart. The symptoms then induced vary with the dose. When the quantity is large, the most prominent symptoms are those of palsy of the heart; and immediately after death that organ is found to have lost its contractility, and to contain arterial blood in its left cavities. When the dose is less the animal perishes after several fits of violent tetanus, which affects the respiratory muscles of the chest in particular, causing spasmodic fixing of the chest and consequent suffocation. When the dose is still less, the spasms are slight or altogether wanting, and death occurs under symptoms of pure narcotism like those caused by opium : the animal appears to sleep away.

This poison acts with violence, and produces nearly the same effects to whatever texture of the body it is applied. It causes death with great rapidity when injected into the sac of the peritonæum, or into that of the pleura; it acts with still greater quickness when injected into a vein; and it also acts when injected into the cellular tissue beneath the skin, but with much less celerity than through any other channel. Eight grains injected into the jugular vein of a dog occasioned almost immediate death : Thirty-three grains injected into the pleura killed another in twelve minutes. The same quan-

* Bulletins de Pharmacie, vi. 87.
† Edin. Med. and Surg Journal, xix. 166.   ‡ Ibid. 169.

tity did not prove fatal, though it caused violent effects, when retained in the stomach by a ligature on the gullet.   One hundred and
sixty grains injected under the skin of the thigh and belly did not
prove fatal for about ten hours.   The symptoms were nearly the same
in every case.*

It is probable from the facts now stated, that oxalic acid, when not
sufficiently concentrated to occasion death by the local injury produced, acts on the nervous system through the medium of the blood.
Nevertheless it is a remarkable circumstance that it cannot be detected
in that fluid.   Mention has already been made of an experiment performed by Dr. Coindet and myself (p. 22), where even after the injection of eight grains of oxalic acid into the femoral vein, and the
consequent death of the animal in thirty seconds, none of the poison
could be detected in the blood of the iliac vein or vena cava.   Similar results have been more lately obtained by Dr. Pommer.   In dogs
killed by the gradual injection of from five to thirty grains into the
femoral vein, he never could detect the poison in the blood of the
right side of the heart or great veins, except in the instance of the
largest doses, where a little could be detected near the opening in
the vein.   Dr. Pommer's experiments likewise agree with those of
Dr. Coindet and myself as to the absence of any change in the
physical qualities of the blood.†   When to these circumstances it is
added that very small quantities of oxalic acid may be detected in
blood, into which it has been introduced immediately after removal
from the body by venesection, it appears reasonable to conclude that
the poison is quickly decomposed in the blood by vital operations.

According to Orfila, however, it may be detected in the urine, in
which crystals of oxalate of lime form on cooling, and more may be
obtained on the addition of hydrochlorate of lime.   Yet he could not
detect any oxalic acid in the liver or spleen.‡

In man the most prominent symptoms hitherto observed have been
those of excessive irritation, because it has been almost always swallowed in a large dose and much concentrated.

It is the most rapid and unerring of all the common poisons.   The
London Courier contains an inquest on the body of a young man who
appears to have survived hardly ten minutes ;§ an equally rapid case
of a young lady, who poisoned herself with a ounce, is mentioned in
the St. James's Chronicle ;‖ and few of those who have died survived
above an hour.   This rule, however, is by no means without exception.   Mr. Hebb has described a case which did not prove
fatal for thirteen hours ;¶ Dr. Arrowsmith of Coventry has favoured
me with the particulars of a very interesting case which lasted for the
same period : and Mr. Frazer has accurately described another, in
which, after the patient seemed to be doing tolerably well, an ex-

* Edin. Med. and Surg. Journal, xix. *passim.*
† Medizinisch-Chirurgische Zeitung, 1828, ii. 203, 219, 235, 254.
‡ Toxicologie Gén. 1843, i. 187.   § London Courier, Feb. 1, 1823.
‖ St. James's Chronicle, August 17, 1826.
¶ London Medical Repository, xxii. 476.

hausting fever, with dyspepsia and singultus, carried him off in twenty-three days.*

Among the fatal cases the smallest dose has been half an ounce ; but there can be little doubt that less would be sufficient to cause death. Dr. Babington of Coleraine has published a case where very severe effects were produced by only two scruples.†

Very few persons have recovered where the quantity was considerable.

In every instance in which the dose was considerable, and the solution concentrated, the first symptoms have been immediate burning pain in the stomach, and generally also in the throat. But when the dose was small, more particularly if the solution was also rather diluted, the pain has sometimes been slight, or slow in commencing. Mr. Hebb's patient, who took only half an ounce dissolved in ten parts of water, and diluted it immediately after with copious draughts of water, had not any pain in the belly for six hours.

In general, violent vomiting follows the accession of pain, either immediately, or in a few minutes ; and it commonly continues till near death. Some, however, have not vomited at all, even when the acid was strong and in a large dose ; and this is still more apt to happen when the poison has been taken much diluted. The man last mentioned did not vomit at all for seven hours, except when emetics were administered. The vomited matter, as in this man's case, and in that of Mr. Frazer's patient, is sometimes bloody. Instant discharge of the poison by vomiting does not always save the patient's life : A woman who swallowed two ounces died in twenty minutes, although she vomited almost immediately after taking the poison.‡

The tongue and mouth occasionally become inflamed if the case lasts long enough. In an instance of recovery, which happened not long ago in St. Thomas's Hospital, London, the tongue was red, swollen, tense and tender, the day after the acid was swallowed.§

Death commonly takes place so soon, that the bowels are seldom much affected. But when life is prolonged a few hours, they are evidently much irritated. Dr. Arrowsmith's patient, who lived thirteen hours, had severe pain in the bowels and frequent inclination to go to stool, and Mr. Hebb's patient, who also lived thirteen hours, had a constant, involuntary discharge of fluid fæces, occasionally mixed with blood. Bloody diarrhœa is very common in dogs.

The signs of depressed circulation are always very striking. In general the pulse fails altogether, it is always very feeble, and the skin is cold and clammy. Contrary to the general fact, however, I once remarked in a dog the pulsation of the heart so strong as to be audible at a distance of several yards.

In some cases nervous symptoms have occurred, but in none so distinctly as in animals that have taken the diluted acid. It should

* Edin. Med. and Surg. Journal, xiv. 606.
† London Medical Gazette, 1842-43, i. 490.
‡ Edin. Med. and Surg. Journal, xix. 187. § London. Med. Gaz. i. 737.

be remarked, however, that few published cases contain good histories of the symptoms ; since they commonly come to an end before being seen by the physician.   Convulsions appear to have occurred in some instances either at the time of death or soon before it.   In the slower cases various nervous affections have been observed.   A girl, who swallowed by mistake about two drachms, and did not vomit till emetics were given, complained much at first of pain, but afterwards chiefly of great lassitude and weakness of the limbs, and next morning of numbness and weakness there as well as in the back. This affection was at first so severe that she could hardly walk up stairs ; but in a few days she recovered entirely.* ʻAnalogous effects took place in Mr. Hebb's patient and in Dr. Arrowsmith's case. The first thing the former complained of was acute pain in the back, gradually extending down the thighs, occasioning ere long great torture, and continuing almost till the moment of death.   Dr. Arrowsmith's patient had the same symptoms, complained more of the pain shooting down from the loins to the limbs than of the pain in the belly, and was constantly seeking relief in a fresh change of posture.   Mr. Frazer's patient had from an early period a peculiar general numbness, approaching to palsy.   Dr. Babington's patient, who took two scruples by mistake for tartaric acid in an effervescing draught, suffered, after the first twenty-four hours, chiefly from headache, extreme feebleness of the pulse, and a sense of numbness and tingling or pricking in the back and thighs.   In a recent case described by Mr. Tapson, which occurred in London, and where it was supposed, but on insufficient grounds,† that so much as two ounces had been taken, violent symptoms of irritation in the alimentary canal came on as usual, but soon afterwards a sense as if the hands were dead, loss of consciousness for eight hours, and then lividity, coldness, and almost complete loss of the power of motion in the legs ; which symptoms were not entirely removed for fifteen days.   In a case related by Mr. Alfred Taylor, where death was caused by seven drachms in fifteen or twenty minutes, there was first violent vomiting, then severe pain in the stomach, and finally clammy perspiration and convulsions, with two or three deep inspirations before death.‡   The effects in this case came very near those generally observed in animals.

In Dr. Arrowsmith's case two symptoms occurred, which I have not seen mentioned in any other.   The first was an eruption or mottled appearance of the skin in circular patches, not unlike the roundish red marks on the arms of stout healthy children, but of a deeper tint.   The second was the poisoning and death of leeches applied to the stomach.   " They were healthy," says Dr. Arrowsmith in the notes with which he obligingly furnished me, " small, and fastened

* Dr. Scott, in Edin. Med. and Surg. Journal, xxiv. 67.
† London Medical Gazette, 1842-43, i. 490.   The quantity could scarcely have been wo ounces, 1, because a penny-worth, which was what the person bought, amounts tonly to two drachms, and 2, because it could not have been dissolved, as the patient said was done, in four ounces of water.   The word *ounces* is probably a misprint for drachms.
‡ Guy's Hospital Reports, 1838, iii, 353.

immediately. On looking at them in a few minutes I remarked that they did not seem to fill, and on touching one it felt hard and immediately fell off, motionless and dead. The others were all in the same state. They had all bitten and the marks were conspicuous; but they had drawn scarcely any blood. They were applied about six hours after the acid was taken." This curious fact illustrates the observations formerly quoted from Vernière's experiments [p. 67]. It will be observed that the leeches were applied several hours after the poison was swallowed, and in a case in which the acid was largely diluted in the stomach; — so that it might have entered the blood and been diffused throughout the body before the observation was made.

SECTION III.— *Of the Morbid Appearances caused by Oxalic Acid.*

The external appearance of the body is commonly natural. In one instance the cellular tissue was distended with gases ten hours after death.* Violent marks of irritation have been commonly found in the stomach; and sometimes that organ has been even perforated.† It is probable that the extensive destruction of the coats noticed by some authors has taken place in part after death from the action of the acid on the dead tissues. — The usual conjunction of morbid appearances is well described by Mr. Hebb. The mucous coat of the throat and gullet looked as if it had been scalded, and that of the gullet could be easily scratched off. The stomach contained a pint of thick fluid. This is commonly dark, like coffee-grounds, as it contains a good deal of blood. The inner coat of the stomach was pulpy, in many points black, in others red. The inner membrane of the intestines was similarly but less violently affected. The outer coat of both stomach and intestines was inflamed. The lining membrane of the windpipe was also very red. — The appearances have also been excellently described in the case published by Mr. Alfred Taylor. The inside of the gullet was pale, as if boiled, strongly corrugated and brittle, and covering a ramification of vessels filled with consolidated blood. The stomach presented externally numerous vessels in the same state; and its villous coat was pale, soft, brittle, but here and there injected with vessels. The duodenum and part of the jejunum were red, the other intestines natural, the liver, spleen, and kidneys congested. The stomach contained a brownish jelly, in which gelatin was detected, as well as oxalic acid. The blood was fluid every where except in the vessels of the gullet and stomach.‡ The consolidated condition of the blood there was evidently owing to the local action of a strong acid, and is the same with what has been observed in poisoning with the mineral acids. — In Mr. Frazer's patient the whole villous coat of the stomach was either softened or removed, as well as the inner membrane of the gullet, so that the muscular coat was exposed; and this coat presented

* London Med. Repository, xi. 20.   † Ibid. vi. 474
‡ Guy's Hospital Reports, 1838, iii. 353,
18*

a dark gangrenous-like appearance, being much thickened and highly injected.

Although these signs of violent irritation are commonly present, it must at the same time be observed, that some cases have occurred where the stomach and intestines were quite healthy.   In a girl who died about thirty minutes after swallowing an ounce of the acid, no morbid appearance whatsoever was to be seen in any part of the alimentary canal.*   In the case of a girl, described by Mr. Anderson, where death took place in twenty minutes, there was no appearance but contraction of the rugæ of the gullet and stomach, one spot of extravasation in the latter and doubtful softening of its villous coat.†

The state of the other organs of the body has not been taken notice of in published cases.   In several instances, as in Mr. Taylor's case, the blood in the veins of the stomach is described as having been black and as it were charred ; probably by the chemical action of the acid after death.

SECTION IV. — *Of the Treatment of Poisoning with Oxalic Acid.*

The chief part of the treatment of this kind of poisoning is obvious.   On account of its dreadful rapidity, remedies cannot be of material use unless they are resorted to immediately after the acid has been swallowed.   Emetics may be given, if vomiting is not already free ; but time should never be lost in administering them if an antidote is at hand.   In particular it is necessary to avoid giving warm water with a view to accelerate vomiting, unless it is given very largely ; for moderate dilution will promote the entrance of the poison into the blood, if it has not the effect of immediately expelling it.

The principal object of the practitioner should be to administer as speedily as possible large doses of magnesia or chalk suspended in water.   Chalk has been given with great advantage in several cases,‡ and magnesia has also been of service.§   As no time should be lost, the plaster of the apartment may be resorted to, when chalk or magnesia is not at hand.   These substances not only neutralize the acid so as to take away its corrosive power, but likewise render it insoluble, so as to prevent it from entering the blood.   There appears no particular reason for using the stomach-pump when antidotes are at hand.   But fashion seems to have authorised the employement of this instrument for every kind of poison.|| Alkalis are inadmissible. As might be inferred from the general statements formerly made on the effect of chemical changes on poisons [p. 28], the alkalis, as they form only soluble salts, will not deprive oxalic acid of its remote or indirect action ; and instances are not wanting of their inutility in actual practice.

* London Med. Repository, iii. 380.
† Lancet, 1838-39, ii. 748.
‡ London Medical Repository, xii. 18.   London Medical Gazette, i. 737.   Edinburgh Medical and Surgical Journal, xxiv. 67.
§ Edin. Med. and Surg. Journal, xiv. 607.
|| London Medical Gazette, i. 737.

Oxalic acid is one of the poisons alluded to under the head of General Poisoning, — of whose operation distinct evidence may sometimes (though certainly not always) be found in the symptoms. If a person, immediately after swallowing a solution of a crystalline salt, which tasted purely and strongly acid, is attacked with burning in the throat, then with burning in the stomach, vomiting particularly of bloody matter, imperceptible pulse and excessive languor, and dies in half an hour, or still more in twenty, fifteen, or ten minutes, I do not know any fallacy which can interfere with the conclusion, that oxalic acid was the cause of death. No parallel disease begins so abruptly and terminates so soon ; and no other crystalline poison has the same effects.

Poisoning with the Oxalates. — Oxalic acid is one of the best examples of a poison that acts throngh all its soluble chemical combinations. Dr. Coindet and I found that the oxalates of potash and ammonia are little inferior in energy to the acid. They do not corrode, indeed, and scarcely ever irritate ; but they produce tetanus and coma, like the diluted acid. Half a drachm of oxalic acid neutralized with potass will kill a rabbit in seventeen minutes ; ninety grains of neutral oxalate of ammonia will kill a strong cat in nine minutes.* The binoxalate of potash, the most familiar of the salts of oxalic acid, was not tried by us. But the preceding facts would leave little doubt of its being a poison.

Since the last edition of this work was published several cases have occurred which amply confirm the results of experimental inquiry. In Dr. Babington's case alluded to above, the greater part of the oxalic acid had been neutralized by bicarbonnte of soda [p. 176]. — Mr. Tripier has communicated the particulars of a case in which half an ounce of the binoxalate of potash was taken by mistake for bitartrate of potash in hot water, and caused death in eight minutes, after an attack of violent pain and convulsions.† — A young woman at Bordeaux was attacked with frequent vomiting after a dose of a drachm and a half of the same salt dissolved in a ptisane. Next morning a similar dose caused bloody vomiting and acute pain at the pit of the stomach ; and a third dose the following day excited delirium, more violent vomiting, and death in the course of an hour.‡ — A girl in London swallowed about an ounce of the same salt dissolved in hot water. Sickness and faintness ensued, with imperceptible pulse, cold, clammy skin, rigors, scalding of the mouth and throat, pain in the back, soreness of the eyes, redness of the conjunctivæ, and dilatation of the pupils. Afterwards there was reaction, with a full frequent pulse, hot skin, flushed countenance, headache, thirst, and tenderness of the abdomen. She recovered under the use of chalk, external heat, ether and opium draughts, leeches and sinapisms to the belly, and carbonate of ammonia.§

* Edinburgh Med. and Surg. Journal, xix. 190.
† Journal de Chim. Med. 1842, 211, and Orfila, Toxicologie Gén. 1843, i. 195.
‡ Annales d'Hyg. Publique, 1842, xxvii. 422.
§ Lond Med. Gazette, 1840-41, i. 480.

No account has yet been published of the morbid appearances in man.

The proper antidote is sulphate of magnesia. Failing this, weak milk of lime may be given with advantage.

Appendix on Tartaric and Citric Acid. — These two acids may be taken in considerable quantities without injury. Dr. Coindet and I gave a drachm of each in solution to cats, without observing that the animals suffered any inconvenience.* Dr. Sibbald, a surgeon of this place, has informed me of an instance in which a patient of his took in twenty-four hours six drachms of tartaric acid, having by mistake omitted the carbonate of potass sent along with the acid to make effervescing draughts; and yet he did not suffer any more inconvenience then the cats on which Dr. Coindet and I experimented.

Pommer, however, found that tartaric acid is scarcely less active than oxalic acid when injected into the blood. When fifteen grains dissolved in half an ounce of water were injected into the femoral vein of a dog in four doses, difficult breathing and discharge of fæces and urine were produced after each operation, and death speedily ensued without any other particular symptom. As in the instance of oxalic acid, the blood in the great veins was not apparently changed in any of its physical qualities. The heart continued contractile long after death, while in the case of oxalic acid its contractility was suddenly extinguished.†

CHAPTER VII.

OF THE ALKALIS AND ALKALINE SALTS.

THE second order of the class of irritants comprehends the alkalis, some of the alkaline salts, and lime. The species which it includes are little allied to one another except in chemical composition; and in particular they are little allied in physiological properties. It appears impossible, however, to make a better arrangement than that proposed by Orfila, which will therefore be here followed.

Most of the poisons of the second order are powerful local irritants. Some of them likewise act indirectly on distant organs; and a few are more distinguished by their remote than by their local effects. This order may be conveniently divided into two groups, — the one embracing the two fixed alkalis with their carbonates, nitrates, and chlorides, and also lime, — the other ammonia, with its salts, and likewise the alkaline sulphurets.

The action of the first group is purely irritant and strictly local. When concentrated, the fixed alkalis and their carbonates produce chemical decomposition, softening the animal tissues, and reducing

* Edin. Med. and Surg. Journal, xix. 185.
† Medizinisch-Chirurgische Zeitung, 1828, ii. 255.

them eventually to a pulpy mass; which change depends on their possessing the power, as chemical agents, of dissolving almost all the soft solids of the body. When much diluted, they produce inflammation, without corroding the textures; and it does not appear that they are even then absorbed in such quantity as to prove injurious to any remote organ. The action of the alkaline nitrates and of lime is that of irritants only; at least their chemical action is obscure and feeble.

Of the Fixed Alkalis and their Carbonates.

SECTION I. — Of their Tests.

Potass in its caustic state, as usually met with in the shops, forms little gray-coloured cylinders or cakes which have a radiated, crystalline fracture, and an excessively acrid caustic taste, and feel soapy if touched with the wet finger. It deliquesces rapidly in moist air, and then attracts carbonic acid from the atmosphere. It is easily fused by heat, and is exceedingly soluble in water. The solution has a strong alkaline reaction on vegetable colours, restoring reddened litmus to blue, turning syrup of violets or infusion or red cabbage to green, and rendering infusion of turmeric brown. It is distinguished from the alkaline earths when in solution, by not precipitating with carbonic or sulphuric acid, and from soda by the tests to be presently mentioned for its carbonate.

Carbonate of potash [subcarbonate, salt of tartar], is usually sold, when pure, in small white grains, formed by melting the salt and stirring it rapidly as it cools. In its impure state it is called in this country potashes, and when somewhat purified, pearl ash. It has then a mixed grayish, yellowish, or bluish colour, and is sold in crumbly lumps of various sizes. In every state it is deliquescent and very caustic. It cannot be crystallized. It gives out carbonic acid gas with the addition of any stronger acid, such as sulphuric, muriatic, or acetic acid. Its solution precipitates yellow with the chloride of platinum, gives a crystalline precipitate with perchloric acid, when the salt forms not less than a fortieth or fiftieth part, — is similarly acted on by a considerable excess of tartaric acid, if the salt constitute about a thirtieth of the fluid, — and yields with the soluble salts of baryta a white precipitate soluble in nitric acid.

Soda resembles potass closely in chemical as well as physiological properties; and the *carbonate* bears the same resemblance to the carbonate of potass. The chief differences are the following. The carbonate of soda is easily crystallized, and effloresces on exposure to the air. A solution in twenty parts of water yields no precipitate with either perchloric acid or an excess of tartaric acid, because there is no sparingly soluble perchlorate or bitartrate, as in the case of potash. Its solution is precipitated by antimoniate of potash, because the antimoniate of soda is very sparingly soluble. All its salts remain unaffected by the chloride of platinum, because their base cannot form like potass an insoluble triple salt with the reagent. The acetate of soda is permanent in the air, while the acetate of potass is one of the most deliquescent salts known. In trying this last test, which is very characteristic, care must be taken to avoid an excess of acid in the acetate of soda by expelling it at a temperature of 212°, otherwise the salt is as deliquescent as the acetate of potass. — Another difference is, that the chloride of sodium, being nearly as soluble in temperate as in boiling water, crystallizes with difficulty and but sparingly by cooling a concentrated boiling solution ; while the chloride of potassium is much more soluble in hot than in cold water, and crystallizes easily and abundantly when a concentrated boiling solution is cooled down.

Process for Potash and its Carbonate in Organic Mixtures. — The following method has been lately recommended for the detection of potash and its carbonate in complex organic mixtures. Ascertain that the mixture is alkaline in its action on litmus-paper and turmeric-paper, and that it is not ammoniacal in odour. Distil to one-third ; ascertain that it has still an alkaline reaction, and evaporate to dryness in a porcelain basin. Agitate the residue, when cold, with absolute alcohol; boil, pour off the liquor, and filter it while hot. Repeat this with the residuum and more alcohol. Distil off most of the alcohol, and evaporate to dryness. Raise the heat to char the residuum, continue the heat as long as vapours come off, remove the charcoaly matter, and incinerate it for forty-five minutes in a silver crucible. Try to separate potash from what remains by means of absolute alcohol ; and if this do not succeed, remove carbonate of potash by boiling water. In either case search for potash by litmus-paper, turmeric-paper, chloride of platinum, and perchloric acid.*

The conclusiveness of this process depends upon the fact, that absolute alcohol cannot dissolve from solid organic substances such a proportion of lactate, tartrate, acetate, sulphate, or phosphate of potash, or chloride of potassium, as to be acted on by chloride of platinum or perchloric acid.† — It is to be observed that carbonate of potash singly is insoluble in absolute alcohol ; but it becomes soluble in that fluid, when it is conjoined with various organic matters. Hence it is that this process, intended fundamentally for caustic potash alone, is applicable to carbonate of potash also.

Process for Soda and its Carbonate in Organic Mixtures. — These substances may be separated by the method just described for potash. If the alcoholic solution of the extract of the suspected matter be alkaline in its action on litmus, and be afterwards found to contain soda or its carbonate, the evidence of these substances having been derived from without is satisfactory, because the carbonate of soda contained in many animal matters cannot be so detached. But if no indications of the presence of soda be thus obtained, it is not enough that soda be found in the alcoholic solution of the incinerated alco-

* Orfila, in Journal de Chimie Médicale, 1842, 145.
† Annales d'Hygiène, Publique, 1842, xxviii. 206.

holic extract, because the natural carbonate of soda of animal matter may be separated in that manner.*

SECTION II. — *Of the Action of the fixed Alkalis, and the Symptoms they cause in Man.*

The action of the two fixed alkalis and their carbonates on the animal system is so nearly the same, that the facts which have been ascertained in respect to one of them will apply to all the rest. The operation of potass and its carbonate has been carefully investigated by Professor Orfila,† and by M. Bretonneau of Tours.‡

When caustic potass is injected in minute portions into the veins, it instantly coagulates the blood. Five grains, according to Orfila, will in this way kill a dog in two minutes. But when small doses either of potash itself, or its carbonate, or indeed any of its salts are used, Mr. Blake found, that without coagulating the blood, they arrested the action of the heart in ten seconds, if injected into the jugular vein; and that when they were injected into the carotid artery, they occasioned in four seconds signs of great obstruction in the capillary circulation, and arrestment of the heart's action in thirty-five minutes, through means of this effect. Next to the salts of baryta he thought the potash salts the most powerful on the heart's action of all those he tried.§ When introduced into the stomach potash acts powerfully as an irritant, and generally corrodes the coats of that organ. Thirty-two grains given by Orfila to a dog caused pain in the gullet, violent vomiting, much anguish, restlessness, and death on the third day. On dissection he found the inner coat of the gullet and stomach black and red; and near the pylorus there was a perforation three-quarters of an inch wide, and surrounded by a hard, elevated margin. The observations of Bretonneau are in some respects different. When potass was swallowed by dogs in the dose of 40 grains, he found that the animals, after suffering for some time from violent vomiting, always died sooner or later of wasting and exhaustion; and that the action of the poison was confined chiefly to the gullet, which was extensively destroyed and ulcerated on its inner surface. But when the gullet was defended by the potass being passed at once into the stomach in a caustic holder, larger doses, even several times repeated, did not prove fatal. The usual violent symptoms of irritation prevailed for two or three days; but on these subsiding, the animals rapidly recovered their appetite and playfulness, appearing in fact to be restored to perfect health. Yet there could be no doubt that the stomach all the while was severely injured; for in some of the animals, which were strangled for the sake of examination several weeks after they took the poison, the villous coat was found extensively removed, and even the muscular and

* Journal de Chimie Médicale, 1842, 197.
† Toxicol. Gén. i. 164, 3me Edition.
‡ Ibid. 166, and also Archives Gén. de Méd. xiii. 373.
§ Edin. Med. and Surg. Journal, li. 335, lvi. 345, lvi. 123.

peritonæal coats were here and there destroyed and cicatrized. Bretonneau farther adds, that ten or fifteen grains introduced into the rectum caused death sooner than three times as much given by the mouth.

The carbonate of potass possesses properties similar in kind, but inferior in degree to those of the caustic alkali. Two drachms given by Orfila to a dog killed it in twenty-five minutes, violent vomiting and great agony having preceded death. The stomach was universally of a deep red colour on its inner surface.

Potash and its carbonate are absorbed in the course of their action, and may be detected by Orfila's process in the liver, kidneys, and urine.*

The actions of soda and its carbonate seem on the whole the same with those of potash; but they are not so energetic. In one respect however soda and its salts differ most materially from those of potash. For while the latter, when admitted directly into a vein, act by arresting the action of the heart, soda and its salts, according to the inquiries of Mr. Blake, have no such effect, but cause death by obstructing the circulation of the pulmonary capillaries, and preventing the return of blood from the lungs to the left side of the heart. This conclusion seems to flow from the following facts. The respiration becomes in a few seconds laborious and soon ceases, whilst the heart continues to beat vigorously: arterial pressure is greatly reduced, while venous pressure is much increased owing to accumulation of blood in the right side of the heart: after death the lungs are found congested and often full of froth: and the heart continues contractile, very turgid in the right side, but quite empty of blood in its left cavities.†

Poisoning with the caustic alkalis is rare. In 1842, a lady suffering from inflammation of the bowels took an ounce of solution of potass by mistake for kali-water, or a solution of bicarbonate of potash surcharged with carbonic acid. She suffered severely at the time, and died in a fortnight, probably of the conjunct effects of her disease and the poison.‡ This is the only case I have found in print of poisoning with a caustic alkali. But the effects of their carbonates have been several times witnessed, and appear to resemble closely those of the concentrated mineral acids.

The symptoms are in the first instance an acrid burning taste, and rapid destruction of the lining membrane of the mouth; then burning and often constriction in the throat and gullet, with difficult and painful deglutition; violent vomiting, often sanguinolent, and tinging vegetable blues green; next acute pain in the stomach and tenderness of the whole belly; subsequently cold sweats, excessive weakness, hiccup, tremors and twitches of the extremities; and ere long violent colic pains, with purging of bloody stools and dark membranous flakes. So far the symptoms are nearly the same in

* Annales d'Hyg. Publique, xxviii. 212.
† Edin. Med. and Surg. Journal, liv. 341.
‡ London Medical Gazette, 1842-43, i. 188.

all cases; but in their subsequent course several varieties may be noticed.

In the worst form of poisoning death ensues at an early period, for example within twenty-four hours, nay even before time enough has elapsed for diarrhœa to begin. A case of this kind, which has been very well described by Mr. Dewar of Dunfermline, and which arose from the patient, a boy, having accidentally swallowed about three ounces of a strong solution of carbonate of potass, proved fatal in twelve hours only.* Here death was owing to the general system or some vital organ being affected through sympathy by the injury sustained by the alimentary canal.

In the mildest form, as in a case related by Plenck† of a man who swallowed an ounce of the carbonate of potass, the symptoms represent pretty nearly an attack of acute gastritis when followed by recovery, — the effects on man being then analogous to those observed by Bretonneau in animals, when the poison was introduced into the stomach without touching the gullet.

But a more common form than either of the preceding is one, similar to the chronic form of poisoning with the mineral acids, in which constant vomiting of food and drink, incessant discharge of fluid, sanguinolent stools, difficulty of swallowing, burning pain from the mouth to the anus, and rapid emaciation, continue for weeks or even months before the patient's strength is exhausted; and where death is evidently owing to starvation, the alimentary canal being no longer capable of assimilating food. Two characteristic examples of this singular affection have been recorded in the Medical Repository,‡ and a third, of which the event has not been mentioned, but which would in all likelihood end fatally, has been communicated by M. Jules Cloquet to Orfila.§ Of the two first cases, which were caused by half an ounce of carbonate of potass having been taken in solution by mistake for a laxative salt, one proved fatal in little more than a month, the other three weeks afterwards. In Cloquet's case, at the end of the sixth week the membrane of the mouth was regenerated; but the gullet continued to discharge pus, and the stools were purulent and bloody.

Another form perhaps equally common with that just described, and not less certainly fatal, commences like the rest with violent symptoms of irritation in the mouth, gullet, and stomach; but the bowels are not affected, and by and by it becomes apparent that the stomach is little injured; dysphagia or even complete inability to swallow, burning pain and constriction in the gullet, hawking and coughing of tough, leathery flakes, are then the leading symptoms; at length the case becomes one of stricture of the œsophagus with or without ulceration; the bougie gives only temporary relief, and the patient eventually expires either of mere starvation, or of that combined with an exhausting fever. Mr. Dewar has related a very striking

* Edin Med. and Surg. Journal, xxx. 310.   † Toxicologia, p. 225.
‡ London Med. Repository, vii. 118.   § Orfila, Toxic. Gén. i. 167.

19

example of this form of poisoning with the alkalis.* His patient, after the first violent symptoms had exhausted themselves, which took place in sixteen or eighteen hours, suffered little for four or five days till the sloughs began to separate from the lining membrane of the mouth, throat, and gullet. The affection of the gullet then became gradually predominant, and terminated in stricture, of which she appears to have been several times so much relieved as to have been thought in a fair way of recovery. After repeatedly disappointing Mr. Dewar's hopes of a successful issue by her intemperance in the use of spirituous liquors, she died of starvation about four months after swallowing the poison. Sir Charles Bell has noticed three parallel cases, and has given delineations of the appearance in the gullet of two of them.† One of his patients did not die till twenty years after swallowing the poison, which in this instance was soap-lees; yet he does not hesitate to ascribe the stricture to that cause, and says death arose purely from starvation.

The carbonate of soda, though a salt in very common use, has not hitherto been the cause of accident, which has found its way into print. It is plainly much less actively corrosive than carbonate of potass, and is therefore probably in every sense less energetic.

SECTION III.— *Of the Morbid Appearances caused by the fixed Alkalis.*

The morbid appearances caused by potass, soda, and their carbonates differ with the nature of the case.

In the boy who died in twelve hours Mr. Dewar found the inner membrane of the throat and gullet almost entirely disorganized and reduced to a pulp, with blood extravasated between it and the muscular coat. The inner coat of the stomach was red, in two round patches destroyed, and the patches covered with a clot of blood ;— its outer coat, as well as all the other abdominal viscera, was sound.

In the two chronic cases mentioned in the Medical Repository the mischief was much more general, the whole peritonæum being condensed, the omentum dark and turgid, the intestines glued together by lymph, the external coats of the stomach thick, the villous coat almost all destroyed, what remained of it red and near the pylorus ulcerated, and the pyloric orifice of the stomach plugged up with lymph so as barely to admit a small probe.

In Mr. Dewar's patient who died of stricture of the gullet the intestines were sound, the inner surface of the stomach red especially towards the cardia, the inner and muscular coats of the gullet thickened and firmly incorporated together by effused lymph, the inner coat here and there wanting, the passage of the gullet every where contracted, and to such a degree about two inches above the cardia as hardly to pass a common probe. In Sir C. Bell's cases the appearances were similar.

Orfila says he is led to conclude from a great number of facts that

* Edin. Med. and Surg. Journ. xxx. 310.
† Surgical Observations, Part i. 82.

of all corrosive poisons potass is the one which most frequently per-forates the stomach.* This appearance, however, has not been mentioned in any case of poisoning in the human subject.

SECTION IV. — *Of the Treatment of Poisoning with the fixed Alkalis.*

In the treatment of poisoning with the alkalis the first object is evidently to neutralize the poison. This may be done either with a weak acid, or with oil. Of the acids the acetic in the form of vinegar is most generally recommended, as it is not itself injurious. A suc-cessful case in very unpromising circumstances, where two ounces and a half of carbonate of potash had been taken by mistake for cream of tartar, and where the antidote was not administered for half an hour, has been related by M. Liégard of Caen. Great relief was experienced to the burning in the throat and stomach, the chilliness, difficult breathing, and frequent efforts to vomit, which were the first symptoms; and after repeated alternations of collapse and reaction, convalescence was established in eight days.† — M. Chereau thinks that for the mineral alkalis and their carbonates fixed oil is a pre-ferable antidote to vinegar ; and he has given the heads of two cases of poisoning with large doses of carbonate of potass, in which the free employment of almond oil prevented the usual fatal consequences. It appears to act partly by rendering the vomiting free and easy, partly by converting the alkali into a soap. It must be given in large quantity, several pounds being commonly required.‡ For the subsequent treatment the reader may consult the paper of Mr. Dewar, which contains many useful hints on the management of the most complex description of cases.

CHAPTER VIII.

OF POISONING WITH NITRATE OF POTASS.

THE *nitrate of potass* [nitre, saltpetre, sal-prunelle], is a dan-gerous poison. It has been often mistaken for the saline laxatives, especially the sulphate of soda, and has thus been the source of fatal accidents.

SECTION I. — *Of the Chemical Tests for Nitrate of Potass.*

It exists in commerce and the arts in two forms, fused and crys-tallized. The fused nitre [sal-prunelle] is sold in little button-shaped masses, spheres of the size of musket-balls, or larger circular cakes, of a snow-white tint. The crystallized salt [sal-pêtre] is sold in whitish, sulcated crystals, which are often regular and large. They

* Toxic. Gén. i. 169. † Bulletin de l'Acad Roy. de Méd. 1836, i. 151.
‡ Journal de Pharmacie, ix. 355, or Med. Repos. xx. 441.

are six-sided prisms, more or lest flattened, and terminated by two converging planes. In both forms nitre has a peculiar, cool, but sharp taste.

Its chemical properties are characteristic. In the solid form, it animates the combustion of burning fuel, and yields nitrous fumes when heated with strong sulphuric acid. In solution it is precipitated yellow by the chloride of platinum, and yields, when not greatly diluted, a crystalline precipitate with perchloric acid. The crude salt of commerce contains chloride of sodium ; and hence the odour disengaged by sulphuric acid may be mixed with that of chlorine or hydrochloric acid gas. When mixed with any vegetable or animal infusion by which it is coloured, crystals may sometimes be easily procured in a state of sufficient purity by filtration and evaporation. But if not, then the same process must be resorted to with that formerly recommended for nitric acid (p. 143), the first step of neutralization with potass being of course dispensed with. — A process nearly the same with this has been suggested by M. Kramer of Milan. He proposes to free the liquid in part of animal matter by adding acetate of lead, transmitting sulphuretted-hydrogen through the filtered fluid to remove any excess of lead, boiling the fluid after another filtration, and then proceeding with acetate of silver to remove chlorides, as in the process I have adopted. In this way he found nitre even in the blood.*

SECTION II. — *Of the Action of Nitrate of Potass and its Symptoms in Man.*

This substance forms an exception to the general law formerly laid down with regard to the effect of chemical neutralization on the local irritants. Both its acid and its alkali are simple irritants ; yet the compound salt, though certainly much inferior in power, is still energetic. Nay, the experiment of Orfila and the particulars of some recently published cases tend even to prove, that the action of its alkali and acid is materially altered in kind by their combination with one another ; for, besides inflaming the part to which it is applied, nitre has at times produced symptoms of a secondary disorder of the brain and nerves.

The experiments of Orfila upon dogs show that on these animals it has a twofold action, the one irritating, the other narcotic. He found that an ounce and a half killed a dog in ninety minutes when the gullet was tied, and a drachm another in twenty-nine hours : that death was preceded by giddiness, slight convulsions, dilated pupil, insensibility and palsy ; that after death the stomach was externally livid, internally reddish-black, and the heart filled in its left cavities with florid blood ; that when the gullet was not tied the animals recovered after several attacks of vomiting, and general indisposition for twenty-four hours ; and that when the salt was applied externally to a wound it excited violent inflammation, passing on to

* Annales d'Hygiène Publique, xxix. 417.

gangrene, but without any symptom which indicated a remote or indirect operation.* Mr. Blake found that this salt, when injected into the veins of a dog in the dose of fifteen grains dissolved in twenty-four parts of water, causes sudden depression and arrestment of the action of the heart, and death in less than a minute ; but that, like other salts of potash, it has no influence on the capillaries of the lungs, though a powerful effect in obstructing the systemic capillary system.† — When taken in the ordinary way, it is absorbed in the course of its action, and has been detected both in the blood and the urine by Kramer of Milan.‡

As to its effects on man, it must first be observed, that considerable doses are necessary to cause serious mischief. In the quantity of one, two, or three scruples, it is given medicinally several times a day without injury ; and Dr. Alexander found by experiments on himself, that an ounce and a half, if largely diluted, might thus be safely administered in the course of twenty-four hours.§ Sometimes, too, even large single doses have been swallowed with impunity. A gentleman of my acquaintance once took nearly an ounce by mistake for Glauber's salt, and retained it above a quarter of an hour : nevertheless, except several attacks of vomiting, no unpleasant symptom was induced. M. Tourtelle has even related an instance where two ounces were retained altogether and caused only moderate griping, with considerable purging and flow of urine.‖ Resting on such facts as these Tourtelle, with some physicians in more recent times,¶ has maintained that nitre is not a worse poison than other saline laxatives ; and some practitioners of the present day have consequently ventured to administer it for the cure of diseases, in the quantity of half an ounce in one dose.** It is not easy to say, why these large doses are at times borne by the stomach without injury, — whether the cause is idiosyncrasy, or a constitutional insensibility engendered by disease, or some difference in the mode of administering the salt. But at all events, the facts which follow will leave no doubt that in general it is a dangerous and rapid poison in the dose of an ounce.

Dr. Alexander found that, in the quantity of a drachm or a drachm and a half, recently dissolved in four ounces of water, and repeated every ninety minutes, the third or fourth dose caused chilliness and stinging pains in the stomach and over the whole body ; and these sensations became so severe with the fourth dose, that he considered it unsafe to attempt a fifth.††

Two cases which were actually fatal have been described in the Journal de Médecine for 1787, the one caused by one ounce, the other by an ounce and a half. In the latter the symptoms were those of the most violent cholera, and the patient died in two days and a

* Toxic. Gén. i. 193. † Edinburgh Med. and Surg. Journal, li. 334, liv. 346.
‡ Annales d'Hygiène Publique, xxix. 415.
§ Experimental Essays, p. 113.
‖ Journal de Médecine, lxxiii. 22.
¶ Tartra sur l'empoisonnement par l'acide nitrique, 136.
** London Med. Repository, xxiii. 523.
†† Experimental Essays, pp. 114, 115.
19*

half;[*] in the former death took place in three hours only, and in addition to the symptoms remarked in the other there were convulsions and twisting of the mouth.[†] In both the pulse failed at the wrist, and a great tendency to fainting prevailed for some time before death. Dr. Geoghegan has communicated to Mr. Taylor a case where an ounce and a half taken by mistake caused severe pain in the stomach, vomiting, and death in two hours.[‡]

Similar effects have been remarked in several cases which have been followed by recovery. A woman in the second month of pregnancy, immediately after taking a handful of nitre in solution, was attacked with pain in the stomach, swelling of the whole body and general pains; she then miscarried, and afterwards had the usual symptoms of gastritis and dysentery, united with great giddiness, ringing in the ears, general tremors and excessive chilliness. She seems to have made a narrow escape, as for three days the discharges by stool were profuse, and composed chiefly of blood and membranous flakes.[§] Dr. Falconer has related another instance, where also the patient's life seems to have been in great danger. The quantity taken was two ounces, and it was swallowed in half a pint of warm water by mistake instead of a laxative salt. Violent pain in the belly was immediately produced, in half an hour frequent vomiting, and in three hours a discharge of about a quart of blood from the stomach. After the administration of gruel and butter the symptoms began to subside; but they receded slowly; and even six months afterwards the man, though otherwise in good health, had frequent pain in the stomach and flatulence.[||] In the case of a female in the second month of pregnancy, described by Dr. Butter, miscarriage did not take place, although the symptoms were very violent and lasting. The quantity taken was two ounces. The symptoms were first bloody vomiting, afterwards dysentery, which continued seven days; and on the tenth day a nervous affection supervened exactly like chorea, and of two months' duration.[¶] The effects of the poison in the latter period of this woman's illness tend to establish the existence of a secondary operation on the nervous system. But this kind of action is more strongly pointed out by the following cases. Three puerperal women in the Obstetric Hospital of Pavia got each an ounce of nitre by mistake for sulphate of magnesia. Two, who vomited immediately, did not suffer. The third, who retained the salt fifteen minutes, had pain in the stomach and vomiting, followed by paleness of the countenance, stiffness of the jaw, some stupor, and convulsive movements of the limbs; which symptoms continued till next day, when she gradually recovered.[**] A German physician, Dr. Geiseler, met with an instance, in which the only disorder pro-

* Souville in Journal de Médecine, lxxiii. 19.
† Laflize in Journ. de Méd. lxxi. 401.
‡ Manual of Medical Jurisprudence, 1844, 130.
§ Alexander, Experimental Essays, p. 109.
|| Memoirs of London Med. Society, iii. 527.
¶ Edin. Med. and Surg. Journ. xiv. 34.
** Annali Univers. di Medicina, 1836, iii. 333.

duced appeared to depend on derangement of the cerebral functions. A woman, after swallowing an ounce of nitre instead of Glauber's salt, lost the use of speech and the power of voluntary motion, then became insensible, and was attacked with tetanic spasms.   This state lasted till next day, when some amelioration was brought about by copious sweating.   It was not, however, till eight days after, that she recovered her speech, or the entire use of her mental faculties ; and the palsy of the limbs continued two months.*   Her case resembles the account given by Orfila of the effects of nitre on animals.

SECTION III. — *Of the Morbid Appearances caused by Nitrate of Potass.*

The morbid appearances observed in man are solely those of violent inflammation of the stomach and intestines.   In Laflize's case, which proved fatal in three hours, the stomach was distended, and the contents deeply tinged with blood ; its peritonæal coat of a dark red colour mottled with black spots ; its villous coat very much inflamed and detached in several places.   The liquid contents gave satisfactory evidence of nitre having been swallowed ; for a portion evaporated to dryness deflagrated with burning charcoal.   In Souville's patient, who lived sixty hours, the stomach was every where red, in many places checkered with black spots, and at the centre of one of these spots the stomach was perforated by a small aperture. The whole intestinal canal was also red.   In Dr. Geoghegan's case, the stomach contained bloody mucus, and its villous coat was brownish-red, and here and there detached.   He could not detect any nitre in it.

CHAPTER IX.

OF POISONING WITH THE ALKALINE AND EARTHY CHLORIDES.

THERE can be little doubt that the *chlorides* of *soda, potass,* and *lime* are active poisons; but the first two have alone been hitherto carefully investigated by physiological experiments.

The two alkaline chlorides are usually seen in the form of colourless solutions.   That of potass is little known in this country ; but that of soda is familiar to all in the shape of Fincham's chloride of soda or bleaching liquid.   The chloride of lime, which is best known of them all, is usually in the form of a dry powder, deliquescent, and acrid, commonly termed bleaching powder.   All these substances are easily known by their peculiar odour of chlorine, and the copious disengagement of that gas on the addition of sulphuric acid.

The action of chloride of soda on the animal body has been examined by Segalas, who infers that it is an irritant poison, which, however, at times occasions symptoms of an affection of the nervous

* Journal der Praktischen, Heilkunde, lvii. i. 124.

system. He remarked that three ounces of the solution, commonly sold in Paris under the name of Labarraque's disinfecting liquid, caused immediate death by coagulating the blood in the heart, when injected into a vein in a dog. Two ounces introduced into the peritonæum excited palpitation, oppressed breathing, constant restlessness, and death in ten minutes ; and three drachms did not prove fatal for some hours, tetanic spasms being produced in the first instance, and peritonæal inflammation being found after death. One ounce introduced into the stomach of a dog excited immediate vomiting, and no farther inconvenience ; and two ounces retained by a ligature on the gullet brought on violent efforts to vomit, from which the animal was gradually recovering, when it was killed in twenty-four hours for the sake of observing the appearances. The stomach was found generally inflamed and interspersed with dark, gangrenous-like spots.*

I am not acquainted with any case of poisoning with these substances in the human subject. But it is probable that symptoms of pure irritation and inflammation will occur, and that moderate doses may prove fatal.

CHAPTER X.

OF POISONING WITH LIME.

Lime, the last poison of the present group, is a substance of little interest to the toxicologist, as its activity is not great.

Its physical and chemical properties need not be minutely described. It is soluble, though sparingly, in water ; and the solution turns the vegetable blues green, restores the purple of reddened litmus, gives a white precipitate with a stream of carbonic acid gas, and with oxalic acid a very insoluble precipitate, which is not redissolved by an excess of the test.

Its action is purely irritant. Orfila has found that a drachm and a half of unslaked lime, given to a little dog, caused vomiting and slight suffering for a day only, but that three drachms killed the same animal in five days, vomiting, languor, and whining being the only symptoms, and redness of the throat, gullet, and stomach, the only morbid appearances.†

Though a feeble poison, it has nevertheless proved fatal in the human subject. Gmelin takes notice of the case of a boy who swallowed some lime in an apple-pie, and died in nine days, affected with thirst, burning in the mouth, burning pain in the belly, and obstinate constipation.‡ A short account of a case of this kind of poisoning is also given by Balthazar Timæus. A young woman, afflicted with pica or depraved appetite, took to the eating of quicklime ; and in consequence she was attacked with pain and gnawing in the

* Journal de Physiologie, iii. 243.   † Toxicol. Gén. i. 174.
‡ Gmelin's Geschichte der Mineralischen Gifte, s. 252.

belly, sore throat, dryness of the mouth, insatiable thirst, difficult breathing and cough; but she recovered.* It is well known that quicklime also inflames the skin or even destroys its texture, apparently by withdrawing the water which forms a component part of all soft animal tissues. When thrown into the eyes it causes acute and obstinate ophthalmia, which may end in loss of sight. On this account it will belong, I presume, to the poisons included in the Scottish act against disfiguring or maiming with corrosives.

CHAPTER XI.

OF POISONING WITH AMMONIA AND ITS SALTS.

THE second group of the order of alkaline poisons, including ammonia with its salts, and the sulphuret of potass, have a double action on the system, analogous to that possessed by many metallic poisons. They are powerful irritants; but they produce besides, through the medium of the blood, a disorder of some part of the nervous system; and their remote is sometimes more dangerous than their local action. The nervous affection produced by ammonia and the sulphuret of potass closely resembles tetanus, and therefore depends probably on irritation of the spinal column.

Of the Chemical tests for the Ammoniacal Salts. — Ammonia is when pure a gaseous body; but as commonly seen, it exists in solution in water, which dissolves it in large quantity. The solution has the usual effects of alkalis on vegetable colours, with the difference, however, — that the changes of colour are not permanent under the action of heat. It forms a yellow precipitate, as potass does, with chloride of platinum. It may at once be distinguished from other fluids by its peculiar pungent odour, which is possessed by no other substance except its carbonate.

Various *carbonates* are known in chemistry, but the only one known in commerce or met with in the shops is the sesqui-carbonate (subcarbonate — smelling salt — volatile salt — hartshorn). It is solid, white, fibrous, and has the same odour as pure ammonia. Its solution differs little in physical properties from the pure liquid ammonia; but, unlike it, is precipitated by the salts of lime.

The *hydrochlorate* (muriate of ammonia — sal ammoniac) — is known by its solid, white, crystalline appearance; its ductility; its volatility; and by the effect of caustic potass and nitrate of silver, the former of which disengages an ammoniacal odour, while the latter causes in a solution of the salt a white precipitate, the chloride of silver.

Of the action of the Ammoniacal Salts, and their effects on man. — To determine the action of ammonia on the animal system, Professor Orfila injected sixty grains of the pure solution into the jugular vein

* Timæi Casus Medicinales, lvii. c. 12.

of a dog. Immediately the whole legs were spasmodically extended ; at times convulsions occurred ; and in ten minutes it died. The chest being laid open instantly, coagulated florid blood was seen in the left ventricle, and black fluid blood in the right ventricle of the heart. No unusual appearance was discernible any where else except complete exhaustion of muscular irritability.* The experiments of Mr. Blake also show that ammonia introduced in large doses into the veins acts by suddenly extinguishing the irritability of the heart. Small doses first lower arterial pressure from debility of the heart's action, and then increase it by obstructing the systemic capillaries. When injected into the aorta from the axillary artery, it causes great increase of arterial pressure, owing to the latter cause ; and then arrests the heart, while the respiration goes on. Four seconds are sufficient for the ammonia to pass from the jugular vein into the heart, so as to be discovered there by muriatic acid causing white fumes.† Half a drachm of a strong solution, introduced by Orfila into the stomach of a dog and secured by a ligature on the gullet, caused at first much agitation. But in five minutes the animal became still and soporose ; after five hours it continued able to walk ; in twenty hours it was found quite comatose ; and death ensued in four hours more. The only morbid appearance was slight mottled redness of the villous coat of the stomach. A third dog, to which two drachms and a half of the common carbonate were given in fine powder, died in twelve minutes. First it vomited ; next it became slightly convulsed ; and the convulsions gradually increased in strength and frequency till the whole body was agitated by dreadful spasms ; then the limbs became rigid, the body and head were bent backwards, and in this state it expired, apparently suffocated in a fit of tetanus.‡

Several cases of poisoning with ammonia or its carbonate have occurred in the human subject. Plenck has noticed shortly a case which proved fatal in four minutes, and which was caused by a little bottleful of ammonia having been poured into the mouth of a man who had been bitten by a mad-dog.§ The symptoms are not mentioned, but it is probable, from the rapidity of the poisoning, that a nervous affection must have been induced. More generally, however, the effects are simply irritant ; and the seat of the irritation will vary with the mode in which the poison is given. If it is swallowed, the stomach and intestines will suffer ; if it is imprudently inhaled in too great quantity, inflammation of the lining membrane of the nostrils and air-passages will ensue. Huxham has related a very interesting example of the former affection, as it occurred in a young man, who had acquired a strange habit of chewing the solid carbonate of the shops. He was seized with great hemorrhage from the nose, gums, and intestines; his teeth dropt out; wasting and hectic fever ensued; and, although he was at length prevailed on to abandon his pernicious habit, he died of extreme exhaustion, after lin-

* Orfila, Toxic. Gén. i. 220.
† Edinburgh Med. and Surg. Journal, li. 336, lvi. 422, liii. 38.
‡ Toxicol. *ut supra*.   § Plenck, Toxicologia, 226.

gering several months.* But the most frequent cases of poisoning with ammonia have arisen from its being inhaled, and thus exciting bronchial inflammation. An instructive instance of the kind has been related by M. Nysten. A medical man, liable to epilepsy, was found in a fit by his servant, who ignorantly tried to rouse him by holding assiduously to his nostrils a handkerchief dipped in ammonia. In this way about two drachms appear to have been consumed. On recovering his senses, the gentleman complained of burning pain from the mouth downwards to the stomach, great difficulty in swallowing, difficult breathing, hard cough, and copious expectoration, profuse mucous discharge from the nostrils, and excoriation of the tongue. The bronchitis increased steadily, and carried him off in the course of the third day, without convulsions or any mental disorder having supervened.† A case precisely similar is related in the Edinburgh Medical and Surgical Journal. A lad, while convalescent from an attack of fever, was seized with epilepsy, for which his attendant applied ammonia under his nose " with such unwearied, but destructive benevolence, that suffocation had almost resulted. As it was, dyspnœa with severe pain of the throat and breast, immediately succeeded ; and death took place forty-eight hours afterwards."‡ A third instance has been recorded of analogous effects produced by the incautious use of ammonia as an antidote for prussic acid. The patient had all the symptoms of a violent bronchitis, accompanied with redness and scattered ulceration of the mouth and throat; but he recovered in thirteen days.§ A fourth case, similar to the preceding, has been related by M. Souchard of Batignolles. A druggist, who inhaled while asleep the fumes of ammonia from a broken carboy, awoke in three-quarters of an hour, with the mucous membrane of the mouth and nostrils corroded, and a bloody discharge from the nose. A severe attack of bronchitis followed, during which he could not speak for six days; but being actively treated with antiphlogistic remedies, he recovered.‖ — An extraordinary case has been published by Mr. Paget of death from injecting ammonia into the blood-vessels. A solution weak enough to allow of the nose being held over it was injected into a nævis in a child two years old. An attack of convulsions immediately followed, and in a minute the child expired.¶

Nysten's case is the only one in the human subject in which the *morbid appearances* were ascertained. The nostrils were blocked up with an albuminous membrane. The whole mucous coat of the larynx, trachea, bronchi, and even of some of the bronchial ramifications, was mottled with patches of lymph. The gullet and stomach showed red streaks here and there; and there was a black eschar on the tongue, and another on the lower lip.

Of Poisoning with Hydrochlorate of Ammonia. — The effects of

* Essay on Fevers, p. 308.
† Bulletins de la Soc. de Méd. 1815, No. viii. T. iv. 352.
‡ Edinburgh Medical and Surgical Journal, xiv. 642.
§ Revue Médicale, xvii. 265.   ‖ Journal de Chimie Médicale, 1840, 499.
¶ London Medical Gazette, 1837, xxi. 529.

the hydrochlorate of ammonia on animals have been examined by Professor Orfila and Dr. Arnold; but I have not yet met with any instance of its operation as a poison on man.   When given to dogs it irritates and inflames the parts it touches, and causes the ordinary symptoms of local irritation.   But it also acts remotely.   For, first, like arsenic, and other poisons of the third order of irritants, it produces inflammation of the stomach, in whatever way it is applied to the body, — Orfila having found that organ affected when the salt was applied to the subcutaneous cellular tissue;[*] and, secondly, according to the experiments of Arnold, it causes, when swallowed, excessive muscular weakness, slow breathing, violent action of the heart, and tetanic spasms, — effects which cannot arise from mere injury of the stomach.   Half a drachm will thus kill a rabbit in eight or ten minutes;[†] and two drachms a small dog in an hour.[‡]

CHAPTER XII.

OF POISONING WITH THE ALKALINE SULPHURETS.

THE liver of sulphur, or sulphuret of potass of the pharmacopœias, the last poison of this order to be mentioned, is allied to the ammoniacal salts in action.   It is of no great consequence in a toxicological point of view in this country, being put to little use ; but several accidents have been caused by it in France, where it is employed for manufacturing artificial sulphureous waters ; and farther, its properties should be accurately ascertained, because till lately it was erroneously resorted to as an antidote for some metallic poisons.

Chemical Tests. — It has a grayish, greenish, or yellowish colour when solid ; its dust smells of sulphuretted hydrogen, which is also copiously disengaged from it by the mineral acids : and it forms with water a yellow solution of the same odour. — In composite fluids it may be detected by heating it with acetic acid, and passing the disengaged gases through solution of acetate of lead, in which a black precipitate of sulphuret of lead is produced, from the action of sulphuretted-hydrogen.[§]

Action and Symptoms. — Orfila found that a solution of six drachms and a half, secured in the stomach of a dog by a ligature on the gullet, caused death by tetanus in seven minutes, without leaving any morbid appearance in the body; that inferior doses caused death in the same manner, but at a later period, and with symptoms of irritation in the alimentary canal, which also was seen red, black, or even ulcerated after death ; that a solution of twenty-two grains injected into the jugular vein killed a dog in two minutes, convulsions having preceded death, and the heart being found paralysed immediately

---

* Orfila, Toxicol Gén. i. 229.
† De salis ammoniaci vi, &c. Heidelberg, 1826. Analysed in Revue Med. 1827, i. 284.   ‡ Orfila, i. 228.
§ Orfila, Annales d'Hygiène Publique, xxviii. 431.

after it; and that a drachm and a half thrust in small fragments under the skin occasioned death in thirteen hours with coma and extensive inflammation of the cellular tissue.* There can be no doubt, therefore, that liver of sulphur is a true narcotic acrid poison. — It is absorbed, and may be detected in the blood, liver, kidneys, and urine by Orfila's process.†

Orfila has collected three cases of poisoning in the human subject with this substance;‡ and a fourth has been related by M. Cayol.§ Of these cases two proved fatal in less than fifteen minutes; and the symptoms were acrid taste, slight vomiting, mortal faintness, and convulsions, with an important chemical sign, the tainting of the air with the odour of sulphuretted-hydrogen. The dose in one case was about three drachms. The two other patients, who recovered, were for some days dangerously ill. The symptoms were burning pain and constriction in the throat, gullet, and stomach; frequent vomiting, at first sulphureous, afterwards sanguinolent; purging, at first sulphureous; sulphureous exhalations from the mouth; pulse at first quick and strong, afterwards feeble, fluttering, and almost imperceptible; in one case sopor; finally severe inflammation of the gullet, stomach and intestines, which abated in three days. One of these patients took four drachms of sulphuret of soda, the other two ounces of sulphuret of potass; but it is probable, that the latter dose was partly decomposed by long keeping.

Morbid Appearances. — The morbid appearances in the two fatal cases were great lividity of the face and extremities, and exhaustion of muscular contractility immediately after death; the stomach was red internally, and lined with sulphur; the duodenum also red; the lungs soft, gorged with black fluid blood, and not crepitant.

Treatment. — The most appropriate treatment consists in the instant administration of any diluent, then of frequent doses of the chloride of soda, and lastly the antiphlogistic mode of subduing inflammation. The chloride of soda or lime decomposes sulphuretted hydrogen, the disengagement of which is the probable cause of death in the quickly fatal cases.‖

CHAPTER XIII.

OF POISONING WITH ARSENIC.

The third order of the irritant class of poisons includes the compounds of the metals. These are of great importance to the medical jurist. They are frequently used for criminal purposes; they give rise to the greatest variety of symptoms; and the medical evidence

---

* Toxic. Gen. i. 177.   † Annales, *ut supra.*
‡ Toxicologie Gen. 1843, i. 269. Two from an Essay by M. Chantourelle, read before the Acad. de Médecine,; and one from M. Lafranque in Ann. de la Méd. Physiolog. Fevrier, 1825.
§ Journ. Universel, xviii. 265.   ‖ See *Poisonous Gases.*

on trials respecting them, while much skill is required on the part of the witness to collect it, is also the most conclusive.

It must not be inferred from their being arranged in the class of irritants that their action is merely local. In fact this is the case with a very few of them only, which produce chemical corrosion. The greater number likewise act indirectly on organs at a distance from the part to which they are applied. Nevertheless the most prominent symptoms generally produced by them are those of violent local irritation; so that they may be justly considered in the place which has been assigned them.

The poisons included in this order are the oxides and salts of arsenic, mercury, copper, antimony, tin, silver, gold, bismuth, iron, chrome, zinc, barium, lead. Many other metals also form poisonous compounds with various acids and other bodies; but these are so rare as to be merely objects of physiological curiosity.

Of all the varieties of death by poison, none is so important to the medical jurist as poisoning with arsenic. On account of the shameful facility with which it may be procured in this country, even by the lowest of the vulgar, and the ease with which it may be secretly administered, it is the poison most frequently chosen for the purpose of committing both suicide and murder. In 1837 and 1838 no fewer than 186 cases of fatal poisoning with arsenic were known to have occurred in England alone (see p. 90). Of 221 cases of murder by poison in France during ten years subsequent to 1829, in which the poison given was ascertained, there were 149 where the substance administered was arsenic.* It is fortunate, therefore, that there are few substances in nature, and perhaps hardly any other poison, whose presence can be detected in such minute quantities and with so great certainty.

SECTION I. — *Of the Chemical Tests for the Compounds of Arsenic.*

Metallic arsenic has an iron-gray colour, a specific gravity of 8·308, and a crystalline fracture. It is very brittle. It has a strong tendency to oxidate, so that it undergoes this change in air, in water, and even in alcohol. In air, particularly when moist, it becomes rapidly tarnished, a black powder being formed, which some have regarded as a regular protoxide.† — When exposed to heat, metallic arsenic is usually said to sublime at the temperature of 356° F.; but according to some late experiments by Dr. Mitchell of Philadelphia this does not happen under a low red heat, luminous in the dark.‡ In close vessels it condenses unchanged; but when heated in the open air, it passes to the state of white oxide, and rises in white

---

* Journal de Chimie Médicale, 1842, p. 656.

† It appears that arsenic does not always undergo this change. Berzelius once kept some fragments in an open phial for three years without observing any change in appearance or weight. [Annales de Chimie et de Physique, xi. 240.] Buchner once made a similar observation, and is inclined to think that oxidation does not occur, if the metal is quite pure. [Repertorium für die Pharmacie, xxi. 29.]

‡ American Journ. of Med. Science, x. 122.

fumes. This substance is a sesquioxide, consisting of two equivalents of metal and three of oxygen. Another oxide likewise exists, which contains two equivalents of metal and five of oxygen, and, possessing strong acid properties, is denominated arsenic acid. The sesquioxide and arsenic acid unite with bases, and produce compounds which, with the exception of those they form with the alkalis, are mostly insoluble. Metallic arsenic unites with sulphur in two proportions, forming an orange-red and a sulphur-yellow compound. The compounds of arsenic have very little chemical action with vegetable and animal principles.

Of the compounds which arsenic thus forms, those which it will be necessary to particularize are the following : — 1. The protoxide of Berzelius, or *fly-powder*. 2. The arsenious acid, or *white arsenic*. 3. The arsenite of copper, or *mineral green*. 4. The arsenite of potass as contained in *Fowler's solution*. 5. The arsenite of potass ; 6. The various sulphurets, pure and impure, namely, *realgar, orpiment*, and *king's-yellow ;* and 7. Arseniuretted-hydrogen gas.

Of the Tests for Fly-powder.

This substance is rarely known as a poison in Britain, but is a familiar poison in France and Germany, under the names of *Poudre à mouches*, and *Fliegenstein*. Of late it has been occasionally used in Scotland for poisoning rats.

It is a fine grayish-black powder, formed by exposing powdered arsenic for a long time to the air ; but it also frequently contains fragments of the metal. It is usually considered by chemists to be a mixture of metallic arsenic and its white oxide.

It is acted on by water, the white oxide being found ere long in solution by its proper tests. Oxidation and solution, however, are also effected upon pure metallic arsenic in the same manner. A thousand grains of water take up a grain in the course of half an hour when boiled on the metal.*

A very simple and decisive test for fly-powder is derived from the effect of heat. If it is heated in a tube two substances are sublimed, first a white crystalline powder, and then a bright metallic crust, the former being the white oxide, the latter the metal. The metallic crust thus formed possesses physical properties, which distinguish arsenic from all other substances, capable of being sublimed by a low heat: The surface next the tube is very like polished steel, being a little darker in colour, but equal in brilliancy and polish ; and the inner surface is either brilliantly crystalline to the naked eye, like the fracture of cast-iron, or has a dull grayish-white colour, but appears crystalline before a common magnifying lens of four or five powers. If these characters be attended to, particularly the appearance of the inner surface, it appears to me scarcely possible to mistake for an arsenical crust any other substance which can be sublimed by any of the methods for subliming arsenic.

* Hahnemann. Uber die Arsenic-vergiftung, 13.

If a farther test should be desired, it is only necessary, as was first proposed by Dr. Turner of London,* to chase the crust up and down the tube with the spirit-lamp flame till it is all oxidated, when little octaedral crystals of adamantine lustre are formed, on which, either with the naked eye or with the aid of a common lens, triangular facettes may be distinguished.

The niceties to be attended to in applying the preceding tests will be considered presently under the head of the next compound, the sesquioxide.

2. Of the Tests for Arsenious Acid.

Arsenious acid, the sesquoixide, or white oxide of arsenic, usually called white arsenic, or simply arsenic, is the most common and important of all the arsenical preparations.

It is met with in the shops in two forms, — as a snow-white gritty powder, and in solid masses generally opaque, but sometimes translucent. When newly sublimed it is in translucent or even almost transparent masses of a vitreous lustre, conchoidal fracture and sharp-edged. By keeping it becomes opaque and white. The nature of the change has not been determined ; but some alteration is certainly effected, for Guibourt, who has examined both varieties with care, found that the opaque variety is more soluble in water than the other. He adds that the former is alkaline, the latter acid, in its action on litmus paper ; but I have always found the opaque variety acid.† The powder soon becomes analogous to the opaque variety of the oxide in mass.

The oxide of arsenic has a specific gravity of 3·729, according to the experiments of Dr. Ure, — of 3·529 when opaque, according to Mr. Alfred Taylor, and 3·798, when translucent. Very incorrect notions prevail as to its taste. It was long universally believed to be acrid,‡ and is described to be so in many systematic works and express treatises ; but in reality it has little or no taste at all. The reader will find some details on this point in a paper I published in the Edinburgh Medical and Surgical Journal.§ In the present work it is sufficient to observe, that I have repeatedly made the trial, and seen it made at my request by several scientific friends, and that, after continuing the experiment as long, and extending the poison along the tongue as far back, as we thought safe, all agreed that it had scarcely any taste at all, — perhaps towards the close a very faint sweetish taste. It appears to me that the experiments made on that occasion might have set at rest the question as to the taste of arsenic, and corrected an important error long committed by systematic authors in chemistry as well as medical jurisprudence. And accordingly in this country the truth is generally known.‖ Professor Orfila, how-

* Edin. Medico-Chirurgical Transactions, ii. 292.
† Journal de Chimie Médicale, ii. 61.
‡ As far back at least as the time of Zacchias. See his Quæstiones Medico-legales, iii. 37, 11.
§ Edin. Med. and Surg. Journal, 1827, xxviii. 96.
‖ Consult among others, Taylor's Manual of Medical Jurisprudence, p. 135.

ever, continues to repeat the error; for even in the last edition of his Toxicologie he says it has " a rough, not corrosive, slightly styptic taste, perceptible not for a few seconds, but persistent, and attended with salivation."* These sensations must be either imaginary or the indications of an organ peculiarly constituted. It is impossible to make satisfactory experiments with safety on its impressions on the back of the palate. But we may rest assured that in general it makes no impression there at all; for it has been often swallowed unknowingly with articles of food. Not a few have in such circumstances noticed merely its grittiness, and thought there was sand in their food. Two instances only am I hitherto acquainted with, where an acrid sensation would seem really to have been experienced in the act of eating or swallowing. In one of these, noticed in Rust's Journal, the individual who was poisoned, could not finish the poisoned dish on account of its unpleasant, very peppery taste.† In the other case, which was lately communicated to me by Mr. Hewson of Lincoln, the individual, who was poisoned by arsenic dissolved in his tea-kettle, — happening in the first instance to wash his mouth with the water, — observed at the time to his daughter, that it had a very odd taste; which subsequently was called a burning taste. These facts, however, are evidently not altogether satisfactory. It is not improbable that, in an *ex post facto* description, the reporters, as others in the same circumstances have clearly done‡, confounded the subsequent inflammation with mere taste in the act of chewing or swallowing. At all events it is absolutely certain that the great majority of people who have been poisoned with arsenic remarked in taking it either no taste at all, or merely a roughness owing to the gritty condition of its powder.

The oxide of arsenic when subjected to heat is sublimed at 380°, or, according to Dr. Mitchell, 425° F.§ and condenses in the form of a crystalline powder, which, if the operation is performed slowly and on a small quantity proportioned to the size of the tube, evidently consists of little, adamantine octaedres. — When it is mixed with carbonaceous matter and heated, it is reduced, and the metal is sublimed. This constitutes the test of reduction, which, when conducted with due care, may be rendered singly a certain proof of the presence of arsenic.

Water dissolves it. Its solubility is a point of some medico-legal importance; for a doubt may arise whether the quantity of a solution that has been swallowed contained a sufficient dose to cause severe symptoms or death. Different statements have gone forth on this head. Klaproth found, that a thousand parts of temperate water take up only two parts and a half, — and that a thousand parts of boiling water take up 77·75 parts or a thirteenth, and retain on cool-

* Toxicologie Gén. 1843, i. 376.
† Magazin für die gesammte Heilkunde, v. 66.
‡ Mr. Blandy, for example, who said he " perceived an extraordinary grittiness in his mouth, attended with a very painful pricking and burning pain in his tongue, throat, stomach, and bowels." [Howell's State Trials, xviii. 1135.]
§ Americal Journal of Medical Science, x. 122.

20*

ing 30 parts or a thirty-third of their weight.* Guibourt found a
difference between the transparent and opaque varieties; for a thousand parts of temperate water dissolved in thirty-six hours 9·6 of the
transparent, 12·5 of the opaque variety; and the same quantity of
boiling water dissolved of the transparent variety 97 parts, retaining
18 when cooled, but of the opaque variety took up 115 and retained
on cooling 29.† More lately Mr. Alfred Taylor observed that temperate water, simply poured on the opaque oxide and left for seventy-two hours, contained one grain in a thousand, but if often agitated,
8·5 grains; that boiling water, occasionally agitated for the same
period, contained 9·27 or 9·54 grains ; that water, boiling gently for
an hour dissolved 31·5, and on cooling and resting for three days
retained 17 ; that with violent ebullition for an hour, it took up 46·3,
and retained 24·7 grains on cooling and resting for three days; that
a saturated boiling solution after six months contained 24 or 26
grains ; and that a saturated boiling solution of the transparent oxide
contained 46 or 47·5 grains, and on cooling and resting for two days
retained 18·7 or 13·4 grains.‡ It is impossible to account for these
discrepancies; for all the experimentalists conducted their investigations with care, and with a view to the medico-legal question stated
above. Hahnemann farther remarked, that at the temperature of the
blood a thousand parts of water dissolve ten parts with the aid of
ten minutes' agitation;§ and Navier, that boiling water kept for an
hour on it, and decanted off in the way an infusion is usually made,
dissolves 12·5 grains in every thousand.‖

Its solubility is impaired by the presence of organic principles.
When mixed with mucus or milk it dissolves, according to Hahnemann, with great difficulty ; and I have found that a cup of tea, left
beside the fire at a temperature of 200° for half an hour upon two
grains of the oxide, does not take up entirely even that small quantity. An important consequence of the fact now mentioned is, that
when swallowed in the solid state, little or no arsenic may be found
in the fluid contents of the stomach. In a case which occurred to
Scheele three grains of solid arsenic were found in the contents, but
hardly a trace in solution.¶ It would be wrong, however, to suppose
that it is never found in the fluid contents. For, not to mention the
observations of others, I have myself often detected it in the fluid
part of the stomach in persons poisoned by arsenic.

The solution of oxide of arsenic in boiling water yields minute
crystals on cooling, which, when their form is defined, are octaedres.
In this state, on account of its whiteness and brilliancy, it exceedingly resembles pounded sugar. By spontaneous evaporation I
have procured in twelve months fine octaedres nearly as large as
peas. These do not become opaque by keeping, like the sublimed
masses.

* Schweigger's Journal der Chemie. vi. 232.
† Journal de Chimie Médicale, ii. 61.
‡ London Philosophical Journal. 1837, ii. 482.
§ Ueber die Arsenic-vergiftung, 10.
‖ Contrepoisons de l'Arsenic du sublimé corrosif, &c. i. 20.
¶ Neues Nordisches Archiv. i.

A difference of opinion prevails as to the action of the oxide on vegetable colours. This is a matter of no great consequence to the medical jurist; but it is right not to leave a disputed point without some notice. Guibourt says the transparent variety faintly reddens litmus, while the opaque variety faintly restores to blue litmus previously reddened.[*] My own experiments are at variance with these statements: I have always found that the solution of the powder, which is of the opaque variety, faintly reddens litmus, and does not alter reddened litmus.

The remaining chemical properties of the oxide, which it is necessary for the medical jurist to know, will be mentioned under what is now to be said of the principal test by which its presence may be ascertained. Under this head will be noticed, first the tests for the solid oxide, secondly, those for its solution, and lastly, the method of detecting it when mingled with vegetable or animal solids and fluids, such as the contents and tissues of the stomach.

Of the Tests for Arsenic in the solid state.

The most characteristic and simple test for oxide of arsenic in its solid state, either pure or mixed or combined with inorganic substances, is its reduction to the metallic state.

Various methods have been at different times proposed for employing the test of reduction. In the ruder periods of analytic chemistry we find Hahnemann recommending a retort as the fittest instrument, and stating ten grains as the least quantity he could detect.[†] Afterwards Dr. Black substituted a small glass tube, coated with clay and heated in a choffer; and in this way he could discover a single grain.[‡] In a paper published in the Edinburgh Medical and Surgical Journal, I showed how to detect a sixteenth of a grain; and afterwards even so minute a quantity as a hundreth part of a grain.[§]

The process is performed in a glass tube; which, when the quantity of the oxide is very small, should not exceed an eighth of an inch in diameter, and may be conveniently used of the form first recommended by Berzelius, and represented in Fig. 3. — The best material for reducing the oxide is recently ignited charcoal, if the quantity of suspected substance be very small. For when any of the ordinary alkaline fluxes is used, more than half of the arsenic is retained, probably in the form of an arseniuret of the alkaline metalloid. But when the quantity of matter for analysis is considerable, charcoal is inconvenient, as it is apt to be projected up the tube on the application of heat; and an alkaline flux is on that account preferable. For this purpose soda-flux, — made by grinding crystals of corbonate of soda with an eighth of their weight of charcoal, and then heating the mixture gradually to redness, so as to drive off all water, — is better than the more familiar black-flux, which con-

* Journal de Chimie Médicale, ii. 61.
† Ueber die Arsenic-vergiftung, 223. ‡ Lectures on Chemistry, ii. 430.
§ Edin. Med. and Surg. Journal, xxii. 82, and Edin. Medico-Chirurgical Transactions, ii. 293.

tains carbonate of potash; because the latter attracts much moisture when kept for some time. — If the quantity operated on is large it should be mixed with the flux before being introduced into the tube; if it is small, it may be dropped into the tube and covered with charcoal. The materials are to be introduced along a little triangular gutter of stiff paper, if the tube is large; but with a small tube it is preferable to use the little glass funnel represented in Fig. 2, to which a wire is previously fitted, for pushing the matter down when it adheres. The material should not be closely impacted. Heat is best applied with the spirit-lamp, first to the upper part of the material, with a small flame, and then to the bottom of the tube, the flame being previously enlarged. A little water, disengaged in the first instance, should be removed with a roll of filtering paper, before a sufficient heat is applied to sublime the metal. As soon as the dark crust begins to form, the tube should be held steady in the same part of the flame. With these precautions a well defined crust will be procured with facility.

The characters of the crust have been mentioned already under the head of fly-powder (p. 199). They are distinct even in crusts weighing only a 300th of a grain. A crust of this weight, a tenth of an inch broad and four times as long, may show characteristically all the physical characters of an arsenical sublimate a hundred times larger.

The fallacies to which the test has been supposed to be liable (excluding at present that part of it which consists in the oxidation of the metal, and which renders it quite unimpeachable), are the following. — Dr. Paris says he has known an instance where a person, " by no means deficient in chemical address, mistook for it a deposit of charcoal,[*] and I have known the same mistake happen in the hands of one of my pupils, a beginner in the study of medico-legal chemistry. The outer surface of a charcoal crust may be mistaken for arsenic by a careless person; but with ordinary care it is quite impossible to err if the inner surface be examined, for that of charcoal is brown, powdery, and perfectly dull. — It has been suggested to me and has been stated in print,[†] that the preparations of antimony yield by reduction a sublimate resembling closely an arsenical crust. But in consequence of repeated trials I am certain that no preparation of antimony, reduced either by charcoal or the black-flux with the fullest red heat of the blowpipe will yield any metallic sublimate; and the same facts were observed by the late Dr. Turner. — It has even been said by Mr. Donovan that the action of the flux on glass which contains lead causes a stain similar to an arsenical crust.[‡] If it be meant by this observation, that the lead contained in the glass usually gives that part of the tube which contains the flux a glimmering appearance and impairs its transparency, the author is correct: but it is impossible that a sublimate can be so formed. — Dr. Mitchell of Philadelphia in an elaborate paper on the process of re-

* Paris and Fonblanque's Medical Jurisprudence, ii. 251.
† Donovan in Dublin Phil. Journal, ii. 402.   ‡ Ibid.

duction seems to consider the crust undistinguishable from that form-ed in similar circumstances by cinnabar.* Crusts of cinnabar, however, do not present the peculiar character possessed by the in-ternal surface of arsenic. — Zinc, it is said, may be sublimed in its metallic state ; but the sublimation of zinc requires a full white heat ; which in the process for arsenic cannot be generated. — Tellu-rium, cadmium, and potassium sublime at a lower heat ; but these metals are so exceedingly rare, that it is quite unnecessary to parti-cularize the characters of their sublimates. — Lastly, it is said that a crust may be produced from arsenic contained in the glass of the tube. A few years ago MM. Ozanam and Idt of Lyons detected arsenic in the remains of a body which had been seven years in-terred ; but subsequently M. Idt imagined he had discovered that the glass used in the analysis contained arsenic, and yielded it by the process of reduction. He accordingly retracted his original opinion ; and the person accused of administering the poison was acquitted. An extended inquiry, however, was in consequence undertaken by the Parisian Academy of Medicine at the request of the French govern-ment. And the result was that no arsenic could be detected in the glass tubes used by MM. Ozanam and Idt ; and that although arsenic is sometimes used in glass-making, and a trace of it may be retained in some opaque glasses or enamels, it cannot be detected by any pro-cess of analysis in any of the clear glass met with in commerce,† the whole arsenic being volatilized during the manufacture of the glass.

It may therefore be safely laid down that the appearances exhibited by a well-formed arsenical crust, even in the minute quantity of a 300th part of a grain, are imitated by no substance in nature which can be sublimed by the process for the reduction of arsenic.

But should farther evidence be required as to the nature of the crust, this may be obtained by subjecting it to oxidation by heat.

The best method of doing so is to heat the ball containing the flux deprived of arsenic, to attach a bit of glass tube to its end, and to draw this gently off in the spirit-flame, taking care to prevent the flux being driven forward on the crust. This being done, the whole crust, or, if it is large, a portion of it, is to be chased up and down the tube with a small spirit-lamp flame till it is all convert-ed into a white powder. In order to show the crystalline form of the powder distinctly, let the flame be reduced to the volume of a pea by drawing in the wick, and let the part of the tube containing the oxide be held half an inch or an inch above it. By repeated trials sparkling crystals will at length be formed, which are octaedres, — the crystalline form of arsenious acid. The triangular facettes of the octaedres may be sometimes seen with the naked eye, though the original crust was only a fiftieth of a grain or even less ; and they may be always seen with a lens of four powers, the tube being held between the eye and a lighted candle or a ray of sunshine, either of

* American Journal of Medical Science, x. 126,
† Annales d'Hyg. Pub. et de Med. Lég. xi. 224,

which is preferable to diffuse daylight for making this observation. —
For the success of the oxidation test it is indispensable that the inside
of the tube be not soiled with an alkaline flux : because the alkali
would unite with the oxide. It is also requisite not to heat the tube
suddenly to redness before the oxide is sublimed ; because then the
oxide is apt to unite with the glass, forming a white, opaque enamel.
The physical characters of the sublimed oxide are so delicate and
precise, that they may be accurately distinguished, even when those
of the metallic crust are obscure, owing to its minuteness. Sometimes too, the metal may be so scanty that it is oxidated at once in
the act of subliming, and never presents the appearance of a metallic
crust. Although the characters of the crystalline oxide in either of
these cases are very precise and distinctive, it may be right to subject
it to a farther test when the metal is not previously exhibited with
its characteristic properties. For this purpose it is sufficient to cut
away with a file the portion of the tube which contains the sublimate, to boil it in another tube with a few drops of distilled water
till the sublimate disappear, and then to test the solution with one of
the fluid tests to be presently described, the ammoniacal nitrate of
silver.

After all that has been recently written as to the old and newer
processes for detecting arsenic, I must nevertheless avow my conviction, that for solid arsenic no test is, for medico-legal purposes, at
once so satisfactory, convenient, and delicate as the test of reduction,
especially with the addition of the supplementary test of oxidation.
That other methods are still more delicate may be readily granted.
But where the suspected substance is in the solid form, what possible
occasion can there be for a method more delicate than one which
will detect a 300th part of a grain?   A method ten times less so would
meet every case in actual practice. — A variety of supplementary tests
have been proposed. But they are all greatly inferior in facility, or
conclusiveness, or both, to the process of oxidation, and ought therefore to be expelled from medico-legal practice, — not even excepting
the alliaceous odour of metallic arsenic in the act of subliming, a
character, the fallaciousness of which was long ago pointed out by
myself as well as others, and to which a preposterous importance has
been attached in some late inquiries.   The reader will find in the last
edition of this work an attempt to estimate the value of various tests
supplementary to that of reduction.   This disquisition is now omitted, as it seems no longer necessary.

Of the Tests for Oxide of Arsenic in Solution.

Oxide of arsenic in a state of solution may be detected in one of
four ways ; by what are called the liquid tests ; by precipitating it
with one of these, and subliming metallic arsenic from the precipitate,
which method is usually termed the reduction process ; by Marsh's
method, which consists in disengaging it in the form of arseniuretted-
hydrogen gas, and decomposing the gas by combustion ; or by the

method of Reinsch, in which metallic arsenic is deposited on the surface of copper, and then separated by heat for farther examination.

Process by Liquid Reagents. — The first method is by the employment of several liquid tests, which cause in the solution peculiar precipitates. Many such tests have been proposed ; but the most characteristic and precise are *hydrosulphuric acid, ammoniacal nitrate of silver*, and *ammoniacal sulphate of copper.* The indications of each of the three tests must concur, otherwise, in a medico-legal case, no one can be entitled to speak with certainty to the existence of arsenic. But when they do concur, the evidence is unimpeachable. When this method of analysis is followed, corresponding experiments ought always to be made with the water that is used for diluting or otherwise preparing the subject of examination, or with distilled water, if the article be already sufficiently aqueous. This precaution is necessary on account of the risk of accidental impregnation of the water or other reagents with arsenic.*

Hydrosulphuric acid [sulphuretted-hydrogen] is obtained by decomposing proto-sulphuret of iron with diluted sulphuric acid in such an apparatus as is represented at Fig. 5. And the gas may be either applied directly to the suspected fluid, or condensed in distilled water, and thus kept in store for occasional use in the liquid shape. Before applying this test, the suspected fluid must be acidulated with acetic or hydrochloric acid ; because an excess of alkali prevents the action. And if an acid be indicated by litmus in the fluid, neutralization, or slight supersaturation, with potash must be effected, before adding acetic or hydrochloric acid ; for if the acidity should happen to be owing to an excess of sulphuric or nitric acid, the test is decomposed, and yellowish-white sulphur deposited. — These precautions being taken, hydrosulphuric acid occasions a sulphur-yellow or lemon-yellow precipitate. If the arsenical solution, however, be very weak, a yellow colour merely is struck, because the precipitate, which is sesqui-sulphuret of arsenic, is dissolved by the excess of the test ; but it separates after ebullition, or a few hours' exposure to the air. Co-existing animal and vegetable principles sometimes enable the fluid to retain a minute portion even after ebullition, so as to acquire a yellow milkiness ; but they do not in any case prevent the test from producing the yellow colour. Acidulation with acetic or hydrochloric acid favours its subsidence in all cases ; and according to Mr. Boutigny, alkaline sulphates, muriates and nitrates have the same effect.†
Hydro-sulphuric acid is so delicate as to act on the oxide in a hundred thousand parts of water. The proper colour of the precipitate

* The only probable source of such impregnation is pyritic sulphur, which is frequently used abroad, and has of late been occasionally employed in this country, for making sulphuric acid. As pyrites commonly contains arsenic, the acid becomes adulterated with oxide of arsenic, and may communicate the same impregnation to various other reagents which are prepared by means of sulphuric acid. The oxide may easily be detected in that acid by a stream of hydrosulphuric acid gas, after moderate dilution with water ; for pure acid is rendered milky ; but an arsenical acid yields a yellow precipitate of sulphuret of arsenic.

† Journal de Chim. Méd. viii. 449.

is lemon or sulphur-yellow ; which, when vegetable or animal matter is present, acquires a shade of white or brown.

It is not liable to any material fallacy. The salts of cadmium yield with it precipitates nearly of the same colour: but they are exceedingly rare ; and the precipitate, unlike sulphuret of arsenic, is insoluble in ammonia. — The salts formed by selenic acid, if decomposed by another acid, also yield yellow precipitates ; but these salts are extremely rare. — The salts of peroxide of tin give a dirty grayish-yellow precipitate ; which however ammonia turns brown. — A lead solution acidulated with hydrochloric acid gives at first a yellow precipitate ; but this becomes brownish-black when more gas is transmitted.* The contents of the human intestines sometimes yield a yellowish precipitate though no arsenic be present ; and it is dissolved, like sulphuret of arsenic, by ammonia.† The tartrate of antimony and potash (tartar-emetic) does not form, as was once thought, any source of fallacy, the antimonial precipitate having always a tint of orange-red ; besides it is not, like sulphuret of arsenic, soluble in carbonate of ammonia. — Other fallacies exist, unless the test be used with the precautions mentioned above. But these need not enumeration here.

Ammoniacal nitrate of silver is prepared by precipitating the oxide of silver by means of ammonia, from a solution of nitrate of silver or lunar caustic in ten parts of water, and then redissolving the precipitate nearly, but not entirely, by adding gradually an excess of ammonia. When thus prepared, it causes, even in a very diluted solution of the oxide of arsenic, a lively lemon-yellow precipitate of arsenite of silver; which passes to dark brown under exposure to the light. — The action of this test is prevented by nitric, acetic, citric, or tartaric acid in excess, particularly by the first and last. It is also prevented by an excess of ammonia ; and in very diluted solutions by the nitrate of ammonia. These facts will suggest the necessity of certain obvious precautions. Its action is obscured by the co-existence of various salts, which singly cause a white precipitate with nitrate of silver ; for the yellow colour is then much lessened in intensity. The only one of these requiring special notice, because it occurs in very many of the fluids which are likely to be subjected to the researches of the medical jurist, is common sea-salt, the chloride of sodium. The best way of getting rid of the difficulty is to use in the first instance, not the ammoniacal nitrate, but the simple nitrate of silver, as long as any white precipitate falls down, to add a slight excess of that test, and then, after subsidence, to drop in ammonia. No arsenic is thrown down by the first steps of this process ; but if any be present, it is subsequently thrown down in the form of the yellow arsenite of silver, on the addition of ammonia. This simple mode of getting rid of chloride of sodium was first proposed by Dr.

---

* Reinsch, in Repertorium für die Pharmacie, lvi. 183.

† This has been occasionally observed by Chevallier [Journal de Chim. Méd. 1840, 434], and once by M. Roturier [Ibidem, 627]. The former met with a medico-legal case where from this circumstance an erroneous opinion was at first formed in favour of poisoning.

Marcet.* — Ammoniacal nitrate of silver is of no use as a test for a moderately diluted solution of the oxide of arsenic, if vegetable or animal matter be present; either the colour of the precipitate is essentially altered, or no precipitate is formed at all.†

If the presence of arsenic is to be inferred only when the full lemon-yellow colour of the precipitate is developed, this test is not liable to any material fallacy. The presence of a phosphate, a serious obstacle according to an old way of using the silver test, is not a source of fallacy in the instance of the ammoniacal nitrate; for the yellow phosphate of silver is so soluble in the ammonia of the test, that it is not thrown down unless the phosphatic solution is very strong. — The silver test, which is extremely delicate, was proposed by Mr. Hume, a chemist of London; and in its improved state was suggested by the late Dr. Marcet. Various foreign authors have fallen into the error of supposing that nitrate of silver without an alkali precipitates oxide of arsenic : without an alkali, pure nitrate of silver gives no precipitate, or at most a bluish-white or yellowish-white haze when both solutions are strong.

Ammoniacal sulphate of copper is prepared by the same process with the last test, sulphate of copper being substituted for nitrate of silver. It is a test of very great delicacy. It causes in solutions of the oxide of arsenic an apple-green or grass-green precipitate of the arsenite of copper. The particular tint is altered apparently by trifling circumstances; but after the precipitate has stood some hours it always assumes a tint intermediate between apple-green and grass-green. The operation of this test is prevented by hydrochloric, nitric, sulphuric, acetic, citric, and tartaric acids in excess; and also by an excess of ammonia. These difficulties are obviated by manifest precautions. It is also prevented, according to Hünefeld, by muriate, nitrate, and sulphate of ammonia;‡ and by almost all vegetable infusions and animal fluids, when the oxide of arsenic is not abundant: these difficulties cannot be obviated. Even when not prevented by such fluids, its operation is often obscured, the precipitate not possessing its characteristic colour.

Ammoniacal sulphate of copper is more open to fallacies than the silver test. Of these the most important is that in some organic fluids it strikes a green precipitate, like the arsenite of copper, though arsenic be not present.§ The solution of bichromate of potass is turned green but not precipitated by it.

On reviewing all that has now been stated regarding the liquid tests for arsenic, it will appear that there is no single test on which absolute reliance can be placed; but that the fallacies to which they are liable are generally remote, and each of them applicable to one test only. Hence if each of the three reagents, applied with due

* London Med. Chirurgical Transactions, iii. 342.
† See a paper by myself in Edin. Med. and Surg. Journal, xxii. 60, where the fallacies to which the liquid tests are liable are investigated at great length.
‡ Horn's Archiv für Medizinische Erfahrung, 1827, i. 230.
§ Edin. Med. and Surg. Journal, xxii. 74.

21

care, gives a precipitate of the characteristic tint, the proof of the presence of arsenic is decisive.

This particular view of the indications of the liquid tests, however obvious it may seem, has been often overlooked by the numerous chemists and medical jurists who have written for and against them. The antagonists of the tests have been content with proving how so many fallacies lie in the way of each, that no dependence can be put in any one of them : They have not considered that the fallacies attached to one are obviated by the conjunct indications of the others.

I am of opinion therefore that the analysis for arsenic by liquid reagents has been unjustly neglected in the present day. It is an exceedingly convenient method, and one of extreme delicacy, because by using small tubes it is easy to operate with precision on very minute portions of a suspected fluid. It is also perfectly conclusive, so far as chemical knowledge now goes. On a remarkable trial a few years ago in this country, a distinguished chemist, who, as witness for the prisoner, was made by counsel to throw discredit on the liquid tests individually, nevertheless admitted to the counsel for the prosecution, that no other substance in nature but arsenic could produce the same effects as it with the whole three tests in succession.

Reduction-process. — The process by reduction of arsenic to the metallic state, as applied to the poison in a state of solution, consists in separating the whole arsenic by a liquid test in such a state as to admit of the precipitated compound being subjected to the process of reduction and sublimation. The best method of the kind is a modification of one described by me in 1824.* This consists in throwing down the whole arsenic in the form of sulphuret by means of hydrosulphuric acid, converting the sulphuret by the process of reduction to the metallic state, and oxidating the metal thus procured. The hydrosulphuric acid is preferred to other liquid reagents, because the precipitate it forms, while possessing a very characteristic colour, is also more bulky than those caused by the other tests, and is therefore more easily collected, — and because its action is not liable to be prevented or obscured by so many disturbing causes. The steps of the process are the following : —

The fluid to be examined must be acidulated with acetic or hydrochloric acid. If the fluid be neutral or alkaline, the acid may be added at once. If on the other hand the fluid redden litmus, and the acid be either unknown or a mineral acid, potash must first be added in a slight excess, and then the alkali must be supersaturated with acetic or hydrochloric acid. The reasons for these precautions are stated under hydrosulphuric acid as a liquid reagent. The fluid being thus prepared, it is subjected to a stream of hydrosulphuric acid gas for ten or fifteen minutes. The first portions of the gas turn the arsenical solution to a bright lemon-yellow colour, and the subsequent portions throw down a yellow flocculent sulphuret of arsenic. If the proportion of oxide in solution is small, a yellow-

* Edinburgh Med. and Surg. Journal, July, 1824.

ness or yellow milkiness only is caused, owing to the sulphuret being soluble in an excess of hydrosulphuric acid. But on expelling that excess by boiling, a distinct precipitate and colourless fluid are produced. The precipitate is then to be collected thus. The precipitate is allowed to subside, and the supernatant fluid being withdrawn, the remainder is poured into a filter. When all the fluid has passed through, the portions of precipitate on the upper part of the filter are washed down to the bottom. The filter is then gently compressed between folds of bibulous paper, and the sulphuret removed with the point of a knife before it dries, and dried in little masses on a watch-glass by the side of a chamber-fire, or still better in a vapour-bath. In this way it is very easy to collect a twenty-fifth part of a grain of the sulphuret. Another method which takes more time, but will enable the least skilful person to collect extremely small quantities, is to allow the sulphuret to subside in the original fluid in which it is formed, to pour off the supernatant liquid, and pour the remainder into a small glass tube, Fig. 7. After the precipitate has thoroughly subsided, the supernatant liquid is to be withdrawn, and its place filled up with boiling water. The operation of alternate subsidence and affusion being repeated a sufficient number of times, the last portions of water should be gently driven off by heat, and wiped off the inside of the tube as the drops condense on it. Finally, the bottom of the tube, with the precipitate attached, is to be cut away with the file, and broken into small fragments with the view of preserving the whole sulphuret for the process of reduction. The sulphuret having been collected in either of these ways, it is now to be dropt into the tube, Fig. 3, and covered by means of the funnel, Fig. 4, with soda-flux. The process in other particulars is the same with that for reducing solid oxide of arsenic.

This method of investigation gives extremely precise results, because it presents the poison successively in three distinct forms, as sulphuret, metal, and crystallized oxide, all of which possess very prominent and characteristic external properties. It is also a method which is capable of detecting very minute quantities of oxide of arsenic. And it has the advantage over the process by liquid reagents of being applicable to organic fluids. It was accordingly followed in most medico-legal researches until the recent discovery of the methods of Marsh and Reinsch.

In order to render it quite satisfactory, it is necessary to go through the steps of the analysis at the same time with distilled water, lest any of the reagents used should accidentally contain arsenic.

Process of Marsh. — This method consists in disengaging arsenic from the solution in the form of arseniuretted-hydrogen gas, burning the gas in such way as to obtain either metallic arsenic or oxide of arsenic, and subjecting the product to various tests.

I have called this beautiful method of analysis Marsh's process, because it appears to me that injustice has been done its discoverer both by himself and those who have since investigated the subject, when they denominated it merely a test. Medico-legal analysis stood in no need of a new test for arsenic, but very much of an easy and infallible method of detaching minute quantities of it in a state of purity from simple and compound fluids, so as to admit of its being accurately examined. It is this important object, and not strictly speaking a new test, that has been attained through means of the discovery of Mr. Marsh.

His discovery consists in the observation, that, if hydrogen gas be disengaged by the action of sulphuric acid or zinc in a fluid containing arsenic dissolved in any form, arseniuretted-hydrogen gas is disengaged along with the hydrogen ; and that if the two gases be burnt together in a fine flame, metallic arsenic is deposited on a white porcelain surface held in the flame, and oxide of arsenic if the porcelain be held immediately above it.[*] The production of a brilliant mirror-like crust in the former case, and of a white powdery one in the other, constituted Marsh's test as originally proposed ; and it was at first conceived to furnish unimpeachable evidence of the detection of arsenic. Afterwards many inquirers, and among them the discoverer himself, became satisfied that certain fallacies stand in the way of a conclusion based on such simple premises. Various supplementary tests were in consequence proposed. And at length it seems to be agreed, that the proper mode of applying Marsh's discovery is to employ a succession of tests, of which that originally pointed out by him is the first. A vast variety of methods of analysis founded on this principle have been proposed by British and continental chemists. It would be tedious and unprofitable to discuss or even to state them here. The reader will probably be satisfied with a reference to the most important of them[†] and with a description of that process, which appears to me, from repeated trials in medico-legal practice, to be at once most convenient, delicate, and conclusive.

Let the liquid to be examined be introduced into a Döbereiner's lamp [Fig 10], or an apparatus constructed with a bottle and a funnel upon the same principle [Fig. 11] ; and dilute the liquid with distilled water, until the lower cavity of the apparatus be nearly full, leaving space however for the tube of the funnel, a fragment of zinc, and some sulphuric acid. Put in a cylinder or rod of zinc, a ; and then add sulphuric acid until a moderate effervescence ensue. Close the junction of the two vessels, and then, allowing a little gas to escape at c, shut the stopcock, and let the gas fill the vessel A, by driving the liquid up into B. Having meanwhile fitted by a cork to the exit-tube, c, the glass tube, d e, which is loosely

* Edinburgh New Philosophical Journal, 1836, xxi. 229.

† Mr. L. Thomson in Lond. Phil. Journal, 1837, i. 353. — Orfila, Journal de Chimie Médicale, 1841, p. 212. — Bischoff, Repertorium für die Pharmacie, lxxv. 411. — Mr. H. H. Watson, Manchester Memoirs, vi. 603. — Pettenkoffer, Repertorium für die Pharmacie, lxxvi. 289. — Berzelius, and a Committee of the French Institute, Journal de Chimie Médicale, 1841, 393. — Flandin and Danger, Ibidem, 1841, 435. — Malapert, Ibidem, 1841, 295. — Lassaigne, Ibidem, 1840, 638.— Mr. Ellis, Lancet, 1843. — A paper of my own, Edinburgh Monthly Journal of Med. Science, iii. 257.

stuffed with raw cotton at the end *d g*, and has a bent plate of copper or tinned iron hung over it at *f*, — open the stop-cock, allow a little gas to escape so as to expel the air in *d e*, and then kindle the gas at *e*, which must be contracted to a capillary opening. Keep the flame low, and hold the surface of a white porcelain vessel across the middle of it for a few seconds. If no stain be produced on the porcelain, there is no arsenic in the fluid. If a stain be formed, regulate the escape of gas by the stop-cock so that the fluid may not rise above the middle of the lower vessel of the apparatus, and apply the heat of a spirit-lamp flame to the tube *d e* on the left hand of the plate *f*, the purpose of which is to prevent the heat being communicated beyond that point. By and by, if there be arsenic in the fluid, a brilliant metallic ring will appear beyond *f*, owing to decomposition of arseniuretted-hydrogen gas. As soon as the crust is thick enough to present its properties characteristically, withdraw the spirit-lamp ; place the tube *e h* so that the flame at *e* shall be completely within the ball, *i* ; let the tube incline very slightly in the direction from *k* to *l* ; and allow a stream of cold water to trickle down upon the portion *k l*, which should be wrapped in a single layer of calico. Oxide of arsenic will gradually condense, partly in white powder or minute sparkling crystals in the ball and between *i* and *k*, and partly between *k* and *l* in the form of a solution, which collects at the bend *l*. The solution which may be increased in quantity by boiling a little distilled water upon the powder in the ball and bend *i k*, is then to be subjected in small portions to the three liquid reagents, ammoniacal nitrate of silver, ammoniacal sulphate of copper, and hydro-sulphuric acid.

Some experience is required to apply this process successfully. But with due attention it furnishes conclusive evidence with great delicacy and precision. A solution containing only a millionth part of oxide of arsenic will part with it readily in the form of arseniuretted-hydrogen ; and the slightest trace of that gas in the hydrogen is indicated by the method recommended above. — The process is compounded of Mr. Marsh's original discovery, the supplementary test of reduction in the exit-tube recommended by Berzelius,* and the formation and examination of the oxide proposed by myself.† — With certain precautions and modes of manipulating, it is applicable to the most complex organic fluids, as well as to simple solutions.

The discovery of Mr. Marsh had not been long made before the test in its original simple form was found liable to divers important fallacies. It appeared, for example, that antimony yields very nearly the same appearance of metallic crust and of white powder, according to the position of the porcelain in the flame ; that some porcelains glazed with oxide of zinc are similarly stained by a flame of simple

* Journal de Chimie Médicale, 1841, 393. Rapport de l'Institut.

† Edinburgh Monthly Journal of Medical Science, 1843, iii. 257.

21*

hydrogen gas; that a great variety of metallic salts, if spirted up into the exit-tube, undergo reduction in the flame, and cause imitative stains on the porcelain; that iron-salts seems to form stains from the same chemical action as what occurs in the case of arsenic; and that certain compounds of phosphorous acid with ammonia and animal matter, or even mere animal matters themselves, will in some circumstances produce a stain more or less similar to that which is occasioned by arsenic.

There is no doubt, that the resemblance of most of these spurious stains to an arsenical crust has been much exaggerated. But still the similarity is sufficient to satisfy every impartial judge, that the mere production of a brilliant metallic, or white powdery stain, or both, upon porcelain, is not conclusive evidence of the detection of arsenic in medico-legal inquiries. It is strong presumptive evidence; and the non-production of such stains is absolute proof that arsenic is not present. But in order to obtain irrefragable proof of its presence, the substance which forms the crusts and stains must be subjected to farther examination. And such is the object of the supplementary methods in the process detailed above. That process is perfectly free of fallacy. No substance yet known but arsenic can yield the succession of phenomena which have been detailed. My opinion farther is, that the process may be safely simplified by withdrawing Berzelius's supplementary test of reduction in the exit-tube, and retaining the test of oxidation only, with the examination of the oxide by liquid reagents. I have retained the former in deference to the opinion expressed by a committee appointed by the French Institute, who examined the whole subject with unwearied zeal, but who, it may be observed, seem never to have had in their view the check-test of oxidation; which, with the consecutive tests, is superior in conclusiveness to the check of reduction only.

Reinsch's process, like the former, has been inconveniently called a new test for arsenic. The fact discovered by Dr. Reinsch is valueless as supplying a mere test; but it forms the ground-work of the best process of all yet proposed for the detection of arsenic in solution. The discovery is, that arsenic in solution is deposited in the metallic state upon copper-leaf, when the fluid is acidulated with hydrochloric acid, and heated till it boils gently or is about to do so; and that by heating the copper gently in a glass tube the arsenic is sublimed from it in the form of oxide or metal according to the quantity present.*

This method is so simple and easy as scarcely to require any detailed explanation. The fluid should contain about a tenth of its volume of hydrochloric acid. It must be heated near ebullition before the copper is introduced, otherwise the copper becomes tarnished, though arsenic be not present. Copper-leaf, or copper-plate worn thin by the action of diluted nitric acid, or fine copper gauze, is the best form for use. In the feeblest solutions ten or fifteen minutes elapse before arsenic is visibly deposited, and forty minutes should

* Journal für Praktischen Chemie, 1842, xxiv. 242.

be allowed for strong deposition; but in strong solutions, the action takes place in a few seconds. The result is a thin, brittle, brilliant, steel like coating of metallic arsenic. As soon as the deposit is formed, the copper is to be removed, dried with a gentle heat, cut into small shreds, and heated with a spirit-lamp in the smallest glass tube that will conveniently contain the whole; upon which a metallic ring of arsenic is sometimes sublimed, but more generally a ring of small sparkling crystals. These are first to be examined as to their form with a common pocket lens; and then dissolved in boiling distilled water, after shaking out the copper, so that a solution may be obtained and subjected to the liquid reagents, especially the ammoniacal nitrate of silver as being the readiest and most delicate. In all medico-legal inquiries it is necessary to perform a preliminary experiment with distilled water and the hydrochloric acid used, lest the acid contain arsenic.

The process here described is one which I have followed with great facility, certainty and despatch in several medico-legal cases.[*] It is extremely delicate; for it will detect at least a 250,000th part of arsenic in solution; and it removes from the fluid every particle of arsenic, because none can be afterwards discovered by means even of Marsh's method. It is not subject to any fallacy. The mere formation of a brilliant coating on the copper is not evidence of arsenic being present; for as Reinsch himself ascertained, solutions of bismuth, tin, zinc, and antimony produce a coating more or less similar to an arsenical one. But the farther steps of the process entirely put aside all these sources of error. The non-formation of a metallic tarnish of copper, however, is perhaps not absolute proof of the absence of arsenic. For, according to a late statement by Drs. Fresenius and Von Babo,[†] " all nitrates, and various salts of mercury and other metals, render the separation of arsenic by copper difficult or even impossible." The authors of this objection, although the paper is otherwise elaborate and detailed, have not given any particulars in illustration of so important a criticism.

Of the Tests for Oxide of Arsenic in Organic Mixtures.

The present is by far the most important of the conditions under which it may be necessary to search for arsenic in medico-legal cases; for in nine cases out of ten the subject of analysis is either some article of food or drink, the contents or tissues of the stomach, or the textures of other organs of the body into which the poison has been carried by absorption.

Accordingly much attention has been paid to this subject for some years past, and many valuable methods of analysis have been suggested, more especially since the recent discovery that arsenic, like many other poisons, undergo absorption, and is diffused by the circulation throughout the body generally. It was proved by me in

* See Edinburgh Monthly Journ. of Med. Science, 1843, iii. 774.
† Annalen der Chimie und Pharmacie, 1844, xlix. 291.

1824,* that the tests for arsenic, at that time in general use, are so fallacious when applied to complex organic mixtures as to be unfit for medico-legal investigations except merely as trial-tests; and a process was proposed, which has since undergone various modifications from others as well as myself. This process, in the form in which it was adopted in the last edition of the present work, is still applicable to a great proportion of cases; and indeed a recent modification of it has been thought by Drs. Fresenius and von Babo to be superior even yet to every other in all circumstances.† But two new methods are at present generally preferred, and probably not without reason. At least they have been much employed and with great success in numerous medico-legal researches, where the quantity of arsenic was to all appearance extremely small, and the subject of examination most complex and troublesome to bring within the sphere of analysis. And in particular they have been successfully employed to detect arsenic in those organs of the human body into which it can obtain admission only through the medium of absorption.

In the following statement I shall describe four processes only, that of Reinsch, by which the arsenic is first separated as a crust on copper, — that of Marsh, who first detaches it in the form of arseniuretted-hydrogen, — my own method, which consists in obtaining in the first instance a sulphuret of arsenic, — and that of Drs. Fresenius and von Babo, which has the same foundation.

Process of Reinsch. — This is the simplest and easiest of all. Remove in the first place any white or gray powder which can be detached from the mixture; and either subject it to the process of reduction by charcoal or soda-flux, as described at p. 203, or dissolve it in boiling distilled water and subject the solution to the three liquid reagents, p. 207, or if there be enough, examine it in both ways. If arsenic be thus obtained, it is seldom necessary to proceed any farther. But if not, cut all soft solids into small fragments, add distilled water if necessary, then add hydrochloric acid to the amount of a tenth of the whole mixture, and more if the subject of analysis be decayed and ammoniacal, so that there may be a decided excess of acid. Boil gently for an hour, or until all soft solids be either dissolved or broken down into fine flakes and grains. Filter through calico; bring the filtered fluid again to the boiling point; and then proceed as described for Reinsch's method in simple arsenical solutions [p. 214].

The only important precaution to be attended to in employing this process is to take care that the water, hydrochloric acid, and calico are free of accidental impregnation with arsenic. This is guarded against by applying the process to them in the first instance. I have lately employed this method of analysis with success in two medico-legal cases where the bodies had been buried for several months, and where the quantity of arsenic must have been very minute. Satis-

* Edinburgh Medical and Surgical Journal, 1824, xxii. 78.
† Annalen der Chemie und Pharmacie, xlix. 308.

factory evidence was obtained from a sixth part of the stomach, and also from the same proportion of the liver.

Process of Marsh. — The chief difficulties in applying the process of Marsh to complex organic mixtures arise from the tendency of oxide of arsenic to adhere with obstinacy to some organic principles in the solid state, and from the liability of the gas disengaged in the apparatus to raise organic fluids in a fine froth, which breaks up slowly, and is therefore apt to pass over into the exit-tube. Many contrivances have been devised, to meet these difficulties, especially by the French chemists and toxicologists, whose attention was turned earnestly to the subject by the investigations carried on in certain late criminal trials of great interest and importance. The various devices now alluded to were subjected to trial in 1841 by a Committee of the French Institute; who came to the opinion that the following method suggested by MM. Flandin and Danger is the most convenient and comprehensive.*

Heat the organic matter with a sixth of its weight of strong sulphuric acid; when complete solution has taken place, concentrate the fluid to a friable almost dry charcoal; add a little concentrated nitric acid gradually to this when cold, and again evaporate to dryness; then act on the residue with boiling distilled water, and a solution of a reddish-brown colour is obtained, which may be used in such an apparatus as that of Döbereiner without risk of obstruction from froth. — The arseniuretted-hydrogen, thus disengaged along with the hydrogen gas, is to be submitted to the succession of tests described in speaking of Marsh's process for detecting arsenic in a state of simple solution [p. 212].

This method of investigation is exceedingly precise and conclusive. The sulphuric acid aided by heat destroys organic matter sufficiently to prevent frothing in the apparatus and dissolves out arsenic from a state of combination with organic principles; and nitric acid afterwards converts any arsenic in the half-charred mass into the soluble arsenic acid. It has been employed with success in various medico-legal proceedings in France. It answers well for detecting oxide of arsenic in the viscera, muscles, and other parts of the body into which the poison has been conveyed through absorption.

Process by Hydrosulphuric Acid. — This method may be employed in two ways, according as the object is merely to prove the presence of oxide of arsenic, or to ascertain also its quantity.

a. If proof of its presence be all that is wanted, cut any soft solids into small pieces, add distilled water if necessary, boil for half an hour, let the decoction cool, and filter it. Add a little acetic acid to the filtered fluid, and if any precipitate form, filter again. Evaporate to dryness, first by ebullition, afterwards over the vapour-bath. Dissolve the residuum again in repeated portions of boiling distilled water, and filter the solution. If it be not acid to litmus-paper add more acetic acid, and transmit hydrosulphuric acid gas through the fluid until an excess be indicated by the sense of smell after agitation.

* Journal de Chimie Médicale, 1841, p. 413.

Then expel the excess of gas by boiling ; and if the precipitate of sulphuret of arsenic do not subside readily add a little of a strong solution of hydrochlorate of ammonia, which will facilitate subsidence. When the precipitate has fallen to the bottom, withdraw the super-natant fluid with the pipette, Fig. 8 ; and replace it with a little boiling distilled water.   Lastly, collect the precipitate on a filter, and proceed as by the reduction-process with soda-flux for oxide of arsenic, in a state of simple solution.

This method answers very well for ordinary cases where the quan-tity of arsenic is not extremely minute.   But I have met with in-stances in medico-legal practice where the process of Reinsch, as well as that of Marsh, succeeded in detecting the poison in sources to which the method by hydro-sulphuric acid had been applied without avail ; because apparently the organic matter existing in so-lution prevented the action of the gas, or, as Orfila thinks, because boiling water will not in all circumstances remove oxide of arsenic from the textures of the animal body which are impregnated with it. In particular I doubt whether this method is sufficiently delicate to detect arsenic in those organs and textures into which it has been conveyed in cases of poisoning through absorption into the blood. — Another objection is its tediousness.   The first filtration, if the sub-stance to be examined be the stomach or its contents, may take two days ; and one way or another the analysis can seldom be completed within four days.   Reinsch's process may be brought to a conclusion in two hours or less, even in the most difficult circumstances.

b. The last process to be mentioned, is one based, like the pre-vious one, upon the precipitation of arsenic in the form of sulphuret, but with very material modifications, the purpose of which is to enable the analyst to separate the whole arsenic in a state of purity, so as to ascertain the exact amount of the poison in the mixture. This method has been recently proposed by Drs. Fresenius and von Babo.*

Cut any soft solids into small pieces, put the whole into a porcelain basin, add as much hydrochloric acid as equals the probable weight of the dry matter in the mixture, and then water enough to form a thin pulp.   Heat the basin over the vapour-bath, adding every five minutes about half a drachm of chlorate of potass, and stirring fre-quently, until the liquid become clear-yellow, homogeneous, and thin.   Add now two drachms more of the chlorate ; filter through linen, washing the residuum on the filter with boiling-water ; con-centrate to a pound ; add a strong solution of sulphurous acid till its odour predominates, and expel the excess of it by heat.   The liquid is now ready for the transmission of hydrosulphuric acid gas, which should be transmitted in a slow stream for twelve hours.   Wash away any sulphuret adhering to the tube by means of ammonia, and add the solution to the principal liquid ; which is next to be left at a gentle heat about 80° F., in a vessel covered with paper, till the sul-phureous smell entirely disappear.   The precipitate, which contains

* Annalen der Chemie und Pharmacie, 1844, Mär 3, xlix. 308.

organic matter as well as sulphuret, is then to be collected on a paper filter, washed, and dried with the filter over the vapour-bath. The animal matter is next destroyed, and the sulphuret converted into arsenic acid, by dropping on it fuming nitrous acid till the whole is moistened, drying the product thoroughly over the vapour-bath, moistening the residuum with concentrated sulphuric acid, heating the mixture again in the vapour-bath for two or three hours, and raising the heat afterwards gradually in a sand-bath to 300° F., till a charred brittle mass be obtained. This is to be heated over the vapour-bath with twenty parts of distilled water, filtered, and washed with boiling water on the filter till what passes through ceases to redden litmus. The solution, which ought to be colourless, is next acidulated with hydrochloric acid, and treated as formerly with hyrosulphuric acid gas. When the sulphuret has been collected on a small filter, diluted ammonia is to be sent through the filter as long as it dissolves any sulphuret, and is to be received in a weighed porcelain basin, in which the ammonia and water are to be driven off at a temperature not exceeding 212°. The sulphuret which is alone left may now be weighed by again weighing the basin ; and one grain of sulphuret is equivalent to 0·803 of a grain of oxide of arsenic. — The authors add an elaborate process for obtaining from this the whole arsenic by reduction. But such a proceeding is unnecessary. It is sufficient in medico-legal inquiries to ascertain by the simpler method given above [p. 204], that it does yield by reduction with soda-flux a true arsenical crust, and that this yields by oxidation white, sparkling crystals with triangular facettes.

Afer a comparative trial of the most esteemed process, Drs. Fresenius and von Babo state that they found the one now described as delicate as any other, and the only method by which the quantity of oxide of arsenic can be ascertained with accuracy. — The hydrochloric acid used at the commencement enables the water to dissolve compounds of arsenic which water alone will not act on ; and it farther facilitates solution by breaking up or dissolving organic textures. The addition of chlorate of potash prevents the escape of oxide of arsenic during the subsequent evaporation ; which is apt to happen when hydrochloric acid is present. The subsequent addition of sulphuric acid converts arsenic acid into arsenious acid, in which shape the sulphuret of arsenic is more readily formed by the action of hydrosulphuric acid gas, when organic matter co-exists in the solution. The steps for destroying organic matter thrown down with the sulphuret at its first formation require no further commentary : They are the most important particulars in the process for its main object, — the determination of the quantity of pure sesquisulphuret, and, through it, of the sesquioxide originally in the subject of analysis.

Of certain alleged Fallacies in the case of Organic Mixtures.

Before taking leave of the detection of arsenic in organic mixtures, it is necessary to notice certain alleged fallacies in the way of every process, arising from arsenic obtaining admission into the subject of analysis through other means than its intentional addition or its introduction as a poison into the body.   This topic, one of paramount importance in medico-legal chemistry, has lately undergone careful investigation during and since the notorious trial of Madame Lafarge. The results are the following : —

It has been alleged that arsenic may obtain accidental admission into the subject of analysis, 1, because the reagents used in the processes may be adulterated with arsenic ; 2, because the material of the apparatus may contain it ; 3, because it may have existed in antidotes administered during life ; 4, because it sometimes forms a constituent part of the human body in the natural state ; and 5, because it exists in the soil of some churchyards.

1. *Arsenic may exist as an adulteration in some reagents.* — It must be apt to occur in *sulphuric acid*, when that substance is prepared with pyritic sulphur, which commonly contains some sulphuret of arsenic ; and it has actually been found in abundance in the acid by various experimentalists, and in England for the first time by Dr. Rees.*   It may be detected by transmitting hydrosulphuric acid gas through the diluted acid ; and it may be effectually removed in the same way,† the acid being afterwards filtered in a funnel whose throat is filled with abestus, and the excess of gas being expelled by heat. — *Hydrochloric acid* may contain arsenic, because it may have been prepared with an arsenicated sulphuric acid.   The impurity may be detected and removed in the same way as in that substance.   Nitric acid seems not apt to be similarly adulterated ;‡ but it may be tested by Marsh's process, after neutralizing the acid with potash, and adding more sulphuric acid than is required to decompose the nitre thus formed.   *Zinc* occasionally contains a little arsenic, which will be evolved in Marsh's process.   Dr. Clark of Aberdeen says zinc is scarcely ever free of a trace of arsenic ; and it has been occasionally detected by others.   Orfila, however, very seldom found so much as to be discoverable by Marsh's test applied continuously for a great length of time.§   A committee of the French Institute came to the same conclusion.‖   M. Jaquelain, acting under the directions of Professor Dumas, could not detect an atom in any French specimen of zinc, or its carbonate or silicated oxide, as met with in commerce.¶ Lastly, Mr. Brett satisfied himself that no British or foreign zinc he could obtain indicated the presence of arsenic by a process capable of detecting a 5000th of that metal in zinc.**   It is an obvious inference from all these inquiries that no difficulty can be experienced in obtaining zinc so pure as to exhibit not a trace of arsenic by Marsh's method.   Neither is there any difficulty in obtaining sulphuric, muriatic, and nitric acid free of that adulteration.

* London Medical Gazette, 1840-41, i. 723.
† Annales de Hygiène Publique, 1839, xxii. 404.
‡ Ibidem, p. 418.
§ Journal de Chimie Médicale, 1839, 452.
‖ Ibidem, 1841, 534.   ¶ Ibidem, 1842, 650.
** London Philosophical Journal, 1842, ii. 403.

But at the same time it is equally obvious, that in medico-legal ana-lyses, unless the reagents used be previously known to be free of arsenic, they ought invariably to be subjected in the first instance to the process, whatever it may be, which the analyst proposes to em-ploy for detecting arsenic in a suspected substance.

2. *Arsenic may be present in some articles of chemical apparatus.* — Arsenic has been detected in the metal of cast-iron pots,* which Orfila and others have proposed to employ in certain analyses on the large scale, as, for example, when the poison is sought for in the whole soft solids of the human body. It is denied, however, that any of that arsenic can be dissolved out of cast-iron by the process which has been followed in such circumstances.†

The primary fact, and the qualification of it, are in my opinion of equally little medico-legal importance. It is not likely that such enormous masses of material will ever be operated on again, as those which were made use of in some late French trials, and for which great iron pots were found indispensable ; — because it has been proved that absorbed arsenic is chiefly to be met with in particular organs or secretions, such as the liver and urine. Besides, a false im-portance has been attached to the enthusiastic analyses of the whole human carcase, with which some French chemists have been astound-ing the minds of the scientific world, as well as the vulgar, on the occasion of certain late trials for poisoning. I confess I could not find fault with a jury, who might decline to put faith in the evidence of poisoning with arsenic, when the analyst, after boiling an entire body, with many gallons of water, in a huge iron cauldron, making use of whole pounds of sulphuric acid, nitric acid, and nitre, and toiling for days and weeks at the process, could do no more than produce minute traces of the poison. What man of common sense will believe, that, with such bulky materials and crude apparatus, it is possible to guard to a certainty against the accidental admission of a little arsenic ? At all events I am much mistaken if any British jury would condemn a prisoner on such evidence, — or any British chemist find fault with them for declining to do so.

3. *Arsenic may have existed in antidotes administered during life.* — It is now generally known, that the only chemical antidote for arsenic is the hydrated sesquioxide of iron. But this substance ap-pears occasionally to contain a little arsenic, obviously derived from the compound of iron whence the oxide is prepared.‡ Such an adul-teration must be rare in what is prepared by the ordinary processes, according to which the oxide of arsenic ought to remain in solution. The only effectual mode, however, of guarding against this source of error, when the antidote has been administered, is to examine a portion of the stock whence the patient was supplied, by dissolving it in an excess of sulphuric acid, and subjecting it to Marsh's test.

4. *Arsenic sometimes exists naturally in the human body.* — This

* Wohler, Journal de Chim. Medicale, 1840, 96.
† Bulletins de l'Acad. Roy. de Médecine, 1839, iii. 1073.
‡ Journal de Chimie Médicale, 1840, 645, and 1841, 242.

22

startling proposition was first advanced by M. Couerbe, and by
Professor Orfila soon afterwards.* The latter subsequently stated,
h at it exists only in the bones, and not in any of the soft solids.†
t is now clear, however, that both of these experimentalists must
have committed an error. Orfila himself admits that his early re-
earches are vitiated by the subsequent discovery of arsenic in some
skinds of sulphuric acid ;‡ and all recent attempts by others to obtain
his results have failed. Thus MM. Flandin and Danger could not
detect arsenic in any part of the human body, when it had not been
administered :§ Pfaff was unable to detect an atom of it in the bones
of man or the lower animals by Orfila's own process :‖ Dr. Rees
was equally unsuccessful :¶ and in 1841 a committee of the
French Institute, who superintended the performance of an analysis in three cases by Orfila, reported that he failed in every instance to find a trace of arsenic, by a process which could detect a
65th part of a grain intentionally mixed with an avoirdupois pound
of bones.**
   There is the strongest possible presumption, therefore, that
human bones never contain any arsenic. And besides, supposing
they did, the source of fallacy would be utterly insignificant ; for,
when it becomes necessary to search for arsenic absorbed into the
textures of the body, it is never necessary to have recourse to the
bones.
   5. *Arsenic mny exist in the soil of churchyards.* — This proposition
too was first announced by Professor Orfila, who found a little in the
churchyard of Villey-sur-Tille, near Dijon, and of the Bicêtre, Mont-
Parnasse, and New Botanic Garden at Paris.†† And although MM.
Flandin and Danger afterwards denied they could ever find any,‡‡
a committee of the Parisian Academy of Medicine reported that
Orfila proved before them the accuracy of his statement.§§ But the
arsenic exists in a state in which it cannot be dissolved out by boiling
water : It has been hitherto separable only by boiling the churchyard
mould with concentrated sulphuric acid. Hence it cannot pass by
percolation through a coffin into a body ; and consequently it becomes
a source of fallacy only when the coffin has been broken up in the
course of time, and the mould lies in actual contact with the organs
to be analysed.‖‖
   It plainly appears, then, that most of the fallacies alleged against the
validity of the evidence derived from the discovery of arsenic within
the human body in cases of poisoning have no real existence ; and
that those which are real can easily be provided against by simple
and obvious precautions.

   * Journ. de Chim. Méd. 1839, 346.
   † Annales d'Hygiène Publique, 1839, xxii.   ‡ Ibidem, 404.
   § Journal de Chimie Médicale, 1841, 223.
   ‖ Repertorium für de Pharmacie, lxxv. 107.
   ¶ Guy's Hospital Reports. 1841, vi. 163.
   ** Journal de Chimie Médicale, 1841, 417, 421, 431.
   †† Annales d'Hygiène Publique, xxii. 450.
   ‡‡ Journal de Chimie Médicale, 1841, 223.
   §§ Ibidem, 1840, 690.   ‖‖ Annales, &c. ut supra.

3. *Arsenite of Copper.*

The arsenite of copper [Scheele's-green, Mineral-green] deserves notice, because it is in use as a pigment, and has actually been used as a poison. Dr. Duncan once detected it in pills, given to a pregnant female with the view of procuring abortion; in Paris it has been detected in sweetmeats, having been used to give them a fine green colour;* and Mr. Ainley of Bingley in Yorkshire informs me he found it to constitute a pigment sold by London pastry-cooks under the name of emerald-green for colouring preserves, and which in his practice had proved poisonous to children who had eaten apple-tarts coloured with it.

It is a compound of arsenious acid and deutoxide of copper, is sold in powder or pulverulent cakes, and has a pale grass-green colour. Its nature may be ascertained by heating it in a glass tube. Crystals of oxide of arsenic sublime, and oxide of copper remains, which, on being dissolved in nitric acid, yields a fine violet-blue solution with ammonia.

The mineral-green of the shops, however, is seldom arsenite of copper. The substance sold in Edinburgh under that name, although believed by colour-men to be a preparation of arsenic, is not the arsenite of copper, but a mixture of hydrated oxide of copper and carbonate of lime; which will be mentioned more particularly under the head of the poisons of copper.

Process for Organic Mixtures. — The suspected mixture is to be heated with a little hydrochloric acid and well stirred. The arsenite being thus dissolved, the solution is to be allowed to cool and then filtered. A stream of hydrosulphuric-acid gas will now cause a dark-brown or yellowish-brown muddiness or precipitate, which is a mixture of sulphuret of copper and sulphuret of arsenic. The precipitate being separated after boiling, and properly cleansed by the process of subsidence and affusion, or if it is large, by washing on a filter, the two sulphurets are to be separated by ammonia, which dissolves sulphuret of arsenic but leaves the sulphuret of copper; and the sulphuret of arsenic may be recovered from the filtered fluid by expelling the ammonia with heat. The sulphuret of arsenic is next to be reduced as directed at page 211; and the sulphuret of copper examined as recommended under the head of copper.

4. *Arsenite of Potass.*

This salt is an object of some importance to the medical jurist, as it forms the basis of a common medicine, Fowler's Solution, or the Tasteless Ague Drop. This preparation contains in every ounce four grains of arsenious acid. It has a brownish-red colour, and an odour of lavender. It is strongly alkaline to litmus. When acidulated with hydrochloric acid, hydrosulphuric-acid gas causes in it a dirty brownish-yellow precipitate; and Reinsch's process will detach arsenic from it upon copper in a state capable of being subjected to the usual tests [see p. 214].

* Revue Médicale. 1827, i. 365,

5. *Arseniate of Potass.*

This substance is so rarely met with as to be an object of little consequence to the medical jurist: nevertheless I have found in the course of reading two instances of poisoning with it. A very dangerous and tedious case has been related by Professor Bernt, which arose from too great a quantity having been given medicinally by an ignorant druggist;* and a case of accidental poisoning with it has been related in the London Medical Repository.† A singular account too has been published of the accidental poisoning of seven horses with it at Paris. They all died, most of them with the symptoms and morbid appearances of well-marked inflammation of the alimentary canal.‡

When solid it forms tetraedral prismatic crystals, acuminated by four planes. It is very soluble in water, fuses at a red heat, and on cooling concretes into a crumbly, foliaceous mass, having a pearly lustre. It is easily known by the effect of the process of reduction — of the nitrate of silver, the salts of copper, and sulphuretted-hydrogen. Heated with charcoal in a tube it gives off metallic arsenic in the usual manner; but a stronger heat is required than for the reduction of the arsenious acid. Dissolved in water and treated with nitrate of silver it yields a brick-red precipitate, the arseniate of silver. With the salts of copper its solution gives a pale bluish-white precipitate, the arseniate of copper. With sulphuretted-hydrogen gas, preceded by acidulation with muriatic acid, and transmitted for a considerable length of time, it yields the yellow sulphuret of arsenic. When in solution it yields arsenic both by Reinsch's process and the method of Marsh.

6. *The Sulphurets of Arsenic.*

In the arts various substances are known which contain a compound of sulphur and arsenic. In the first place, two pure sulphurets are known in chemistry and in painting, the one of a fine orange colour, and known by the name of realgar, the other of a rich sulphur-yellow, and termed orpiment. Secondly, the name of orpiment is familiarly given to a pigment in more general use than either of the former, which has a less lively colour, and consists of pure orpiment with a large admixture of arsenious acid. Lastly, orpiment also forms a great proportion of another common pigment, King's yellow.

The orange-red sulphuret (realgar, risigallum, Σανδαϱαχη), sandaracha), is chiefly a natural production. It is solid, of a bright orange-red colour, and composed of small shining scales, so soft as to be scratched with the nail. It is composed of one equivalent of metal and one of sulphur. Its best chemical characters are the disengagement of metallic arsenic when it is heated in a tube with potass or the black flux; and its undergoing sublimation unchanged when heated alone in a tube.

The yellow sulphuret (orpiment, auripigmentum, αϱσενικον), is both

* Beiträge zur gerichtlichen Arzneikunde, iv. 221.   † January, 1819.
‡ Annales d'Hygiène Publ. et de Med. Legale, xii. 393.

a natural production, and the result of many chemical operations. The sulphuret thrown down from solutions of arsenic by sulphuretted-hydrogen is quite conformable in physical and chemical characters with the natural orpiment. Natural orpiment, when in mass, consists of broad scales of much brilliancy and of a rich yellow colour. It is composed of two equivalents of metal and three of sulphur. Its most striking chemical characters are the same with those of realgar, from which it is distinguished chiefly by its colour.

It has been stated by Hahnemann in his elaborate work on Arsenic, that the pure sulphurets are somewhat soluble in water, — that native orpiment is soluble in 5000 parts of water with the aid of ebullition, and that artificial orpiment by precipitation is soluble in 600 parts.[*] Hahnemann, however, was mistaken in supposing that the water dissolved these sulphurets. It does not dissolve, but decomposes them. Very lately M. Decourdemanche has found that, by slow action in cold water, and much more quickly with the aid of heat, the arsenical sulphuret is decomposed by virtue of a simultaneous decomposition of the water, hydrosulphuric acid being evolved and an oxide of arsenic remaining in solution. And he has farther remarked, that this change is promoted by the presence of animal and vegetable principles dissolved in water.[†] These facts are interesting, as they explain certain apparent anomalies to be noticed presently in the physiological properties of the sulphurets.

The common orpiment of the shops is not a pure sulphuret like the natural orpiment, but a much more active substance, a mixture of orpiment and arsenious acid. It is made by subliming in close vessels a mixture of sulphur and oxide of arsenic. It is met with in the shops in two forms, in that of a fine powder possessing a yellow colour with a faint tint of orange, and in that of concave masses composed of layers of various tints of white, yellow and orange, commonly also lined internally with tetraedral white pyramidal crystals. Till lately it was accounted a variety of sulphurèt, and some ingenious conjectures were made as to the cause of its superior energy over the other sulphurets as a poison. But M. Guibourt has proved that it always contains oxide of arsenic, and is commonly impregnated with it to a very large amount, some parcels containing so much as 96 per cent.[‡] The inner surface I have often seen lined with large crystals of pure oxide. In a very interesting account by Dr. Symonds of Bristol, describing the case of Mrs. Smith, for whose murder a woman Burdock was executed in that city a few years ago, it is stated that artificial orpiment was the poison given, that death took place in a very few hours, and that a sample from the druggist's shop where the poison was bought contained on an average 79 per cent. of oxide of arsenic.[§]

Another impure sulphuret, a good deal used in painting, and a favourite poison in this country for killing flies, is King's yellow. It

* Ueber die Arsenic-vergiftung, pp. 14, 45.　　† Journal de Pharmacie, xiii. 207.
‡ Journal de Chim. Med. ii. 113.
§ Trans. of Provincial Med. and Surg. Association, iii. 465.
22*

is sold in the form of a light powder or in loose conical cakes. It has an intense sulphur-yellow colour. This substance is soluble, though not entirely, in water, both cold and warm, and forms a colourless solution, from which, on cooling, or by evaporation, a yellow powder separates. In this respect it differs essentially from the pure sulphurets. The solution is not acted on by reagents in the same way as the solution of arsenious acid. Lime-water and hydrosulphuric acid have no effect on it, the ammoniacal nitrate of silver causes a copious dirty brown, and the ammoniacal sulphate of copper a scanty, dirty lemon-yellow precipitate. I have not seen any account of the mode of preparing it or an analysis of its composition. But according to my own experiments it contains a large proportion of sulphuret of arsenic, a considerable proportion of lime, and about 16 per cent. of sulphur. Its nature is best shown by the following method of analysis. Let the powder be agitated in diluted ammonia till the colour becomes white. The filtered fluid contains the sulphuret of arsenic, which, on addition of an acid, falls down, and may be separated and reduced in a tube with the black flux. The remaining white powder, well freed from adhering sulphuret by washing, is next to be agitated in diluted acetate or hydrochloric acid and again filtered. The solution on being neutralized precipitates abundantly with oxalate of ammonia and the alkaline carbonates, showing that lime was taken up by the acid : and, as the acid operates without effervescence, the lime must have been in the caustic state. The powder which remains after the action of the acid will be found to fuse with a gentle heat and to burn almost entirely away with a blue flame, emitting sulphureous vapours. These experiments make it obvious that King's yellow contains sulphuret of arsenic, caustic lime, and free sulphur ; and in all probability the lime exists in the form of a triple sulphuret of lime and arsenic.

All the preparations containing the sulphuret of arsenic are interesting to the medical jurist, but particularly the two impure sulphurets last mentioned. The King's yellow above all should be carefully studied, because on account of its frequent employment as a fly-poison it has been the source of fatal accidents. It was likewise taken intentionally a few years ago in this city, and proved fatal in thirty-six hours. Dr. Duncan also, while he was Professor of Medical Jurisprudence, met with an instance of an attempt to poison by mixing King's yellow with tea; and at the Glasgow Spring Circuit of 1822 a woman was tried for poisoning her child with it.

Process for Organic Mixtures. — If sulphuret of arsenic be present in such mixtures in appreciable quantity, the particles, owing to their intense yellow colour, will be visible in any mass which has not the same tint. From this state of admixture they may be removed by adding caustic ammonia which dissolves sulphuret of arsenic; and the solution, on being acidulated with muriatic acid, will deposit the sulphuret sufficiently pure for undergoing the process of reduction.

Sulphuret of arsenic sometimes exists in small quantity in the stomach, although the poison was given in the form of oxide ; for a portion of the oxide is subject to be converted into the sulphuret by hydrosulphuric acid gas evolved in the stomach after death.* In every instance of the kind yet carefully examined a large proportion of the oxide has remained unacted on, although the intense colour of the mixed sulphuret makes it appear as if that were the only compound present.

7. *Arseniuretted-Hydrogen.*

This compound presents the form of a colourless gas, possessing a fetid garlicky odour, a density of nearly 2·7, and great virulence as a poison. It is mentioned here, because accidental poisoning with it has happened occasionally within a few years, chiefly owing to the occasional adulteration of sulphuric acid with arsenic, and the liability of the arsenic to form arseniuretted-hydrogen when such sulphuric acid is used to prepare hydrogen gas. Dr. O'Reilly has mentioned a melancholy instance of a young chemist losing his life in this way.† Dr. Schlinder of Greifenberg has related another, which did not prove fatal.‡ And it is well known that the German chemis Gehlen lost his life by accidentally breathing arseniuretted-hydrogen while engaged in examining its chemical properties.§ It is an inflammable body; and its presence in any other gas is easily detected by burning it according to the method of Marsh.

SECTION II. — *Of the Action of Arsenic and the Symptoms it excites in Man.*

It is now generally admitted that arsenic produces in the living body two classes of phenomena, — or that, like the narcotico-acrids, it has a twofold action. One action is purely irritant, by virtue of which it induces inflammation in the alimentary canal and elsewhere. The other, although it seldom occasions symptoms of narcotism properly so called, yet obviously consists in a disorder of parts or organs remote from the seat of its application.

It is also the general opinion of toxicologists, that arsenic occasions death more frequently through means of its remote effects than in consequence of the local inflammation it excites. In some cases indeed no symptoms of inflammation occur at all; and in many, although inflammation is obviously produced, death takes place long before it has had time to cause material organic injury. Nevertheless in some, though certainly in comparatively few instances, the local action, it must be admitted, predominates so much, that the morbid changes of the part primarily acted on are alone adequate to account for death.

Its chief operation being on organs remote from the part to which it is applied, a natural object of inquiry is, whether this action re-

* See subsequently *Morbid Appearances.*
† Dublin Journal of the Med. Sciences, xx. 422.
‡ Repertorium fur die Pharmacie, lxix. 271.
§ Buchner's Toxicologie, 476.

sults from the poison entering the blood, and so passing to the remote organs acted on, or simply arises from the organ remotely affected sympathizing through the medium of the nerves with the impression made on the organ which is affected primarily. On this question precise experiments are still wanted. The general opinion has for some time been that it acts through the blood. And this view has of late been strengthened by indisputable evidence, that the poison does enter the blood, and is diffused by it throughout the body.

For a long period chemists sought in vain for arsenic in the animal tissues and secretions at a distance from the alimentary canal. Such was the position of matters at the date of the last edition of this work; in which the failure was ascribed to the methods of analysis then known not being delicate enough to discover the small quantity of arsenic which disappears by absorption in cases of poisoning.* That statement is now referred to, because in a late controversy in France an attempt was made, by an erroneous quotation of this work, to deprive Professor Orfila of the honour, which is due to him alone, of having recently been the first to demonstrate the possibility of detecting arsenic throughout the organs and secretions generally of the bodies of men and animals poisoned with it.

This most important discovery, pregnant alike with interesting physiological deductions and valuable medico-legal applications, was first announced by him to the Parisian Academy of Medicine in January, 1839; when he stated that arsenic is absorbed in such quantity in cases of poisoning as to admit of being discovered by an improved process of analysis in various organs and fluids of the body, such as the liver, spleen, kidneys, muscles, blood, and urine.† In November, 1840, he proved these facts to the satisfaction of a committee of the academy.‡ And since then they have been confirmed by others, not merely in express experiments, but likewise in the familiar experience of medico-legal practice. The situations where arsenic is met with in largest quantity are the liver, the spleen, and the urine, but above all the liver. The precise circumstances in which it may be found in one or another of these quarters have not yet been determined. But in most cases of acute arsenical poisoning where the search has been made at all, it has proved successful in the liver. In two late instances I have readily found arsenic by the process of Marsh or Reinsch in the liver after four months' interment.

Since arsenic then is clearly absorbed into the blood, it becomes an interesting question whether the organization of the blood is thereby changed. This question cannot be answered with confidence. But in all probability the blood does undergo some change in its *crasis;* for in most cases of acute poisoning that fluid is found after death in a remarkable state of fluidity [see Section on the Morbid Appearances]; and Mr. James observed that if venous or arterial

* Treatise on Poisons, third edition, pp. 270, 271.
† Bulletins de l'Acad. Roy. de Médecine, 1839, iii. 426.
‡ Journal de Chimie Médicale, 1840, p. 690.

blood be received into a solution of arsenic, instead of coagulating in the usual way, a viscous jelly first forms, and lumpy clots separate afterwards.*

Our knowledge of the affection induced by the remote action of arsenic is in some respects vague. Toxicologists have for the most part been satisfied with calling it a disorder of the general nervous system. When employed to designate the state of collapse which accompanies or forms the chief feature of acute cases of poisoning with arsenic, this term is misapplied. The whole train of symptoms is that not of a general nervous disorder, but simply of depressed action of the heart. That this is the chief organ remotely acted on in such cases farther appears probable from certain physiological experiments, in which it has been remarked, that immediately after rapid death from arsenic the irritability of the heart was exhausted or nearly so, while that of the intestines, gullet, and voluntary muscles continued as usual.† As to the singular symptoms which often arise in the advanced stage of lingering cases, the term, disorder of the general nervous system, is more appropriately applied to them. They clearly indicate a deranged state sometimes of the brain, sometimes of particular nerves.

Arsenic belongs to those poisons which act with nearly the same energy whatever be the organ or texture to which they are applied. The experiments of Sproegel,‡ repeated by Jaeger,§ and by Sir Benjamin Brodie,‖ leave no doubt, that when applied to a fresh wound it acts with at least equal rapidity as when swallowed. Although in such circumstances the signs of irritation are often distinct, yet the symptoms are on the other hand sometimes more purely narcotic than by any other mode of administering it, — Sir B. Brodie in particular having observed loss of sense and motion to be induced, along with occasional convulsions. Arsenic likewise acts with energy when applied to the conjunctiva of the eye, as was proved by Dr. Campbell. It acts too with great energy when inhaled in the state of vapour into the lungs, or in the form of arseniuretted-hydrogen. It farther acts with violence through the mucous membrane of the vagina, producing local inflammation, and the usual constitutional collapse. These facts were determined experimentally by the Medical Inspectors of Copenhagen on the occasion of a singular trial which will be noticed afterwards. Arsenic also acts, as may easily be conceived, when injected into the rectum. And farther, it acts as a poison, when it is applied to the surface of ulcers, yet certainly not under all circumstances. Its power of act-

* Gazette Médicale, 1839, No. 20.

† In a rabbit killed by arsenic applied to a wound Sir B. Brodie found the heart contracting feebly after death; and in a dog there were tremulous contractions incapable of supporting circulation. Sproegel found the peristaltic motion of the intestines and gullet vigorous in a dog an hour after death. [Diss. Inaug. in Halleri Disput. Med. Prac. vi. Exp. 31.] Orfila in some experiments found the heart apparently inflamed and its irritability destroyed. [Arch. Gén. de Med. i. 147.]

‡ Haller's Disput. Med. Pract. vi. Exp. 35.

§ Diss. Inaug. Tubing. 1808. De effectibus Arsenici in var. organismos.

‖ Phil. Trans. cii. 211.

ing through the unbroken skin has been questioned. Jaeger found that, when it was merely applied and not rubbed on the skin of animals, it had no effect.[*] But some cases will be afterwards mentioned which tend to show that the reverse probably holds in regard to man. According to the last-mentioned author. who is the only experimentalist that has hitherto examined the subject consecutively, arsenic is most active when injected into a vein, or applied to a fresh wound, or introduced into the sac of the peritonæum; it is less powerful when taken into the stomach; it is still less energetic when introduced into the rectum; and it is quite inert when applied to the nerves.

It is a striking fact in the action of that poison that, whatever be the texture in the body to which it is applied, provided death do not ensue quickly, it almost always produces symptoms of inflammation in the stomach; and on inspection after death traces of inflammation are found in that organ. In some instances of death caused by its outward application, the inflamed appearance of the stomach has been greater than in many cases where it had been swallowed. Sproegel met with a good example of this in a dog killed by a drachm applied to wounds. The whole stomach and intestines, outwardly and inwardly, were of a deep-red colour, blood was extravasated between the membranes, and clots were even found in the stomach.[†]

Of the different preparations of arsenic, it may be said in general terms, that those are most active which are most soluble. In conformity with what appears to be a general law in toxicology, the metal itself is inert. It is difficult to put this fairly to the test, because it is not easy to pulverize the metal without a sufficient quantity being oxidated to cause poisonous effects. Bayen and Deyeux, however, found that a drachm carefully prepared might be given in fragments to dogs without injuring them; and they once gave a cat half an ounce without any other consequence than temporary loss of flesh.[‡] Its alloys are also inert. The same experimentalists found it inactive when combined with tin; and Renault likewise found it inactive when united with sulphur and iron in the ore mispickel, or arsenical pyrites.[§]

It is probable that all the other preparations of arsenic are more or less deleterious.

A difference of opinion prevails as to the power of the sulphurets. Various statements have been published on the subject. But it may be sufficient to observe, that in consequence of the poisonous properties of the sulphurets having been imputed to the oxide, with which they are often adulterated, — Professor Orfila made some experiments with native orpiment and realgar, and with the sulphuret procured by sulphuretted-hydrogen gas (which are all pure sulphurets); and he found that in doses varying from 40 to 70 grains they all caused death in two, three, or six days, whether they were ap-

* Jaeger, p. 28.　　　　　　　　　　　† Halleri Disput., &c., Exp. 36.
‡ Renault sur les Contrepoisons de l'Arsénic, p. 42.　§ Ibidem, 45.

plied to a wound, or introduced into the stomach.* It may appear at first view singular that the sulphurets, being insoluble, should be poisonous; but the apparent anomaly vanishes on considering the experiments of M. Decourdemanche formerly noticed; which prove that in animal fluids the sulphurets are rapidly changed into the oxide (see p. 225). The sulphurets, however, are much less active than the preparations in which the metal exists already oxidated. Yet in sufficient doses they will prove rapidly fatal. In the Acta Germanica there is the case of a woman who was killed in a few hours by realgar, mixed by her step-daughter in red-cabbage soup.† The common artificial orpiment procured by sublimation is very active, in consequence of the oxide mixed with it. Renault found three grains killed a dog in nine hours.‡

Among the less active preparations of arsenic may also be enumerated such of the arsenites and arseniates as are not soluble in water. They have not indeed been actually tried. But there can be little doubt that they will prove poisonous; because, though insoluble in water, they are probably somewhat soluble in the animal juices. We may infer from their sparing solubility, even in these menstrua, that they will be less active than the preparations now to be mentioned, which are more soluble.

These are the alkaline arsenites and arseniates, arsenic acid, arsenious acid, the black oxide or fly-powder, and arseniuretted-hydrogen. With regard to arsenic acid, and the alkaline arseniates and arsenites, it is probable, from their effects in medicinal doses, that they are as active as the white oxide, if not more so. But they have not been particularly examined, as they are not objects of great interest to the medical jurist.

The fly-powder or black oxide is very active. Renault found that four grains killed a middle-sized dog in ten hours.§ It has been likewise known to prove quickly fatal to man. In a French journal there is a case related which ended fatally in sixteen hours;‖ and in the Acta Germanica is an account of four persons, who died in consequence of eating a dish of stewed pears poisoned with it, and of whom three died within eighteen hours.¶ The dose is not mentioned; but it is probable from the collateral circumstances that it was not considerable.

Arseniuretted-hydrogen is probably the most active of all arsenical compounds. The celebrated German chemist Gehlen, having accidentally inhaled a small portion of it, died in nine days with the usual symptoms of arsenical poisoning. In Dr. O'Reilly's case, which proved fatal in seven days, it was computed that the equivalent of twelve grains of oxide had been inhaled. And Dr. Schlinder's patient had inhaled a quantity of gas corresponding with only

* Journal de Chim. Méd. ii. 153.   † Acta Germanica, v. Observ. 102.
‡ Sur les Contrepoisons de l'Arsénic, p. 57.
§ Sur les Contrepoisons de l'Arsénic, p. 48.
‖ Nov. Bibliothèque Méd. 1827, ii 59.
¶ Acta Germanica, v. Observ. 102.

an eighth of a grain of sesquioxide ; yet he appears to have made a narrow escape.*

It is of some consequence to settle with precision the power of the white oxide. Witnesses are often asked on trials how small a quantity will occasion death ? It is obvious that this question admits only of a vague answer : It can be answered at all only in reference to concomitant circumstances, and even then but presumptively. Nevertheless, it is right to be aware what facts are known on the subject.

It has been stated by various systematic authors that the white oxide will prove fatal to man in the dose of two grains. Hahnemann says in more special terms, that in circumstances favourable to its action four grains may cause death within twenty-four hours, and one or two grains in a few days.† But neither he nor any of the other authors alluded to have referred to actual cases. Foderé knew half a grain cause colic pains in the stomach and dysenteric flux, which continued obstinately for eight days ;‡ and I have related an instance where six persons, after taking each a grain in wine during dinner, were seriously and violently affected for twelve hours.§ Mr. Alfred Taylor mentions three similar cases occasioned by arsenic accidentally taken in port-wine after dinner, — one, an infant of sixteen months who got about a third of a grain, another, a lady who took a grain and a half, and the third, a gentleman, who had two grains and a half, — in all of whom violent vomiting, and prostration, without pain, occurred for three or four hours ; and the gentleman of the party did not recover for several days.‖ M. Lachèse mentions his having met with a number of cases of poisoning from small doses taken in bread or soup ; whence he concludes, that an eighth of a grain taken in food may cause vomiting ; — that a quarter of a grain or twice as much taken once only causes vomiting, colic, and prostration, — that the same quantity repeated next day renews these symptoms in such force as to render the individual unfit for work till three or four days afterwards, — and that four such doses, taken at intervals during two days, that is between one and a half and two grains in all, excite acute gastro-enteritis and may prove fatal, since two individuals who had taken this much died, one in seven weeks, the other three weeks later.¶ The smallest fatal dose I have found recorded elsewhere is four grains and a half ; and death ensued in six hours only.** But the subject was a child, four years old, and the poison was taken in solution. Alberti mentions the case of a man who died from taking six grains ; but I am unacquainted with the particulars, not having seen the original account.†† Two children, whose cases are

* For the references to these cases, see p. 227.
† Ueber Arsenic-Vergiftung, p. 53-4.　　　　‡ Journal Complémentaire, i. 107.
§ Edin. Med. and Surg. Journal, xxxiii. 67.
‖ Guy's Hospital Reports, 1841, vi. 29.
¶ Annales d'Hygiène Publique, 1837, xvi. 336, 345.
** Rust's Magazin für die gesammte Heilkunde, xx. 492.
†† Wibmer. Die Wirkung der Arzneimittel und Gifte, i. 257. From Alberti, Jurisp. Med. v. 619, cas. 24.

alluded to in the Proceedings of the Academy of Medicine of Paris, died, the one in two days, the other a day later, after taking rather less than sixteen grains. The former was four years and a half old, the latter seven years.* Valentini alludes to a case where thirty grains of the oxide in powder killed an adult in six days.† The effects of medicinal doses, which seldom exceed a quarter of a grain without causing irritation of the stomach, and the fatal effects of somewhat larger doses on animals, Renault having found that a single grain in solution killed a large dog in four hours,‡ must convince every one that the general statement of Hahnemann cannot be very wide of the truth. Mr. Taylor thinks his own cases mentioned above throw doubt over this inference. But it must be remembered, that his patients had dined just before taking the poison.

It is not improbable that the activity of oxide of arsenic is impaired by admixture with other insoluble powders. M. Bertrand, conceiving from some experiments on animals that he had found an antidote for arsenic in charcoal powder, took no less than five grains of the oxide mixed with that substance, and he did not suffer any injury, although his stomach was empty at the time, and he did not vomit.§ But Orfila afterwards showed, that other insoluble powders, such as clay, have the same effect; that no such powder can be of any use if not introduced into the stomach till after the arsenic is swallowed; and that they appear to act solely by enveloping the arsenical powder and preventing it from touching the membrane of the alimentary canal.‖ Although M. Bertrand's discovery will not supply the physician with an antidote, the medical jurist will not lose sight of the interesting fact, that, by certain mechanical admixtures, arsenic in moderate doses may be entirely deprived of its poisonous quality. A singular case of recovery from no less a dose than sixty grains, which happened in the case of an American physician, probably comes under the same head with the experiments of Bertrand, —a large quantity of powder of cinchona-bark having been swallowed along with the arsenic. In this case, however, the symptoms were severe for three days.¶

The tendency of habit to modify the action of arsenic is questionable. So far as authentic facts go, habit has no power of familiarizing the constitution to its use. One no doubt may hear now and then of mountebanks who swallow without injury entire scruples or drachms of arsenic, and vague accounts have reached me of patients who took unusually large doses for medicinal purposes. But as to facts of the former kind, it is clear that no importance can be attached to them; for it is impossible to know how much of the feat is genuine, and how much legerdemain. With respect to the latter facts, I have never

* Bulletins de l'Académie Roy. de Médecine, 1841, v. 145.

† Valentini Pandectæ Med.-legales, I, iii. c. 24

‡ Sur les Contrepoisons de l'Arsénic, p. 62.

§ Foderé, in Journal Complémentaire, i. 107, from Bertrand, Manuel Medico-legal des Poisons, p. 185.

‖ Toxicologie Gén. i, 429.   ¶ American Journal of Med. Science, xi. 61.

been able to ascertain any precise instance of the kind ; and so far
as my own experience goes, the habit of taking arsenic in medicinal doses has quite an opposite effect from familiarizing the stomach
to it.

Oxide of arsenic being sparingly soluble, its operation is often
much influenced by the condition of the stomach as to food at the
time it is swallowed.   If the stomach be empty, it adheres with
tenacity to the villous coat and acts with energy.   If the stomach
be full at the time, the first portions that come in contact with
the inner membrane may cause vomiting before it can be diffused,
so that the whole or greater part is discharged.   One remarkable case of this nature has been quoted in page 29.   In another,
where severe symptoms did supervene, and recovery was ascribed
to the use of magnesia as an antidote, the favourable result seems to
have been really owing to the circumstance, that the patient had
supped heartily not long before taking the arsenic.*   An extraordinary case related by Mr. Kerr, in which nearly three-quarters of an
ounce were retained for two hours without causing any serious mischief, probably comes under the same category ; for the arsenic was
taken immediately after a meal, and the stomach was cleared out by
emetics.†

In the following detail of the symptoms caused by arsenic in man,
its effects when swallowed will be first noticed ; and then some remarks will be added on the phenomena observed when it is introduced through other channels.

The symptoms of poisoning with arsenic may be advantageously
considered under three heads.   In one set of cases there are signs of
violent irritation of the alimentary canal and sometimes of the other
mucous membranes also, accompanied with excessive general depression, but not with distinct disorder of the nervous system.   When
such cases prove fatal, which they generally do, they terminate for
the most part in from twenty-four hours to three days.   In a second
and very singular set of cases there is little sign of irritation in any
part of the alimentary canal ; perhaps trivial vomiting or slight pain
in the stomach, but sometimes neither ; the patient is chiefly or solely
affected with excessive prostration of strength and frequent fainting ;
and death is seldom delayed beyond the fifth or sixth hour.   In a
third set of cases life is commonly prolonged at least six days, sometimes much longer, or recovery may even take place after a tedious
illness ; and the signs of inflammation in the alimentary canal are
succeeded or become accompanied, about the second or fourth day
or later, by symptoms of irritation in the other mucous passages, and
more particularly by symptoms indicating a derangement of the
nervous system, such as palsy or epilepsy.   The distinctions now laid
down will be found in practice to be well defined, and useful
for estimating in criminal cases the weight of the evidence from
symptoms.

1. In one order of cases, then, arsenic produces symptoms of

---

* Mr. Hume, London Medical and Physical Journal, xlvi. 467.
† Edinburgh Med. and Surg. Journal, xxxvi. 94.

irritation or inflammation along the course of the alimentary canal. Such cases are the most frequent of all. The person commonly survives twenty-four hours, seldom more than three days; but instances of the kind have sometimes proved fatal in a few hours, and others have lasted for weeks. On the whole, however, if the case is much shorter than twenty-four hours, or longer than three days, its complexion is apt to be altered. In the mildest examples of the present variety recovery takes place after a few attacks of vomiting, and slight general indisposition for a day or two.

In regard to the ordinary progress of the symptoms, the first of a decisive character are sickness and faintness. It is generally thought indeed that the first symptom is an acrid taste; but this notion has been already shown to be erroneous. For some account of the sensations felt in the act of swallowing the poison, the reader may refer to what has been stated in p. 200. There is no doubt, that in the way in which arsenic is usually given with a criminal intent, namely, mixed with articles of food, it seldom makes any impression at all upon the senses during the act of swallowing.

In some instances the sickness and faintness, particularly when the poison was taken in solution, have begun a few minutes after it was swallowed. Thus in a case mentioned by Bernt, in which a solution of arseniate of potass was taken, the symptoms began violently in fifteen minutes;[*] in one related by Wildberg, where the oxide was given in coffee, the person was affected immediately on taking the second cup;[†] in one related by Mr. Edwards, the patient was taken ill in eight minutes,[‡] in one mentioned by M. Lachèse of Angers, violent symptoms commenced within ten minutes after the poison was swallowed with prunes;[§] in a case communicated to me by Mr. J. H. Stallard of Leicester, the symptoms set in with violence ten minutes after it was taken dissolved in tea; nay, in a case of poisoning with orpiment in soup, mentioned by Valentini, the man felt unwell before he had finished his soup, and set it aside as disagreeable.[‖] It is a mistake therefore to suppose, as I have known some do, that arsenic never begins to operate for at least half an hour. Nevertheless it must be admitted, that in general arsenic does not act for half an hour after it is swallowed. — On the other hand, its operation is seldom delayed beyond an hour. The following, however, are exceptions to this rule. Lachèse in the paper quoted above mentions an instance where the interval was two hours, and where the issue was eventually fatal. The arsenic had been in very coarse powder. Mr. Macaulay of Leicester has communicated to me a case where the individual took the poison at eight in the evening, went to bed at half-past nine, and slept till eleven, when he awoke with slight pain in the stomach, vomiting, and cold sweats. In this instance the dose was seven drachms, and death took place in nine hours. M. Dever-

* Beiträge zur gerichtlichen Arzneikunde, iv. 221.
† Praktisches Handbuch für Physiker, iii. 298.
‡ London Med. and Phys. Journal, xlix 117.
§ Annales d'Hygiène Publique, xvii. 338.
‖ Pandectæ Medico-legales, P. i. s. iii. cas. xxvi. pp. 134, 135.

gie has related a similar case of poisoning with the sulphuret, where
the symptoms did not begin for three hours; and here too the patient
fell asleep immediately after swallowing the poison.* Professor
Orfila has noticed an instance, to be quoted afterwards, where there appears to have been scarcely any symptom at all for five hours† (p. 243).
I suspect we must also consider as an instance of the same kind the
case which gave occasion to the trial of Mrs. Smith here in 1827. A
white draught was administered in a suspicious manner at ten in the
evening; the girl immediately went to bed; and no symptoms appeared till six next morning, from which time her illness went on
uninterruptedly.‡ In three of the preceding cases it will be remarked
that sleep intervened between the taking of the poison and the invasion of the symptoms; and it is therefore not improbable that the
reason of the retardation is the comparative inactivity of the animal
system during sleep. — In voluntary poisoning, as in a case related
by Dr. Roget, a slight attack of sickness or vomiting occasionally
ensues immediately after solid arsenic is swallowed, and some time
before the symptoms commence regularly.§

The observations now made will often prove important for deciding accusations of poisoning; for pointed evidence may be derived
from the commencement of the symptoms, after a suspected meal,
corresponding or not corresponding with the interval which is known
to elapse in ascertained cases. The reader will see the effect of such
evidence in attaching guilt to the prisoner in the case of Margaret
Wishart, which I have detailed elsewhere.|| In the trial of Mrs.
Smith, the want of the correspondence just mentioned contributed
greatly to her acquittal; for the symptoms of poisoning did not begin
till more than eight hours after the only occasion on which the prisoner
was proved to have administered any thing in a suspicious manner.
As I was not at the time acquainted with any parallel case except that
recorded by Orfila, I hesitated to ascribe the symptoms to the draught;
and consequently, as the other medical witnesses felt the same hesitation on the same account, the proof of administration was considered to have failed. I am not sure that I should have now felt the
same difficulty. The intervening state of sleep probably affords an
explanation of the long interval; and the cases noticed by Mr.
Macaulay and M. Devergie are parallel, though the interval in them
was certainly not so great. — There is a limit, however, to the possible
interval in such cases. It seems impossible that the action of the
poison shall be suspended for three entire days. Yet death has been
ascribed to arsenic in such circumstances. A child $3\frac{1}{2}$ years old
having swallowed eight grains with bread and butter, but being soon

---

* Diction. de Méd. et de Chir. Pratique, Art. Arsenic, iii. 340.

† Archives Gén. de Médecine, vii. 14. — Another case somewhat analogous has been
related by Tonnelier in Corvisart's Journal de Médecine (iv. 15). The person, a girl
nineteen years of age, took the poison at eleven, dined pretty heartily at two, and concealed her sufferings till seven. Even before dinner, however, she had been observed
occasionally to change countenance, as if uneasy.

‡ Edin. Med. and Surg. Journal, xxvii. 450.

§ London Med. Chir. Trans. ii. 134.

|| Edin. Med. and Surg. Journal, xxix. 23. See also above, p. 77.

made to vomit forcibly by emetics, presented no decided symptom at the time, or for three days more; but on the fourth day difficult breathing ensued, with anxiety of expression, frequency of the pulse, and heat of the skin; and next day death took place. There was no morbid appearance found in the body.* I do not know of any parallel instance of death from arsenic, and cannot admit that the poison was the cause of the symptoms and fatal event.

Soon after the sickness begins, or about the same time, the region of the stomach feels painful, the pain being commonly of a burning kind, and much aggravated by pressure. Violent fits of vomiting and retching then speedily ensue, especially when drink is taken. There is often also a sense of dryness, heat, and tightness in the throat, creating an incessant desire for drink; and this affection often precedes the vomiting. Occasionally it is wanting, at other times so severe as to be attended with suffocation and convulsive vomiting at the sight of fluids.† Hoarseness and difficulty of speech are commonly combined with it. The matter vomited is greenish or yellowish; but sometimes streaked or mixed with blood, particularly when the case lasts longer than a day.

In no long time after the first illness diarrhœa generally makes its appearance, but not always. In some cases, instead of it, the patient is tormented by frequent, ineffectual calls: in others the great intestines are scarcely affected. About this time the pain in the stomach is excruciating, and is often likened by the sufferer to a fire burning within him. It likewise extends more or less downwards, particularly when the diarrhœa or tenesmus is severe; and the belly is commonly tense and tender, sometimes also swollen, though not frequently, — sometimes even on the contrary drawn in at the navel.‡ When the diarrhœa is severe, the anus is commonly excoriated and affected with burning pain.§ In such cases the burning pain may extend along the whole course of the alimentary canal from the throat to the anus. Nay at times the mouth and lips are also inflamed, presenting dark specks or blisters.‖

Sometimes there are likewise present signs of irritation of the lungs and air-passages, — almost always shortness of breath (which, however, is chiefly owing to the tenderness of the belly), — often a sense of tightness across the bottom of the chest, and more rarely decided pain in the same quarter, darting also through the upper part of the chest. Sometimes pneumonia has appeared a prominent affection during life, and been distinctly traced in the dead body.¶

In many instances, too, the urinary passages are affected, the patient being harassed with frequent, painful and difficult micturition, swelling of the penis, and pain in the region of the bladder, or, if a female,

---

* Mr. Page, Lancet, 1836-37, ii. 626.
† Wendland in Augustin's Archiv der Staatsarzneikunde, ii. 34.
‡ Pyl's Aufsätze und Beob. i. 55.
§ Bachmann. See subsequently, p. 260. State Trials, xviii. Case of Miss Blandy.
‖ Wepfer, Historia Cicutæ, 276.
¶ In a case by Schlegel. See Henke's Zeitschrift für die Staatsarzneikunde, i. 81.

23*

with burning pain of the vagina and excoriation of the labia.* Sometimes the irritation of the urinary organs is so great as to be attended
with total suppression of urine, as in a case related by Guilbert of
Montpellier, in which this symptom continued several days.† During the late contentions among chemists, physiologists, and physicians,
occasioned by the case of Madame Lafarge, it was alleged by Flandin
and Danger that in animals the urine is always suppressed, by Orfila
that it is always secreted, by Professor Delafond of the Alfort Veterinary School, that it is never suppressed, but always diminished, and
sometimes even to a sixth of the natural quantity.‡ There is, however, no invariable rule in the matter. And in fact, urinary symptoms
are seldom present unless the lower bowels are likewise strongly
irritated; but are then seldom altogether wanting. They are rarely
well marked in cases of the present variety, unless life is prolonged
three days or more.

When symptoms of irritation of the alimentary canal have subsisted
a few hours, convulsive motions often occur. They commence on
the trunk, afterwards extend over the whole body, are seldom violent,
and generally consist of nothing else than tremors and twitches.
Cramps of the legs and arms, a possible concomitant of every kind
of diarrhœa, is peculiarly severe and frequent in that caused by
arsenic.

The general system always sympathizes acutely with the local
derangement. The pulse commonly becomes very small, feeble and
rapid soon after the vomiting sets in ; and in no long time it is often
imperceptible. This state is naturally attended with great coldness,
clammy sweats, and lividity of the feet and hands. Another symptom referrible to the circulation which has been observed, though,
very rarely, is palpitation.§

The countenance is commonly collapsed from an early period, and
almost always expressive of great torture and extreme anxiety or
despair ; the eyes are red and sparkling ; the conjunctiva often so injected as to seem inflamed ; the tongue and mouth parched ; and the
velum and palate sometimes covered with little white ulcers.

Delirium sometimes accompanies the advanced stage, and stupor
also is not unfrequent. Coma occasionally precedes death, as in Mr.
Stallard's case (p. 235), in which the symptoms of irritation, at first
very violent, gradually gave place in two hours to complete insensibility, proving fatal in two hours more. Very often, however, the
patient remains quite sensible to the last. Death in general comes
on calmly, but is sometimes preceded by a paroxysm of convulsions.||
In some cases it takes place quite unexpectedly, as if from sudden
deliquium, as in a case mentioned by Dr. Dymock of this city. The
patient, a girl who had taken two ounces intentionally, rose from her

* Buchmann, p. 40.   † Journal de Médecine, iv. 383.
‡ Journal de Chimie Med. 1842, p. 580.
§ Pyl's Aufsätze und Beob. i. 55.
|| Metzger's Materialien für die Staatsarzneikunde, ii. 96. — Lond. Med. Phys. Journ.
xxviii. 345 — and Wildberg's Praktisches Handbuch, iii. 235-390.

bed without help two hours and a half afterwards, went to a chair at the fireside, and had scarce sat down when she expired.*

Various eruptions have at times been observed, especially in those who survive several days ; but they are more frequent in the kind of cases to be considered afterwards, in which life is prolonged for a week or more. The eruptions have been variously described as resembling petechiæ, or measles, or red miliaria, or small-pox. In the case already quoted from Guilbert a copious eruption of miliary vesicles appeared on the fifth day, and for fifteen days afterwards. They were attended with perspiration and abatement of the other symptoms, and followed with desquamation of the cuticle. Another external affection which may be noticed is general swelling of the body. Several cases of this nature have been described by Dr. Schlegel of Meiningen ; and in one of them the swelling, particularly round the eyes, appears to have been considerable.†

In some cases of the kind now under consideration a short remission or even a total intermission of all the distressing symptoms has been witnessed, particularly when death is retarded till the close of the second or third day.‡ This remission, which is accompanied with dozing stupor, is most generally observed about the beginning of the second day. It is merely temporary, the symptoms speedily returning with equal or increased violence. Sometimes the remission occurs oftener than once, as in a case related in the London Medical and Physical Journal. The patient, a child seven years old, lived thirty-six hours in a state of alternate calm and excitement ; and during the state of calm no pulse was to be felt at the wrists.§ — So far as at present appears a long intermission is impossible.

In cases such as those now described death often occurs about twenty-four hours after the poison is swallowed, and generally before the close of the third day. But on the one hand life has been sometimes prolonged, without the supervention of the symptoms belonging to a different variety of cases, for five or six days,‖ nay perhaps even for several weeks. And, on the other hand, the symptoms of irritation of the alimentary canal are sometimes distinct, although death takes place in a much shorter period than twenty-four hours. Metzger has related a striking case, fatal in six hours, in which the symptoms were acute colic pain, violent vomiting, and profuse diarrhœa ;¶ and Wildberg has related a similar case fatal in the same time.** Hohnbaum describes another fatal in five hours ;†† and I met with as brief a case in this city in 1843, where all the usual symptoms of irritation in the stomach and bowels were violent. These symptoms were also present at first in Mr. Stallard's case, which was fatal in four hours ;

* Edinburgh Med. and Surg. Journal, lix. 350.
† Henke's Zeitschrift für die Staatsarzneikunde, i. 29.
‡ Tonnelier's case. Corvisart's Journal de Médecine, iv. — Roget's case. Med. Chir. Transactions, ii.
§ Med. and Phys. Journal, xxviii. 347.   ‖ Henke's Zeitschrift, i. 31.
¶ De Veneficio caute dijudicando. Schlegel's Opusc. iv. 22.
** Praktisches Handbuch für Physiker, iii. 298.
†† Zeitschrift für die Staatsarzneikunde, ii. 307.

Pyl has recorded one, where all the signs of irritation in the stomach and intestines were present, except vomiting, and which proved fatal in three hours ;* and Dr. Dymock met here with a similar instance which lasted only two hours and a half.† This is one of the shortest undoubted cases of poisoning from arsenic I have hitherto found in authentic records. Dr. Male mentions one, which was fatal in four hours ;‡ Wepfer another equally short ;§ Johnston another fatal in three hours and a half ;‖ and I shall presently mention others without symptoms of irritation which ended fatally in two, five, or six hours [p. 242].¶ Wibmer has even quoted a case fatal in half an hour ; but there seems to have been some doubt whether the poison taken was arsenic.**

Such is an account of the symptoms of poisoning by arsenic in their most frequent form. It will of course be understood, that they are liable to a great variety as to violence, as well as their mode of combination in actual cases ; — and that they are by no means all present in every instance. The most remarkable and least variable of them all, pain and vomiting, are sometimes wanting. A case, in which pain was not felt in the stomach, even on pressure, although the other symptoms of inflammation were present, has been briefly described in the Medical Repository.†† A smilar case fatal in fourteen hours and a half, where there was much vomiting and some heat in the stomach, but no pain or tenderness, has been related by Dr. E. Gairdner.‡‡ Another very striking example of this anomalous

* Aufsätze und Beobachtungen, v. 106.
† Edinburgh Med. and Surg. Journal, 1843, lix. 350.
‡ Elements of Juridical Medicine, 68.
§ Historia Cicutæ, p. 282.
‖ Essay on Mineral Poisons, 1795, p. 30.
¶ These facts are important, because they will enable the medical jurist in some circumstances to decide a question which may be started as to the possibility of arsenic having been the cause of death when it is very rapid. I have dwelt on them more particularly than may appear necessary, because some loose statements on the subject were made in a controversy on the occasion of a trial of some note, that of Hannah Russell and Daniel Leny, at Lewes Summer Assizes 1826, for the murder of the husband of the former. Arsenic was decidedly detected in the stomach, and it was proved that the deceased did not live above three hours after the only meal at which the prisoners could have administered the poison. Now during the controversy which arose after the execution of one of the prisoners, it was alleged by one of the parties, among other reasons for believing arsenic not to have been the cause of death, that this poison never proves fatal so soon as in three hours, — that Sir Astley Cooper and Mr. Stanley of London had never known a case prove fatal in less than seven hours — and that Dr. Male's case mentioned above is the shortest on record. The instances quoted above overthrow this whole line of statement. It was mentioned by Mr. Evans, the chief crown witness, but I know not on what authority, that, on the trial of Samuel Smith for poisoning, held at Warwick Summer Assizes 1826, the deceased was proved to have expired in two hours after taking a quarter of an ounce of arsenic. I have examined with some care the documents in the Lewes case, which were obligingly communicated to me by Mr. Evans ; and I have been quite unable to discover any reason for questioning the reality of poisoning, or for the ferment which it seems the subsequent controversy excited. The case seems to have been satisfactorily made out by Mr. Evans in the first instance ; and no sound medical jurist would for a moment suffer a shadow of doubt to be thrown over his mind by the criticisms of Mr. Evans's antagonist.
** Die Wirkung der Arzneimittel und Gifte, i. 271.
†† London Medical Repository, ii. 270.
‡‡ Edinburgh Med. and Surg. Journal, xxxii. 305.

deficiency has been detailed by Dr. Yellowly. A lad sixteen years old died twenty-one hours after swallowing half an ounce of the white oxide; and the presence of inflammation was denoted all along by sickness, vomiting, purging, and heat in the tongue; yet he never complained of pain, neither did he ever seem to his friends to suffer any. Another anomaly in the case was, that the pulse, contrary to what is usual, was very slow : twelve hours after he took the poison, the pulse was 40, and two hours before death it was so slow as 30.* These deviations from the ordinary course of the symptoms are taken notice of merely to put the practitioner on his guard, and prevent the medical jurist from drawing hasty conclusions. Upon the whole, they are rare ; and the symptoms of poisoning by arsenic are in general very uniform.

2. The second variety of poisoning with arsenic includes a few cases in which the signs of inflammation are far from violent or even altogether wanting, and in which death ensues in five or six hours or a little more, — at a period too early for inflammation to be always properly developed. The symptoms are then generally obscure, and are referrible chiefly to the mode of action, which is probably the cause of death in most cases, — a powerful debilitating influence on the circulation, or on the nervous system.

These symptoms occasionally amount to absolute narcotism, as in some of the animals on which Sir B. Brodie experimented. Thus, when he injected a solution of the oxide into the stomach of a dog, the pulse was rendered slow and intermitting ; the animal became palsied in the hind-legs, lethargic, and in no long time insensible, with dilated pupils ; and soon afterwards it was seized with convulsions, amidst which it died, fifty minutes after the poison was administered.† In man the symptoms very seldom resembled so closely those of the narcotic poisons. In Mr. Stallard's case, however, formerly mentioned, the symptoms of irritation which appeared at first speedily gave place to complete insensibility for two hours before death (pp. 235, 238), a similar instance has been related in Henke's Journal. A young man who got an arsenical solution from an old woman to cure ague, was attacked after taking it with vomiting and loud cries, afterwards with incoherent talking, then fell into a deep sleep, and finally perished in convulsions in five hours.‡

In some cases of the kind now under consideration, one or two attacks of vomiting occur at the usual interval after the taking of the poison; but it seldom continues. The most uniform and remarkable affection is extreme faintness, amounting at times to deliquium. Occasionally there is some stupor, or rather oppression, and often slight convulsions. Pain in the stomach is generally present ; but it is slight, and seldom accompanied with other signs of internal inflammation. Death commonly takes place in a few hours. Yet, even when it is retarded till the beginning of the second day, the faintness and stupor are sometimes more striking features in the case than the symptoms of inflammation in the stomach.

* Ibidem, v. 389.   † Philos. Transactions, 1812, p. 212.
‡ Henke's Zeitschrift für die Staatsarzneikunde, v. 410.

This variety of poisoning has been hitherto observed only under the three following circumstances, — when the dose of poison was large, — when it was in little masses, — or when it was in a state of solution. The mode in which the first and last circumstances operate is evident ; they facilitate the absorption of a large quantity of arsenic in a short space of time, so that its remote action begins before local inflammation is fully developed. But it is not easy to see how any such effect can flow from the arsenic being in little masses. It is also to be observed that none of the circumstances here mentioned is invariable in its operation. An instance is related in Rust's Magazine, of the customary signs of irritation having been produced even by the solution.*

On the whole, the present variety of poisoning is rather uncommon, and indeed, although the attention of the profession was pointedly called to it even in the first edition of the present work, its existence does not seem to be so generally known as it ought to be.† It may be right therefore to specify the cases which have been published.

In the Medical and Philosophical Journal of New York,‡ is related the case of a druggist, who swallowed an ounce of powdered arsenic at once, and died in eight hours, after two or three fits of vomiting, with slight pain and heat in the stomach. — A similar case has been related by Metzger. A young woman died in a few hours, after suffering from trivial diarrhœa, pain in the stomach and strangury ; her death was immediately preceded by slight convulsions and fits of suffocation ; and on dissection the stomach and intestines were found quite healthy. Half an ounce of arsenic was found in the stomach.§ — A third case similar in its particulars to the two preceding was submitted to me for investigation by the sheriff of this county in 1825. The subject, a girl fourteen years of age, took about ninety grains, and died in five hours, having vomited once or twice, complained of some little pain in the belly, and been affected towards the close with great faintness and weakness. The stomach and intestines were healthy.‖ — A fourth case allied to these is succinctly told in the Medical and Physical Journal. The person expired in five hours; and vomiting never occurred, even though emetics were given.¶ — A fifth has been related by M. Gérard of Beauvais. The subject was a man so addicted to drinking, that his daily allowance was a pint of brandy. When first seen, there was so much tranquillity, that doubts were entertained whether arsenic had really been swallowed ; but at length he was discovered actually chewing it. This state continued

* Magazin für die gesammte Heilkunde, xxii. 483.

† This statement might be excellently illustrated by the particulars of an English trial in 1842, where the prisoner escaped, though arsenic was found in the stomach of the deceased, because the judge, resting on the medical evidence, urged that arsenic caused so much pain in the stomach as generally to make the person shriek with agony, while in this case there was no uneasiness except pain in the head. As the case, however, was by no means creditable to the parties concerned in it, I shall rest satisfied with the present allusion.

‡ Vol. iii. quoted in Kopp's Jahrbuch, vii. 401.

§ Materialien für die Staatsarzneikunde, ii. 95.

‖ Edin. Med. Chir. Transactions, ii. 298.

¶ Lond. Med. Phys. Journal, xxxiv.

for nearly five hours, when some vomiting ensued : coldness of the extremities and spasmodic flexion of the legs soon followed ; and in a few minutes more he expired.* — A sixth and very singular case of the same kind has been described by Orfila. The individual having swallowed three drachms at eight in the morning, went about for two hours bidding adieu to his friends and telling what he had done. He was then prevailed on to take emetics and diluents, which caused free, easy vomiting. He suffered very little till one, when he became affected with constricting pain and burning in the stomach, feeble pulse, cold sweats, and cadaverous expression, under which symptoms he died four hours later.† Orfila justly designates this case as the most extraordinary instance of poisoning with arsenic that has come under his notice. — A seventh is related by Mr. Holland of Manchester where death took place in the course of eight or nine hours, and the symptoms were at first some vomiting, afterwards little else but faintness, sickness, a sullen expression, and a general appearance which led those around to suppose the individual intoxicated.‡ — Professor Chaussier has described a still more striking case than any yet mentioned. A stout middle-aged man swallowed a large quantity of arsenic in fragments and died in a few hours. He experienced nothing but great feebleness and frequent tendency to fainting. The stomach and intestines were not in the slightest degree affected during life ; and no morbid appearance could be discovered in them after death.§ — A similar instance not less remarkable has been communicated to me by Mr. Macauley of Leicester, where the individual died with narcotic symptoms only within two hours after taking nearly a quarter of a pound of arsenic. — Another fatal in four hours has been described by Mr. Wright, where the symptoms were vomiting under the use of emetics, great exhaustion, feeble hurried pulse, cold sweating, drowsiness and finally stupor. In this case the quantity of arsenic taken was about an ounce.‖ — Another of the same nature is recorded by Morgagni. An old woman stole and ate a cake, which had been poisoned with arsenic for rats. She died in twelve hours, suffering, says Morgagni, rather from excessive prostration of strength than from pain or convulsions.¶ — The following case related by M. Laborde is most remarkable in its circumstances. A young woman was caught in the act of swallowing little fragments of arsenic, and it afterwards appeared that she had been employed most of the day in literally cracking and chewing lumps of it. When the physician first saw her the countenance expressed chagrin and melancholy, but not suffering. After being forced to drink she vomited a good deal, but without uneasiness. Two hours afterwards her countenance was anxious ; but she did not make any complaint, and very soon resumed her tranquillity. Five hours after the last portions of the poison were taken she became drowsy, then remained perfectly calm for four hours more, and at

* Revue Médicale, 1822, vii. 105.
† Archives Gén. de Médecine, vii. 14.
‡ London Medical Gazette, xv. 828.   § Orfila, Toxicologie Gen. i. 397.
‖ Lancet, xvi. 612.   ¶ Epist. Anat. lix. 3.

length on trying to sit up in bed, complained of slight pain in the stomach, and expired without agony. A clot of blood was found in the stomach.* — Dr. Platner of Pavia describes a case, fatal probably in five hours, where the symptoms were a tranquil, melancholic expression, great coldness, paleness of the features, slow languid pulse, retarded respiration, and suppression of urine, but no pain or swelling of the belly, and no diarrhœa till near death, when there was one copious fluid evacuation.† — Lastly, Dr. Choulant has related the case of an elderly female who got a thimbleful of arsenic in soup, and died in eleven hours, affected with occasional, easy vomiting, uneasiness, thirst, and undefinable uneasiness in the chest, but without pain of any kind, or any other complaint.‡

The cases of which an abstract has here been given, will, it is apprehended, be sufficient to correct the erroneous impression of many, — that arsenic, when it proves fatal, always produces violent and well-marked symptoms. It will of course be understood that cases of the present kind pass by insensible shades into those of the first class, — the following, for example, being intermediate between the two. A young man had frequent vomiting and diarrhœa, which were supposed to depend on indigestion merely, as the countenance was calm, without any appearance of suffering, the appetite tolerable, and the abdomen quite free of tenderness. The pulse, however, quickly sunk, the voice failed, and death took place in eleven hours; and on dissection about twenty grains of arsenic were found in the stomach with strong signs of inflammation.§ — In a case communicated to me by a former pupil, Mr. Adams of Glasgow, that of a woman who died five hours after taking six drachms of arsenic, there was some vomiting not long after she swallowed it; but subsequently she presented no prominent symptoms except a ghastly expression, redness of the eyes, a fluttering pulse and extreme prostration, until within half an hour before death, when the action of an emetic and the stomach pump was followed by severe burning pain.

3. The third variety of poisoning with arsenic places in a clear point of view its occasional action on the nervous system. This occurs chiefly in persons who, from having taken but a small quantity, or from having vomited soon after, are eventually rescued from destruction; but it has also been met with in some cases where death ensued after a protracted illness.

In such cases the progress of the poisoning may be divided into two stages. The first train of symptoms is exactly that of the first or inflammatory variety, and is commonly developed in a very perfect and violent form. In the second stage the symptoms are referrible to nervous irritation.

These generally come on when the former begin to recede; yet sometimes they make their appearance earlier, while the signs of in-

---

* Journal de Médecine, lxx. 89.
† Annali Universali di Medicina, 1836, ii. 43.
‡ Zeitschrift für die Staatsarzneikunde, xlii. 402.
§ Journal Hebdomadaire, 1832, viii. 476.

flammation in the alimentary canal continue violent; and more rarely both classes of symptoms begin about the same period. The nervous affection varies in different individuals. The most formidable is coma; the slightest, a peculiar, imperfect palsy of the arms or legs, resembling what is occasioned by the poison of lead; and between these extremes have been observed epileptic fits, or tetanus, or an affection resembling hysteria, or mania. As these affections are of much interest, in respect to the evidence of poisoning from symptoms, it may be well to relate in abstract a few characteristic examples of each.

A good example of epilepsy supervening on the ordinary symptoms of inflammation has been minutely related by Dr. Roget. A girl swallowed a drachm of arsenic, and was in consequence attacked violently with the usual symptoms of irritation in the whole alimentary canal. After being ill about twenty-four hours, she experienced several distinct remissions and had some repose, attended with fainting. In twelve hours more she began to improve rapidly; the pain subsided, her strength and spirits returned, and the stomach became capable of retaining liquids. So far this patient laboured under the common effects of arsenic. But a new train of symptoms then gradually approached. Towards the close of the second day she was harassed with frightful dreams, starting from sleep, and tendency to faint; next morning with coldness along the spine, giddiness, and intolerance of light; and on the fourth day with aching of the extremities and tingling of the whole skin. These symptoms continued till the close of the sixth day, when she was suddenly seized with convulsions of the left side, foaming at the mouth, and total insensibility. The convulsions endured two hours, the insensibility throughout the whole night. Next evening she had another and a similar fit. A third, but slighter fit occurred on the morning of the tenth; another next day at noon; and they continued to return occasionally till the nineteenth day. For some time longer she was affected with tightness across the chest and stomach complaints; but she was eventually restored to perfect health.*

A characteristic set of similar cases, which occurred in London in 1815, has been related in a treatise on arsenic by Mr. Marshall.† They were the subject of investigation on the trial of Eliza Fenning, a maid-servant, who attempted to poison the whole of her master's family by mixing arsenic with a dumpling, and whose condemnation excited an extraordinary sensation at the time, as many persons believed her to be innocent. Five individuals partook of the poisoned dish, and they were all violently seized with the usual inflammatory symptoms. But farther, one had an epileptic fit on the first day, which returned on the second, and he had besides frequent twitches of the muscles of the trunk, a feeling of numbness in one side, and heat and tingling of the feet and hands. Another had tremors of the right arm and leg on the first day, and several epileptic fits in the

* London Med. Chir. Transactions, ii. 134.
† See also a full abstract in Edin. Med. and Surg. Journal, xiii. 507.

24

course of the night. During the next fifteen days he had a paroxysm every evening about the same hour; which returned after
an intermission of eight days, and frequently for several months afterwards.

In the following set of cases the nervous symptoms exhibited a
singular combination of delirium, convulsions, tetanus, and coma,
such as is frequently met with in paroxysms of hysteria; but the
cases are probably not pure examples of poisoning with arsenic, for
liver of sulphur was administered as a remedy to a considerable
amount. Three servant girls in one of the Hebrides ate a mixture
of lard, sugar, and arsenic, which had been laid for destroying rats.
The ordinary signs of irritation in the stomach ensued, but on the
following morning were greatly mitigated. They were then ordered
twelve grains of liver of sulphur every other hour. Soon afterwards
the inflammatory symptoms became more severe, the root of the
tongue swelled and inflamed, and in the afternoon two of them lost
the power of speech and swallowing, and were attacked with locked-
jaw and general convulsions. The third had not locked-jaw, but
was otherwise similarly affected. On the morning of the third day
one of the two former was found comatose, with continuance of the
locked-jaw and occasional return of convulsions; and on being roused
by venesection and the cold affusion, she complained of headache and
heat in the throat. The sulphuret of potass, which had been discontinued on account of the locked-jaw, was then resumed. On the
evening of the fourth day the headache increased, and the patient
became delirious and unmanageable. The cold affusion, however,
soon restored her again to her senses, and from that time her recovery
was progressive. In the other patients the symptoms were similar,
but less violent. In these instances the evidence of an injury of the
nervous system was decisive; but it may be doubted whether the
symptoms were not, in part at least, owing to the sulphuret of
potass, which has been already described as an active poison, capable of inducing convulsions and tetanus. Its properties were not
generally known in this country at the time the cases in question
happened.*

Sometimes the convulsions caused by arsenic assume the form of
pure tetanus. At least a case of this affection is noticed by Portal.†
He has given only a mere announcement of it; and I have not hitherto
met with a parallel instance in authors.

A common nervous affection in the advanced stage of the more
tedious cases of poisoning with arsenic is partial palsy. Palsy in the
form of incomplete paraplegia is a very common symptom even of
the early stage in animals, and has been also sometimes observed
during that stage in man. The paralytic affection, however, is more
frequent in the advanced stage; and in those persons who recover, an
incomplete paralysis of one or more of the extremities, resembling
lead-palsy, is often the last symptom which continues.

* Edin. Med. and Surg. Journal, xv. 553.
† Traitement des Asphyxiés, 135.

Dehaen relates a distinct example of this disorder occurring in a female who took a small quantity of arsenic by mistake. The ordinary signs of inflammation were soon subdued, and for three days she did well; but on the fourth she was attacked with cramps, tenderness, and weakness of the feet, legs and arms, increasing gradually till the whole extremities became at length almost completely palsied. At the same time the cuticle desquamated. But the other functions continued entire. The power of motion returned first in the hands, then in the arms, and she eventually recovered ; but eleven months passed before she could quit the hospital where Dehaen treated her.*

An excellent account of a set of similar cases has been given by Dr. Murray of Aberdeen. They became the subject of judicial inquiry on the trial of George Thom, who was condemned in 1821 at the Aberdeen autumn circuit for poisoning his brother-in-law. Four persons were simultaneously affected about an hour after breakfast with the primary symptoms of poisoning with arsenic, and some in a very violent degree. But besides these symptoms, in all of them the muscular debility was great; and in two it amounted to true partial palsy. One of them lost altogether the power of the left arm, and six months after, when the account of the cases was published, he was unable to bend the arm at the elbow-joint. The other had also great general debility and long-continued numbness and pains of the legs.†

An interesting case of the same nature with these was lately submitted to me on the part of the crown. A man after taking arsenic was attacked with vomiting, purging, and other symptoms of abdominal irritation, which were mistaken for dysentery. Five days afterwards he began to suffer also from feebleness of the limbs; amounting almost to palsy. Subsequently an improvement slowly took place ; but he continued to suffer under irritative fever, diarrhœa, and faintness. Several weeks later the diarrhœa abated, but he had great stiffness, numbness, and loss of power in the joints of the hands and feet. Two months after he first took ill, and while he was slowly recovering from this paralytic affection, arsenic was again administered and proved fatal in eighteen hours.

Another, somewhat similar to the preceding, has been related by M. Lachèse of Angers. Two people took about half a grain in soup twice a day for two days, and were attacked with the usual primary symptoms. One of them died in ten weeks, gradually worn out, but without any particular nervous affection. The other was seized with convulsions, and afterwards with almost complete palsy of the limbs.‡ — A well-marked case of the same nature has been noticed by Professor Bernt. It was the case formerly alluded to as arising from an overdose of the arseniate of potass. The paralytic affection consisted in the loss of sensation and of the power of motion in the hands, and of the loss of motion in the feet, with contraction of the

* Ratio Medendi, iii. 113. † Edin. Med. and Surg. Journal, xviii. 167.
‡ Annales d'Hygiène Publique, xvii. 336.

knee-joints. The issue of the case is not mentioned.* — Dr. Falconer observes in his essay on Palsy, that he had repeatedly witnessed local palsy after poisoning with arsenic, and alludes to one instance in which the hands only were paralysed, and to two others in which the palsy spread gradually from the fingers upwards till the whole arms were affected.† — On the whole, then, local palsy is the most frequent of the secondary effects of arsenic.

It is sometimes very obstinate, as the cases related by Dehaen and Murray will show. But it even appears to be sometimes incurable. For in the German Ephemerides there is related the case of a cook, who after suffering from the usual inflammatory symptoms, was attacked with perfect palsy of the limbs, and had not any use of them during the rest of her life, which was not a short one.‡

Occasionally, instead of being palsied, the limbs are rigidly bent and cannot be extended.§ They were contracted, as well as palsied in the case noticed by Bernt.

The last nervous affection to be mentioned is mania. The only instance I have hitherto found of that disease arising from arsenic is related by Amatus Lusitanus. He has not recorded the particulars of the case, but merely observes that the individual became so outrageously mad as to burst his fetters and jump out of the window of his apartment.‖ According to Zacchias, Amatus was not very scrupulous in his adherence to fact in recording cases.

The preceding remarks contain all that is known with certainty of the effect of arsenic on man when it is swallowed. Independently of the obvious nervous disorders which succeed the acute symptoms, other morbid affections of a more obscure character and chronic in their nature have been sometimes observed or supposed to arise from this poison. — Among these the most unequivocal is dyspepsia. Irritability of the stomach, attended with constant vomiting of food, has been occasionally noticed for a long time after. Wepfer has described two cases in which the primary symptoms were followed, in one by dyspepsia of three years' standing, in the other by emaciation and an anomalous fever, which ended fatally in three years.¶ — Hahnemann farther adds, that in the advanced stage the hair sometimes drops out, and the cuticle desquamates, accompanied occasionally with great tenderness of the skin;** and Wibmer mentions a case of the kind, where not the cuticle and hair only, but likewise even the nails, fell off.†† Desquamation of the cuticle and dropping of the nails are at times produced by the continued use of arsenic in medicinal doses. — Other effects have likewise been ascribed to its employment medicinally. Thus passing over what was stated by its

* Beiträge zur gerichtlichen Arzneikunde, iv. 221.
† Mem. of London Medical Society, ii. 224.
‡ Nova Acta Naturæ Curiosorum, iii. 532.
§ Hahnemann über die Arsenic-Vergiftung, 59.
‖ Curationes Medicinales. Cent. ii. Obs. 33.
¶ Cicutæ Aquaticæ Historia et Noxæ, 280.
** Ueber die Arsenic-Vergiftung, 61.
†† Die Wirkung der Arzneimittel und Gifte, i. 266.

opponents at the time when its introduction into the materia medica was made the subject of controversy over Europe, Broussais maintained that it causes chronic inflammation of the stomach or intestines;[*] and Dr. Astbury inferred, from an instance which fell under his notice, that it may bring on dropsy.[†] Neither of these ideas is supported by the general experience of the profession ; and although some persons even of late have alleged that those, who take it medicinally to any material amount, invariably die soon after of some chronic disease,[‡] there cannot be a doubt, that, under proper restriction, it is both an effectual and a safe remedy. — A case where salivation, with fetor and superficial ulceration of the gums, seemed to have been produced by arsenic, was lately published in an English Journal.[§]

In the present place may also be considered the supposed effects of the celebrated *Aqua Toffana* or *Acquetta di Napoli*, a slow poison, which in the sixteenth century, was believed to possess the property of causing death at any determinate period, after months for example, or even years of ill health, according to the will of the poisoner.

The most authentic description of the aqua Toffana ascribes its properties to arsenic. According to a letter addressed to Hoffman by Garelli, physician to Charles the Sixth of Austria, that Emperor told Garelli, that, being governor of Naples at the time the aqua Toffana was the dread of every noble family in the city, and when the subject was investigated legally, he had an opportunity of examining all the documents, — and that he found the poison was a solution of arsenic in *aqua cymbalariæ*.[||] The dose was said to be from four to six drops. It was colourless, transparent, and tasteless, like water.

Its alleged effects are thus eloquently described by Behrends, a writer in Uden and Pyl's Magazin. " A certain indescribable change is felt in the whole body, which leads the person to complain to his physician. The physician examines and reflects, but finds no symptom, either external or internal, — no constipation, no vomiting, no inflammation, no fever. In short, he can advise only patience, strict regimen, and laxatives. The malady, however, creeps on ; and the physician is again sent for. Still he cannot detect any symptom of note. He infers that there is some stagnation or corruption of the humours, and again advises laxatives. Meanwhile the poison takes firmer hold of the system ; languor, wearisomeness and loathing of food continue ; the nobler organs gradually become torpid, and the lungs in particular at length begin to suffer. In a word, the malady is from the first incurable ; the unhappy victim pines away insensibly, even in the hands of his physician ; and thus is he brought to a miserable end through months or years, according to his enemy's desire."[¶] An equally vigorous and somewhat clearer account of the

* Dict. des Sciences Méd. ii. 307.
† Edin. Med. and Surg. Journal, xv. 415.
‡ Cadet de Gassicourt. Article Arsenic in Dict. des Sc. Méd.
§ London Medical Gazette, 1839-40, p. 266.
|| Hoffman, Medicina Rationalis Systematica, i 198.
¶ Magazin für die gerichtlichen Arnzeikunde, ii. 473.

24*

symptoms is given by Hahnemann. " They are," says he, " a gradual sinking of the powers of life, without any violent symptom, —
a nameless feeling of illness, failure of the strength, slight feverishness, want of sleep, lividity of the countenance, and an aversion to
food and drink and all the other enjoyments of life. Dropsy closes
the scene, along with black miliary eruptions, and convulsions, or
colliquative perspiration and purging."*

Whatever were its real effects, there appears no doubt it was
long used secretly in Italy to a fearful extent, the monster who has
given her name to it having confessed that she was instrumental in
the death of no less than six hundred persons. It has been already
stated, however [p. 40], that she owed her success rather to the ignorance of the age than to her own dexterity. At all events, the art
of secret poisoning cannot now be easily practised. Indeed even the
vulgar dread of it is almost extinct. Partly on account of the improvement in general knowledge and chiefly in consequence of the
subtility and precision, which the refinement of modern physic and
chemistry have introduced into medico-legal inquiries, it is rare that
the suspicious scrutiny of the world now " recognizes in the accounts
of the last illness of popes and princes the effects of poison insidiously
introduced into the body."†

I may add in conclusion, that I was consulted a few years ago on
the part of the crown in a case which considerably resembled the
effects ascribed in former times to the aqua Toffana, except that it
was more acute in its character and swifter in its progress. As this
case will probably be found to represent pretty nearly the usual
effects of moderate doses frequently repeated, it is here given in some
detail.

A woman of indifferent character married a young man in circumstances which led to a breach between him and his relatives ; but
the pair appeared to live on good terms with one another. Eighteen
months after the marriage she was attacked with sickness and faintness ; and on the fourth day of this illness, while she was recovering,
the symptoms unexpectedly increased, and she seemed very unwell.
On the fifth day she became extremely weak, and suffered much
from yellow vomiting. On the seventh, when she was first visited
by a medical man, she had frequent vomiting, burning in the stomach, a yellow tongue, flushed countenance, hot skin, and hurried
pulse. On the ninth the throat was sore and red, and the expression
anxious ; and next day the soreness was greater, affected the nose
and mouth also, and was attended with excoriation of the lips and
nostrils, swelling of the glands of the throat, dimness of sight, and
great exhaustion. On the eleventh day, while previously again getting better, she became much worse, and suffered greatly from excessive vomiting, pain in the stomach, and an increase of the other
symptoms. On the thirteenth she was very hoarse, and despaired of

* Ueber die Arsenic-Vergiftung, 63.

† Gmelin's Geschichte der Mineralischen Gifte. Gmelin attempts to show from
symptoms, that the Popes Pius Third and Clement Fourteenth died of arsenic secretly
and gradually given, p. 107.

recovery. Next day she was occasionally incoherent, and had twitches of the facial muscles; the hands and face were swelled, the eyelids dingy, the conjunctivæ injected, and the nails blue. On the morning of the fifteenth there was for two hours violent delirium and fierce maniacal excitement, which were succeeded by coma, and this by death in the course of the evening. There was no diarrhœa, or urinary complaint, and no paralysis or eruption on the skin. A variety of circumstances of a general nature, which it would be out of place to enumerate here, — the detection of arsenic in various articles of which the woman had partaken, and in which the arsenic had been dissolved sometimes simply, sometimes with the aid of an alkali, — together with the fact, that the body five months after death was found preserved from decay, as it is now well known to be in most cases of arsenical poisoning, — left little doubt that the woman died of the effects of arsenic taken in several small doses at distant intervals, although none could be detected in the stomach or intestines. The case did not go to trial, owing to the death of an essential witness.

The effects of arsenic on man, when introduced into the living body through other channels besides the stomach, will now require some observations. It is necessary for the medical jurist to be well acquainted with them, because there is hardly an accessible part of the human body to which this poison has not been applied either accidentally or by design. When some account was given of its comparative action on the different tissues of animals, it was observed that arsenic acts when applied to a wound or ulcer, to the peritonæal membrane, to the eye, and to the vagina. On man it has been known to act through an ulcer or wound, the inner membrane of the rectum, the membrane of the vagina, the membrane of the air-tubes, the membrane of the nose, and even the sound skin.

Many persons have been poisoned by the application of arsenic to surfaces deprived of the cuticle, such as blistered surfaces, eruptions, ulcers, or wounds. When applied in this manner it commonly induces both local inflammation and constitutional symptoms. Amatus Lusitanus relates the case of a young man, who, against the advice of his physician, anointed an itchy eruption of the skin with an arsenical ointment, and next day was found dead in bed.[*] A similar case, not so rapidly fatal, has been recorded by Wepfer. A girl, affected with psoriasis of the scalp, had it rubbed with a liniment of butter and arsenic. In a short time she was seized with acute pain and swelling of the whole head, fainting-fits, restlessness, fever, delirium, and she died in six days.[†] Zitmann has noticed the cases of two children, eight and ten years of age, who were killed by the application of an arsenical solution to a similar eruption of the head.[‡] And Belloc relates the case of a woman who, trying to cure an inveterate itch with an arsenical lotion, was attacked in consequence with severe erysipelas of the whole body, succeeded by tremors and

[*] Curat. Medic. C. ii. Obs. 33.　　　　[†] De Cicuta, p. 289.
[‡] Quoted by Hahnemann, über die Arsenic-Vergiftung, p. 41.

gradual exhaustion of the vital powers, ending fatally in two years.*
M. Errard of Injurieux in France lately met with two cases, where,
in consequence of a freshly blistered surface being dressed with a
cerate made with the stearine of arsenicated candles (see p. 256),
local pain, nausea, pain in the stomach, urgent thirst, redness of the
tongue, involuntary contractions of the muscles of the extremities,
and weakness and irregularity of the pulse came on ; and one person
died within twenty-four hours, while the other recovered, chiefly
because the dressing caused so much pain that the patient could not
keep it on long.†

Next as to ulcers ; M. Roux has noticed the case of a girl, who
was killed by the application of the arsenical paste to an ulcer of the
breast, and in whom the constitutional symptoms were strongly
marked, although the quantity of the poison must have been very
small. The preparation used, which contains only a twenty-fourth
of its weight of arsenic, was applied for a single night on a surface
not exceeding an inch and a half in diameter. Yet she complained
next day of violent colic and vomited frequently, the countenance
soon became collapsed, and she died two days afterwards in great
anguish.‡ Another instance of the like kind is related in the Annales d'Hygiène, where death arose from an arsenical ointment ignorantly applied for scirrhous breast over a large surface of the skin
stripped of the cuticle by a blister. The particular symptoms and
their duration are not stated ; but there was violent irritation of the
stomach.§ Another fatal case, related by Dr. Küchler, arose from
the application of Frère Cosme's powder to a soft fungoid tumour on
the temple, which discharged serum usually and blood upon slight
pressure. About a drachm and a half of arsenic mixed with fifteen
grains of other powders was applied. Severe inflammation spread
round the tumour next day ; and soon afterwards, the patient was
attacked with great difficulty of breathing, thirst, pains in the belly,
and purging, then with difficulty in swallowing from swelling of the
base of the tongue, delirium, cold sweating, and extreme debility ;
and death ensued in four days.‖

There is a singular uncertainty in the effects of arsenic when applied to ulcerated surfaces. Some persons, like Roux's patient, are
obviously affected by a single application ; while others have had it
applied for a long time without experiencing any other consequences
than the formation of an eschar at the part. Two causes have been
assigned for these differences, and probably both are founded on fact.
One, which has been assigned by Mr. Blackadder, is the relative
quantity of arsenic applied. He says he never witnessed but one
instance of its acting constitutionally, although he often applied it to
sores ; and he imputes this success to his having always used a large
quantity. For he considers that by so doing the organization of the

* Cours de Médecine Légale, p. 121.
† London Medical Gazette, 1842-43, i. 351 ; from Gazette Médicale, 1842, Nov. 5.
‡ Elémens de Médecine Opératoire.
§ Annales d'Hyg. Publ. et de Méd. Lég. xi. 461.
‖ Journ. de Chimie Médicale, 1836, 482.

part is quickly destroyed, and absorption prevented, — but that if the quantity be small, as in the mode practised by Roux, it will cause little local injury and readily enter the absorbing vessels.* Another unequivocal cause is pointed out by Harles in his treatise on arsenic. While treating of its therapeutic properties, and noticing the controversy that prevailed last century throughout Europe repecting the propriety of its outward application, he remarks that it may be applied with safety to the abraded skin, to common ulcers, to wounded surfaces, and to malignant glandular ulcers, even when highly irritable, provided the part be not recently wounded, so as to pour out blood.† The reason of this is obvious ; the application of the poison to open-mouthed vessels is the next thing to its direct introduction into a vein. It is some confirmation of Harles's opinion, that Roux, whose patient was so easily affected, recommends that before arsenic is applied to an ulcer, a fresh surface be made by paring away the granulations ; and that Küchler's patient had an ulcer which did not discharge pus, but serum, and was easily made to bleed.

In the cases related above it will be remarked that the symptoms vary in their nature. Sometimes the chief disorder is inflammation, spreading over and around the eruption or ulcer, sometimes inflammation of the alimentary canal, sometimes an affection of the nervous system. In general the sufferings of the patient both from the local inflammation and constitutional symptoms are very severe. But this rule has its exceptions. In Pyl's Memoirs there is the history of a child who died four days after an itchy eruption of the whole body had been washed with an arsenical solution, and signs of vivid inflammation were found after death in many parts ; yet she appears to have complained only of headache.‡ Occasionally too, without exciting either inflammation of the part, or disorder of the stomach, or a general injury of the nervous system, it seems to give rise to partial palsy of the muscles adjoining the seat of its application. An extraordinary case is noticed in an American Journal, in which the prolonged use of an arsenical preparation for destroying a tumour on the right side of the neck, was followed by complete palsy of the muscles of the neck and arm of that side.

In the next place, poisoning has been perpetrated by introducing arsenic into the fundament with an injection.§ Foderé has noticed a case of this kind, which happened in France, and was communicated to him by a physician of Thoulouse. A lady under medical treatment for some trifling illness, died unexpectedly under symptoms of poisoning ; and it was discovered that her servant, after unsuccessfully attempting to despatch her by dissolving arsenic in her soup, had ultimately succeeded by administering it repeatedly in injections.‖ There is no doubt that by this mode all the usual effects of arsenic may be induced ; and on account of the facility

* On Phagedæna Gangrænosa, or Med. Phys. Journal, xl. 238.
† De Arsenici usu in Medicina, p. 158.
‡ Aufsätze und Beobachtungen, i. 43.
§ Paris and Fonblanque, ii. 222.   ‖ Médecine, Légale, iv. 226.

with which the colon and rectum may be evacuated, it is not likely that the poison will be found in the gut after death, if the individual did not die in a few hours after its administration.

In the third place, women have also died of poisoning by arsenic introduced into the vagina. Two examples of this revolting crime are on record. One of them occurred in 1799, in the Department of the Ourthe in France. A middle-aged female was seized with vomiting, diarrhœa, swelling of the genitals and uterine discharge ; and she expired not long after. Before her death she told two of her neighbours, that her husband had some time before tried to poison her by putting arsenic in her coffee, and had at length succeeded by introducing a powder into her vagina while in the act of enjoying his nuptial rights. The vulva and vagina were gangrenous, the belly distended with gases, and the intestines inflamed.*

The other case, which happened in Finland in 1786, gave rise to an excellent dissertation on the subject by Dr. Mangor, at that time medical inspector for Copenhagen. A farmer near Copenhagen lost his wife suddenly under suspicious circumstances, and six weeks afterwards married his maid-servant. In a few years he transferred his affections to another maid-servant, with whose aid he endeavoured to poison his second wife. For some time his attempts proved abortive ; till at last one morning, after coïtion, he introduced a mixture of arsenic and flour on the point of his finger into the vagina. She took ill at mid-day and expired next morning ; and the murderer soon after married his guilty paramour. But a few years had not elapsed before he got tired of her also ; and one morning, after the conjugal embrace, he administered arsenic to her in the same way as to her predecessor. About three in the afternoon, while enjoying good health, she was suddenly seized with shivering and heat in the vagina. The remembrance of her former wickedness soon awoke the suspicions of the unhappy woman, and she wrung from her husband a confession of his crime. Means were resorted to for saving her life, but in vain : She was attacked with acute pain in her stomach and incessant vomiting, then became delirious, and died in twenty-one hours. After death grains of arsenic were found in the vagina, although frequent lotions had been used in the treatment. The labia were swollen and red, the vagina gaping and flaccid, the os uteri gangrenous, the duodenum inflamed, the stomach natural. In the course of the judicial proceedings which arose out of these two cases, Dr. Mangor made experiments on mares, with the view of settling the doubts which were entertained as to the likelihood of arsenic proving fatal in the manner alleged ; and the results clearly showed that, when applied to the vagina of these animals, it produces violent local inflammation and fatal constitutional derangement.†

In the fourth place, poisoning by arsenic through the bronchial

* Ansiaulx, Clinique Chirurgicale, and Henke's Zeitschrift für die Staatsarzneikunde, ii. 188.
† Acta Hafniensia, iii. 178.

membrane or membrane of the air passages is a comparatively rare accident, which can take place only in consequence of arsenical gases or vapours being incautiously breathed. The effects of oxide of arsenic when introduced in this way are described from personal experience by Otto Tachenius, a chemist of the sixteenth century. " Once," said he, " when I happened to breathe incautiously the fumes of arsenic, I was surprised to find my palate impressed with a sweet, mild, grateful taste, such as I never experienced before. But in half an hour I was attacked with pain and tightness in the stomach, then with general convulsions, difficult breathing, an un- speakable sense of heat, bloody and painful micturition, and finally with such an acute colic as contracted my whole body for half an hour." By the use of oleaginous drinks he recovered from these alarming symptoms; but during all the succeeding winter he had a low hectic fever.*

Balthazar Timæus relates a similar case which came under his no- tice. An apothecary of Colberg, while subliming arsenic, had not been careful enough to avoid the fumes; and was soon after seized with frequent fainting, tightness in the præcordia, difficult breathing, inextinguishable thirst, parched throat, great restlessness, watching, and pains in the feet. He had afterwards profuse daily perspiration and palsy of the legs; and several months elapsed before he got en- tirely well.† The same author says that the famous Paracelsus, being one day put out of temper by an acquaintance, made him hold his nose over an alembic in which arsenic was subliming; and that the object of this severe joke nearly lost his life in consequence. Wib- mer quotes the heads of several cases where swelling of the tongue, headache and giddiness, nausea, and an oppressive sense of constric- tion in the throat, were occasioned by the incautious inhalation of arsenical fumes.‡ The following extraordinary case, closely allied to malignant cholera in its early stage, has been ascribed by the re- porter Dr. Welper of Berlin to the inspiration of arsenical fumes, — with what probability I am not prepared to say. A stout healthy man, who in the forenoon had freely and for some time exposed him- self to the steam from a vessel where he was boiling several ounces of orpiment in water, was attacked at night with sickness, and next morning with extreme weakness and some difficulty of breathing. These symptoms were greatly relieved by an emetic. But towards evening the extremities became ice-cold and very stiff, the breathing much oppressed, the pulse very hurried, and imperceptible except in the neck, the mouth and throat dry, and the tongue rigid; but the mind remained clear, though anxious and afraid of impending disso- lution. His state of collapse was removed in twelve hours by fo- mentations, and in no long time he recovered entirely except from the dyspnœa, which continued more or less till a few years after- wards, when he died of hydrothorax.§

* Hippocrates Chymicus, c. 24. p. 213.
† Casus Medicinales, lib. vii. cas. 11.
‡ Die Wirkung der Arzneimittel und Gifte, i. 299.
§ Journal der Praktischen Heilkunde, lxxii. v. 134.

The slighter effects of arsenic are said to have been repeatedly observed of late in this country from inhaling the products of the combustion of arsenicated candles, — an article of recent invention, in which arsenic, to the extent of three or four grains and a half in each candle, is introduced for the purpose of hardening the stearine chiefly used in manufacturing them. It is unnecessary to say, that such candles are prejudicial and ought to be prohibited. In a set of experiments made to try their effects by Messrs. Everitt, Bird, and Phillips in 1838, birds were killed in no long time, and small quadrupeds were severely affected, when kept in an apartment lighted with them.*

Analogous to the effects of inhaling oxide of arsenic are those lately observed from the incautious inhalation of arseniuretted-hydrogen gas. Gehlen the chemist died of this accident, but no particular account has been published of the symptoms he suffered. Two cases, however, have been detailed within a few years. In one of these, which has been related by Dr. Schlinder, of Greifensberg, the individual inhaled in forty minutes about half a cubic inch of the gas, which is equivalent to about an eighth of a grain of arsenic. In three hours he became affected with giddiness, and soon afterwards with an uneasy sense of pressure in the region of the kidney, passing gradually into acute pain there and upwards along the back. General shivering ensued, with coldness of the extremities, and gouty-like pains in the knees, shoulders, and elbows. The hands and lower half of the fore-arms, the feet and legs nearly to the knees, the nose and region of the eyebrows, felt as if quite dead, but without any diminution of muscular power. There was also acute pain in the stomach and belly generally, painful eructation of gas, and occasional vomiting of bitter, greenish-yellow mucus. The most tormenting symptom, however, was the pain in the kidneys, which soon became attended with constant desire to pass water, and the discharge of deep reddish-brown urine, mixed with clots of blood. The whole expression of the countenance was altered, the skin becoming dark brown, and the eyeballs sunk, yellow, and surrounded by a broad livid ring. Warm drink brought out a copious sweat and removed the sense of numbness; but next day there was little change otherwise in the symptoms, except that the urine was no longer mixed with clots, and that the hair on the benumbed parts had become white. On the third day the pains had abated, and the urine became clear; but there was hiccup, an excited state of the mind, and a feeling as if a great stone lay in the lower belly. In seven days he was much better. In the third week the whole glans and prepuce became covered with little pustules which were followed by small ulcers. It was not till the close of the seventh week that he recovered completely.† Dr. O'Reilly has related the following case, which arose from the inhalation of hydrogen gas impregnated with arseniuretted-hydrogen in consequence of the sulphuric acid used

* London Medical Gazette, 1837-38, i. 585.
† Buchner's Repertorium für die Pharmacie, lxix. 271.

for dissolving zinc having contained arsenic. Mr. Brittan, a Dublin chemist, wishing to ascertain the effects of hydrogen on the body, proceeded to inhale 150 cubic inches of it. Immediately after the second inhalation, he was seized with confusion, faintness, giddiness and shivering, and passed a stool, as well as two ounces of bloody urine, but without any pain. Pain in the limbs followed, and in two hours frequent vomiting and dull pain in the stomach. The pulse at this time was 90, the skin cold, and the voice feeble. Ammonia, laudanum, and emollient clysters gave him little relief. During the subsequent night there was frequent vomiting and no urine; the face became copper-coloured, and the rest of the body greenish; there was tenderness of the epigastrium and hiccup; but he was free of fever. On the third day there was diarrhœa and still no urine; but the jaundice had disappeared. On the fourth the breath was ammoniacal, and somnolency had set in. On the fifth the skin became again deeply jaundiced, and the face was œdematous; no urine had yet been discharged, and the bladder, examined with the catheter, was found empty. On the evening of the seventh day he expired. On examination of the body, two pints of red serum were found in the pleural cavities; the lungs were sound, the heart pale and flaccid, the liver indigo-blue, the gall-bladder distended with bile, the kidneys also indigo-blue, the stomach empty, and its villous coat brittle, with here and there inflamed-like spots on it, the bladder empty, the brain bloodless, the cellular tissue generally anasarcous. Arsenic was detected in the pleural serum. By an approximate calculation it was supposed that the hydrogen this gentleman inhaled had contained the equivalent arsenic of twelve grains of the oxide.*

It would appear that arsenic acts with great rapidity and force when respired in any form.

Poisoning through the lining membrane of the nostrils is a still rarer accident than that last mentioned. There is a distinct example of it in the German Ephemerides, which arose from an arsenical solution having been used by mistake as a lotion for a chronic discharge from the nostrils. The individual was attacked with a profuse discharge from the nostrils, and then with stupor approaching to coma. Weakness of sight and of memory continued after sensibility returned; and he died two years afterwards, death having been preceded for some time by convulsions.†

Arsenic when applied to the sound skin of animals does not easily affect them. The experiments of Jaeger formerly noticed prove that no effect is produced, if the poison is simply placed in contact with the skin. Nay even when rubbed into it with fatty matters it does not operate with energy; for in that case, according to the experiments of Renault, it causes sometimes a pustular eruption, sometimes an eschar, but never any constitutional disorder.‡   It is more ener-

* Dublin Journal of the Medical Sciences, xx. 422.
† Eph. Curios. Naturæ, Dec. iii. An. 9 and 10, Obs. 220.
‡ Sur les Contrepoisons de l'Arsénic, p. 112.

25

getic, however, when applied to the more delicate skin of the human subject. Some experiments were made by Mr. Sherwen on himself with the view of proving this ;* but they are not satisfactory. The following facts, however, will show that it may produce through the sound skin all the ordinary signs of poisoning. Desgranges, a good authority, relates the case of a woman who anointed her head with an arsenical ointment to kill lice, and, after using it several days, was attacked with erysipelas of the head and face, attended with ulceration of the scalp, swelling of the salivary and cervical glands, and inflammation of the eyes. There were likewise violent constitutional symptoms, — much fever, fainting, giddiness, vomiting and pain in the stomach, tenesmus, and ardor urinæ, tremors of the limbs, and even occasional delirium. Afterwards the whole body became covered with an eruption of white papulæ, which dried and dropt off in forty-eight hours. She recovered gradually ; but appears to have made a narrow escape. Her hair fell out during convalescence.†
A similar instance is recorded in the Acta Germanica for 1730. A schoolboy having found in the street a parcel of arsenic, his mother mistook it for hair powder ; and as he had to deliver a valedictory speech at school next day, she advised him to powder himself well with it in the morning. This he accordingly did. In the middle of his speech he was attacked with acute pain of the face ; and a fertile crop of pustules soon broke out upon it. The head afterwards swelled much, and the pustules spread all around it ; he was tormented with intolerable heat in the scalp ; and the hair became matted with the discharge into a thick scabby crust. This crust separated in a few weeks, and he soon recovered completely.‡ Schulze, a German physician, has related no fewer than five cases of the same description, all arising from arsenic having been mistaken for hair-powder ; aud one of them proved fatal. Two of the cases were slight. The other persons had the same violent inflammation of the head as Desgranges's patient and the German schoolboy. In the fatal case death took place in twenty-one days; and on dissection, besides other morbid appearances, the scalp was found gangrenous and infiltered with fluid blood, and the stomach much inflamed.§ The two survivors, who were severely ill, it is well to add, were not attacked with the erysipelas of the scalp till six days after they powdered themselves. Sproegel mentions a fatal case from fly-powder having been applied in like manner to the head ; and Wibmer quotes another, but not fatal, where from the same cause great swelling of the head and face arose, followed by erysipelas of the face, neck, and belly, and a papular eruption on the hands which continued five days.‖

From the statements now made, it is evident that arsenic applied to various parts of the external surface and natural apertures of the

* Mem. of London Medical Society, ii. 397.
† Recueil Périod. de la Soc. de Med. vi. 22.
‡ Acta Germanica, ii. 33.
§ Knape und Hecker's Kritische Annalen der Staatsarzneikunde, i. 143-159.
‖ Die Wirkung der Arzneimittel und Gifte, i. 241.

body, will prove poisonous, and will often act with a certainty and rapidity not surpassed by its effects when taken internally. Many of the cases furnish a striking confirmation of a circumstance formerly noticed with respect to its action, — namely, that it produces signs of irritation in the stomach, in whatever manner it is introduced into the body. In some instances, indeed, the signs of inflammation in the stomach were quite as distinct as in the cases previously described, where the poison was taken internally.

The subject of the symptoms caused by arsenic will now be concluded with a few remarks on the strength of the evidence which they supply.

The present doctrine of toxicologists and medical jurists seems generally to be, that symptoms alone can never supply decisive proof of the administration of arsenic. This opinion is certainly quite correct when applied to what may be called a common case of poisoning with arsenic, the symptoms of which are little else than burning pain in the stomach and bowels, vomiting and purging, feeble circulation, excessive debility, and speedy death. All these symptoms may be caused by natural disease, more particularly by cholera ; and consequently every sound medical jurist will join in condemning unreservedly the practice which prevailed last century of deciding questions of poisoning in such circumstances from symptoms alone. But modern authors appear to have overstepped the mark, when they hold that the rule against deciding from symptoms does not admit of any exceptions. For there are cases of poisoning with arsenic, not numerous certainly, yet not very uncommon neither, which can hardly be confounded with natural disease; and, what is of some consequence, they are precisely those in which the power of deciding from symptoms alone is most required, because chemical evidence is almost always wanting. Either the peculiar combination of the symptoms is such as cannot arise from natural causes, so far at least as physicians are acquainted with them : or these symptoms occur under collateral circumstances, which put natural causes almost or altogether out of the question.

Thus, let the medical jurist consider in the first place, the symptoms occasionally observed in those who survive five, six or ten days ; let him exclude for the present the secondary nervous affections ; and instead of a compounded description, which may be objected to as apt to convey a false and exaggerated idea of the facts, let him take an actual example. In a paper by Dr. Bachmann on some cases of poisoning with arsenic, there is a minute account of the case of a lady who was poisoned by her maid with fly-powder and white arsenic, and whose symptoms were those of universal inflammation of the mucous membranes. After suffering two days from retching and vomiting, colic pains and purging, these symptoms suddenly became more violent, and attended with oppressed breathing and hoarseness so that she could hardly make herself be heard,—with vesicles on the palate, burning pain in the throat, and excessive difficulty in swallowing, — with spasm and pain of the bladder in passing water, — and with extreme feebleness of the pulse. Three days afterwards the symptoms increased still more. She complained of intolerable burning and spasms of the throat, which, as well as the mouth, was excessively inflamed, — of violent burning pain in the stomach and bowels, — of burning in the fundament and genitals, both of which were inflamed even to gangrene, — of indescribable anxiety and anguish about the heart ; and she died the following day, death being proceded by subsultus, delirium, and insensibility.* Or take the case in the trial of Miss Blandy. On two successive evenings, immediately after taking some gruel which had been prepared by the prisoner, Mr. Blandy was attacked with pricking and burning of the tongue, throat, stomach, and bowels, and with vomiting and purging. Five days after, when the symptoms were fully formed, he had inflamed pimples round the lips, and a sense of burning in the mouth ; the nostrils were similarly affected ; the eyes were bloodshot and affected with burning pain ; the tongue was swollen, the throat red and excoriated, and in both there was a tormenting sense of burning ; he had likewise swelling, with pricking and burning pain of the belly ; excoriations and ulcers around the anus and intolerable burning there ; vomiting and bloody diarrhœa ; a low, tremulous pulse, laborious respiration, and great difficulty in speaking and swallowing. In this state he lingered several days, death supervening nine days after the first suspected basin of gruel was taken.† Can the symptoms, in these two cases, attacking, as they did, at one and the same time, the whole mucous membranes, be imitated by any natural combination of symptoms ? Viewing the endless variety and wonderful complexity of the phenomena of disease, the practitioner will probably, and with justice, reply that a natural combination of the kind is possible. But if his attention is confined, as in strictures it ought to real occurrences, — if he is required to speak only from actual experience, personal or derived, it is exceedingly questionable whether any one could say he had ever seen or read of such a case. At all events, if a medical witness had to give his opinion from symptoms only in such a case as that of Mr. Blandy, or that described by Bachmann, he would certainly be justified in declaring that poisoning was highly probable; and, admitting general poisoning to be proved, he would, it is likely, fix on arsenic as the substance which could most easily produce the effects.

Let him next, however, take also into consideration the nervous affections that sometimes either immediately follow the inflammation of the mucous membranes, or become united with it when it has existed a few days; and confining his attention still to actual occurrences, let him reflect on the symptoms in Dr. Roget's case, in which there was first violent inflammation of the whole alimentary canal, and then regular and obstinate epilepsy (p. 245), or on those in Dehaen's patient, in whom the nervous disorder was partial palsy (p. 247). On reconsidering these narratives, still greater reason will appear for

* Einige auserlesene Medizinisch-gerichtliche abhandlungen von Schmitt, Bach-mann, &c. p. 40.
† State Trials, xviii.

doubting whether such a combination of simultaneous, and in the present instance also consecutive symptoms, ever arise from natural causes. It is difficult to conceive a fortuitous concurrence of natural diseases producing at the same moment that variety and complexity of disorder which occur in the primary stage of the cases alluded to; and it would surely be a still more extraordinary combination which should farther add the supevention of epilepsy or partial palsy from a natural cause, at the exact period at which it appears as the secondary stage of poisoning with arsenic. All that any practitioner could say is, that a concurrence of the kind is within the bounds of possibility. He must be compelled to admit that it is in the highest degree improbable, and likewise that it could hardly take place from natural causes without the real causes of the symptoms being clearly indicated.

But to conclude, there are likewise collateral circumstances connected with the symptoms, which, taken along with the symptoms themselves, will sometimes place the fact of poisoning with arsenic beyond the reach of a doubt. Thus, if a person were taken several times ill with symptoms of general inflammation of the mucous membranes, after partaking each time of a suspected article of food or drink, the proof of the administration of arsenic would be very strong indeed ; and it would be unimpeachable if at length a nervous affection succeeded at the usual period. Or above all, suppose several persons, who have partaken of the same dish, are seized about the same time with nearly the same symptoms of irritation of the mucous membranes. The proof of general poisoning would then be unequivocal. And if one or more of them should afterwards suffer from a nervous disorder, little hesitation ought to be felt in declaring that arsenic is the only poison which could have caused their complaints.

These views are of more practical consequence than may at first sight be thought. The doctrine which has been here espoused might have been applied to decide two criminal cases which at the time made a great noise in this country. One was the case of Eliza Fenning (p. 245). Here five persons were simultaneously attacked with symptoms, more or less violent, of inflammation of the whole alimentary canal; and in two of them epileptic convulsions appeared before the inflammatory symptoms departed. The other was the case of George Thom (p. 247). Here four persons were at one and the same time seized with the primary symptoms in an aggravated form ; and in two of them, as these symptoms abated, obstinate partial palsy came on. On both trials, then, it might have been stated from the symptoms alone that poison had been given, and that arsenic was the only poison hitherto known to be capable of producing such effects.

In applying this doctrine to parallel instances two precautions must be attended to. On the one hand, care must be taken to ascertain, as may always be done, that the simultaneous symptoms of general irritation in the alimentary canal, arising soon after a meal, are not owing to unsound meat having been used in preparing it. And on

25*

the other hand, which is of more consequence, the symptoms on which so important an opinion is founded, must be strongly marked and well ascertained by a competent person. The signs of irritation in the mucous membranes must be really general and unequivocal ; and those of a disorder of the nervous system must be likewise developed characteristically. Care must be taken in particular to distinguish symptoms of the latter class from others which approach to them in nature, and are the ordinary sequels of natural disease : for example, the true palsy caused by arsenic must not be confounded with the numbness and racking pains in the limbs, which occasionally succeed cholera.

With these precautions the evidence from symptoms may in certain cases be decisive of the question of poisoning with arsenic. And it is of moment to observe, as has been already hinted, that, although such cases are numerous, they are precisely of the kind in which it is most essential to the ends of justice that the symptoms should, if possible, supply evidence enough to direct the judgment ; for the characteristic symptoms referred to occur chiefly when the patient either recovers or survives many days, and where consequently the chemical evidence, usually procured from the examination of the contents of the stomach, is almost always wanting.

SECTION III. — *Of the Morbid Appearances caused by Arsenic.*

The morbid appearances caused by arsenic will next require some details. In treating of them the same plan will be pursued as in the preceding section : the various morbid appearances left by it will first be mentioned in their order ; and the subject will then be wound up with some remarks on the force of the evidence from these appearances, as they are usually combined in actual cases.

In the first instance, there are some cases in which little or no morbid appearance is to be seen at all. These all belong to the second variety of poisoning, which is characterized by the absence of local imflammation, and the presence of symptoms indicating an action on the heart, or some other remote organ. In such circumstances death takes place before a sufficient interval has elapsed for inflammation to be developed.

Several examples of the absence of diseased appearances in the dead body are to be found in authors. Thus in Chaussier's case formerly quoted (p. 243), in that related by Metzger (p. 242), in another related by Etmuller, which was fatal in twelve hours,* and in a fourth related by Professor Wagner of Berlin, where life was also prolonged for twelve hours under incessant vomiting,† there was positively no morbid alteration at all. Such was also the state of the whole alimentary canal in the extraordinary case related by Orfila (p. 243). In the case quoted from the Medical and Physical Journal (p. 242), there was merely a slight redness at the pyloric end of the

---

* Ephem. Academ. Cæsareo-Leopoldinæ, 1715. Obs. cxxvi.
† Horn's Archiv für Medizinische Erfahrung, 1834, 755.

stomach. In the case of the American grocer too, there was only a little redness. In Mr. Wright's case (p. 243), there was scarcely any morbid appearance, — nothing more than two small vascular spots and a minute ecchymosis. In that which fell under my own notice (p. 242), the villous coat of the stomach was of natural firmness, and had an exceedingly faint mottled-cherry-red tint, barely perceptible in a strong light; and the rest of the alimentary canal, as well as the body generally, was quite healthy.

Although in these examples the morbid appearances were trifling or undistinguishable, it must not be supposed that the same happens in all cases of rapid death from arsenic. In Gérard's case, where the usual irritant symptoms were wanting, and which proved fatal in five hours, there was dark redness of the whole villous coat of the stomach. In Mr. Holland's case, fatal in eight or nine hours (p. 243), the stomach was of an intense purple colour at its pyloric end, and contained bloody mucus ; and the mucous coat of the cœcum presented extensive softening and congestion. Mr. Alfred Taylor refers to three cases observed by Mr. Forster of Huntingdon, in which the mucous coat of the stomach was highly inflamed, though death took place in $6\frac{1}{2}$, $3\frac{1}{2}$, and 2 hours only :[*] in Mr. Hewson's case, fatal in five hours, the whole stomach was exceedingly vascular, and presented both spots of extravasation, and several small erosions (p. 201). In a case alluded to at p. 239 as having fallen under my own observation, and which was also fatal in five hours, the whole villous coat of the stomach was intensely red, except where the folds of the rugæ protected it from contact with the poison ; and the prominences of the rugæ presented corroded spots of ecchymosis. In Dr. Dymock's case, fatal in two hours and a half, the stomach, which I had an opportunity of examining, presented on its mucous coat many scarlet patches, and here and there a purplish appearance (p. 240). Lastly, an instance is related by Pyl of this poison proving fatal in three hours, and leaving nevertheless in the dead body distinct signs of inflammation in the stomach.[†]

In the ordinary cases in which death is delayed till the second day or later, a considerable variety of diseased appearances has been observed. They are the different changes of structure arising from inflammation in the alimentary canal, in the organs of the chest, and in the organs of generation — together with certain alterations in the state of the blood and condition of the body generally.

The first set of appearances to be mentioned are those indicating inflammation of the alimentary canal, viz., redness of the throat and gullet, — redness of the villous and peritonæal coats of the stomach, blackness of its villous coat from extravasation of blood into it, softening of the villous coat, ulceration of that as well as of the other coats, effusion of coagulable lymph on the inner surface of the stomach, extravasation of blood among its contents, — finally, redness and ulceration of the duodenum and other parts of the intestinal

[*] Guy's Hospital Reports, 1841, vi. 278.
[†] Aufsätze und Beobachtungen, i. 53, and v. 107.

canal, and more particularly of the rectum ; to which may also be added, though not properly a morbid phenomenon, certain appearances put on by the arsenic which remains undischarged.

Redness of the throat and gullet is not common, at least it does not often occur in the descriptions of cases. Jaeger, however, says that in his experiments he usually found redness at the upper and purplish stripes at the lower end of the gullet :[*] and Dr. Campbell likewise found the gullet red in animals.[†] Similar appearances have also been remarked in man. In the case of a man who lived eight days, Dr. Murray found the gullet very red ;[‡] in that of a woman who lived scarce seven hours, Dr. Booth observed the gullet inflamed downwards very nearly to the cardia ;[§] and Wildberg has reported two cases of the same nature, in one of which it is worthy of remark that the poisoning lasted only six hours.[||]   On the whole, it appears probable that inflammation of the throat and gullet would be found more frequently in the reports of cases, if it was more carefully look- ed for.

Redness of the inner coat of the stomach is a pretty constant effect of arsenic, when the case is not very rapid.   All the varieties of red- ness, formerly mentioned among the effects of the irritant poisons generally, may be produced by arsenic.   There is nothing, however, in the redness caused by this poison, any more than in the redness of inflammation generally, by which it is to be distinguished from the pseudo-morbid varieties. (See p. 110.)

It is singular, that, however severe the inflammation of the inner membrane of the stomach may be, inflammatory redness of the peri- tonæal coat is seldom found.   Yet inflammatory vascularity does occur sometimes on the peritonæal coat.   Sproegel found it in ani- mals;[¶] and it was present in the case of the girl Warden, whose death gave rise to the trial of Mrs. Smith.[**]   Dr. Nissen, a Danish physi- cian, has related another case in which the external coat of the sto- mach appeared as if minutely injected with wax.   But the patient had been attacked with incarcerated hernia during the progress of his illness, and the whole peritonæal membrane was in consequence inflamed.[††]   A common appearance when the internal inflammation is well marked, and one often unwarily put down as inflammation of the peritonæum, is turgescence of the external veins, sometimes so great as to make the stomach look livid.

Blackness of the villous coat from effusion of altered blood into its texture is sometimes met with.   When the colour is brownish-black, or grayish-black, not merely reddish-black, when the inner mem- brane is elevated into firm knots or ridges by the effusion, and the black spots are surrounded by vascularity or other signs of reaction,

* Diss. Inaug. Tubingæ, 1808, de Effectibus Arsenici in varios organismos, p. 39.
† Diss. Inaug. Edin. 1813, de Venen. Mineralibus, pp. 5, 6, 12.
‡ Edin. Med. and Surg. Journal, xviii. 171.
§ London Medical Gazette, xiv. 62.
‖ Praktisches Handbuch, iii. 232 and 304.   ¶ Dissert. Exp. 36.
** Edin. Med. and Surg. Journal, xxvii. 453.
†† Nordisches Archiv, i. 334.

the appearances strongly indicate violent irritation. I have already said that such appearances are never imitated by any pseudo-morbid phenomenon.

One of the most remarkable appearances occasionally observed in the stomach in those instances where the body has been buried for at least some weeks before examination, is the presence of bright yellow patches, of various sizes, which appear as if painted with gamboge, and obviously arise from the oxide of arsenic diffused throughout the tissues having been decomposed and converted into sulphuret of arsenic by the sulphuretted-hydrogen disengaged during putrefaction. I have witnessed this appearance in several cases. In the case mentioned at p. 247, where the body had been buried twenty days, numerous brilliant yellow patches were visible on the villous coat of the stomach. In the case of a female who was poisoned about the same time with that man, and, as was suspected, by the same individual, the body was not examined till three months after interment; and here broad, bright, yellow patches, disappearing under the action of ammonia, were found under the peritonæal coat of the left end of the stomach, the adjoining great intestine, and also the muscular parietes of the abdomen. In the case of Mr. Gilmour, for whose murder his wife was tried a few months ago in this city, but acquitted, — and who undoubtedly died of poisoning with arsenic, howsoever administered, — there were found fourteen weeks after death numerous yellow streaks and patches both on the inner surface of the stomach, on its outer surface under the peritonæum, on the adjoining transverse colon, and on the small intestines in contact with the stomach. From these and other parallel facts which have been occasionally noticed by the periodical press, it seems probable that the appearance in question is common in bodies which have been some time buried. It is an extremely important part of the pathological evidence. I doubt whether natural causes can occasion any appearance similar to it. And indeed, what is it but the effect of a chemical test applied to the poison by nature?

The next appearance which may be mentioned is unnatural softness of the villous coat of the stomach. This coat has certainly been often found, after death from arsenic, unusually soft, brittle, and easily separable with the nail.* But the same state occurs in dead bodies so often and so unconnected with previous symptoms of irritation in the stomach, that it cannot with any certainty be assumed as the effect of irritation when it is found subsequently to such symptoms. So far from softening and brittleness being a necessary effect of the irritation produced by arsenic, it is a fact that a condition precisely the reverse has been also noticed. In a case which I examined, the villous coat, except where it had been disintegrated by effused blood and ulceration, was strong and firm; and the rugæ were thickened, raised and corrugated, as if seared with a hot iron.† Metzger once found the mucous membrane dense, thickened, and the rugæ like thick cords.‡ Pyl too once met with the same appear-

* Jaeger, p. 40.   † Edin. Med. and Surg. Journal, xxvii. 453.
‡ Schlegel, Collect. Opusc. &c. 423.

ance, and ascribes the thickening to gorging of vessels ;* and in a
case related by Dr. Wood of Dumfries, where I had an opportunity
of examining the stomach, this appearance was present in a remarkable degree, and it clearly arose from elevation of the villous coat by effusion of blood under it.† Remer, in his edition
of Metzger's Medical Jurisprudence, says he once met with an
instance where the stomach was shrivelled like a bladder subjected to boiling water.‡

Sometimes the villous and also more rarely the other coats of the
stomach are found actually destroyed and removed in scattered spots
and patches. This loss of substance is occasionally owing to the
same action which causes softening and brittleness of the villous coat,
— the action, however, having been so intense as to cause gelatinization. That such is the nature of the process appears from the breach
in the membrane being surrounded by gelatinized tissue, and not by
an areola of inflammatory redness. Of this species of destruction
of the coats I have seen a characteristic example.§ But in other
cases the loss of substance is owing to a process of ordinary ulceration, as is proved by the little cavities having a notched irregular
shape, and being surrounded both by a red areola and a margin of
firm tissue. This was the character of the ulcers in the case of
Warden, which I have described elsewhere.‖ Destruction of the
coats of the stomach by ulceration is not a very common consequence
of poisoning with arsenic, as death frequently takes place before
that process can be established. It does not often occur, unless the patient survive nearly two days. Mr. Alfred Taylor, however, mentions a case fatal in seventeen hours where he found ulceration of the stomach, and another fatal in ten hours where several
small ulcers were seen on the lesser curvature, and two nearly circular ones as big as a sixpence.¶ Mr. Hewson too informs me he found
many eroded spots even in his case which proved fatal in five hours (p.
56). I suspect, however, that spots of healthy membrane surrounded by
vascular redness are sometimes mistaken for ulcers in such cases ;
for indeed nothing can more exactly resemble them. In many general works on Medical Jurisprudence, and in some express treatises
on arsenic, it is stated that this poison may cause complete perforation of the stomach.** But this effect is exceedingly rare. I have
related one distinct example of it ;†† Professor Foderé has briefly alluded to a case he witnessed which proved fatal in two days and a
half ;‡‡ I have likewise found in an account of a trial in North America, an instance in which the stomach was perforated by numerous
small holes, so that when held before the light it appeared as if rid-

* Aufsätze und Beobachtungen, i. 58.
† Edinburgh Med. and Surg. Journal, xxxiii. 66.
‡ Metzger's System der gerichtlichen Arzneikunde, von Remer, 1820, p. 257.
§ Edin. Med. and Surg. Journal, xxix. 25.
‖ Edin. Med. and Surg. Journal, xxvii. 453.
¶ Guy's Hospital Reports, 1837, ii. 29, and 1841, vi. 266.
** Gmelin's Geschichte der Mineralischen Gifte, 124. Foderé, Médecine-Légale, iv.
127. Sallin, Journal Gén. de Médecine, iv.
†† Edin. Med. and Surg. Journal, xxix. 25.
‡‡ Journal Complémentaire, i. 106.

dled like a sieve ;* but I have not been able to find in medical authors any farther authority for the general statement. Destruction of the coats of the stomach as produced by arsenic has been variously described by authors under the terms erosion, corrosion, dissolution, ulceration. But the correct mode of describing it appears to be by the terms gelatinization, or ulceration, according to the nature of the diseased action by which it is induced. At all events it is necessary to beware of being misled by the terms erosion, corrosion, and the like, which all convey the idea of a chemical action; while it is well ascertained that a chemical action either does not exist at all between arsenic and the animal tissues, or, if it has existence, tends to harden and condense rather than to dissolve or corrode them. Arsenic is not a corrosive.

Another species of destruction of the coats of the stomach, which will require a little notice, is sloughing or gangrene. This appearance occurs frequently in the narratives of the older writers; but it has not been enumerated in the list of morbid appearances at the commencement of this section, because its existence as one of the effects of arsenic is problematical. It has not been witnessed so far as I know by any recent good authority. Those who have mentioned it have probably been misled by the appearance put on by the black extravasated patches, when they are accompanied by disintegration of the villous coat and effusion of clots of black blood on its surface — an appearance which resembles gangrene closely in every thing but the fetor. Sir B. Brodie has stated that Mr. John Hunter has preserved in his museum, as an example of a slough of the villous coat caused by arsenic, which turned out on examination to be nothing else than an adhering clot.† It is clear too, that, when Mr. James speaks of having found " several gangrenous patches" on the villous coat of the stomach, and " patches of sphacelus" in the intestines, on examining the body of a notorious French criminal, Soufflard, who poisoned himself with arsenic in prison in 1839, he mistook for gangrene what was merely extravasation ; for the man lived only twelve hours.‡

Various secretions have been found on the inner surface of the stomach. The mucous secretion of the inner membrane is generally increased in quantity. Frequently it is thin, but viscid, as in its natural state ; but sometimes it is both abundant and solid, as if coagulated ; and then it forms either a uniform attached pellicle, or loose shreds floating among the contents.§ In both forms it has been mistaken for the mucous membrane itself. I believe this increased secretion and preternatural firmness of the gastric mucus cannot take place without some irritating agent being applied to the stomach. Both may occur without any other sign of inflammation in the mucous membrane. In a case of suicide after seduction which came under

* Trial of Medad Mackay at Allegany, 1821. The prisoner was found not guilty. But the presence of arsenic in the stomach was proved by several tests.

† Philosophical Transactions, cii. 216.

‡ Archives Gén. de Médecine, l. 107.

§ Harles de Arsenico, 153, and Renault sur les Contrepoisons de l'Arsénic.

my notice in this city in 1843, and which proved fatal in five hours [p. 239], the mucus in the stomach, which was very abundant, put on the appearance of curdled milk, owing to its being rendered opaque and white by the large quantity of finely powdered arsenic diffused through it; and it was actually mistaken for curdled milk by several medical men. — Sometimes the matter effused is true coagulable lymph. This is rarely seen as the effect of arsenic. I have remarked it, however, very distinctly in dogs, and Dr. Baillie saw it once in the human subject.* It is of course quite decisive of the presence of inflammation. It is known from tough mucus, to which it bears some resemblance, by its reticulated disposition, and by the threads of the reticulation corresponding with inflamed lines on the stomach beneath.

Another very common appearance is the presence of a sanguinolent fluid, or even actual blood in the cavity of the stomach. In several of the cases which have come under my own notice, the subject of analysis was a thick, dirty brownish-red fluid, evidently containing a large proportion of blood ; and many other examples of the same nature are on record.† In Laborde's case formerly mentioned actual clots were found among the contents ; in the instance of a woman who died in five days, as related by Zittmann, half a pound of coagulated blood was found in the stomach ;‡ and in another case mentioned by Professor Bernt, the stomach contained no less than three pounds of black ichor mixed with clots of blood.§ A good deal of reliance has been placed on bloody effusion in proof of the administration of arsenic or some other active irritant. It is of some importance, as it appears not to be an effect of that irritation which causes cholera.

Among the appearances observed in the stomach the presence of arsenic may be included, though not properly speaking a morbid appearance. Under the head of the medical evidence of poisoning generally it was stated, that many causes conspire to remove from the stomach during life poisons which have actually caused death. In addition to the illustrative cases there alluded to, I may here also refer to an interesting case communicated to me by Mr. J. H. Stallard, and already noticed for a different purpose [p. 235]. Arsenic in no large quantity had been swallowed in tea, and death took place in four hours only. Here none of the poison could be detected by Marsh's process, either in the contents of the stomach, or in its tissues, or in the liver. — In the instance of arsenic, however, the operation of the causes which tend to remove the poison is prevented by various circumstances, in particular by its insolubility and firm adhesion to the stomach. Hence it happens, that even after long continued vomiting a portion still generally remains behind, either in the contents of the stomach or in its tissues. Sometimes the arsenic exists

* Morbid Anatomy, p. 128.
† Metzger in Schlegel's Opuscula, iv. 23. Pyl's Aufs. und Beob. i. 60. Platner, Quæstiones Medicinæ Forenses, 206.
‡ Medicina Forensis, Cent. v. Cas. 45, quoted by Wibmer.
§ Beiträge zur gerichtlichen Arzneikunde, iv. 221.

dissolved in the contents ; more commonly it is present there in the solid form ; and is then either in loose particles, or enveloped in coagulated mucus,* or in little clots of blood,† or is wrapped up in the more solid parts of the contents.‡ Frequently it adheres to the coats of the stomach, and is then either scattered in the form of fine dust or collected in little knots. The adhering particles are always covered by mucus ; they are often surrounded by redness of the membrane or by effused blood ; and sometimes they are imbedded in little ulcers. — A remarkable appearance which the arsenic sometimes puts on is a brilliant yellowness of its surface, owing to its conversion into the sulphuret. This appearance existed in six cases which have come under my own notice, first in one related in the Edinburgh Medico-Chirurgical Transactions,§ next in the instance of Margaret Warden,‖ again in the case of a young woman whose death gave rise to the trial of John Lovie held at Aberdeen in the Autumn Circuit of 1827, again in a case described by Dr. Wood, which I had an opportunity of examining ;¶ and lastly, in two others which I had occasion to examine in 1842 and 1843. In one of these, the case of Mr. Gilmour, adverted to at p. 265, Drs. Wylie and M'Kinlay, who examined the body in the country, found the inner surface of the stomach thickly sprinkled with small yellow particles, some of which were very bright. In all of these cases oxide was found, as well as the sulphuret of arsenic. In the case related by Dr. Nissen [p. 264], a similar yellow appearance, observed on the surface of the arsenic, was ascribed with justice to the action of sulphuretted hydrogen-water, which had been given as an antidote during life.** In a very important case examined here a few years ago by my colleague Dr. Traill, and which will be noticed more particularly for a different purpose afterwards, this conversion of the oxide into sulphuret had taken place to a great extent [p. 277]. In every instance of the kind yet examined, however, the conversion has been only partial, so that a large proportion of oxide could easily be detected by the usual process.

Care must be taken not hastily to consider as arsenic every white powder which may be found lining the inside of the stomach. Many other white powders may obtain entrance from without; and besides, small, white, shining, pulverulent scales, not unlike finely powdered arsenic, but rarely composed of animal matter, sometimes form naturally on the mucous coat of the stomach and intestines. In a medico-legal report published a few years ago, Professor Orfila has noticed two instances in which these scales were mistaken for arsenic;†† in another published not long after he mentions that he found white particles which crackled when bruised, and appeared brilliant before the microscope, and which nevertheless were not arsenic.‡‡ Buchner

---

* Bernt, Beiträge zur gerichtlichen Arzneikunde, iv. 221.
† Metzger's Materialien für die Staatsarzneikunde, ii. 95. ‡ ii. 284.
§ Edin. Med. and Surg. Journal, xxvii. 457. ‖ Ibid. xxxiii. 66.
¶ Sproegel's Dissert. Exp. xxxi.
** Pfaff and Scheele's Nordisches Archiv. i. 345.
†† Archives Gén. de Med. vii. 1. ‡‡ Ibidem, vii. 285.

too says he is acquainted with an instance where, in a medical in-spection on account of a suspicion of poisoning, the villous coat of the stomach was found lined with a white granular substance which presented the properties of a fat and contained no mineral ad-mixture;* and in the case of Warden I remarked a similar ap-pearance, which, as arsenic was found in the stomach, I was disposed to consider a sprinkling of that poison, until the contrary was ascer-tained by analysis. The present caution, therefore, is not superfluous.

In a few cases the stomach is the only situation where morbid ap-pearances are visible, even though life has been prolonged for so much as two days. This state of matters is well exemplified by a French case of death in forty-three hours, where the stomach pre-sented much redness and extravasated patches, but where the in-testines, the larynx and the contents of the head and chest were in a natural condition.† Such limitation, however, of the diseased ap-pearances are rare.

Redness of the mucous membrane of the intestines is often present when the stomach is much inflamed. Dissolution of the mucous coat is much less frequent in the intestines than in the stomach. Ul-ceration occasionally occurs in lingering cases. In the case of Mitchell, which has been several times alluded to, the inner coat of the duodenum was dark-red, pulpy, thickened, easily separable ; and on a spot as big as a crown-piece, both the inner and the muscular coats were wanting.‡ Perforation of the small intestine was found in a case communicated to me by Mr. Sandell, and detailed at page 277. But as the person survived only eight hours, and had laboured under symptoms of disease in the bowels for some days before taking the arsenic, it is unlikely that this appearance, which has not been observed, to my knowledge, in any other instance, arose from the action of the poison.

The signs of inflammation are seldom distinct in the small intes-tines much lower down than the extremity of the duodenum ; and they do not often affect the colon. But the rectum is sometimes much in-flamed, though the colon, and more particularly the small intestines, are not. Dr. Male mentions, than in man he has found the rectum abraded, ulcerated, and even redder than the stomach itself ;§ and Dr. Baillie also notices two cases in which the lower end of the rec-tum was ulcerated.‖ A common appearance in lingering cases is excoriation of the anus,¶ and it is said that even gangrene has been produced.**

A late writer draws attention to the fact that in the only two fatal cases he had seen the whole colon was contracted to an extraordinary degree ;†† and this state is mentioned in other cases. The appear-

* Repertorium für die Pharmacie, xxiv. 144.
† Archives Gén. de Méd ii. 58.
‡ Edin. Med. and Surg. Journal, xviii. 171.
§ Elements of Juridical Medicine, 76.   ‖ Morbid Anatomy, p. 128.
¶ Case of Mr. Blandy, State Trials, xviii.
** Bachmann's Essay (see p. 259)
†† Houlton in London Med. Gazette, xiv. 712.

ance deserves notice ; but of course whatever empties the colon thoroughly will have the same effect.

The chief appearances in the alimentary canal have now been mentioned. The next quarter in which deceased appearances are to be met with is the cavity of the chest. Here are sometimes seen redness of the pleura, redness and congestion of the lungs, redness of the inner surface of the heart, and redness of the lining membrane of the windpipe.

Redness of the diaphragmatic part of the pleura, or even of the whole of that membrane, has been at times observed ; as one would expect, indeed, from the pectoral symptoms which occasionally prevail during life. Inflammation of the lungs themselves has also been noticed. Dr. Campbell twice found great congestion of blood in the lungs of animals poisoned by the application of arsenic outwardly.* Sproegel likewise found the pleura, pericardium, and whole lungs deeply inflamed in animals.† Dr. Venables found the pleura of a bright crimson colour in some poultry maliciously poisoned with arsenic, — more redness there indeed than in the stomach.‡ Mr. James says that in his experiments on animals he constantly found the lungs much gorged with blood, unless when death occurred quickly ; but that he could see no evidence of the congestion being inflammatory.§ A distinct example of advanced pneumonia in man is related in Pyl's Magazine : the patient died after vomiting and purging incessantly for eight days ; and on dissection the lungs were found "in the highest state of inflammation ; and so congested as to resemble a lump of clotted blood."‖ A distinct case of the same nature is related in Henke's Journal ; this patient had obvious pneumonic symptoms during life ; and in the dead body the lungs were found so gorged, that, on being cut into, nothing could be seen but clotted blood in their cellular structure.¶ In a case formerly adverted to [p. 252] of death from arsenic applied externally for scirrhus, excessive congestion was found in the lungs, " both lungs being completely gorged with blood, and presenting all the characters of pulmonary apoplexy."** In another described by Dr. Booth of Birmingham, where death occurred in seven hours only, the lungs presented sufficient congestion to have completely impeded respiration.††

It has been alleged that the inner surface of the heart has been found red from inflammation. In a case examined judicially at Paris by Orfila, the left cavities of the heart were of a mottled red hue, and in the ventricle were seen many small crimson specks which penetrated into the muscular part of the parietes. The right cavities had a deep reddish-black tint, and the ventricle of that side contained specks like those in the other, but more faint. Orfila adds,

* Diss. Inaug. Edin. 1813, pp. 11 and 12.
† Diss. in Haller's Disp. de Morbis, vi. Exp. xxxvi.
‡ London Med. Gazette, x. 115.
§ Gazette Médicale de Paris, 1839, No. 20.   ‖ Neues Magazin, I. iii. 508.
¶ Zeitschrift für die Staatsarzneikunde, i. 32.
** Annales d'Hyg. Publique, xi. 461.
†† London Med. Gazette, xiv. 62.

that he had previously seen the same appearance in animals.* These observations are not satisfactory. There is no evidence that the observer drew the distinction between the redness of inflammation, and that produced by the dyeing of the membrane with blood after death. The subject was afterwards brought before the Royal Academy of Medicine at Paris by M. Godard, who had also observed the appearance in question in a person killed by arsenic, and who dwelt strongly on it as characteristic of this species of poisoning. It was distinctly proved, however, by many members present that the appearance arises from various other causes.†

The inner membrane of the windpipe is said to be sometimes affected with inflammatory redness. Jaeger found it so in animals ;‡ and the symptoms referrible to the windpipe during life would lead us to expect the same thing in man.

The organs of generation are occasionally affected. The penis in the male and the labia in the female have been found distended and black ; in an interesting case related by Bachmann the external parts of generation (in a female) were surrounded by gangrene ;§ and in a case related in Pyl's collection the inside of the uterus and Fallopian tubes was inflamed.‖ It is probable that signs of inflammation in the internal organs of generation will be found if there have been corresponding symptoms during life. But in truth this part of the pathology of poisoning with arsenic has not been particularly attended to.

To complete this account of the morbid appearances of the mucous membranes, it may be added that the conjunctiva of the eyes frequently presents vascularity and spots of extravasation.¶

It now only remains, under the head of the morbid appearances produced by arsenic, to mention certain alterations that are said to take place in the state of the blood and general condition of the body.

With regard to the state of the blood Sir B. Brodie observes in general terms, that in animals killed by arsenic it is commonly fluid.** Harles, on the authority of Wepfer, Sproegel, and Jaeger, says it is black, semi-gelatinous, and sometimes pultaceous.†† Novati alleges that the blood after death is without exception black and liquid as after cholera, of a blackish-purple tint that colours linen reddish-brown, viscid, opaque, and without any trace of coagulation.‡‡ In a fatal case related by Wildberg the blood was everywhere fluid.§§ This condition, however, is not uniform ; for Dr. Campbell found the blood coagulated in the heart of a rabbit ;‖‖ and Wepfer found it also coagulated in the dog.¶¶

* Archives Gén. i. 147.   † Nouvelle Bibliothêque Médicale, 1829, i. 395.
‡ Jaeger, de Effectibus Arsenici, p. 40.
§ Bachmann's Essay, p. 41, or above, p. 259.
‖ Aufsätze und Beobachtungen, i. 50.
¶ Wibmer. Die Wirkung der Arzneimittel und Gifte, i. 281, 283.
** Phil. Trans. cii. 214.   †† De Arsenici usu in Medicina, 1811, p. 154.
‡‡ Journal de Chimie Médicale, 1839, p. 127.
§§ Practisches Handbuch, iii. 229.
‖‖ De Venenis Mineralibus. Diss. Inaug. Edinburgi, 1813.
¶¶ Historia Circutæ, 288.

It has been stated by some authors in medical jurisprudence that the dead body occasionally exhales an aliaceous odour, resembling that of sublimed arsenic. This is a very questionable statement. The only fact of the kind worth mentioning is one brought forward by Dr. Klanck, as occurring in the course of certain experiments, which will presently be noticed, on the antiseptic virtues of arsenic. Several animals which had been killed with arsenic are said to have exhaled an odour like that of sublimed arsenic from three to eight weeks after death.*

A great discordance of opinion at one time prevailed among authors, as to the influence of arsenic on the putrefactive process in the bodies of those poisoned with it   The vulgar idea, borrowed probably from the ancient classics, that the bodies of those who have been poisoned decay rapidly, was till lately the prevalent doctrine of medical men, and even of medical jurists ; and it was applied to arsenic as well as other poisons.   Even so lately as 1776 we find Gmelin stating in his History of Mineral Poisons, that the bodies of those who have died of arsenic pass rapidly into putrefaction, that the nails and hair often fall off the day after death, and that almost the whole body quickly liquefies into a pulp.†   A similar statement has been made in 1795 by a respectable author, Dr. John Johnstone.‡ It appears that this rapid or premature decay does really occur in some instances.   Thus in a case related by Plattner of death from arsenic administered as a seasoning for mushrooms, the body had a very putrid odour the day after death.§   Loebel also asserts he found by experiments on animals, that after death from arsenic putrefaction took place rapidly, even in very cold weather.‖

In other instances the body probably decays in the usual manner. For example, in Rust's Magazin is related the case of a child who died in six hours of poisoning with arsenic, and in whose body, fourteen days after death, the integuments were found considerably advanced in putrefaction, and the liver and kidneys beginning to soften.¶   In the case of a man who died in two days, and in whose body arsenic was found by MM. Chapeau and Parisel throughout many of the tissues, " putrefaction was so far advanced eight days after death as to render the examination of parts obscure."**   And in the course of some experiments on dogs poisoned with the oxide Dr. Seeman found the usual changes after five months' interment.††

But it has been proved in recent times that in general arsenic has rather the contrary tendency, — that, besides the antiseptic virtues which it has been long known to exert when directly applied in moderate quantity to animal substances, it also possesses the singular

* Augustin's Repertorium.   Neue Entdeckungen betreffend die Kennzeichen der Arsenic-vergiftung, I. i. 30.
† Geschichte der Mineralischen Gifte.   ‡ Essay on Mineral Poisons, 36.
§ Quæst. 'Medicinæ Forenses, 206.
‖ Jaeger, de Effectibus Arsenici, p. 47.
¶ Magazin für die gesammte Heilkunde, xx. 485.
** Bulletins de l'Acad. Roy. de Méd. v. 137.
†† Geiger's Magazin für Pharmacie, xxxii. 301, from Seeman's Dissert. Inaug. Berolini, 1824.

property of enabling the bodies of men and animals poisoned with it both to resist decay unusually long, and to decay in an unusual manner. The observations and inquiries which have been made abroad on this subject were little known any where else than in Germany before the publication of the earlier editions of the present work; but parallel examples have been since met with both in Britain and France; and in this country the importance of the subject is generally appreciated.

The first occasion on which the antiseptic property of arsenic was brought under public notice was about the beginning of the present century, in the course of the trial of the widow of a certain state-councillor, Ursinus of Berlin. Some time before that Dr. Welper, then medical inspector in the Prussian capital, having remarked that the body of a person poisoned with arsenic remained quite fresh for a whole week in summer, he attended carefully to the subject at every opportunity, and invariably, he says, found that the body resisted putrefaction. Not long after making this remark, he was concerned in 1803, by virtue of his office, in the investigations in the case of the widow Ursinus. This lady having been discovered in an attempt to poison her servant, suspicions arose regarding the previous sudden death of three persons in her family, her husband, a young officer who had carried on an amour with her, and an aunt from whom she derived an inheritance. They had all died in mysterious circumstances, and the lady had been their only nurse. Dr. Welper disinterred the bodies of the husband and aunt, which had been buried, the former two years and a half before at Berlin, the latter half a year afterwards at Charlottenberg; and he found them not putrid, but dried up; and specks of an appearance, which is described as being gangrene, but which was probably warty extravasation, were visible in the stomach. Arsenic could not be detected.

He afterwards got Dr. Klanck, his acquaintance, to make some express experiments on animals; and the results were strikingly conformable. In dogs poisoned with arsenic and left for two months sometimes buried in a damp cellar, sometimes exposed to the air of the cellar, the flesh and alimentary canal were red and fresh, as if pickled; and though the place where the carcases were subsequently buried again was flooded for eight months after, the intestines were eventually found entire and red, the fat converted into adipocire, and most of the muscles unaltered, — those only being soft and greasy which were directly acted on by the water. From a set of comparative experiments which were made on dogs killed by blows, or poisoned by corrosive sublimate, or by opium, Klanck found, that, after being buried in the same place, and for the same space of time the whole soft parts of the carcases were converted into a greasy mass. In a subsequent year he repeated his experiments, the bodies, however, being this time left exposed to the air of the cellar. The experiments were commenced in the month of August. In ten days there appeared slight signs of incipient putrefaction; a faint putrid smell was exhaled, and all flies that settled on the carcase died.

This state continued for eight or ten weeks without increasing. After that the soft parts began to grow firmer and drier, and at the same time the putrid odour was succeeded by a smell like that of garlic, which became insupportably strong when the carcases were removed into warm air. The bodies, three years afterwards, still continued dry and undecayed.*

A similar set of facts was again brought before the public between 1809 and 1811, during the criminal proceedings in a case like that of the widow Ursinus, tried first at Bayreuth and afterwards by appeal at Munich. A lady near Bayreuth died of five days' illness, under symptoms of violent general irritation of the alimentary canal. Some months afterwards a variety of circumstances having raised a suspicion that she had been poisoned by her maid, Margaretha Zwanziger, a judicial investigation was set on foot; the consequence of which was, that the same woman came under suspicion of having also previously poisoned another lady and a gentleman with whom she had been successively in service. The bodies of the three people were accordingly disinterred, one of them five months, another six months, and the third fourteen months after death. In all of them the external parts were not properly speaking putrid, but hard, cheesy, or adipocirous; in the last two the stomach and intestines were so entire as to allow of their being tied, taken out, cut up, and handled; and in one a sloughy spot was found in the region of the pylorus. Arsenic was detected in two of the bodies by Rose's process of analysis.†

The next example to the same effect which will be mentioned is perhaps the most satisfactory of all, because it was the result of an express experiment on the human subject. Dr. Kelch of Königsberg buried the internal organs of a man who had died of arsenic, and whose body had remained without burial till the external parts had begun to decay; and on examining the stomach and intestines five months after, he found that the hamper in which they were contained was very rotten; but that " they had a peculiar smell, quite different from that of putrid bowels, were not yet acted on by putrefaction, but as fresh as when first taken from the body, and might have served to make preparations. They had lost nothing of their colour, glimmer, or firmness. The inflamed spots on the stomach had not disappeared, and the small intestines also showed in some places the inflammatory redness unaltered."‡

In a recent French case, although the degree of preservation was less remarkable, the other circumstances are so striking as to render it well worthy of notice. In this instance the body was disinterred after having been seven years in the ground, in a high situation and

* For an excellent analysis of the case of Ursinus and the experiments of Klanck, see Augustin — Neue Entdeckungen betreffend die Kennzeichen der Arsenic-vergiftung und Berichtigung älterer Angaben über diesen Gegenstand, — in Augustin's Repertorium, I. i. 36.

† Bachmann, Einige auserlesene gerichtlich-medizinische abhanlungen, von Schmidt, Bachmann, und Küttlinger. Nürnberg, 1813.

‡ Hufeland's Journal, xix. iv. 11, and xxii. i. 166.

sandy soil. The coffin, which was of oak, had become dry and brittle, and no moisture appeared on the inside. The body was entire : the head, trunk, and limbs retained their situation; but the organs of the chest and belly were converted into a brown soft mass of the consistence of plaster, which lay on each side of the spine. In this mass MM. Ozanam and Idt, the medical inspectors, succeeded in discovering by chemical analysis a considerable quantity of arsenic.[*]

M. Ollivier describes another French case, where the body had been burried for three years, and was found so completely dried up that the trunk weighed only two pounds. The integuments were entire, dark-brown, and of a faint odour like decayed wood. The organs of the chest and belly were confounded together in a foliaceous membranous mass, in which the liver only could be distinguished, but in an exceedingly shrivelled state. Arsenic was detected in the membranous matter by MM. Barruel and Henri. The preservative power of the arsenic was promoted in this case by the sandy nature of the soil.[†]

In the case of the girl Warden, which has been several times alluded to, the internal organs were also preserved somewhat in the same manner as in the German cases. The body had been buried three weeks ; yet the mucous coat of the stomach and intestines, except on its mere surface, was very firm, and all the morbid appearances were consequently quite distinct. Nay, three weeks after disinterment, except that the vascularity had disappeared, the membranes and the appearances in them remained in the same state.[‡] A similar case has been recorded by Metzger. It is that of an old man who died of six hours' illness, and in whose stomach three drachms of arsenic were found. The body had been kept ten days in February before burial, and was disinterred eight days after that ; yet there was not the slightest sign of putrefaction any where.[§] A parallel case was described by myself in the Edinburgh Medico-Chirurgical Transactions ;[||] and I have met with three others of the same kind since.

In a very important case, that of Mrs. Smith, which was made the subject of investigation at Bristol in December, 1834, the body was also found in a state of great preservation, modified, however, by adipocirous decomposition, owing to the presence of water in the coffin. The body had been fourteen months interred. The internal parts, especially of the head and neck, were here and there decayed somewhat or converted into adipocire, the muscles and internal organs entire, though more or less shrivelled, the alimentary tube remarkably preserved, " every part being almost as distinct as if the inspection had been made at a very short period after death,"

* Archives Gén de Med. xxi. 615, or Revue Médicale, 1830, i. 165.
† Annales d'Hygiène Publique, 1837, xviii. 466 ; and Journal de Pharmacie, 1837, 386.
‡ Edin. Med. and Surg. Journal, xxvii. 457.
§ De veneficio caute dijudicando, in Schlegel's Opuscula, iv. 23.
|| Edin. Med. Chir. Trans. ii. 284.

" the mucous membrane sufficiently tenacious to be lifted by the forceps in as large flakes as usual ;" and the reporters, Drs. Riley and Symonds, Messrs. Herapath and Kelson, seem to have had no difficulty in ascertaining the absence of vascularity, extravasation, or even abrasion of the inner membrane. Artificial orpiment, the preparation proved to have been given [see p. 225], was found in the stomach by Mr. Herapath, and the quantity appeared to be about half a drachm.*

A similar instance, very remarkable in all its circumstances, was investigated here in 1834 by my colleague Dr. Traill to whom I am indebted for the particulars. The master of a foreign vessel died in about twenty-four hours, apparently of malignant cholera, at a small port in the neighbourhood of Edinburgh : and the body was forth-with buried. A suspicion, however, having arisen in his native country that he had been poisoned by his mate, an inquiry was in-stituted at the request of the foreign government ; and the body was disinterred five months after death. The face and neck was swollen, black, and decayed ; but the rest of the body was quite free of the usual signs of putrefaction. The skin was white and firm, the muscles fresh, the lungs crepitating, the liver and spleen much shri-velled, the stomach and intestines entire throughout their whole tissues, and capable of being handled freely without injury. On the mucous coat of the stomach several dark patches of extravasa-tion were found, likewise several spots and large patches which presented on their surface a firmly adhering bright-yellow crust ; and the contents of the stomach consisted of a considerable quan-tity of yellow sandy matter of the consistence of paste. The con-tents and adhering crusts were found to consist chiefly of oxide of arsenic partially converted into sulphuret. In this instance, as in that last described, the coffin contained water, owing to its having laid in a sandy soil resting on clay.

An important case of the same nature was communicated to me in 1843 by Mr. Sandell of Potton, Bedfordshire, and afterwards pub-lished by Mr. Hedly of Bedford. A man Dazley at Wrestlingford, affected with symptoms of gastro-enteric irritation for five or six days, was seized with sickness, vomiting, heat and constriction in the throat, and great weakness, about an hour after getting a white powder from his wife ; and in eight hours he expired, without any suspicion of unfair usage arising at the time. Suspicions, however, being entertained afterwards, the body which had not been exa-mined at first, was disinterred in five months, during the month of March. The countenance was so entire as to be recognisable. Adi-pocire had been formed in many places. The stomach and intes-tines were " in a most perfect state of preservation," as if death had taken place only a few days previously. The stomach pre-sented yellow patches on its outer and inner surface, — was gener-ally red over its villous coat, which had also been abraded near the

* Dr. Symonds's Account of the Examination, &c., Trans. of Provincial Med. and Surg· Association, iii. 432.

cardiac end, — and, together with the small intestines, was lined with white powder and contained more of it enveloped in much red mucus. This powder proved to be arsenic. About the middle of the small intestines a small ulcerated opening was found, through which some arsenic had escaped.*

The following cases which have come under my own notice during the last five years are also worthy of observation. In a case submitted to me on the part of the crown in 1841, which has been adverted to above for another purpose [p. 265], the body after being three months interred was found with the head and face decayed and putrid; but the muscular substance was little changed; and the inspectors were particularly struck with the state of preservation of the body, and also with the very distinct state of inflammation seen over almost the whole external and internal surfaces of the alimentary canal," — a description, the accuracy of which I had afterwards an opportunity of verifying. In the case of Mr. Gilmour (p. 265), whose body had been buried 101 days, the external parts were more decayed; but the alimentary canal appeared equally entire both to the original inspectors, Drs. M'Kinlay and Wylie, and likewise to myself three weeks later. But the following instance, in which I was consulted in 1839, is the most remarkable one of the kind that has hitherto occurred to me; because the observations then made were the result of an express experiment in a medico-legal investigation. The history of this case, which arose from small doses of arsenic frequently administered, has been already given above in some detail [p. 250]. Arsenic not having been detected in the contents or tissues of the stomach, and the trial of the individual suspected of giving the poison being necessarily postponed for some months, I recommended that a third examination of the body, — for it had been twice disinterred for inspection within ten days after death, — should be made at as distant an interval as possible, in order to ascertain whether it underwent preservation from decay. It was accordingly disinterred again, five months after death. It had an ammoniacal, but not a putrid odour. The skin was here and there covered with a thin sebaceous matter, at one or two places stripped of the epidermis, but for the most part natural in appearance, firm, and elastic. The nails were loose. The muscles of the head and near the tops of the scapulæ were adipocirous, on the chest and abdomen obscurely fibrous in texture and hardened, but elsewhere unaltered, and " in the lower extremities so perfect that they might have been used for an anatomical demonstration." The liver and lungs were also in a state of good preservation, and the latter crepitated when cut. The other viscera had been removed at the previous examinations.

It may be added that the experiments of Klanck on dogs adverted to above have been more recently repeated by Hünefeld on rabbits and mice, with precisely the same results. The animals were sometimes left in the air, at other times buried, and generally in a moist place. In every instance putrefaction made more or less progress

* Lancet, 1843-44, ii. 801.

at first; but in a few days a peculiar garlicky odour arose, from which time the progress of decay seemed to be arrested; and the bodies underwent a process of hardening and desiccation which completely preserved them.*

On considering attentively the illustrations now given, the toxicologist can hardly doubt that in some cases arsenic has appeared both to retard and to modify putrefaction in the bodies of persons poisoned with it.

Assuming arsenic to have been the cause of the preservation of the bodies, it becomes a point of consequence to account for its effect, and more particularly to reconcile that effect with what has certainly been noticed in other cases of poisoning with the same substance, namely, ordinary rapidity of decay, if not actually an increased tendency to putrefaction.

At the outset of this part of the inquiry some light may be thrown upon it by separating the local from the general operation of arsenic.

Arsenic is a good preservative of animal textures when it is directly applied to them in sufficient quantity. This is well known to stuffers of birds and beasts, was experimentally ascertained by Guyton Morveau,† and has come also under my observation.‡ It is now likewise known to be an excellent substance for preserving bodies, when injected in the form of solution into the blood-vessels.

Hence, if in a case of poisoning the arsenic be not discharged by vomiting, and the patient die soon, it will act as an antiseptic on the stomach at least, perhaps on the intestines also; while the rest of the body may decay in the usual manner. This is very well shown in a case examined by Dr. Borges, medical inspector at Minden, fourteen weeks after death. The stomach and intestines were firm, of a grayish-white colour, and contained crumbs of bread, while all the other organs in the belly were pulpy, and the external parts adipocirous.§ It is also equally well exemplified in a case that happened at Chemnitz so early as 1726, and which was examined five weeks after burial. The skin was every where very putrid, but the stomach and intestines were perfectly fresh.‖ In the case of Warden the appearances were precisely the same. Three weeks after burial the Dundee inspectors found the external parts much decayed, yet three weeks later the stomach and intestines were found by myself in a state of almost perfect preservation. A striking experiment performed by Dr. Borges on a rabbit will likewise illustrate clearly the fact now under consideration. The rabbit was killed in less than a day with ten grains of arsenic, and its body was buried for thirteen months in a moist place under the eaves of a house. At the end of this period it was found, that "the skin, muscles, cellular tissue, ligaments and all the viscera, except the alimentary canal, had

* Dissertatio de vera Chemiæ Organicæ notione, additis experimentis de vi Arsenici in corpore organico mortuo. 1822. Quoted fully by Wibmer, die Wirkung der Arzneimittel und Gifte, i. 312.

† Elemens de Chymie, ii. 343.   ‡ See this work, First Ed. 1829, p. 258.
§ Kopp's Jahrbuch, ii. 226.
‖ Bernt's Beiträge zur gerichtlichen Arzneikunde, iv. 219.

disappeared, without leaving a trace ; but the alimentary canal from the throat to the anus, along with the hair and the bare bones, was quite entire.*

In all of these cases arsenic was found in the body. In the rabbit experimented on by Dr. Borges, above five grains of arsenic were separated in the form of a metallic sublimate.

But, on the contrary, if the arsenic is all or nearly all discharged by vomiting, not only the body generally, but likewise even the stomach and intestines, may follow the usual course of decay. Accordingly, in the case of the child formerly quoted [273], where the body putrified in the usual manner, only four grains and a half of arsenic had been taken ; and as it was swallowed in a state of solution and caused violent vomiting, it must have been almost all ejected. Nay, in such circumstances, the alimentary canal, in consequence of its unnatural supply of moisture and incipient disorganization, may decay somewhat faster than other parts. Thus Dr. Murray observed in the case of a man formerly mentioned (264), who lived under violent gastric symptoms for seven days, and vomited much, that the stomach, which was removed for more minute examination, decayed so rapidly that in twenty-four hours an examination was impracticable, while the body in general rather resisted putrefaction.†

The preceding statements on the differences in the state of preservation of the body after poisoning with arsenic are not then incapable of some explanation. Nevertheless, it must be granted that the reasons assigned will not account for all the apparent cases of the preservative powers of arsenic. And especially they will not explain how the whole body has sometimes resisted decay altogether, and become as it were mummified. It is impossible to ascribe this preservation to the anstiseptic power of the arsenic diffused throughout the body in the blood ; the quantity there being extremely small. Consequently if the preservation of the bodies is not occasioned by some accidental collateral cause (a mode of accounting for the phenomena which seems inadmissible), this property of arsenic must depend on its causing, by some operation on the living body, a different disposition and affinity among the ultimate elements of organized matter, and so altering the operation of physical laws on it. There appears no sound reason for rejecting this supposition, especially as it is necessary to admit an analogous change of affinities as the only mode of accounting for a still more incomprehensible violation of the ordinary laws of nature, — the spontaneous combustion, or preternatural combustibility, of the human body.

The following judicious observations by Harles on this subject are worthy of attention : — " In regard," says he, " to this singular property of arsenic, now no longer doubtful, it should be remembered that certain circumstances will limit or impair it, while others will favour or increase it ; — circumstances, for example, connected with

* Ueber eine Vergiftung durch weissen Arsenic — Rust's Magazin für die gesammte Heilkunde, v. 61.
† Edin. Med. and Surg. Journal, xviii. 172.

the soil of the burying-ground, or the air of the vaults where the bodies are deposited. Different soils and different conditions of the air will materially affect the decomposition of all bodies indiscriminately, and will therefore affect likewise the anaseptic properties of arsenic. For it would be absurd to ascribe to arsenic the power of preventing putrefaction in all circumstances whatsoever, — a power which those who make use of it for preserving skins know very well it does not possess, and a power possessed by no antiseptic whatever, not even by alcohol."*

An important consequence of the preservative tendency of arsenic is, that in many instances the body in this kind of poisoning may be found long after death in so perfect a state as to admit of an accurate medico-legal inspection and a successful chemical analysis. In one of his cases Dr. Bachmann detected arsenic in the stomach fourteen months after interment; Dr. Borges had no difficulty in detecting it in an animal after thirteen months; Mr. Herapath discovered it after fourteen months in the human body; M. Henry detected it after three years and a half, and obtained no less than seven grains of metallic arsenic from the shrivelled viscera;† and MM. Ozanam and Idt found it after the long interval of seven years. — The late experiments of Orfila and Lesueur confirm the fact that arsenic may remain long in contact with decaying animal matter, and yet continue in such a state as to be easily detected.‡ It might be supposed that the poison would pass off partly in the gaseous state by being converted into arseniuretted-hydrogen, partly in the liquid state by becoming arsenite of ammonia, a very soluble compound. But the fact nevertheless is, that, notwithstanding these reasons for its disappearance, it may be detected after the lapse of several years.

Under the head of the diseased appearances left by arsenic in the dead body, every change of structure has now been described which has been mentioned by authors and supported by trustworthy statements. Another set of appearances may still be noticed; but they are here separated from the rest, because the author who first notices them has not been supported in the statement by any special observations of his own, or by an adequate number of facts observed by others. In an elaborate essay on a case of poisoning by Professor Seiler of Wittemberg, it is said in general terms that arsenic may cause gorging of the vessels of the brain, effusion of serum into the ventricles, inflammation of the brain, and even extravasation of blood.§ Turgescence of vessels is mentioned in several published cases, and I have myself met with it. But it is seldom so considerable as to attract attention. In the following instance, however, which has been related by Dr. Hofer of Biberach the evidence of cerebral congestion was unequivocal. A man addicted to intoxication, but enjoying good health otherwise, was attacked after supper with

* De usu Arsenici, 164.   † Journal de Pharmacie, 1837, p. 386.
† Revue Médicale, 1828, ii. 470.
§ Knape und Hecker's Kritische Jahrbücher, ii. 76.
27

sickness, vomiting, and pain in the belly.   On going to bed he fell
soon quiet ; and six hours after he took ill, he was found dead.
Arsenic was detected in the stomach, and in what he vomited ; and
considerable redness was seen on the villous coat of the stomach.
But the most remarkable appearances were gorging of the cerebral
vessels, adhesion of the dura mater to the membranes beneath, and
the effusion of eight ounces of serosity into the lateral ventricles.*
The only instance I am acquainted with to justify the opinion that
extravasation of blood into the brain may occur from poisoning with
arsenic, is the remarkable case of apparent death from eating poultry
poisoned with arsenic, which was communicated to me by Mr. Jamieson of Aberdeen.   The individual, after suffering under the usual
primary symptoms, became apoplectic after a fit of sneezing, and
died three days afterwards ; and in the dead body, besides other signs
of disease in the brain, a recent clot of blood was found in the right
anterior lobe. (See p. 69.)

It is quite unnecessary to notice lividity of the skin among the signs
of poisoning with arsenic, except for the mere purpose of reminding
the medical jurist that, although it has been sometimes much relied
on as a sign of death from arsenic, it is not of the slightest importance as a sign either of that or of any other kind of poisoning.
(See p. 51.)

The action of arsenic on the alimentary canal after death will now
require a few remarks ; the purpose of which is to prepare the medical
inspector for investigating attempts to impute the crime of poisoning
to innocent persons, by introducing arsenic into the dead body.   Such
attempts, according to Orfila, have been made ; but I am not acquainted with any actual instance.

The action of arsenic on dead intestine has been fully examined
by the last mentioned author.   If it is introduced into the anus immediately after death, and allowed to remain there twenty-four hours,
the mucous membrane in contact with it becomes of a lively red
colour, with darker interspersed patches as if from extravasation.
The other coats are natural; and so is the mucous membrane itself
wherever the poison does not actually touch it.   Consequently the
margin of the coloration is abrupt and well-defined.   When the arsenic is not introduced till twenty-four hours after death, the part to
which it is actually applied presents dark patches, while the rest of
the membrane is quite healthy.†

The appearance of redness in the former case is probably the result
of lingering vitality.   The cause of the dark appearance in the latter
it is not easy to comprehend.

When arsenic has been applied during life, the redness, if it has
had time to begin at all, extends to some distance from the points
with which the poison has been in contact, and passes by degrees
into the healthy colour of the surrounding membrane.

On reviewing what has been said of the pathological appearances

* Henke's Zeitschrift für die Staatsarzneikunde, xxxix. 176.
† Toxicologie Générale, ii.

caused by arsenic, it must appear that the medical jurist can never be supplied from this source alone with satisfactory evidence of the cause of death.   But in some circumstances the evidence may amount to a strong probability of one variety or another of irritant poisoning. Mere redness, conjoined or not with softening of the mucous membrane, may justify suspicion only.   But if there should be found in the body of a person who has died of a few days' illness, redness, black warty extravasation, and circumscribed ulcers of the villous coat of the stomach, — effusion of blood or bloody clots among the contents of that organ, — also redness of the intestines, more especially redness and ulceration of the colon and rectum, — and redness of the pharynx, or of this along with the gullet, — the proof of poisoning with some irritant will amount to a strong presumption.   At least it is difficult to mention any natural disease which could produce in so short a time such a conjunction of appearances as this ; which arsenic and other analogous poisons sometimes occasion.

Section IV. — *On the Treatment of Poisoning with Arsenic.*

It was formerly proved that arsenic acts in all its forms of chemical combination, which have been hitherto tried, and nearly in the ratio of their solubility.   This general fact is conformable with the law laid down as to the influence of chemical changes on the energy of poisons which enter the blood [p. 37].   Hence every supposed chemical antidote must be useless, which does not render the arsenic insoluble not only in water, but likewise in the contents and secretions of the stomach.

The antidotes chiefly trusted to until recent times, such as vinegar, sugar, butter and other oily substances, lime-water, bitter decoctions, and the like, have now justly fallen into disuse.   The liver of sulphur or sulphuret of potassium, which maintained its character for some time longer on account of its chemical action with oxide of arsenic in solution, is not more efficacious.   The experiments of Renault on the counterpoisons for arsenic, confirmed by the subsequent researches of Orfila, have proved that the arsenical sulphuret formed by solutions of the liver of sulphur is scarcely less active than the oxide itself.*

It appears that fine impalpable powders, though inert as physiological agents, and destitute of any true chemical action with oxide of arsenic, may nevertheless prove useful in certain limited circumstances. Thus Mr. Hume of London and others have apparently found some advantage in the administration of large doses of magnesia.†   If this substance be of any use at all, which is doubtful, it can act only by covering the arsenical particles with its fine insoluble powder, and so preventing them from coming in contact with the surface of the stomach ; for in its state of magnesia it has no chemical action with oxide

* Sur les Contrepoisons de l'Arsénic, pp. 33, 35.
† London Med. and Phys. Journal, xlvi. 466, 545.   Mr. Edwards, Ibidem, xlix. 117. Mr. Buchanan, London Med. Repository, xix. 288.

of arsenic.   Another remedy of the same nature is charcoal powder, which was proposed in 1813 with much confidence by M. Bertrand.* That it has some efficacy when swallowed along with the poison seems to admit of no doubt ; for the proposer of it himself swallowed five grains of arsenic in one dose along with charcoal in a state of emulsion, and sustained little inconvenience of any kind.   In all probability it acts merely by enveloping the particles of arsenic.   But it may possibly be also of service, if recently exposed to heat, by the superficial attraction it exerts over substances in solution ; through means of which property it will remove many soluble substances from a fluid, and render them insoluble.   Charcoal, however, has been proved to be destitute of all efficacy when not administered till after the arsenic is swallowed.   The one must be given along with the other, otherwise it is useless.†

For some time past the formation of an insoluble arsenite has been aimed at by most experimentalists who have endeavoured to discover an antidote for arsenic.   But in general the arsenites, though very insoluble in water, are sufficiently so in weak acids or in organic fluids, so that they are soluble enough in the juices of the stomach to enter the blood in such quantity as to prove fatal.   The only exception now admitted to exist is the arsenite produced when a solution of oxide of arsenic is brought in contact with the hydrated sesquioxide of iron.   The compound thus formed is held to be insoluble in the secretions of the stomach ; and consequently the hydrated sesquioxide of iron is usually regarded as a true antidote.

The substance, the Ferrugo of the Edinburgh Pharmacopœia, — a compound which differs little from the older preparation, the rust of iron, when not deprived of its combined water, — was announced in 1834 by Drs. Bunsen and Berthold as an effectual remedy even when given some time after the arsenic is swallowed.‡   Their experiments were repeated with variable success.   Similar results were obtained by MM. Soubeiran and Miquel, as well as MM. Orfila and Lesueur, in some experiments on dogs, and by M. Boullay on the horse.§ The last experimentalist found that the effects of a dose adequate to occasion death are almost entirely prevented in the horse by giving the oxide of iron either immediately after the poison, or within four hours.   Results of the same nature were obtained in this country by Mr. Donald Mackenzie.∥   Others, however, such as Mr. Brett¶ and Mr. Orton,** have failed to observe any antidotal virtues, and even deny that the sesquioxide of iron can remove oxide of arsenic from a state of solution.   But in 1840 the causes of these discrepant statements were explained by Dr. Douglas Maclagan,†† who found,

* Journal Gén. de Médecine, 1813 and 1815, p. 363.
† Toxicologie Gén. i. 429.
‡ Das Eisenoxydhydrat, ein Gegengift der Arsenigen saüre, Göttingen, 1834.
§ Annales d'Hygiène Publique. xiv. 134.
∥ Probationary Essay, Edin. Roy. Coll. of Surgeons, 1839.
¶ London Medical Gazette, xv. 220.
** Lancet, 1834-35, p. 232.
†† Edinburgh Medical and Surgical Journal, liv. 108.

in corroboration of the remarks of Drs. Bunsen and Berthold, as well as various French authorities, that the oxide must be given in large quantity, and that the failures of some were owing to the quantity used having been too small. He ascertained, that, in order to remove one part of arsenic from a state of solution, twelve parts of oxide of iron in the moist state are necessary, and sixty parts if it be previously dried ; that the arsenic so appropriated is with difficulty removed from the insoluble matter even by boiling ; and that, as the discoverers of this antidote first stated, the preparation made by precipitating the sesquioxide of iron by means of ammonia, is a more active form than any other. As the oxide prepared in this way always contains ammonia, and the proportion necessary for removing the arsenic is far greater than what is required to constitute a simple arsenite of iron, it is reasonable to infer that the ammonia forms a part of the insoluble compound actually produced. At all events the action of the antidote would appear to be chemical, and not mechanical, as has been thought by many, and as was stated to be probable in the last edition of this work. In confirmation of these views, and as a fact worthy of farther investigation on its own account, it is worthy of notice, that, according to Dr. Duflos, the acetate of sesquioxide of iron answers equally well as an antidote with the sesquioxide itself. It precipitates both arsenious and arsenic acid from every state of solution, and always the more quickly the more the solution is diluted ; and the co-existence of acetic acid is no obstacle to this action taking place.* — More recently Professor Orfila has called in question the absolute efficacy generally ascribed to the sesquioxide of iron. He alleges that the arsenical compound formed, though insoluble in water, is soluble to some extent in the gastric juices, and is consequently a poison to animals ; that the sesquioxide is therefore only partial in its operation as a remedy ; but yet that the influence of the animal fluids in the stomach in counteracting it may be overcome by giving it in excess, so that, as fast as the compound is dissolved, it is thrown down again.†

The cases of the successful employment of this antidote in the human subject, which have appeared in the periodical press during the last eight years, are so numerous, that its utility can scarcely be called in question, whatsoever may be its precise mode of action. The hydrated sesquioxide of iron ought therefore to be kept in readiness in every druggist's establishment; for it cannot be prepared when wanted without great loss of time. The quickest way to make it is to dissolve the common anhydrous sesquioxide, formerly miscalled carbonate of iron, in diluted sulphuric acid aided with a gentle heat ; to decompose the hot solution with an excess of strong ammonia; to filter off the fluid by means of a cloth filter and wash the precipitate well with warm water ; and then to let it drain thoroughly and to squeeze out more of the water by expression. It should be kept in this state, and not allowed to dry.

* Buchner's Repertorium für die Pharmacie, lxvi. 126.
† Journal de Chimie Médicale, 1841, p. 240.

In regard to all antidotes for arsenic, it must be observed, that they can seldom be otherwise employed than in unfavourable circumstances. If, as most generally happens, the poison has been taken some time before medical aid is obtained, its powder is diffused over the surface of the stomach, adheres with tenacity to the villous coat, and excites the secretion of tough mucus, through which it is with difficulty reached by any antidote possessing a chemical action with it. In all cases, therefore, it is advisable to promote vomiting occasionally, if not already full and free, so as to aid the stomach in clearing itself of the secreted mucus.

If the existence of a chemical antidote for arsenic be doubtful, much less is there any one known of that rarer denomination which operates by exciting in the system a action contrary to that established by the poison.

A good deal, however, may be done by general medical treatment to improve the chance of recovery. If vomiting should be delayed, as often happens, for half an hour or more, advantage ought to be taken of the opportunity to administer an emetic of the sulphate of zinc, with the view of withdrawing the powder in mass before it is diffused over the stomach ; and for the same purpose milk should be drunk both before and after vomiting has begun, as it appears to be the best substance for enveloping the powder, and so procuring its discharge. The patient should never be allowed to exhaust his strength in retching without a little milk or other fluid in his stomach to act on. At the same time, there is probably some justice in the opinion expressed by a late writer on this subject, that large draughts of diluents are injurious ; and that, unless the stomach is allowed to contract fully and frequently on itself, it cannot discharge from its surface the mucous secretion, in which the powder of arsenic is in general closely enveloped.* The stomach-pump, although it has been applied to cases of poisoning with arsenic, does not possess any advantage whatever over emetics or the natural efforts of nature, and is less effectual in expelling the mucus which envelopes the poison. Even emetics are unnecessary, when full vomiting is caused by the poison itself. If milk in sufficient quantity cannot be procured, strong farinaceous decoctions will probably prove useful.

Supposing the poison to have been removed from the stomach, or that the patient has been put on the course which appears best fitted to accomplish that end, — two objects remain to be accomplished, namely, to allay the inflammation of the alimentary canal, and to support the system under that extraordinary depression which it undergoes in the generality of cases. Were it not for the latter of these objects, the treatment would be both obvious and frequently successful. But it is highly probable that the active remedies, to which the physician trusts in internal inflammations generally, and which are urgently called for by the inflammation caused by arsenic, cannot be enforced with the requisite vigour, on account of the remote depressing effects also produced by this poison on the body.

* Mr. Kerr in Edin. Med. and Surg. Journal, xxxvi. 97.

Nevertheless, it is certain that in a few even very aggravated cases the purest and most vigorous antiphlogistic treatment has been resorted to with success. Dr. Roget's patient, whose case was formerly referred to for another purpose, seems to have been saved by venesection; and at all events, the amelioration effected was unequivocal. In the Medical Repository there is another good example of the beneficial effects of blood-letting carried even to a greater extent than in Roget's case;[*] and in the Medical and Physical Journal[†] a third instance will be found, which after the first twenty-four hours assumed the form of pure gastritis, and was treated as such with success. Blood-letting ought not to be practised till the poison is nearly all' discharged from the stomach, because it promotes absorption by causing emptiness of the blood-vessels.

Orfila has lately advocated the use of blood-letting, on the ground that it tends to remove from the system a portion of the poison which circulates with the blood, and is the main source of danger to life. He has endeavoured to show by experiments on animals, that doses adequate to cause death may be given without this result flowing, if depletion be vigorously enforced along with other treatment. And he has related a case of recovery in the human subject under unfavourable circumstances, where blood-letting was practised five times, and on every occasion with marked relief.[‡]

It is not probable that any material advantage will be derived' from topical blood-letting, at least in the early stage, because if depletion is to be of use at all, it must be carried at once to a far greater extent than it is possible to attain by local evacuants. Blisters on the abdomen will prove useful auxiliaries in the advanced stage.

While many have advocated the employment of blood-letting and' other antiphlogistics, and have used them with apparent advantage, Rasori was of opinion, and more recently Giacomini has strenuously maintained that the proper treatment in all cases of arsenical poisoning is the purely stimulant method. The remedy recommended by the latter is a mixture of eight ounces of beef-tea and two ounces of wine. These notions are evidently dictated by the prevailing pathological delusions of the Italian school. Although upheld in some measure by a Report of the Parisian Academy of Medicine upon some experiments by M. Rognetta on this subject,[§] Professor Orfila subsequently proved, that the practice recommended is utterly useless, if not even hurtful.[||] At the same time no one who has ever seen a case of poisoning by arsenic can doubt that it is often necessary to counteract the overwhelming languor of the circulation by the moderate use of stimulants.

Opium in repeated doses will prove useful, when the poison has been removed, and the inflammation subdued by blood-letting. And I conceive that to the form of gastritis, caused by arsenic, may be:

[*] London Med. Repository, ix. 456.
[†] Med. and Phys. Journal, xxix.
[‡] Journal de Chimie Médicale, 1839, p. 189.
[§] Bulletins de l'Acad. Roy. de Méd. iii. 1124. [||] Ibidem, 1840, vi. 135.

applied a method of treatment by anodynes, which has been success-fully used in acute inflammation generally, — the free administration of opium immediately after copious depletion. For the safe em-ployment of this method, however, it is essential that the arsenic be completely removed from the stomach and intestines. And from the results of many cases there must always be great reason to apprehend, that, before the treatment can be with propriety resorted to, the pa-tient's strength will be exhausted.

The harassing fits of vomiting which often continue long after the poison has been discharged from the stomach are best removed by opium in the form of clyster, or rubbed over the inside of the rectum in the form of ointment with the finger.

The use of laxatives is particularly required in all cases in which there is tenesmus instead of diarrhœa, or where, in the latter stages, diarrhœa is succeeded by constipation ; and castor oil is the laxative generally preferred. While diarrhœa is present, and the evacuations are profuse or the intestines have been thoroughly emptied, laxatives are unnecessary or even hurtful ; but emollient clysters are advisable, and opium in the form of enema or suppository. In short, so far as regards the intestinal affection, the treatment of the acute stage of dysentery is to be enforced.

Professor Orfila lays great stress on the employment of diuretics after the stomach has been cleared out, and founds this practice on his observations which show that arsenic is absorbed into the blood, and gradually discharged by the secretions, especially the urine. Experience seems to confirm theory. Dogs, after receiving a small dose, adequate to occasion death, recovered under the active ad-ministration of diuretics. Having ascertained that this animal was constantly killed in a period varying from thirty to forty-eight hours by two grains applied to a wound, provided no remedies were em-ployed, he tried the diuretic method with six which had been thus poisoned ; and all of them recovered.* The diuretic he recommends is a mixture of ten pounds of water, five of white [French] wine, a bottle of Selzer water, and three ounces of nitre ; the dose of which is two wine-glassfuls frequently.† This method has been followed with success in the human subject. M. Augouard relates a case where 230 grains produced in half an hour all the usual symptoms, which he immediately proceeded to treat by administering a grain and a half of tartar-emetic, to excite full vomiting. Having accom-plished this object, he gave frequent doses of decoction of mallow " strongly salpetred," which in seven hours excited so profuse a diuresis that in the ensuing ten hours no less than eighteen imperial pints was discharged. At the close of this period a material amend-ment took place, and recovery was complete in fifteen days.‡ It may be observed, however, that it is sometimes impossible to excite diuresis.§

* Bulletins de l'Académie Roy. de Médecine, 1840, vi. 136.
† Journal de Chimie Médicale, 1840, p. 711.
‡ Ibidem, 1843, p. 265.   § Ibidem, 1841, p. 258.

Little need be said of the practice to be pursued in the advanced stages of poisoning with arsenic, when convalescence has begun. The principal object is to support the system by mild nourishment, avoiding at the same time stimulant diet of every kind, but especially spirituous and vinous liquors. Whatever may be the difference of results obtained with the antiphlogistic mode of cure, the opposite system has been invariably detrimental in the advanced stage.

The treatment of the nervous and dyspeptic affections, which may supervene after the symptoms of local inflammation have ceased, is not a fit object of review in this work, as it would lead to great details.

CHAPTER XIV.

OF POISONING WITH MERCURY.

THE next genus of the metallic poisons includes the preparations of mercury. Some of these are hardly less important than the arsenical compounds. They act with equal energy, produce the same violent symptoms, and cause death with the same rapidity. They have therefore been often given with a criminal intent; and have thus become the subject of inquiry upon trials. In another respect, too, they claim the regard of the medical jurist: their effects on the body, when insidiously introduced in the practice of the arts in which mercury is used, form a branch of that department of medical police, which treats of the influence of trades on the health.

SECTION I. — *Of the Chemical History and Tests for the preparations of Mercury.*

Mercury is a fluid metal, exceedingly brilliant, of a silver-white colour, and of the specific gravity 13·568.

When heated to about 660° F. it sublimes, and on cooling it condenses unchanged. If this experiment is made in a small glass tube, the metal forms a white ring of brilliant globules, which may be made to coalesce into a single large one. In this way its physical properties may be recognised, though the quantity is exceedingly minute.

Two oxides of this metal, a protoxide and peroxide, exist in combination with acids. A bluish-gray or grayish-black protoxide is separated from the salts of the protoxide by the fixed alkalis. The peroxide has an orange-red colour, and is the common red precipitate of the apothecary. Mercury unites with sulphur in two proportions. The protosulphuret, which is black, is formed from the salts of the protoxide by the action of sulphuretted-hydrogen: the bisulphuret is the well known pigment, cinnabar or vermilion. Mercury likewise unites with chlorine in two proportions, forming an insoluble protochloride and a soluble bichloride, the former calomel, the latter corrosive sublimate. It likewise unites with cyanogen. Mercury also unites in the state of protoxide and peroxide with the acids. Several compound salts are known to the chemist, but few occur in commerce or the arts.

Among the compounds resulting from the action of this metal with other substances, those which require notice in a toxicological treatise are the following:— 1. The binoxide or *red precipitate ;* 2. The bisulphuret or *vermilion;* 3. The protochloride or *calomel;* 4. The bichloride or *corrosive sublimate;* 5. The sulphate or *Turbith mineral ;* 6. The *bicyanide* or prussiate of mercury ; and 7. The *nitrates* of mercury. Its other compounds are of little consequence to the toxicologist.

1. *Of Red Precipitate.*

Red precipitate, when well prepared, is in the form of fine powder or small, brilliant, heavy scales of a scarlet or orange colour. It consists of 101 mercury and 8 oxygen. It is insoluble in water.

It is easily distinguished from all other substances by the action of heat. If a little of it is heated in a small glass tube, it becomes dark brown, and on cooling recovers its original colour. But if the heat be raised higher, metallic globules are sublimed, and oxygen gas is disengaged. The escape of oxygen may be ascertained by plunging to the bottom a small bit of burning wood, when the combustion will be observed to be enlivened.

2. *Of Cinnabar.*

Cinnabar or vermilion, the bisulphuret of mercury, usually exists in the arts in the form of a fine, heavy, red powder, of a peculiar tint, which is termed from this substance vermilion-red. In mass its structure is coarsely-fibrous, and its colour reddish-brown ; and it has some lustre. When thrown down from a solution of corrosive sublimate by sulphuretted-hydrogen, or the alkaline hydrosulphates, it forms a black powder, which acquires a red tint by being sublimed. It is composed of 101 metal and 16 sulphur.

It is distinguished from other substances by the operation of heat, and by the effects of reduction with iron filings. Heated alone in a tube it sublimes without change. Its colour, indeed, which is fugacious under heat unless particular manipulations are used, becomes darker and dingy ; but its lustre and crystalline texture are retained. Heated with iron filings in a tube, it gives off globules of mercury ; and the existence of sulphuret of iron in what remains may be proved by the escape of sulphuretted-hydrogen on the addition of diluted sulphuric acid.

3. *Of Turbith Mineral.*

The Turbith mineral, or subsulphate of the binoxide of mercury, exists in the form of a bright lemon-yellow, heavy powder. It is soluble in 2000 parts of water, and has an acrid taste.

It may be known by the effects of heat. When heated in a tube, globules of mercury are sublimed, and at the same time sulphurous acid gas is disengaged, as may be ascertained by the smell. But a better method of proving the existence of sulphuric acid in it is to expose it to the action of a solution of caustic potass: The potass separates from it the brownish-yellow peroxide, and appropriates the sulphuric acid, which may be found in the solution by acidulating with nitric acid, and then adding hydrochlorate of baryta, when a heavy, snow-white precipitate of sulphate of baryta will form. The nitric acid used in this process must be quite pure, and free of sulphuric acid, which the acid of commerce often contains.

4. Of Calomel.

Calomel (muriate, mild muriate, chloride, protochloride of mercury), is commonly met with in the shops in the form of a heavy powder, having a faint yellowish-white colour, and no taste or smell. In mass it forms compact, fibrous, translucent, shining cakes of great density. It is insoluble in water.

It is distinguished by the effects of heat, and those of the solution of caustic potass. Heated in a tube it sublimes unchanged, and condenses in a crystalline or crumbly mass. The solution of caustic potass or soda turns it at once black, disengaging protoxide of mercury and acquiring hydrochloric acid, the presence of which is proved by neutralizing the solution with nitric acid, and adding nitrate of silver, when a heavy white precipitate is formed, the chloride of silver. In applying this process, care must be taken to employ potass quite free of muriates, and nitric acid free of muriatic acid. Ammonia also renders calomel powder black, but the action and product are much more complex in their nature.

5. Of Corrosive Sublimate.

Corrosive sublimate (oxymuriate, corrosive muriate, bichloride of mercury), is by far the most important of the mercurial poisons, as it is both the most active of them, and the one most frequently used for criminal purposes. It is commonly met with in the form of a heavy, snow-white powder, or of small, broken crystals, or in white, compact, concave, crystalline cakes. It is permanent in the air; but in the sunshine is slowly decomposed, a gray insoluble powder being formed. It readily crystallizes, and the common form of the crystals is the quadrangular prism. Its specific gravity is 5·2. Its taste is strongly styptic, metallic, acrid, and persistent; and its dust powerfully irritates the nostrils. It is soluble, according to Thenard, in 20, according to Orfila, in 11 parts of temperate water, and in thrice its weight of boiling water. Its solution faintly reddens litmus. It is more soluble in alcohol than in water, boiling alcohol dissolving its own weight, and retaining when it cools, a fourth part. It is also very soluble in ether, so that ether will remove it from its aqueous

solution. Corrosive sublimate may become the subject of a medico-
legal analysis in three states. It may be in the solid form; it may
be dissolved in water along with other mineral substances; and it
may be mixed with vegetable and animal fluids or solids.

Of the Tests for Corrosive Sublimate in the solid state.

Corrosive sublimate in the solid state is distinguished from other
substances by the action of the heat, and the effects of solution of
caustic potass. Subjected to heat alone it sublimes in white acrid
fumes; and if the experiment is made in a little tube, it condenses
again unaltered in a crystalline cake. Treated with solution of caustic potass, it becomes yellow, the binoxide being disengaged, and
hydrochloric acid uniting with the potass, as may be proved by nitrate of silver, after filtration and neutralization with nitric acid.
The yellow colour of the binoxide which is separated in this process
distinguishes corrosive sublimate from calomel, which is also decomposed by the potass solution, but yields a black protoxide. Caustic
soda has the same effect. Not so caustic ammonia: Ammonia
blackens calomel, but does not change the colour of corrosive sublimate, as it forms with it a white triple salt, commonly called white
precipitate.

The process here described is the best and simplest method of determining chemically the nature of corrosive sublimate in its solid
state. But two other tests may also be mentioned, as they have been
a good deal used. A very good test is the process of reduction with
potass, by which globules of mercury are sublimed, and a chloride of
potassium left in the flux, as may be proved by the action of nitrate
of silver on the solution of the flux previously neutralized with nitric
acid. This test alone will not distinguish corrosive sublimate from
calomel: The solubility of the former must be taken into account. —
Another satisfactory test is the solution of protochloride of tin. Corrosive sublimate, when left for some time in this solution, first becomes grayish-black, and ere long its place is supplied by globules
of mercury, — the chlorine being entirely abstracted by the protochloride of tin, which consequently passes to the state of a bichloride.
Calomel is similarly affected.

Of the Tests for Corrosive Sublimate in a state of Solution.

Two processes may be mentioned for the detection of corrosive
sublimate in mineral solutions, — a process by reduction, and a process by liquid tests.

Reduction process. — In order to procure mercury in its characteristic metallic state from a solution of corrosive sublimate, the following plan of procedure will be found the most delicate and convenient.
Add to the solution, previously acidulated with hydrochloric acid if
very weak, a little of the protochloride of tin, which will be seen
presently to be a liquid reagent of great delicacy. If the solution is
not darkened there is not present an appreciable quantity of mercury.

If mercury is present a bluish-gray or grayish-black precipitate falls down, owing to the chemical action already particularized. After ebullition, this precipitate is to be allowed to subside, first in a tall glass vessel suited to the quantity of the solution, and afterwards in the small glass tube, Fig. 7, the superincumbent fluid being previously decanted off as far as possible. After it has subsided in the tube, the remaining fluid is withdrawn with the pipette, Fig. 8; water is poured over it; and this is withdrawn again after the precipitate has subsided a third time. The bottom of the tube is then cut off with a file, and the moisture which remains is driven off with a gentle heat. When this is accomplished, the powder, which is nothing else than metallic mercury, sometimes runs into globules. Should it not do so, the bit of tube is to be broken in pieces and heated in the tube, Fig. 1, when a brilliant ring of fine globules will be formed. If the globules are too minute to be visible to the naked eye, the tube is to be cut off with the file close to the ring ; and the globules may then be easily made to coalesce into one or more of visible magnitude by scraping the inside of the tube with the point of a penknife.

This process is not recommended as preferable to the plan by liquid reagents which is next to be mentioned, and which is both more easily put in practice, and at the same time quite as satisfactory. It is related chiefly because it forms the groundwork of a process for detecting mercury in mixed animal or vegetable fluids. It will be remarked that the process does not prove with what acid the mercury was combined in the solution. But this is a defect of little consequence ; for the only other soluble salts of mercury ever met with in the arts, namely, the nitrate, acetate, and cyanide, are too rare to be the source of any material fallacy ; and are besides all equally poisonous with corrosive sublimate.

Process by Liquid Tests. — The process by liquid reagents consists in the application of several tests to separate portions of the solution. The tests which appear to me the most satisfactory are hydrosulphuric acid gas, hydriodate of potass, protochloride of tin, and nitrate of silver.

1. *Hydrosulphuric acid gas* transmitted in a stream through a solution of corrosive sublimate causes a dark, brownish-black precipitate, the bisulphuret of mercury. When the solution is not very diluted, the gas forms a whitish or yellowish precipitate before the blackening commences, — an effect which, according to Pfaff, distinguishes the salts of the peroxide of mercury from all other metals that are thrown down black from their solutions by sulphuretted-hydrogen.* The cause of this is that the particles of sulphuret first formed acquire a thin covering of corrosive sublimate by that property which chemists of late have termed superficial attraction. Hydrosulphuric acid is a very delicate test of the presence of mercury. It will detect corrosive sublimate, where its proportion is only a 35000th of the solution.†

* Kopp's Jahrbuch der Staatsarzneikunde, iv. 354.
† Devergie. Annales d'Hyg. Publ. xi. 418.

This test is not alone sufficient, unless reliance be placed on Pfaff's criterion, which is rather a trivial one; for hydrosulphuric acid occasions a black precipitate in other metallic solutions, for example, in solutions of lead, copper, bismuth and silver. In mixed organic fluids its action is not liable to be prevented; but the precipitate formed is often kept intimately suspended, as in the instance of milk. It may be conveniently used in the form of hydrosulphate of ammonia. This test produces a dark-brown precipitate, which is said to pass slowly to a bright cinnabar red; but I have not been able to observe any transformation of the kind.

Hydriodate of Potass causes in solutions of corrosive sublimate a beautiful pale scarlet precipitate, which rapidly deepens in tint. The precipitate is the biniodide of mercury. This is a test of great delicacy when skilfully used, as it acts where the salt forms only a 7000th of the solution (Devergie). Care must be taken, however, not to add too much of the test, because the precipitate is soluble in an excess of the hydriodate, or too little, because the precipitate is also soluble in a considerable excess of corrosive sublimate.

The action of hydriodate of potass is not liable to any important ambiguity: no other iodide resembles in colour the biniodide of mercury. It is not a certain test, however, when other salts exist in solution along with corrosive sublimate. Chloride of sodium, nitrate of potass, and probably also other neutral salts possess the power of dissolving the precipitate. Sulphuric and nitric acids, even considerably diluted, oxidate and dissolve the mercury, and disengage iodine, which colours the fluid reddish-brown. When corrosive sublimate is dissolved in coloured vegetable infusions or animal fluids, the hydriodate of potass cannot be relied on, the colour of the precipitate being altered, as in infusion of galls, or the action of the test being suspended altogether, as by milk.

Protochloride of Tin causes first a white precipitate, which, when more of the test is added, gives place to a grayish-black one. In very diluted solutions the colour struck is grayish or grayish-black from the beginning. In such solutions Devergie has found it useful to acidulate with hydrochloric acid before adding the test. The chemical action here is peculiar. The white powder thrown down at first is protochloride of mercury; a part of the chlorine of the bichloride of mercury having been abstracted by the protochloride of tin, which becomes in consequence the bichloride. On more of the test being added these changes are repeated, the chlorine is removed from the protochloride of mercury, and metallic mercury falls down. This test is one of extreme delicacy, affecting solutions which contain only an 80,000th of salt. It is prepared by acting on tin powder or tinfoil with strong hydrochloric acid aided by a gentle heat. The solution must be kept carefully excluded from the air; otherwise bichloride of tin is formed, which does not act at all on the solution of corrosive sublimate.

The protochloride of tin is not liable to any fallacy. Neither is it liable to be suspended in its action by the co-existence of other saline substances. It causes precipitates with almost all animal and most vegetable fluids. But when corrosive sublimate is present, even in very small proportion, the precipitate is always darker than when no mercurial salt exists in solution, and frequently has its proper grayish-black tint. This property, as will presently be seen, is the foundation of a process for the detection of mercury in all states of admixture with organic matters.

Nitrate of Silver causes a heavy white precipitate, the chloride of silver, which darkens under exposure to light. This is a test for the chlorine of the corrosive sublimate, but not for the mercury, and is a necessary addition to the three former tests in order to determine how the mercury is kept in solution. It acts with very great delicacy.

It is of no use, however, when chlorine or hydrochloric acid is present either free or combined with other bases. It is not of use, therefore, in animal fluids and vegetable infusions, because very many of them, besides organic principles which form white precipitates with this test, contain a sensible proportion of hydrochlorate of soda.

Although the preceding liquid reagents when employed conjunctly are amply sufficient for determining the presence of corrosive sublimate in a fluid, many other tests hardly less characteristic and delicate have been used by medical jurists. These will now be shortly mentioned.

1. *Lime-Water* throws down the binoxide of mercury in the form of a heavy yellow powder. The precipitate first thrown down is lemon-yellow, an additional quantity of the test gives it a reddish-yellow tint, and a still larger quantity restores the lemon-yellow. This test is characteristic, but not so delicate as those already mentioned. — 2. *Caustic Potass* has precisely the same effect as lime-water, except that the tint of the precipitate is always yellow — 3. *Caustic Ammonia* causes a fine, white, flocculent precipitate of intricate composition, commonly called precipitate. It is a very delicate test; but ammonia likewise causes a white precipitate in other metallic solutions. — 4. *Carbonate of Potass* causes a brisk-red precipitate, by virtue of a double decomposition, the precipitate being carbonate of mercury. — 5. The *Ferro-cyanate of Potass* causes at first a white precipitate, the ferro-cyanide of mercury. The precipitate becomes slowly yellowish, and at length pale-blue, owing, it is believed, to the admixture of a small quantity of iron with the corrosive sublimate. — 6. *A polished plate of Copper* immersed in a solution of corrosive sublimate becomes in a few seconds tarnished and brownish ; and in the course of half an hour a grayish-white powder is formed on its surface. This powder, according to Orfila,* is a mixture of calomel, mercury, and a copper amalgam. If it is wiped off, and the plate then rubbed briskly where tarnished, it assumes a white argentine appearance. — 7. *A little Mercury* put into a solution of corrosive sublimate is instantly tarnished on the surface ; the solution in a few

* Toxicologie Gén. i. 241.

seconds becomes turbid, a heavy grayish precipitate is formed, and in no long time with the aid of agitation the whole corrosive sublimate is removed from the solution.   The powdery precipitate is a mixture of finely divided mercury and calomel; the former being derived from the surface of the mercury, and the latter produced by the corrosive sublimate uniting with a larger proportion of the metal to form the protochloride. — 8. *A solution of Albumen* causes a white precipitate, which is soluble in a considerable excess of the reagent. The nature of this precipitate will be discussed presently. — A *slip of Gold* aided by galvanism, becomes silver-white in the solution, in consequence of the formation of an amalgam.   When the solution is concentrated, it may be thus tested by simply putting a few drops on a bit of gold, and touching the gold through the solution with an iron point, as recommended by Mr. Sylvester and Dr. Paris.*   When the solution is very weak, a different method is necessary, and a process for the purpose has been proposed by M. Devergie, which appears so delicate, accurate, and at the same time simple a mode of detecting traces of mercury in very weak solutions, as to deserve detailed notice.   A thin plate of gold, and another of tin, a few lines broad, and two or three inches long, being closely applied to one another by silk threads at the ends, and then twisted spirally, this galvanic pile is left for twenty-four or thirty-six hours in the solution previously acidulated with muriatic acid ; upon which the gold is found whitened, and mercury may be obtained in globules by heating the gold in a tube.   Distinct indications may be obtained by this method, where the corrosive sublimate forms but an 80,000th of the water.†   For facility of application, an important condition is, that the quantity of fluid should not exceed three or four ounces, because in a larger quantity the pile of the size stated above cannot remove the whole mercury.   Somewhat similar to this is the galvanic method of Mr. Davy of Dublin.   He proposes to place the suspected solution in a platinum crucible with hydrochloric acid, diluted with its own weight of water, to excite galvanic action by immersing in the fluid a plate of zinc, and to sublime and collect the reduced mercury, by washing the crucible, heating it over a spirit-lamp, and condensing the mercurial vapours on a plate of glass placed over the mouth of the crucible.‡

Of the Tests for Corrosive Sublimate when mixed with Organic Fluids and Solids.

The process for detecting corrosive sublimate in mixtures of organic fluids and solids, such as the contents of the stomach, is now to be described.   But some remarks are previously required on the chemical relations subsisting between this poison and various principles of the vegetable and animal kingdoms.

* Medical Jurisprudence, ii. 208.
† Annales d'Hyg. Publ. et de Méd Lég. xi. 411.
‡ Philosophical Transaction, 1831, cxxi. 155, 160.

These relations are important in a medico-legal point of view on several grounds. On the one hand, the chemical changes which corrosive sublimate undergoes often alter so much the action of its tests, as to render necessary a process of analysis materally different from any hitherto described. And on the other hand, these chemical changes, of which some take place rapidly, others slowly, will hinder the corrosive sublimate, more or less completely, from exerting its usual operation on the animal system; so that it may thus either accidentally fail to act as intended, or be checked in its operation by antidotes administered for the purpose.

It appears from the researches of M. Boullay, confirmed by those of Professor Orfila, that various vegetable fluids, extracts, fixed oils, volatile oils and resins, possess the power of decomposing corrosive sublimate. According to M. Boullay, a part of the chlorine is gradually disengaged in the form of hydrochloric acid, and the salt is consequently converted into calomel, which is deposited in a state of mixture or combination with vegetable matter.* Some vegetable fluids produce this change at once, others not for some hours, others not for days, and only when aided by a temperature approaching ebullition. For example, a strong infusion of tea, mixed with a solution of a few grains of corrosive sublimate, becomes immediately muddy, and an insoluble cloud separates in half an hour. But the remaining fluid slowly becomes muddy again, and in eight days a considerable precipitate is formed. Both precipitates contain mercury; the former, I find, contains 31 per cent. On the other hand, an infusion of galls in like circumstances does not become muddy for six or seven hours. A solution of sugar does not undergo any change after being mixed with a solution of corrosive sublimate for months at the ordinary temperature of the atmosphere; but at the temperature of ebullition Boullay has found that the usual changes ensue, though to no great extent.

The experiments of Professor Taddei of Florence have farther shown, that the property of decomposing corrosive sublimate is possessed in an eminent degree by one of the vegetable solids, gluten. If the salt in solution is properly mixed with a due proportion of gluten of wheat, that is, about four times its weight, the water will be found no longer to contain any mercury, while the gluten becomes whitish, brittle, hard, and not prone to putrefaction. A ternary compound is formed, the protochloride of mercury and gluten.† This change is effected with rapidity.

The researches of Berthollet,‡ repeated and extended by Professor Orfila,§ have also shown that the same property is possessed by most animal fluids and solids. Among the soluble animal principles, albumen, caesin, osmazôme, and gelatin possess it in a high degree, but above all albumen, the action of which has been examined with

* Annales de Chimie, xliv. 176, and Orfila, Toxicol. Gén. i. 243.
† Taddei, Recherches sur un nouvel Antidote contre le sublimé corrosif.
‡ Berthollet, sur la Causticité des sels Métalliques. Mém, de l'Acad. 1780.
§ Toxic. Gén. i. 245,

some care, as it supplies the physician with the most convenient and effectual antidote against the effects of the poison.

If a solution of albumen, for example that procured by beating white of eggs in water, is dropped by degrees into a solution of corrosive sublimate, a white flaky precipitate is immediately thrown down, which when separated and dried forms horny masses, hard, brittle, and pulverizable. The precipitate is soluble in a considerable excess of albumen; so that wherever albumen abounds in any fluid, to which corrosive sublimate has been added, a portion of the mercury will always be found in solution. The precipitate is also soluble in a considerable excess of corrosive sublimate. The dry precipitate I have found to contain 6 per cent. of metallic mercury.

The action of casein as it exists in milk is precisely the same. A solution of corrosive sublimate, poured into a large quantity of milk, causes no change ; but if the proportion of salt be considerable, a flaky coagulum is formed, and the milk becomes clear. The principles, osmazôme and gelatin, are similar in their effects, though not quite so powerful. Urea has no chemical action with corrosive sublimate. Of the compound animal fluids, blood and serum have the same effects as albumen.

Many insoluble animal principles, as well as all the soft solids of the animal body, act in the same manner with vegetable gluten. Fibrin, for example, coagulated albumen, or coagulated casein, acts precisely in the same way. Muscular fibre, the mucous and serous membranes, the fibrous textures, and the brain, have all the same effect : they become firmer, brittle, white, and a white powder detaches itself from their surface, which contains mercury and animal matter. This chemical action, which Taddei has proved to take place in the living[*] as well as in the dead dody, is the source of the corrosive property of the poison, as was first pointed out by Berthollet in his essay formerly quoted.

In all of the compounds thus formed by vegetable and animal substances, the presence of mercury is easily proved by boiling the powder in a solution of caustic potass. The organized matter is dissolved; a heavy, grayish-black powder is formed, which is protoxide of mercury; and if this be collected in the way formerly described, it forms running quicksilver when heated.

A difference of opinion prevails as to the nature of the changes effected by the mutual action of corrosive sublimate and organic matter. For example, in the instance of the action of albumen, which has been most carefully examined, Berzelius and Lassaigne[†] regard the precipitate as a compound of bichloride of mercury with albumen. Professor Rose and Dr. Geoghegan[‡] have proved it, in their opinion, to be a compound of binoxide of mercury and albumen without any chlorine. And according to Boullay it is composed of albumen

---

[*] Recherches, &c. p. 60.   [†] Journal de Chimie Médicale, 1837, p. 161.
[‡] Poggendorff's Annalen der Physik und Chemie, xxviii. 135.

in union with calomel.* Lassaigne says he has found it to be a compound of ten equivalents of albumen with one of mercury, or 93·33 per cent. of the former, and 6·67 of the latter.† The compound with fibrin he considers to be analogous in composition.

With regard to the changes induced by these effects of organized matter on the operation of the liquid tests for corrosive sublimate, it will in the first place be manifest that the poison may thus be wholly removed from their sphere of action : it may be thrown down as an insoluble substance, on which any process by liquid tests hitherto mentioned will of course fail to act. But secondly, even when a moderate quantity does remain in solution, the operation of the liquid tests, as formerly noticed under the head of each, will be materially modified. It is of some moment for the medical jurist to remember, that by reason of the slowness with which the changes in question sometimes takes place, the poison may exist abundantly in solution at one time, and yet be present only in small quantity after an interval of some hours or days.

Process for Organic Mixtures. — Various processes have been proposed for detecting corrosive sublimate in organic mixtures. The first I shall mention is one proposed by myself in former editions of this work. It is a double one ; of which sometimes the first part, sometimes the second, sometimes both may be required. The first removes the corrosive sublimate undecomposed from the mixture, which may be accomplished when its proportion is considerable ; the second, when the proportion of corrosive sublimate is too small to admit of being so removed, separates from the mixture metallic mercury ; and the analyst will know which of the two to employ by using the protochloride of tin as a trial-test in the following manner.

A fluid mixture being in the first instance made, if necessary, by dividing and bruising all soft solids into very small fragments, and boiling the mass in distilled water, a small portion is to be filtered for the trial. If the protochloride of tin causes a pretty deep ash-gray or grayish-black colour, the first process may prove successful ; if the shade acquired is not deep, that process may be neglected, and the second put in practice at once.

First branch of the Process. — In order to remove the corrosive sublimate undecomposed, the mixture, without filtration, is to be agitated for a few minutes with about a fourth part of its volume of sulphuric ether ; which possesses the property of abstracting the salt from its aqueous solution. On remaining at rest for half a minute or a little more, the etherial solution rises to the surface, and may then be removed by suction with the pipette (Fig. 8). It is next to be filtered if requisite, evaporated to dryness, and the residue treated with boiling water ; upon which a solution is procured that will present the properties formerly mentioned as belonging to corrosive sublimate in its dissolved state. This branch of the process is derived from one of Orfila's methods.

Second branch of the Process. — If the preceding method should

* Annalen der Pharmacie, xxiv. 36.   † Annales de Chimie, xliv. 176.

fail, or shall have been judged inapplicable, as will very generally be the case, the mixture is to be treated in the following manner. In the first place, all particles of seeds, leaves, and other fibrous matter of a vegetable nature, are to be removed as carefully as possible. This being done, the mixture, without undergoing filtration, is to be treated with protochloride of tin as long as any precipitate or coagulum is formed. If there were solid animal matters in the mixture, besides being cut and carefully bruised as directed above, they should also be brought thoroughly in contact with the salt of tin by trituration. The mixture, even if it contains but a very minute proportion of mercury, will acquire a slate-gray tint, and become easily separable into a liquid and coagulum. The coagulum is to be collected, washed and drained on a filter; from which it is then to be removed without being dried; and care should be taken not to tear away with it any fibres of the paper, as these would obstruct the succeeding operations. The mercury exists in it in the metallic state for reasons formerly mentioned.

The precipitate is next to be boiled in a moderately strong solution of caustic potass contained in a glass flask, or still better in a smooth porcelain vessel glazed with porcelain; and the ebullition is to be continued till all the lumps disappear. The animal and vegetable matter, and oxide of tin united with them, will thus be dissolved; and on the solution being allowed to remain at rest, a heavy grayish-black powder will begin to fall down in a few seconds. This is chiefly metallic mercury, of which, indeed, globules may sometimes be discerned with the naked eye or with a small magnifier.

In order to separate it, leave the solution at rest under a temperature a little short of ebullition for fifteen or twenty minutes, or longer, if necessary. Fill up the vessel gently with hot water without disturbing the precipitate, so that a fatty matter, which rises to the surface in the case of most animal mixtures, may be skimmed off first with a spoon, and afterwards with filtering paper. Then withdraw the whole supernatant fluid, which is easily done on account of the great density of the black powder. Transfer the powder into a small glass tube, and wash it by the process of affusion and subsidence till the washings do not taste alkaline. Any fibrous matter which may have escaped notice at the commencement of the process, and any lumpy matter which may have escaped solution by the potass, should now be picked out. The black powder is the only part which should be preserved. If the quantity of powder is very minute, an interval of twelve hours should be allowed for each subsidence, and the tube represented in Fig. 7 should be used.

Lastly, the powder is to be removed, heated, and sublimed, as in the last stage of the process described in page 293, for detecting corrosive sublimate in a pure solution.

The second branch of this process is very delicate. I have detected by it a quarter of a grain of corrosive sublimate mixed with two ounces of beef, or with five ounces of new milk, or porter, or tea made with a liberal allowance of cream and sugar. I have also detected a tenth part of a grain in four ounces of the last mixture, that is in 19,200 times its weight.

It may be applied successfully and without difficulty to a very large majority of medico-legal cases. The only difficulty in the way of applying it to all organic mixtures whatever arises from the occasional presence of some vegetable matters, such as seeds, leaves, ligneous fibre and the like, which are insoluble in caustic potass, and which may therefore be left behind with the mercurial precipitate, and obstruct the subsequent sublimation of the metal. This difficulty may be sometimes got rid of, as recommended above, by picking such matters out of the mixture before the protochloride of tin is added. No mercury is lost by so doing, for none of it is united with these vegetable matters : corrosive sublimate does not form any chemical compound with them as it does with other vegetable matters soluble in caustic potass, and with the soft animal solids. When the particles are too small to admit of being thus removed, or cannot be afterwards removed during the process of washing the black powder, which is left after the action of potass — the analyst must be content with the increased facility of sublimation derived from the abstraction of other vegetable and animal admixtures, and take care to use a tube of greater length and with a larger ball than usual. If the sublimate is too much obscured by empyreumatized matter to exhibit distinctly its metallic, globular appearance, the portion of the tube is to be broken off, and scraped, washed, and boiled with a little rectified spirit in a tube. If the globules do not then become visible, a second sublimation will render them distinct. This supplemental operation, however, will be very seldom required ; and the process given above will be found to apply to a great majority of instances.

Various objections brought against this process by reviewers and others were noticed in previous editions of this work. The result of the investigation is, that, though not by any means a perfect process, it is one of the most convenient and certain, and least fallacious of all yet proposed. The first step for separating corrosive sublimate by ether in the undecomposed state, — which is borrowed from a suggestion of Professor Orfila, will seldom succeed ; for the poison is seldom present in sufficient quantity.

It must be observed that this as well as every other method yet proposed for discovering corrosive sublimate in compound mixtures merely indicates the presence of mercury, and does not point out its state of combination. More especially, in the case of the contents of the stomach, if mercury be not obtained from the filtered fluid, it is impossible to know whether what is detected in the solid matter only may not have proceeded from calomel given medicinally. This objection can be obviated solely by sufficient evidence that calomel was not administered ; at least the different criterions laid down by Professor Orfila for distinguishing calomel in the alimentary canal from the products of the decomposition of corrosive sublimate do not appear sufficiently precise, or commonly applicable.[*]

* Toxicologie Générale, i. 301.

Various processes for detecting corrosive sublimate in organic mixtures have been proposed by others. But none of these seem to me preferable to the method detailed above, with the exception of one which has been lately proposed by Professor Orfila, and which is particularly deserving of notice, because, although complex, he has found it sufficiently manageable and delicate for detecting mercury in the animal textures and secretions, into which it has obtained admission through the medium of absorption in cases of poisoning with the compounds of mercury. Like the previous process, however, it merely detects mercury, and cannot point out the state of combination in which mercury was administered, or mixed with the substance examined.

If the suspected matter be sufficiently liquid, boil for a few minutes and filter; acidulate the product with a few drops of hydrochloric acid; and immerse some slips of copper-leaf in it for a few hours. Should they be tarnished, dissolve oxide and chloride of copper from the surface by means of ammonia; wash them and press them between folds of filtering-paper; cut them in pieces, and heat these in a glass tube. Globules of mercury may be obtained or not. In either case, let the liquid, in which the plates were first immersed, be evaporated to dryness over the vapour-bath; add to the residue a sixth of sulphuric acid in a retort with a receiver; and heat gently till a nearly dry carbonaceous mass be obtained. Boil this with an ounce and a half of nitro-hydrochloric acid [Edin. Pharm.], until the charcoal be again nearly dry. Heat what remains with boiling distilled water, filter, apply to a small part of the liquid the copper test as just described, and try whether corrosive sublimate can be detached from the remainder by means of sulphuric ether (p. 299). The distilled fluid in the receiver may contain corrosive sublimate in considerable proportion, relatively to what existed in the subject of analysis. In order to discover it, boil the liquid for fifteen minutes with nitro-hydrochloric acid; transmit chlorine gas for an hour, filter, and evaporate to dryness over the vapour-bath; dissolve the residue in water, and search for corrosive sublimate both by copper plates, and by agitation with ether.

If mercury be not thus detected, proceed to the solid matter left on the filter, by which the subject of analysis was in the first instance separated into a liquid and solid part. Examine this by evaporation to dryness over the vapour-bath, and charring with sulphuric acid in a retort with a receiver attached; and then subject the product to the same steps as those detailed above for the dried residuum of the liquid part.

If the materials for analysis be soft solids, especially the stomach, intestines, liver, and the like, commence at once with the process of charring with sulphuric acid. In the case of the urine, examine both the liquid and sediment. Filter the liquid, transmit chlorine to excess, let the product rest twenty-four hours, filter, evaporate to dryness, dissolve the residue in water acidulated with hydrochloric acid, and test the solution both with copper-leaf and by agitation with ether. Heat the sediment with nitro-hydrochloric acid as directed above, and then proceed as with the liquid portion of the urine.*

Some other processes, but probably inferior to that of Professor Orfila, will be found in the last edition of this work. It seems unnecessary to reproduce them here.

6. *Of Bicyanide of Mercury.*

The bicyanide of mercury is a compound of mercury and cyanogen. It is usually sold in the form of white, opaque, heavy, crystals, which are rhomboidal prisms. It has a disagreeable, corrosive, metallic taste. It is easily known from every other substance by the effects of heat. If a small quantity of it, previously well dried, be introduced into a glass phial to which a small tube is fitted by means of a cork, on the application of heat the salt becomes black; mercury is sublimed, and condenses in globules on the upper part of the phial; and a gas escapes, which has the odour of prussic acid, and burns with a beautiful rose-red flame.

7. *Of the Nitrates of Mercury.*

The nitrates of mercury are used in some of the arts, but have so rarely been the cause of injury to man that they are of little medicolegal importance. I am acquainted with only one case of poisoning with them.†

There are two nitrates, the protonitrate and pernitrate. 1. The protonitrate is in transparent colourless crystals, entirely soluble in water with the aid of a slight excess of nitric acid; and the solution is precipitated black by the alkalis, black by sulphuretted-hydrogen, white by muriatic acid, and yellow by hydriodate of potass. The crystals when heated discharge fumes of nitrous acid, and when the whole acid is driven off the red oxide is left, which by farther heat is converted into metallic mercury. 2. The pernitrate is similarly affected by heat. Its crystals form white or yellowish needles. Water decomposes them, separating an insoluble yellowish subnitrate, and dissolving a supernitrate, which is precipitated yellow by the alkalis, black by sulphuretted-hydrogen, carmine-red by the hydriodate of potass. Copper separates mercury from both nitrates; and so does gold or platinum when aided by a galvanic current.

SECTION II. — *Of the mode of Action of Mercury and the Symptoms it excites in Man.*

The effects of mercury on the animal body are more diversified than those of any other poison. It acts on a great number of important organs, and in consequence the phenomena of its action are proportionately various. It is not surprising, therefore, that some

* Annales d'Hygiène Publique, xxviii. 424.
† Dr. Bigsby in London Medical Gazette, vii. 329.

ambiguity still prevails as to its mode of action and the circumstances by which the action is regulated.

The attention of toxicologists in their physiological researches has been chiefly turned to the more active preparations of mercury, and especially to corrosive sublimate, when given in such quantity as to prove fatal in a few days at farthest. The more immediate and prominent properties of corrosive sublimate have consequently received some elucidation. But its qualities as a slow poison, as well as the analogous operation of the less active compounds of mercury, have not been experimentally examined with the same care : indeed it is questionable whether the phenomena of the latter description as they occur in man can be studied with much advantage by means of experiments on animals. — In treating of the mode in which the compounds of mercury act, the most convenient method will be to consider at present its action in the form of corrosive sublimate in large doses as ascertained by late experiments. and to reserve the consideration of the general action of mercurial poisons at large till their effects on man have been fully described.

The mode of action of corrosive sublimate has been examined particularly by Sir B. Brodie in 1812 ;* by Dr. Campbell in 1813.† by M. Smith in 1815,‡ by M. Gaspard in 1821,§ and more lately by Professor Orfila.‖ The following is a short analysis of their experiments and results.

The leading phenomena remarked by Sir B. Brodie, on large doses being introduced into the stomach, were very rapid death, corrosion of the stomach, and paralysis of the heart. In rabbits and cats, from six to twenty grains, injected in a state of solution into the stomach, produced in a few minutes insensibility and laborious breathing, then convulsions, and death immediately afterwards, — the whole duration of the poisoning varying from five to twenty-five minutes. After death the inner membrane of the stomach was gray, brittle, and here and there pulpy, — changes precisely the same with those produced by corrosive sublimate on the dead stomach. When the chest was opened immediately after death, the heart was found either motionless or contracting feebly ; and in both circumstances the blood in its left cavities was arterial.

These experiments make it evident that the brain was acted on as well as the heart, and that the immediate cause of death was stoppage of the heart's action. But they do not show whether the action takes place through absorption, or by a primary nervous impression transmitted along the nerves.

I am not acquainted with any other experiments of consequence on the operation of corrosive sublimate when introduced into the alimentary canal. But some interesting observations have been made by Campbell, Smith, Gaspard, and Orfila severally as to its effects

* Philosophical Transactions, cii. 222.
† Tentamen Inaugurale de Venenis Mineralibus, Edinb. 1813, p. 36.
‡ Orfila, Toxicologie Gén. i. 257.
§ Journal de Physiologie, i. 165 and 242.   ‖ Toxicologie, i. 261.

when applied to the cellular tissue or injected at once into the blood of a vein. It follows from their researches, taken along with those of Sir B. Brodie, that, like arsenic, corrosive sublimate is an active poison, to whatever part or tissue in the body it is applied.

Campbell, Smith, and Orfila all agree in assigning to it dangerous properties, when it is applied to a wound or the cellular tissue of animals. Even in the solid state, and in the dose of three, four, or five grains only, it causes death in the course of the second, third, fourth, or fifth day. The symptoms antecedent to death are generally those of dysentery; and corresponding appearances are found after death, namely, redness, blackness, or even ulceration of the villous coat of the stomach and rectum, the intermediate part of the alimentary canal being sound. This poison, therefore, has, like arsenic, the singular power of inflaming the stomach and intestines, even when it is introduced into the system through a wound.

But this is not its only property in such circumstances. According to Smith and Orfila, it also possesses the power of inflaming both the lungs and the heart. Orfila found the lungs unusually compact and œdematous in some parts; and Smith observed on their anterior surface black spots, elevated in the centre, evidently the consequence of effusion of blood. As to the heart, in one of Smith's experiments black spots were found in its substance, immediately beneath the lining membrane of the ventricles; and Orfila invariably found in one part or another of the lining membrane, most commonly on the valves, little spots of a cherry-red or almost black colour; nay, on one occasion he observed these spots so soft that slight friction made little cavities. The production of pneumonia by corrosive sublimate when applied to a wound appears well established; but the appearances assumed as indications of carditis are equivocal, since they may have arisen simply from dyeing of the membrane of the heart in the fluid part of the blood after death.

The researches of Gaspard were confined to the effects of the poison when injected at once into the blood. They show still more clearly its tendency to cause inflammation of the lungs; and they prove that through the channel of the blood, as through the cellular tissue, it is apt to cause inflammation of the stomach and rectum. The symptoms were vomiting, bloody diarrhœa, difficult breathing, apparent pain of chest, and bloody sputa; and death took place in a few seconds or in three or four days, according to the dose, which varied from one to five grains. The appearances in the dead body were principally redness in the mucous membrane of the intestines; and in the lungs, according to the length of time the animal survived, either black ecchymosed spots, or black tubercular masses, some inflamed, others gangrenous, others suppurated, or finally, regular abscesses separated from one another by healthy pulmonary tissue.*

Besides the effects mentioned in the preceding abstract, two of the experimentalists referred to have likewise observed in animals the same remarkable operation on the salivary organs which forms so

* Journal de Physiologie, i. 165.

conspicuous a feature in the action of the compounds of mercury on man. Dr. Campbell observed mercurial fetor, and M. Gaspard mercurial salivation. Another writer, Zeller, found that dogs might be made to salivate, but not graminivorous animals.* Schubarth, however, remarked profuse salivation in a horse, to which twenty-four ounces of strong mercurial ointment were administered in the way of friction in sixteen days:† and I observed the same symptoms in a rabbit on the sixth day after the commencement of daily mercurial inunction.

The result of the preceding inquiry is, that corrosive sublimate causes, when swallowed, corrosion of the stomach, and in whatever way it obtains entrance into the body, irritation of that organ and of the rectum, inflammation of the lungs, depressed action and perhaps also inflammation of the heart, oppression of the functions of the brain, inflammation of the salivary glands. These phenomena are diversified enough. But it will presently be found that other organs still are implicated in its effects on man.

Before proceeding, however, to its effects on man, some notice may be taken of a question, connected with its mode of action, which has long been the subject of controversy. The experiments already quoted render it probable that corrosive sublimate, before it can exert its remote action, must enter the blood ; and the facts to be enumerated under the next head of the present section will render it probable that the milder compounds of mercury used in medicine also act in a similar manner. Physicians and chemists, therefore, long sought to discover this metal in the solids and fluids of the body while under its influence ; and the failure of some attempts to detect it has naturally led to its presence throughout the system being called in question by many. This inquiry, besides its interest in a physiological point of view, is highly important in respect to medico-legal practice, since it forms a material branch of the general questions which at present occupy the attention of medical jurists, — whether poisons that act through the blood should be sought for by chemical analysis in other parts of the body besides the stomach, intestines, or other organ to which they have been directly applied — and in what particular quarters the search should be principally made.

In the case of mercury, the evidence of the absorption of the poison, and of its entering the tissues and secretions of the body, is now unimpeachable. This is chiefly derived from observations and experiments made on man and animals after the long-continued use of the milder preparations of mercury ; it being imagined that if the poison enters the blood at all, the greatest quantity will be found under these circumstances. The facts may be arranged under three heads. Some relate to the discharge of metallic mercury from the living body during a mercurial course for medicinal purposes; others to the discovery of metallic mercury in the dead body after a mercurial

* Autenrieth und Zeller, über das Daseyn von Quecksilber in der Blutmasse der Thiere. Reil's Archiv für die Physiologie, viii. 216.
† Horn's Archiv für Medizinische Erfahrung, 1823, ii. 417.

course, and others to the detection of mercury by a careful chemical analysis in the fluids and solids during life or after death.

Many stories are related by the older authors of the discharge of running quicksilver from the living body during a mercurial course. Some of the most authentic of them have been collected by Zeller. In his list of cases it is stated that Schenkius met with an instance of the discharge of a spoonful of quicksilver by vomiting; that Rhodius twice remarked quicksilver pass with the urine; and that Hochstetter once saw it exhaled with the sweat.* Fallopius likewise states, that in people who had used mercurial inunction for three years, and who had the bones of the leg laid bare by suppurating nodes, he had seen quicksilver collected in globules on the tibia; and he speaks of its being the practice in his day to draw the mercury from the body, when overloaded with it, by successively amalgamating a bit of gold in the mouth and heating the amalgam to expel the mercury.† With regard to these statements of the older authors it may be observed that, although their singularity renders them questionable, they ought not to be rejected at once, as some have done, merely because corresponding facts have not been witnessed in modern times; for no one can now-a-days have such opportunities for observation as were enjoyed by Fallopius and his contemporaries. The experiment of amalgamating gold in the mouth of a person under a course of mercury has always failed in modern times. But who can now have an opportunity of making the experiment during a mercurial course of three years? Besides, the statements quoted above are not all destitute of modern confirmation. Thus Fourcroy has noticed the case of a gilder attacked with an eruption of little boils, in each of which was contained a globule of quicksilver. Bruckmann mentions the case of a lady who subsequently to a course of mercury remarked after a dance many small black stains on her breast, and minute globules of quicksilver in the folds of her shift.‡ And Dr. Jourda has described in a late French periodical a case where fluid mercury was passed by the urine. The last fact appears satisfactory in all its circumstances. A patient had been taking corrosive sublimate for a month in the dose of a grain, besides using for the first sixteen days a gargle containing metallic mercury finely divided. Towards the close of the month he observed on the sill of the window, on which he used to turn up his chamber-pot after using it, many little globules of mercury, amounting in all to four grains. Dr. Jourda on learning this observation of his patient collected some of the urine with care, and after it had stood some time found in it a black, powdery sediment, which, when separated and dried, formed little globules of mercury.§

The next class of facts in favour of the entrance of mercury into

* Diss. Inaug. Tubingæ, 1808, sistens experimenta quædam circa effectus hydrargyr in animalia viva, pp. 25, 31, also Reil's Archiv, *ut supra*.

† Tract. de Morb. Gall. in Opera Omnia, pp. 728, 729.

‡ Archiv für Medizinische Erfahrung, 1810, ii. 252.

§ Corvisart's Journ. de Méd. xxvii. 244.

the blood are derived from the discovery of the metal in the bodies of persons who had undergone a long mercurial course recently before death. In the German-Ephemerides it is said that no less than a pound of it was found in the brain and two ounces in the skull-cap of one who had been long salivated.* This is certainly too marvellous a story. But analogous observations have been made lately. In Hufeland's Journal it is mentioned that a skull found in a churchyard contained running quicksilver in the texture of its bones, and that there is preserved in the Lubben cabinet of midwifery a pelvis infiltered with mercury, and taken from a young woman who died of syphilis.† An unequivocal fact of the same nature has been related by Mr. Rigby Brodbelt. In a body of which he could not learn the history he found mercurial globules as big as a pin-head lying on the os hyoides, laryngeal car-, tilages, frontal bone, sternum, and tibia.‡ Another equally unquestionable fact of the kind has been supplied by Dr. Otto. On scraping the periosteum of several of the bones of a man who had laboured under syphilis, he remarked minute globules issuing from the osseous substance : in some places globules were deposited between the bone and periosteum, where the latter had been detached in the progress of putrefaction; and in other places, when the bones were struck, a shower of fine globules fell from them.§ Wibmer observes that Fricke, surgeon to the Hamburg Infirmary, has obtained mercury by boiling the bones of persons who had been long under a course of mercurial inunction.‖

The third and most satisfactory class of facts are the result of actual chemical analysis. These results were long variable. On the one hand, Mayer, Marabelli,¶ and Devergie,** failed to detect mercury in the fluids of people under a mercurial course ; and I myself,†† as well as Dr. Samuel Wright,‡‡ had no better success in some experiments on animals. On the other hand, Zeller detected it after death in the blood and bile, Cantu procured it from the urine, Buchner found it in the blood, saliva, and urine, and Schubarth extracted it from the blood. The first experimentalist found that in the blood and bile of animals killed by mercurial inunction, mercury could be detected by destructive distillation, but not by any fluid tests.§§ Cantu, by operating on sixty pounds of urine, taken from persons under the action of mercury, procured no less than twenty grains of the metal from the sediment.‖‖ The experiments of Buchner are very satisfactory. By destructive distillation of the crassamentum of seven ounces of blood taken from a patient who was salivated by mercury, he ob-

* Dec. I. Ann. i. Obs. 8.   † Journ. der Prakt. Heilkunde, li. 5, p. 117.
‡ Mem. of Lond. Med. Soc. v. 112.
§ Seltene Beobachtungen zur Anat. Physiol. und Pathol. Berlin, 1824, ii. 36. Quoted by Marx, die Lehre von den Giften, I. ii. 163.
‖ Die Wirkung der Arzneimittel und Gifte, iii. 86.
¶ Zeller, in Reil's Archiv. viii. 233.
** Nouvelle Bibliothèque Médicale, 1828, iv. 17 and 18.
†† See the last Edition of this work, p. 366.
‡‡ See my Dispensatory, 1842, p. 507.   §§ Reil's Archiv, viii. 223.
‖‖ Journal der Praktischen Heilkunde, lx. 115.

tained rather more than a quarter of a grain of globules ; two pounds of saliva yielded in the same way a 200th of a grain ; and the urine contained so much that it became brownish-black with sulphuretted-hydrogen.* Buchner likewise adds, that Professor Pickel of Würzburg procured mercury by destructive distillation from the brain of a venereal patient who had long taken corrosive sublimate.† Not less satisfactory are the experiments of Dr. Schubarth. A horse after being rubbed for twenty-nine days with mercurial ointment to the total amount of eighty ounces, died of fever, emaciation, diarrhœa, and ptyalism. On the sixteenth day, when ptyalism had set in, a quart of blood was drawn from the jugular vein, and after death another quart was collected from the heart, great vessels and lungs, — extreme care being taken to collect it perfectly pure. In each specimen there was procured by destructive distillation a liquor, in which minute metallic globules were visible. A copper coin agitated in the liquor was whitened ; and when the oily matter was separated by filtration and boiling in alcohol, the residue gave with nitric acid a solution, which produced an orange precipitate with hydriodate of potass.

These researches were considered adequate to prove the strong probability of the absorption of mercurial preparations when introduced into the animal. But the frequency with which negative results were obtained by competent inquirers, and in circumstances apparently favourable, threw an air of doubt over the positive facts, however clear they seem to be in themselves, — till at length Professor Orfila proved by a series of careful experiments that the cause of failure must generally have been the want of a process sufficiently delicate : for in all ordinary circumstances, by using his process described above, he succeeded in obtaining mercury in the urine and liver of animals poisoned with corrosive sublimate, as well as in the urine of patients who were taking that salt in medicinal doses. He could not detect it, however, in the blood.‡ Since these investigations, Professor Landerer of Athens detected mercury in the brain, liver, lungs and spinal cord of a man who poisoned himself with two ounces and a half of corrosive sublimate ;§ and M. Audouard has twice found it in the urine and once in the saliva of persons salivated with mercury, by simply transmitting chlorine, exposing the liquid to the air for a day, evaporating it nearly to dryness, dissolving the residue in water slightly acidulated with hydrochloric acid, immersing copper-leaf for twenty-four hours, and heating the stained portions in a tube.‖

The cases of poisoning with the preparations of mercury, which have been observed in the human subject, may be conveniently arranged under three varieties. In one variety the sole or leading symptoms are those of violent irritation of the alimentary canal.

---

* Toxicologie 3te Auflage, 539.　　　　　　　† Ibidem, 433.
‡ Journal de Chimie Médicale, 1842, p. 428.
§ Buchner's Repertorium für die Pharmacie, lxxvi. 249.
‖ Journal de Chimie Médicale, 1843, p. 137.

In another the symptoms are at first the same as in the former, but subsequently become united with salivation and inflammation of the mouth, or some of the other disorders incident to mercurial erethysm, as it is called. In a third variety the preliminary stage of irritation in the alimentary canal is wanting, and the symptoms are from beginning to end those of mercurial erethysm in one or another of its multifarious forms.

The first variety of poisoning with mercury is remarked only in those who have taken considerable doses of its soluble salts, particularly corrosive sublimate. The second is produced by the same preparations. The third may be caused by any mercurial compound.

1. The symptoms in the first variety are very like what occur in the ordinary cases of poisoning with arsenic, — namely, vomiting, especially when any thing is swallowed, violent pain in the pit of the stomach, as well as over the whole belly, and profuse diarrhœa. But there exist between the effects of the two poisons some shades of difference which it is necessary to attend to.

In the first place, — taking corrosive sublimate as the best example of the preparations which cause this variety of poisoning with mercury, — the symptoms generally begin much sooner than those caused by arsenic. The symptoms of irritation in the throat may begin immediately, nay, even during the very act of swallowing;[*] and those in the stomach may appear either immediately,[†] or within five minutes.[‡]

Secondly, the taste is much more unequivocal and strong. Even a small quantity of corrosive sublimate, either in the solid or fluid state, and considerably diluted, has so strong and so horrible a taste, that no one could swallow it in a form capable of causing much irritation in the stomach, without being at once made sensible by the taste that he had taken something unusual and injurious. Occasionally, indeed, persons thus warned of their danger while in the act of swallowing the poison, have stopped in time to escape fatal consequences.[§]

Thirdly, the sense of acridity which it excites in the gullet during the act of deglutition, and throughout the whole course of the subsequent inflammation of the alimentary canal, is usually much stronger. If the dose be not small, or largely diluted, or in the solid form, the sense of tightness, acridity, or burning in the throat and gullet during deglutition is often far greater than ever occurs at any stage in the instance of arsenic; and sometimes it is very severe even when corrosive sublimate is taken in the solid form.[‖]   The tightness and

---

* Hodgson's Trial, Edin. Med. and Surg. Journal, xxii. 439, also a case by Mr. Black-lock, Ibid. xxxvi. 92.

† Case by Ollivier in Archives Gén. de Méd. ix. 100; also one by Mr. Valentine, Edin. Med. and Surg. Journal, xiv. 471.

‡ Case by Fontenelle, Arch. Gén de Méd v. 345; also Hodgson's Trial.

§ Hodgson's Trial; also Orfila, Tox. Gén. i. 263 : and Mr. Valentine's 5th case, the only survivor.

‖ Hodgson's Trial ; also Mr. Buchanan's case in Lond. Med. Repos. xix. 374.

burning in the throat often continue throughout the whole duration of the poisoning; and may be so excessive as to cause complete inability to swallow,[*] or even to speak.[†] Occasionally the affection of the throat is the only material injury inflicted by the poison, as in a case related by Dr. J. Johnstone of a young woman, who tried to swallow two drachms of corrosive sublimate in the solid state, but was unable to force it down on account of the constriction it caused in the gullet. She died in six days of mortification of the throat.[‡] The greater violence of the action of corrosive sublimate on the throat, compared with that of arsenic, is evidently owing to its greater solubility and powerful chemical operation on the animal textures.

Fourthly, instead of the contracted ghastly countenance observed in cases of poisoning with arsenic (but which, it will be remembered, is not invariable in that kind of poisoning), those who are suffering under the primary effects of corrosive sublimate have frequently the countenance much flushed, and even swelled.[§]

Corrosive sublimate seems to occasion more frequently than arsenic the discharge of blood by vomiting and purging, — obviously because it is a more powerful local irritant.

It likewise gives rise more frequently to irritation of the urinary passages. This irritation generally consists in frequent, painful micturition; but the secretion of urine is often suppressed altogether. Instances of this kind have been related by Mr. Valentine,[‖] by my colleague, Professor Syme,[¶] by an anonymous writer in the Medical and Physical Journal,[**] by Dr. Venables,[††] by Mr. Blacklock,[‡‡] and by M. Ollivier, in whose case, however, the poison was the bicyanide of mercury.[§§] In the last three cases the suppression was total, and continued till death; which did not ensue, in one till eight, in the next till five, and in the last till nine days after the poison was taken. Sometimes, as in Ollivier's case, the urinary irritation is attended with symptoms of excitement of the external parts, such as swelling and blackness of the scrotum and erection of the penis.

Another distinction seems to be that corrosive sublimate is more apt than arsenic to cause nervous affections during the first inflammatory stage. The tendency to doze, which sometimes interrupts the inflammatory symptoms caused by arsenic, has been more frequently observed in cases of poisoning with corrosive sublimate.[‖‖] The same may be said of tremors and twitches of the extremities. Sometimes the stupor approaches even to absolute coma;[¶¶] and the twitches occasionally amount to distinct, nay violent convulsions.[***] In other instances paraplegia has been witnessed.[†††]

* Mr. Valentine's Cases, Edin. Med. and Surg. Journal, xiv. 470.
† Mr. Anderson's case in Edin. Med. and Surg. Journal, xiv. 474.
‡ Essay on Mineral Poisons, p. 52.
§ Dumonceau in Journ de Med. lxix. 36; Orfila, Tox. Gén. i. 264; and Blacklock's case.

‖ Edin. Med. and Surg. Journal, xiv. 468.   ¶ Ibid. xliv. 26.   ** xli. 204.
†† London Medical Gazette, viii. 616.
‡‡ Edin. Med. and Surg. Journal, xxxvi. 92.   §§ Archives Gén. de Méd. ix. 99.
‖‖ Orfila, Tox. Gen. i. 265.   ¶¶ Mr. Valentine's cases.
*** Ollivier's case, and Fontenelle's.
††† Case by Devergie in Arch. Gén. de Méd. ix. 463.

Another difference is, that the effects of mercurial irritants are fully more curable than those of arsenic. Recovery has taken place even after half an ounce was swallowed, with the effect of inducing both bloody vomiting and purging.* This may depend in part on the greater solubility of mercurial preparations, so that they are more easily discharged than arsenic, which often remains in the stomach after days of continual vomiting, — and in part on corrosive sublimate and other soluble salts of mercury being converted, in no long time and much more easily, into comparatively innocuous compounds, either by antidotes intentionally given for the purpose, or by animal principles in the secretions and accidental contents of the alimentary canal.

Lastly, deviations from the ordinary course and combination of the symptoms appear to be more rare in the instance of corrosive sublimate than in that of arsenic.

To these general statements, it may be right to add the heads of one or two actual cases, lest an exaggerated idea be conveyed of the combination of the symptoms as they usually occur. For this purpose it will be sufficient to refer to a fatal case related by M. Devergie, to an instance of recovery, without salivation having supervened, which is contained in Orfila's Toxicology, and to another by Dr. Vautier, presenting the mildest possible symptoms of this variety. In Devergie's case, the patient, a female, swallowed three drachms of corrosive sublimate in solution, and was soon after seized with vomiting, purging, and pain in the belly. In five hours, when she was first seen by Devergie, the skin was cold and damp, the limbs relaxed, the face pale, the eyes dull, and the expression that of horror and anxiety. The lips and tongue were white and shrivelled; and she had dreadful fits of pain and spasm in the throat whenever she attempted to swallow liquids, also burning and pricking along the course of the gullet, and increase of pain in these parts on pressure. There was likewise frequent vomiting of mucous and bilious matter, with burning pain in the stomach and tenderness of the epigastrium on the slightest pressure. She had farther profuse diarrhœa, with pricking pain and tenesmus. The pulsation of the heart was deep and slow, the pulse at the wrist almost imperceptible, and the breathing much retarded. In eighteen hours these symptoms continued without any material change; but the limbs were also then insensible. In twenty-three hours she died in a fit of fainting, the mind having been entire to the last.† — Orfila's case was that of a gentleman who drank by mistake an alcoholic solution of corrosive sublimate, but fortunately was so much alarmed by its taste while drinking it, that he did not finish the poisonous draught. Nevertheless, he was instantly attacked with a sense of tightness in the throat and burning in the stomach, and then with vomiting and purging. Two hours after the accident Orfila found him with the face very full and red, the eyes sparkling and restless, the pupils contracted, and the lips dry and cracked. There was also acute pain along the whole

* Houlston, in London Med Journal, vi. 271.
† Arch. Gén. de Méd. ix. 463.

course of the alimentary canal, particularly in the throat.   The belly was swelled, and so tender that he could not bear the weight of fo-mentation-cloths.   The pulse was 112, small and sharp; the skin intensely hot and pungent; micturition scanty, frequent, and difficult; the breathing very much oppressed ; the purging bilious.   The pa-tient had likewise a tendency to doze, and was affected with occa-sional convulsive twitches of the face and extremities, and with con-stant cramps in the limbs.   Next morning all the symptoms were sensibly mitigated; and they went on decreasing till convalescence was established in eight days.   In the course of a few weeks he re-covered his usual health, without suffering salivation.* — In Vautier's case, where sixteen grains had been swallowed, the patient was im-mediately attacked with pain in the throat and stomach, cold extre-mities, trembling of the arms and legs, vomiting, paleness of the fea-tures, and great feebleness of the pulse.   Vomiting being promoted by frequent draughts of warm water, and white of egg given subse-quently, no further symptoms ensued, those first excited slowly sub-sided, and in a few days recovery took place, without any salivation. Yet it was upwards of half an hour before any measures could be taken for his relief.†

The only material and common symptom which was wanting in the case now related was blood in the stools and in the matter vomit-ed.   In other respects they are good examples of the ordinary train of symptoms in cases of the present variety.   For other examples of the same nature the reader may refer particularly to the paper of Mr. Valentine, who has described five cases that happened at one time in the same family, the mother having attempted to poison herself and four children.‡

It may sometimes be necessary to know the usual duration of this variety of mercurial poisoning, and also the extremes of its duration. On these points I have not hitherto had opportunities of consulting a sufficient number of cases to be able to lay down the general rule with precision.   But, so far as my inquiries go, the ordinary dura-tion in fatal cases is from twenty-four to thirty-six hours.   It is pro-bable that a few may last three days,§ but only one instance has come under my notice where the duration was greater; and in that instance, which is described by Dr. Venables, life was prolonged under great agony from pain of the belly, bloody vomiting, diarrhœa and suppression of urine, but without salivation, for no less than eight days.‖   In cases of recovery the symptoms of irritation may continue very long, and nevertheless not pass into the second variety of this kind of poisoning, — a transition, however, which on the whole is uncommon.   In the case of which an analysis has been given from Orfila's narrative, and likewise in one of Mr. Valentine's patients who recovered, the symptoms all along were those of irritation in the

* Toxicol. Gén. i. 263.   † Journal de Chimie Médicale, 1842, p. 294.
‡ Edin. Med. and Surg. Journal, xiv. 468.
§ Mr. Valentine's 4th case.
‖ London Medical Gazette, viii. 616.

alimentary canal ; there was not any ptyalism, or other symptom of proper mercurial erethysm. — The shortest duration yet recorded is two hours and a half. This was in a case related by Dr. Bigsby of Newark-on-Trent, where a tea-spoonful of a concentrated solution of nitrate of mercury was swallowed by a lad sixteen years old, and were the chief symptoms were burning pain from the mouth to the stomach, tenderness of the whole belly, mucous vomiting, and feculent purging.* In a case which occurred in London, and which has been published succinctly by Mr. Illingworth, death must have occurred either as soon, or very shortly afterwards. The dose of corrosive sublimate, though not positively ascertained, was large.† Next to this the shortest case recorded proved fatal in eleven hours.‡

2. The second variety of poisoning with mercury comprehends the cases, which begin, like the former, with irritation in the alimentary canal, but in which the symptoms of what is called mercurial erethysm gradually supervene. In fatal cases of this description death sometimes arises from the primary action of the poison, exactly as in the previous variety ; but in other instances it is owing to general disturbance of the constitution, or the local devastation, brought on by the secondary effects.

It is unnecessary to describe here the several forms of mercurial erethysm which may thus be developed, because they will immediately be considered under the third variety of mercurial poisoning. It is sufficient to state in passing that the leading affection is inflammation of the organs in and adjoining the mouth, and more particularly of the salivary glands.

But it may be right to endeavour in the present place to fix the period of the poisoning at which these secondary affections may and usually do commence. This cannot be done so satisfactorily as might be wished, because the cases already published which I have been able to examine do not form a large enough induction. Among the recorded cases I have hitherto seen, salivation has never been retarded beyond the third day ;§ but in an instance of suicide by corrosive sublimate which happened in the Castle of Edinburgh in 1826, and which was communicated to me by the late Dr. Shortt, the salivation did not begin till the fourth. Salivation seldom comes on sooner than the beginning of the second ;‖ and the most usual date of its commencement is towards the close of the second day. There is little doubt that it may be retarded till a period considerably later than I have yet found recorded. It is doubtful whether true mercurial salivation ever begins much sooner than after the first twenty-four hours. Occasionally, however, corrosive sublimate produces salivation of a different kind, which has been mistaken for the specific variety caused by mercury. Thus in a paper on the cure of gonor-

* London Medical Gazette, vii. 329.
† Ibidem, 1842-43, i. 556.   ‡ Mr. Valentine's case 1st.
§ Case in Med. and Phys. Journal, xli.
‖ Case by Dr. Anderson in Edin. Med. and Surg. Journal, vii. 437.

rhœa by corrosive sublimate in single large doses, communicated by Mr. Addington of West Bromwich to Dr. Beddoes, it is stated that a grain and a half, taken at once in half an ounce of rectified spirit, causes immediately " a great burning in the throat and stomach, and quickly afterwards a copious salivation, lasting between an hour and a half and two hours, and amounting frequently to more than a quart."* These facts have been appealed to by authors in medical jurisprudence as proving the rapid production of mercurial salivation. But the effect produced is not the specific ptyalism of mercury ; for its brief duration is scarcely consistent with this supposition. And farther, the author goes on to observe, that, if the dose be taken on going to bed, the latter part of the night is passed quietly, and no inconvenience is felt afterwards, even when the dose is taken five or six times at intervals of three or four days. The effects here observed is a sympathetic phenomenon depending on the topical action of the poison. And such, I have no doubt, has been the nature of the salivation in several cases of poisoning with corrosive sublimate, which have been supposed to be at variance with the general rule, that this affection does not begin till about twenty-four hours have elapsed. Such seems to have been the nature of the salivation in a case published by Dr. Perry,† that of a girl who was attacked with swelling of the cheeks and lower lip, burning in the throat, flushed face, feeble, pulse, and cold, clammy extremities after swallowing corrosive sublimate, and who had a copious flow of saliva in an hour and a half ; for there is no mention made of fetor, and the girl was well enough to leave the hospital in a few days, — which could scarcely happen if she had been affected with ptyalism from the constitutional action of mercury. — In like manner Dr. Alexander Wood has related a case, fatal in fourteen days, in which the patient said salivation came on in seven hours.‡ But, notwithstanding Dr. Wood's argument in support of the patient's statement, — for he did not see him till nine days after the poison was taken, — there is no satisfactory evidence that the salivation was the true constitutional salivation of mercury, and not simply the result of its topical action, which seems to have been very severe. — Farther, in an instance related by Dr. H. Anderson of Belfast, where salivation appeared to him to begin in nineteen hours, it seems not improbable that he mistook for mercurial ptyalism the common salivation arising from inability to swallow on account of sore throat ; for this patient too was quite convalescent in three days.§ — Mr. Alfred Taylor alludes to a case in Guy's Hospital of salivation occurring in four hours ; but so briefly, that its true influence on the present question cannot be judged of.‖ — On the whole, then, although it is clear that ptyalism of one kind or another may occur very soon after corrosive sublimate is swallowed, it remains a matter of doubt, whether the true, specific ptyalism, depending on the con-

* Beddoes' Contributions to Physical and Medical Knowledge, 1799, p. 231.
† London Medical Gazette, 1842-43, i. 941.
‡ Edinburgh Med. and Surg. Journal, li. 114.   § Ibidem, xiv. 474.
‖ Manual of Medical Jurisprudence, 162.

stitutional action of the poison begins sooner than after an interval of above twenty-four hours.

As to the total duration of this variety in fatal cases, I have found an instance fatal on the fourth day, salivation having begun on the second;* and Orfila quotes a case from Degner, in which the gastro-enteritic symptoms were succeeded by ptyalism about the same period, and which proved fatal in fifteen days.† These periods, however, probably do not form the extremes; for in such cases as the former death is the consequence of the primary affection, and may therefore ensue immediately after the secondary stage has begun to develope itself; and when death arises from profuse salivation, as in Degner's patient, or from the ravages committed by ulceration and gangrene, it may be delayed almost as long as in cases of the third variety of mercurial poisoning, in which there is no precursory stage of inflammation in the alimentary canal.

Death may arise, not only from the primary action of the poison, or from the exhaustion caused by mercurial erethysm, but likewise from incidental occurrences. Thus, in Dr. Alexander Wood's case, referred to above, death arose directly from sudden profuse hemorrhage from the bowels, to the amount of six pounds.

The present variety of poisoning with corrosive sublimate may be concluded with the heads of an excellent example related in the Medical and Physical Journal. The patient, a stout young girl, swallowed soon after supper a drachm of corrosive sublimate dissolved in beer, and in a few minutes she was found on her knees in great torture. All the primary symptoms of this kind of poisoning were present in their most violent form, — burning in the stomach, extending towards the throat and mouth, followed in no long time by violent vomiting of a matter at first mucous, afterwards bilious and bloody; by purging of a brownish, fetid fluid; suppression of urine and much tenderness of the urethra and bladder; small, contracted, frequent pulse, anxious countenance, and considerable stupor, interrupted frequently by fits of increased pain. All these symptoms were developed in four hours. Subsequently the pain in the stomach became much easier, but that in the throat much worse. At length in the course of the second day, the teeth became loose, the gums tender, the saliva more abundant than natural; profuse ptyalism and great fetor of the breath ensued, and the patient expired towards the close of the fourth day.‡

3. The third variety of poisoning with mercury comprehends all the forms of what is called mercurial erethysm. Without endeavouring to settle the precise meaning of this term, which is now used in rather a vague sense, I shall consider under the present head all the secondary and chronic effects of mercury. These may be caused by any of its preparations, but are most frequently seen as

* Lond. Med. and Phys. Journal, xli.
† Toxic. Générale, i. 282, from Degneri Historia Med. de Dysent. Bilios. Contag. 250.
‡ Lond Med. and Phys. Journal, xli. 204.

the consequence of its milder compounds, either given medicinally in frequent small doses, or applied continuously to the bodies of workmen who are exposed by their trade to its fumes.

The secondary and chronic effects of mercury are multifarious enough in reality ; but if credit were given to all that has been written, and is still sometimes maintained on this subject, almost every disease in the nosology might be enumerated under the present head ; for there is scarcely a disease of common occurrence, which has not been imputed by one author or another to the direct or indirect operation of mercury. The present remarks, however, will be confined as much as possible to what is well ascertained, and bears on the medical evidence of poisoning with mercury, or is important in regard to medical police. With this view, salivation and its concomitants, the most usual of the secondary effects of mercury, will first be treated of. Some observations will then be made on the shaking palsy, or mercurial tremor, which is caused in those who work with mercury. And in conclusion, a short view will be taken of the other diseases which are more indirectly induced by this poison, as well as some which have been ascribed to it on insufficient grounds. This being done, the mode of action of mercurial poisons will be resumed, and a description given of their relative effects when introduced by different channels and in different chemical forms.

Of Mercurial Salivation. — Mercurial salivation may be caused by any of the preparations of mercury, and either by a single dose or by frequently repeated small doses. It may be caused by corrosive sublimate as the secondary stage of a case which commenced with inflammation in the alimentary canal ; or it may be the first sign of mercurial action, as in the medicinal mode of administering calomel and blue pill. Even in the latter case a single dose, and that not large, may be sufficient to induce pytalism of the most violent kind. When induced by a single dose it usually commences between the beginning of the second and end of the third day, rarely within twenty-four hours. But an extraordinary case is mentioned by Dr. Bright, where five grains, put on the tongue in apoplexy and not washed over, excited in three hours most violent salivation, with such swelling of the tongue that scarifications became necessary.* It commences with a brassy taste and tenderness of the mouth, swelling, redness, and subeequently ulceration of the gums ; peculiar fetor of the breath ; and at last an augmentation is observed in the flow of the saliva, commonly accompanied with fulness around the lower jaw. These symptoms increase more or less rapidly. Sometimes they are very mild ; nay, this form of the secondary effects of mercury may consist in nothing else than brassy taste, tenderness of the mouth, redness of the gums, and fetor. On the other hand, the symptoms are often very violent, the salivation being profuse, the face swelled so as to close the eyes, and almost fill up the space between the jaw and clavicles, the tongue swollen so as to threaten

* Reports of Medical Cases, ii. 337.

30

suffocation, the inside of the mouth ulcerated, nay gangrenous, and at times the gangrene extends over the face. It is not uncommon to observe severe and extensive ulceration without particular increase of the saliva.

These local affections are almost always accompanied with more or less constitutional disorder. If severe, they are attended with the symptomatic fever proper to inflammation and gangrene, from whatever cause they spring. But independently of that, mercurial salivation is accompanied, and indeed commonly preceded, by a constitutional disorder or symptomatic fever of its own, which occasionally exhibits some peculiarities. The mildest affection of the mouth and salivary glands is very generally preceded by some exaltation of the pulse and temperature, and other symptoms of fever. But when the local disorder begins violently, and above all when this takes place by idiosyncrasy from small doses of mild preparations, there is often great rapidity of the pulse, irregular action of the heart, and various nervous disorders possessing the hysteric character, — all of which, except the quick pulse, will sometimes gradually abate or even disappear, when the salivation is fairly established.

The phenomena of ordinary mercurial salivation being familiar to every practitioner, it is unnecessary to quote here any illustrative example; but the following instance may be given to exemplify its most malignant forms. A patient of Mr. Potter of Chipping-Ongar, in Essex, after taking eighteen grains of blue pill in divided doses during three days, was seized with excessive salivation and great constitutional disturbance, indicated by offensive evacuations, copious sweating, bleeding from the nose, purple spots on the skin, dilated pupils, and such severe local disease that the teeth dropped out, and he expired six days after mercurial action set in.[*]

As the phenomena of mercurial salivation have been often known to lead to important evidence and much contrariety of opinion upon trials, it will be necessary to dwell at some length on some parts of the subject.

In the first instance, then, the dose which is required to bring on salivation may be noticed. It is needless to mention the ordinary quantity required in mercurial courses. A more useful object of consideration is the departure from the ordinary rule. One of the most common and important of these deviations is excessive sensibility to the action of mercury, in consequence of which the individuals who have this idiosyncrasy may be profusely salivated by one or two small doses even of the mildest preparations. Three grains of corrosive sublimate divided into three doses have caused violent ptyalism.[†] Fifteen grains of blue pill, taken in three doses, one every night, have excited fatal salivation.[‡] Nay, two grains of calomel have caused ptyalism, extensive ulceration of the throat, exfoliation of the lower jaw, and death.[§] Three drachms of mercurial ointment

* Lancet, 1838-39, i. 215.
† M. Colson in Arch. Gén. de Méd. xii. 84.
‡ Dr. Ramsbotham in Lond. Med. Gazette, i. 775.
§ Dr. Crampton, Trans. Dublin College of Physicians, iv. 91.

applied externally have caused violent ptyalism and death in eight days. On the other hand, it is well known that some constitutions resist the action of mercurials very obstinately, so as even sometimes to appear incapable of being salivated at all. I have more than once met with cases of the last description, where mercurial courses had been continued for three months and upwards without avail. It may be added, that, except in constitutions naturally predisposed to suffer from a few small doses, a few large doses do not appear apt to excite severe salivation, or even to cause any at all. This has been clearly shown in the course of the practice lately introduced of administering calomel in doses of a scruple. On that subject more will be said by and by. At present I may mention, that, in conformity with the practice alluded to, I have several times, in various diseases, given eight or ten grains of calomel five or six times a day for two or three days together, without observing that ptyalism was apt to ensue.

The next point to be considered is, whether mercurial salivation can be confounded with any other affection. In a very difficult case of poisoning which was tried here in 1817, that of William Patterson for murdering his wife,* it appeared probable that he had given her repeatedly large doses of calomel. But the proof of this was circumstantial only, and an important circumstance in the chain of evidence was a deposition to the occurrence of salivation during the woman's illness. This fact, however, rested on the skill and testimony of a quack-doctor only ; and the admissibility of such a person to decide on a point of this nature, will depend on the facility with which the true mercurial form of salivation can be recognised. This statement will show the practical object of what is to follow.

Many other causes may excite a preternatural flow of saliva. Several other poisons may have that effect, for example, preparations of gold, preparations of copper, antimony, croton-oil, and foxglove : foxglove has been known to cause violent salivation for three weeks.† Opium too has occasionally excited salivation,‡ and also hydrocyanic acid and iodide of potassium.

Even a common sore throat, if the swelling and pain are so great as to render swallowing very difficult and distressing, may be accompanied, as every physician must have remarked, with a profuse flow of saliva ; and in the ulcerative stage there is also often a fetor that is hardly distinguishable from the mercurial kind. In the ulceration of the mouth called *cancrum oris* there is some salivation with great fetor of the breath.

Salivation likewise forms an idiopathic disease, and may then be both profuse and obstinate. Mr. Davies has described a case of spontaneous ptyalism which had lasted for a fortnight before he was called to see the patient ; and during all that time the quantity of saliva discharged was two or three pints daily. How long it endured afterwards he does not mention ; but it must have continued for some time, because during his attendance first one physician and

---

* See page 335.   † Rust's Magazin, xxv. 578.
‡ Journal der Praktischen Heilkunde, ix. ii. 201.

then another were called into consultation with him. Laxatives slowly removed it. Mr. Davies has not described the state of the mouth ; but the first physician mistook the salivation for a mercurial one.* In the same journal which contains this case another has been related which lasted four months.† Another very remarkable case has been recorded by Mr. Power. The patient, a young lady, discharged for more than two years from sixteen to forty ounces of saliva daily. In the last two cases the mouth was not affected.‡ Two other instances have been related by M. Bayle, in one of which the patient was cured after spitting five pounds daily for nine years and a half; while the other continued to be affected after spitting profusely for three years. In neither was there any ulceration of the mouth.§ An instance has been related by an Italian physician, Dr. Petrunti, where, in the course of various nervous affections of the hysteric character, the patient became affected with heat and tightness in the throat, and so profuse a salivation for two months, that between three and four pounds were discharged daily.|| A case somewhat similar is related in Rust's Magazin of a man who suffered upwards of two years from a daily salivation alternating occasionally with a mucous discharge from the bowels or lungs.¶ M. Guibourt describes the case of a lady who had an attack of profuse salivation every thirty, forty, or fifty days, lasting between twenty-four and forty-eight hours, and unaccompanied with any other affection of the mouth or adjoining parts except a sense of tightness in the throat.** M. Gorham relates an interesting case of a lady who in three successive pregnancies was attacked soon after impregnation with excessive ptyalism, which continued to the extent of between two and four quarts daily until the period of quickening on two occasions, and on the third till her delivery ; but there was never any fetor or any affection of the gums.†† I have likewise met with a singular case where spontaneous ptyalism accompanied an ulcerated sore throat of the mercurio-syphilitic kind. The patient had taken mercury to salivation about six months before coming under my care, and got completely rid of both the sore throat and salivation. But the sore throat returned, together with the salivation, two months before I saw him, and the salivation continued for two months longer to the extent of twenty or even thirty ounces daily,—the ulcer of the throat during that interval being sometimes healed up, and again returning as severely as ever. In three weeks more the discharge rapidly diminished, and ceased. During all the time he was under my care there was no fetor of the breath, and no redness, ulceration, or sponginess of the gums. A singular account of an epidemic salivation which occurred in connection with a continued tertian fever,

* Lond. Med. and Phys. Journal, xxvi. 452.   † Ibid. xxvii. 275.

‡ Trans. Lond. Coll. Phys. i. 34.

§ Revue Medicale, 1828, iv. 76.

|| Ibidem, 1829, i. 467, from Osservatore Medico di Napoli, Febb. 1829.

¶ Dr. Tott, in Rust's Magazin für die gesammte Heilkunde, xxxv. 50.

** Journ. de Chem. Med. ix. 197.

†† London Medical Gazette, 1837-38, ii. 578.

has been given in an inaugural dissertation contained in one of Haller's Collections. The author, Quelmalz, says that the ptyalism sometimes continued for three weeks, that it was in one instance as great in extent as the most violent mercurial salivation, and that it was accompanied by fetor, superficial ulceration of the mouth, pustules on the tongue, relaxation of the gums, and looseness of the teeth.*

Salivation may likewise be produced by the influence of the imagination. I have seen a singular example of this. A woman who had a great aversion to calomel was taking it with digitalis for a dropsical complaint. Some one having told her what she was using, she immediately began to complain of soreness of the mouth, salivated profusely, and even put on the expression of countenance of a salivating person, although she had taken only two grains. On being persuaded, however, that she had been misinformed, the discharge ceased gradually in the course of one night. Two days afterwards she was again told on good authority that calomel was contained in her medicines, upon which the salivation began again and was profuse. It did not last above twenty-four hours; but the symptoms during that period resembled a commencing mercurial salivation in every thing but the want of fetor and redness of the gums.

In general, mercurial salivation may be easily distinguished from all the preceding varieties by an experienced practitioner. If its progress has been traced from the first appearance of brassy taste and fetor to the formation of ulcers and supervention of ptyalism, no attentive person can run any risk of mistaking it. Its characters are also quite distinct at the time salivation just begins. The fetor of the breath and sponginess and ulceration of the gums at this stage distinguish it from every other affection. But if the state of the mouth is not examined till the ulcers have existed several days, the characters of the mercurial disorder are much more equivocal. They cannot be distinguished, for example, from some forms of idiopathic ulceration of the mouth connected with unsoundness of the constitution, and characterized by extensive sloughing, ptyalism, and gangrenous fetor.† In particular they cannot be distinguished from the effects of the disease called *cancrum oris*. A few years ago indeed a London physician was charged, in consequence of this resemblance, with having killed, by mercurial salivation, a patient to whom it was proved that he had not given a particle of mercury, and who clearly died of the disease in question;‡ and a similar case, where fatal mercurial salivation was suspected, but which was clearly proved on a Coroner's Inquest to have been also a case of cancrum oris, has been more lately published by Mr. Dunn.§

For distinguishing these and such other affections from mercurial

* De Ptyalismo Febrili. Diss. Inaug. Lipsiæ, in Halleri Disput. de Morb. Histor. i. 469.

† See Evidence of Mr. Bromfield on the Trial of Miss Butterfield for the murder of Mr. Scawen, p. 40.

‡ London Medical Gazette, 1839-40, ii. 875.

§ Lancet, 1843-44, i. 60.

30*

salivation Dr. Davidson of Glasgow has lately proposed a character, the exact scope of which cannot yet be appreciated, — namely, that in true mercurial salivation there is never any sulphocyanic acid in the saliva; so that sesquichloride of iron does not render it red. The presence of sulphocyanic acid may possibly prove that salivation is not mercurial; but the converse does not hold good, because other causes tend to deprive human saliva of its sulphocyanic acid.[*]

The next point to be noticed regarding mercurial salivation is, that a long interval may elapse after the administration of the mercury has been abandoned, before the effect on the salivary glands and mouth begins, — mercury in small doses being what is called a cumulative poison, or a poison whose influence accumulates silently for some time in the body before its symptoms break forth. Swédiaur has met with instances where the interval was several months,[†] Cullerier with a case in which it was three months.[‡] It will at once be seen how strongly such facts may bear on the evidence in a criminal case, where the administration of mercury in medicinal doses, which have been long abandoned, is brought forward to account for salivation, appearing weeks or months after, and giving rise, in conjunction with other circumstances, to a suspicion of mercurial poisoning of more recent date.

Another question which has been made the subject of discussion is the duration of mercurial ptyalism. The medical witness may be required to give his opinion how long this affection may last after the administration of mercury has been abandoned. The present question may be cut short by stating, that there appears to be hardly any limit to its possible duration. Linnæus met with an instance of its continuing inveterately for a whole year;[§] Swédiaur says he has known persons languish for months and years from its effects;[‖] and M. Colson knew an individual who had been salivated for six years.[¶] These, however, are very rare incidents. After an ordinary mercurial course the mouth and salivary glands generally return to the healthy state in the course of a fortnight or three weeks.

A fifth question, whether the ptyalism, or, speaking in general terms, the erethysm of mercury, is susceptible of a complete intermission, formed a material subject of inquiry, and the cause of much contradictory statement on a noted criminal trial, that of Miss Butterfield in 1775 for the murder of her master, Mr. Scawen. She was accused of administering corrosive sublimate; and it was alleged in her defence, that the salivation and consequent sloughing of which he died might have arisen, without the fresh administration of mercury, from the renewal of a previous ptyalism, which had been brought on by a common mercurial course, and had ceased two months before the second salivation began. It appeared that Mr. Scawen was salivated with a quack medicine from the beginning till

[*] London Medical Gazette, 1841-42, i. 338.
[†] Swediaur on Venereal Diseases, ii. 251.
[‡] Colson in Arch. Gén. de Méd. xii. 99.   [§] Flora Suecica.
[‖] On the Venereal Disease, ii. 143.
[¶] Colson in Arch. Gén. de Méd. xii. 99.

the middle of April ; and that about the middle of June he was again seized with violent salivation, of which he died. It was rendered very improbable, that during the interval between the two salivations any more mercury had been taken medicinally. The question then was, whether the original ptyalism could have reappeared after so long an interval, without the fresh administration of mercury? The witnesses for the prosecution, gentlemen in extensive practice, said it could not. 'But one of the prisoner's witnesses, Mr. Bloomfield of the London Lock Hospital, said he had repeatedly known salivation reappear after a long intermission; that it was quite common for hospital patients to have a second salivation, when thought well enough to go out the next dismissal day ;* that in one case the interval was three months ; and that one of his patients was attacked periodically with salivation at intervals of six weeks or a month for a whole year. Mr. Howard, another surgeon of the Lock Hospital, deposed to the same effect ; and the prisoner was acquitted, apparently upon their evidence.†

Notwithstanding what was said by these gentlemen, I believe the recurrence of mercurial salivation after so long an interval, without the repetition of mercury, is exceedingly rare. Dr. Gordon Smith, in alluding to the trial of Miss Butterfield, has mentioned a case which occurred to the late Dr. Hamilton of this University, and used to be related by him in his lectures. The interval was so great as four months.‡ Mr. Green of Bristol has lately described another unequivocal case, where the interval was six weeks.§ Dr. Mead says he met with an instance where the interval was six months;‖ and Dr. Male mentions another where mercury brought on moderate salivation in March, and after a long interval excited a fresh salivation in October, of which his patient died in a few weeks.¶ M. Louyer-Villermé met with a case, where, in consequence of exposure to cold, a sudden attack of salivation was caused a twelvemonth after the removal of syphilis by mercury.** Some other cases not less wonderful have been recorded by M. Colson in his paper on the effects of mercury. He quotes Dr. Fordyce for the case of a man who had repeated attacks of salivation, with metallic taste, which lasted for three weeks, although mercury had not been taken for twelve years ; and Colson himself knew a surgeon who had a regular and violent attack of all the symptoms of mercurialism eight years after he had ceased to take mercury.†† It is impossible to attach credit to such marvellous stories as the last two. Granting the ptyalism to be really mercurial, it would require much better evidence than any practitioner could procure, to determine the fact that mercury had not been given again during the supposed interval. This objection indeed will apply more or less even to the instances where the alleged interval did not exceed a few months.

* The exact time is not mentioned.
† Trial by Gurney and Blanchard, pp. 39, 47.
‡ Principles of Forensic Medicine, 2d Ed. 118.
§ Trans. of the Prov. Med. and Surg. Association, ii. 262.
‖ Mead's Medical Works, p. 202.   ¶ Male's Juridical Medicine, 89.
** Archives Gén. de Méd. xl. 254.   †† Ibid. xii. 100.

The last point to be noticed regarding mercurial salivation is the manner in which it proves fatal. Death may ensue from the mildest preparations, and from the smallest doses, in consequence of severe salivation being produced by them in peculiar habits. Two instances have been already mentioned which illustrate both of these statements, and others might easily be referred to were the fact not familiar.

Death may be owing to a variety of causes. Some of those which have been assigned are direct and unquestionable in their operation; others indirect and more doubtful.

The most direct and obvious manner is by extensive spreading gangrene of the throat, mouth, face, and neck. The late happy changes, introduced into the treatment of syphilis and other diseases which are benefited by mercury, render this mode of death rare in the present day. Yet I may mention that I have seen an example of it in a woman who was salivated to death, because her medical attendant, a firm believer in the powers of mercury as an antidote, forgot that the antidote is itself a poison, if not given in moderation. In general, when gangrene is the cause of death, it begins within the mouth or in the throat, and spreads from that till it even reaches the face. But sometimes it begins at once on the external surface, at a distance from the primary ulcers. An example of such a progress of the symptoms has been related by Dr. Grattan. A child ten years old was violently salivated by twenty grains of calomel given in six days. On the fifth day of the salivation, a little vesicle appeared on the skin near the mouth on each side, and was the commencement of a gangrenous ulcer, which spread over the whole cheek, and proved fatal eight days after its appearance.*

Another cause of death appears to be exhaustion from profuse and protracted discharge of saliva, without material injury of the mouth or adjoining organs.

A third manner of death which I have witnessed is exhaustion from laryngeal phthisis; and from the circumstances of the case, I have little doubt but, in the state to which patients are then sometimes reduced, death may also take place suddenly from suffocation. My patient had undergone before I saw him five long salivations for a venereal complaint, and had latterly been attacked with symptoms of ulceration of the glottis. This affection went on slowly increasing, and he died of exhaustion after many weeks of suffering. During this period he was repeatedly attacked with alarming fits of suffocation, which were relieved by the hawking of mucous flakes. The symptoms were explained on dissection by the appearance of extensive ulceration and thickening of the glottis, and almost total destruction of the epiglottis.

The other causes of death are more indirect, and will be mentioned presently. They depend on the pre-existence of other diseases, on which mercury acts deleteriously during the state of erethysm excited by it in the constitution.

Of Mercurial Tremor. — The second division of the secondary

----
* Trans, Dublin Coll. Physicians, iii. 236.

effects of mercury comprehends the palsy or tremor, with the collateral disorders induced in miners, gilders, and other workmen, whose trade exposes them to the operation of this poison. Under the present head, which might be treated at considerable length as an important branch of medical police, I shall confine myself chiefly to an analysis of an interesting essay by Mérat on the *Tremblement Metallique*, and to some remarks by Jussieu on the health of the quicksilver miners of Almaden in Spain.

Mérat's account of the shaking palsy induced by mercury is very interesting.[*] The disease, he states, may sometimes begin suddenly; but in general it makes its approaches by slow steps. The first symptom is unsteadiness of the arms, then quivering, finally tremors, the several movements of which become more and more extensive till they resemble convulsions, and render it difficult or impossible for the patient to walk, to speak, or even to chew. All voluntary motions, such as carrying a morsel to the mouth, are effected by several violent starts. The arms are generally attacked first and also most severely. If the man does not now quit work, loss of memory, sleeplessness, delirium, and death ensue. But as the nature of the disease soon renders working almost impossible, he cannot well continue ; and in that case death is rare. The concomitant symptoms of the trembling are a peculiar brown tint of the whole body, dry skin, flatus, but no colic, no disorder of respiration, and, except in very old cases, no wasting or impaired digestion. The pulse is almost always slow. — This description agrees with a somewhat later account of the disease by Dr. Bateman, as he observed it in mirror-silverers ;[†] and also with some interesting cases recently published by Dr. Bright.[‡]

In general the tremors are cured easily, though slowly, several months being commonly required. One of Dr. Bright's patients got almost well in little more than a fortnight under the use of sulphate of zinc. Sometimes, however, the trembling is incurable.[§] I have said the disease is rarely fatal. Mérat quotes three cases only, in one of which death was owing to profuse salivation and gangrene, in the others to marasmus. On the whole, those who are liable to the shaking palsy do not appear liable to salivation. Yet the two affections are sometimes conjoined, as in three of the cases described by Dr. Bright, and in some noticed by Mr. Mitchell among the mirror-silverers of London.[‖] Gilders, miners, and barometer-makers are all subject to the disease. Even those who undergo mercurial frictions may have it, according to Mérat; and M. Colson, who confirms this statement, quotes Swédiaur as another authority for it.[¶] It is not merely long-continued exposure to mercurial preparations that causes the shaking palsy : a single strong exposure may be sufficient;

* Appendix to his Traité de la Colique Metallique, p. 275.
† Edin. Med. and Surg. Journal, viii. 376, and ix. 180.
‡ Reports of Medical Cases, ii. 495.
§ Fernelius, de Lues Ven. Curat. c. vii.
‖ London Med. and Phys. Journal, lxvii. 394.
¶ Arch. Gén. de Méd. xiv. 109.

and the same exposure may cause tremor in one and salivation in another.   Professor Haidinger of Vienna some time ago mentioned to me an accident a barometer-maker of his acquaintance met with, which illustrates both of these statements.   This man and one of his workmen were exposed one night during sleep to the vapours of mercury from a pot on a stove, in which a fire had been accidentally kindled.   They were both most severely affected, the latter with salivation, which caused the loss of all his teeth, the former with shaking palsy, which lasted his whole life.

In regard to all such workmen, it is exceedingly probable that with proper care the evils of their trade may be materially diminished. This appears at least to be the result of the observations made long ago by Jussieu on the miners of Almaden in La Mancha.   Most quicksilver mines are noted for great mortality among the workmen. But Jussieu maintains that the trade is not by any means so neces- sarily or so dreadfully unhealthy as is represented, or as it really is in some places.   The free workmen at Almaden, he says, by taking care on leaving the mine to change their whole dress, particularly their shoes, preserved their health, and lived as long as other people ; but the poor slaves, who could not afford a change of raiment, and who took their meals in the mine. generally without even washing their hands, were subject to swelling of the parotids, aphthous sore throat, salivation, pustular eruptions, and tremors.*

Of the indirect effects of mercurial erethysm. — The last division of the secondary effects of mercury relates to its indirect action when concurring with other diseases or predispositions to disease.

Of these effects there are some of which the poison appears to be the chief, if not even the sole cause.   Thus, during the symptomatic fever which precedes salivation there are sometimes remarked imita- tive inflammations, or coma, or affections of the heart, which go off as salivation is established.

Other effects require the distinct co-operation of collateral causes. Many inflammatory diseases, not easily excited in ordinary circum- stances, arise readily from improper exposures during salivation, for example dropsy, pneumonia, phrenitis, iritis, erysipelas, and various chronic eruptions.

Other effects again require the co-operation of disease, such as sloughing gangrene supervening on ordinary ulcers during the action of mercury, — a not uncommon accident.   This appears most likely to happen when the ulcers are constitutional.

Lastly, in conjunction with other diseased morbid actions, either going on at the same time, or immediately preceding mercurial ere- thysm, this poison is apt to occasion some modifications of disease which are rarely otherwise witnessed.   Modifications of the kind have already been traced in the instances of lues venerea and scro- fula ; but there is reason to believe that the same singular property may also exist in relation to other constitutional disorders.

These observations conclude the inquiry into the symptoms caused

* Mém. de l'Acad. des Sciences, 1719, p. 474.

in man by mercurial poisons generally. Returning now to its mode of action, we have to examine its relative effects through the different animal textures, and in its various chemical forms.

The result of the previous remarks as to its action on animals, it will be remembered, was, that its soluble preparations cause when swallowed corrosion of the stomach, and in whatever way it enters the body irritation of the stomach and rectum, inflammation of the lungs, depressed action and perhaps inflammation of the heart, oppression of the functions of the brain, and inflammation of the salivary glands. All of these effects have likewise been mentioned in the preceding sketch, as occurring in a greater or less degree in consequence of its operation on man.

Mercury acts as a poison on man in whatever way it is introduced into the body, — whether it be swallowed, or inhaled in the form of vapour, or applied to a wound, or even simply rubbed or placed on the sound skin. But the kind of action excited differs according to the channel by which it is introduced.

The most ordinary and dangerous cases of poisoning arise from the introduction of corrosive sublimate into the stomach. The poison then kills by corroding or inflaming the alimentary canal, or by causing salivation and its concomitants.

When applied to a wound or ulcer corrosive sublimate does not often occasion dangerous symptoms. Yet it is sometims a hazardous remedy. It is not a convenient escharotic even in a concentrated state ; for its escharotic action is not incompatible with its absorption ; at all events it certainly sometimes acts constitutionally through the surface of wounds and ulcers, and the symptoms brought on in this way are generally violent. They are the symptoms of mercurial salivation, accompanied at times with well-marked inflammation of the alimentary canal. When applied to sores in a diluted state it has also been known to cause dangerous effects if too long persevered in. A case of the kind has been related by Mr. Robertson, an army-surgeon. After anointing an itchy eruption of the arms for seven days with a solution of corrosive sublimate containing five grains to the ounce, his patient was attacked with fever, inflammation of the stomach and bowels, and in two days more with violent salivation.[*] A case of the same nature has been related by Mr. Sutleffe.[†] His patient, a child, in consequence of having an eruption of the head washed with a solution of corrosive sublimate, was attacked with violent salivation, which proved fatal in a few days. Pibrac has recorded three fatal cases from the free application of corrosive sublimate to ulcerated surfaces. One of these proved fatal in five days, another in twenty-four hours, and a third during the night after the poison was applied. The symptoms generally indicated violent action on the alimentary canal.[‡] In an instance mentioned by Degner, fatal in twenty-five days, there was also violent irritation

* Edin. Med. and Surg. Journal, viii. !95.
† London Medical Repository, xvi. 458.
‡ Mémoires de l'Acad. de Chirurgie, iv. 154.

of the stomach ; but the chief affection was excessive swelling of the face and throat, together with profuse ptyalism.*

One of the readiest modes of bringing the system under the poisonous action of mercury is by introducing its preparations into the lungs. It appears from some experiments by Schlöpfer that the fluid preparations act rapidly through the lining membrane of the air-passages. Six grains of corrosive sublimate in solution will thus kill a rabbit in five minutes.† But the effects of mercury through this channel are much better exemplified when its preparations are inhaled in the form of vapour. Corrosive sublimate when incautiously sublimed in chemical experiments has been known to cause serious effects. Dr. Coldstream of Leith informs me, that while subliming about twenty-four grains of it with the blowpipe when a student, he and several of his fellow-apprentices were seized with painful constriction of the throat, several had headache, and one had sickness and vomiting. The phenomena produced by the various preparations of mercury in more violent cases, are sometimes protracted tremors,‡ sometimes severe ptyalism and tedious dysentery,§ sometimes salivation and gangrene of the mouth ending fatally.‖ This last form was produced remarkably in a chimney-sweeper, after cleaning a gilder's chimney, during which operation he felt a disagreeable sense of tightness in the throat.

Several extraordinary instances have happened of poisoning from long-continued inhalation of the vapours which arise from metallic mercury. That vapours do arise from metallic mercury of the ordinary temperature of the atmosphere has been fully proved by Mr. Faraday ; who found, that when a bit of gold was suspended from the top of a phial, the bottom being covered with a little mercury, the gold soon became amalgamated.¶ The vapours thus discharged may produce the worst species of mercurialism, if they are diffused through an apartment insufficiently ventilated. One of the most striking examples known of the baneful effects of mercury thus gradually insinuated into the system, occurred in a well-known accident which befel the ships Triumph and Phipps. These vessels were carrying home in 1810 a large quantity of quicksilver saved from the wreck of a ship near Cadiz, when by some accident several of the bags were burst and the mercury spilled. On the voyage home the whole crews of both vessels were more or less severely salivated, two died, many were dangerously ill, all the copper articles on board became amalgamated, all the rats, mice, cockroaches, and other insects, as well as a canary-bird and several fowls, and all larger animals, such as cats, dogs, goats, and sheep were destroyed.**

The action of mercury is often violently excited when it is applied to the skin even not deprived of the cuticle. The effects of

* Wibmer. Die Wirkung der Arzneimittel und Gifte, iii. 46.
† Diss. Inaug. de Effectibus Liquidorum in vias aëriferas applicatorum, p. 35.
‡ Hufeland's Jour.al, xlii.   § Mr. Hill in Edin. Med. Ess. iv. 38.
‖ Corvisart's Journal, xxv. 209.   ¶ London Journal, of Science, x. 354.
** Edin. Med. and Surg. Journal, vi. 513, and London Medical and Physical Journal, xxvi. 29.

mercurial inunction form a well-known and satisfactory proof of this. Even without the aid of infriction, the soluble preparations of mercury will excite mercurial action by being put simply in contact with the skin. Thus it has been shown by a German physician, Dr. Guerard, that pytalism may be induced by a warm-bath of corrosive sublimate in the proportion of an ounce to 48 quarts of water, and that the effect commonly begins after the third bath with an interval of three days between them.* It is not so generally known that the more active preparations, such as corrosive sublimate or nitrate of mercury, may, like arsenic, cause through the sound skin effects almost as violent as through the alimentary canal. The following pointed illustration is related by Dr. Anderson. A gentleman affected with rheumatism, was persuaded by a friend to use a nostrum, which was nothing else than a solution of half a drachm of corrosive sublimate in an ounce of rum. This was rubbed on the affected part for several minutes before going to bed. Ere the friction was ended, he felt a sensation of heat in the part, to which, however, he paid little attention. But during the night he was attacked with pain in the stomach, sickness, and vomiting, and soon after with purging and tenesmus. In the morning Dr. Anderson found him very weak and vomiting incessantly. The arm up to the shoulder was prodigiously swelled, red, and blistered. Next day he complained of brassy taste and tenderness of the gums, and regular salivation soon succeeded.† Another case of much interest has been described by my colleague, Professor Syme, where a solution of the nitrate was rubbed by mistake upon the hip and thigh instead of camphorated oil. Intense pain immediately followed, and afterwards shivering; the urine was suppressed for five days, without any insensibility, and during its suppression urea was detected in the blood ; pytalism appeared on the third day, became very profuse, and was followed by exfoliation of the alveolar portion of the lower jaw, but recovery nevertheless slowly took place.‡

The mere carrying of mercurial preparations for a length of time near the skin, though not in direct contact with it, may be sufficient to induce the peculiar effects of the poison, as the following example will show. A man applied to a German physician, Dr. Scheel, affected with violent salivation evidently mercurial which proved fatal, but which it was impossible to trace to its real cause till after death, when a little leathern bag containing a few drachms of mercury was found hanging at his breast ; and it was then discovered that he had been in the practice of carrying this bag for six years as a protection against itch and vermin, and during that period had frequent occasion to renew the mercury.§

The effects of mercury as a poison differ with the chemical form in which it is introduced into the system.

In its metallic state it is probably inactive. This fact is a material

* Horn's Archiv für Medizinische Erfahrung, 1831, 519.
† Edin. Med. and Surg. Journal, vii. 437.　‡ Ibidem, xliv. 26.
§ Medizinisch-Chirurgische Zeitung, 1833, iv. 330.

31

one for the medical jurist to determine precisely; for running quicksilver has been given with a criminal intent. A case of the kind forms the subject of a medico-legal report in Pyl's Repertory;* and another is mentioned in Klein's Annals.†

It is well ascertained that large quantities of fluid mercury have been repeatedly swallowed, without any injury or peculiar effect having followed. In neither of the German cases now referred to was any bad effect produced; and it has proved equally harmless when given medicinally to remove obstruction in the intestines. Farther, M. Gaspard mentions in his paper quoted in a former page, that he has left large quantities shut up for many hours in the various cavities of the body in animals, without observing any other result than at times inflammation, which was evidently owing to the mere presence of a foreign body, and not to the action of an irritant poison.‡

It has been already stated, however, that the vapours of metallic mercury, even at the temperature of the air, produce mercurialism when inhaled. But then, in all likelihood, some of the metal is oxidated before being inhaled. At least the chemist knows that the surface of a mercurial trough soon tarnishes, especially when the mercury is not pure.

But it may be said that the blue ointment, which is made with running quicksilver, will not act as a mercurial when rubbed upon the skin. Here too, however, some oxidation takes place in the making of the ointment. Mr. Donovan endeavoured to prove that some of the mercury is always oxidated;§ and I have generally found a sufficient quantity of oxide to account for the effects.‖

It has been farther said, in proof of the poisonous action of quicksilver in its metallic state, — that patients, who have taken it for obstructed bowels, have sometimes been salivated. This accident has, I believe, happened in a few instances where the mercury was retained long in the body. But such cases are undoubtedly very rare. Zwinger mentions the case of a man, who took four ounces for colic, and was seized in seven days with salivation.¶ Laborde relates the particulars of another instance where seven ounces taken in fourteen days excited ptyalism, ulceration of the mouth, and great feebleness of the limbs.** In the days of Dr. Dover, when the administration of large doses of fluid mercury was a fashionable practice for a variety of purposes, it was alleged to have even sometimes proved fatal; and the case of an actor is specially mentioned, to whom, when convalescent from ague, Dover gave mercury to the amount of two pounds in five days, and who at the close of that period was seized with headache, colic, restlessness, and costiveness, proving fatal in two days; and the whole lower intestines were found black and

* Repertorium für die öffentl. und gerichtl. Arzneiwissenschaft, i. 223.
† Annalen der Gesetz-gebung, iii. 55.
‡ Journ. de Physiologie, i.
§ Annals of Philos. xiv. 241, 321.   ‖ See my Dispensatory, 1842, p. 500.
¶ Acta Naturæ Curiosorum, Dec. ii. Ann. vi. Obs. 231.
** Journal de Médecine, l. 3.

lined with minute metallic globules.* Perhaps then it must be admitted that fluid mercury is not altogether inactive, speaking medicolegally. But this admission is no argument in favour of the metal being physiologically a poison; because in the course of the cases referred to, a part is in all likelihood oxidated by the oxygen in the intestinal gases. It is said to have been taken in the dose of an ounce daily for nine months, without either good or harm resulting.†

The question regarding the poisonous qualities of running quicksilver was carefully investigated some years ago by the Berlin College of Physicians in a report on the case in Pyl's Repertory.‡ They observe that the opinion of Pliny, Galen, Hippocrates, Dioscorides, and many of the earlier moderns, including even Zacchias, had led to the popular belief in the deadly properties of fluid mercury; but that this belief is erroneous; for many surgeons, and among the rest Ambrose Paré, had given without injury to their patients several pounds of it to cure obstructed bowels; and in 1515 the Margrave of Brandenburg, overheated on his marriage night with love and wine, and rising to quench his thirst, drank by mistake a large draught of quicksilver without suffering any harm. Fallopius mentions that he had known instances of women swallowing pounds of mercury, for the purpose of procuring miscarriage, and who did not suffer any injury.§

The sulphurets of mercury, like the metal, are not possessed of any deleterious action on the animal body. Orfila found that half an ounce of the sulphuret, formed in a solution of corrosive sublimate by sulphuretted-hydrogen, and half an ounce or six drachms of cinnabar, had no effect whatever on dogs.‖ The sulphurets which have appeared injurious in the hands of Smith¶ and other previous experimentalists must therefore have been impure.

Of the compounds of mercury, the red-precipitate and Turbith-mineral act as irritants, besides possessing the property common to all mercurial compounds, of causing mercurial erethysm. But they are not escharotics, though generally termed such. That is, they do not chemically corrode the animal textures. The effects of red-precipitate have been variable. Mr. Allison relates the case of a girl who in a fit of jealousy swallowed thirty grains of it. Being immediately detected, an emetic was given, which operated freely, and subsequently the stomach-pump was used; but on neither occasion was any red powder brought away. She was attacked with burning pain in the stomach, which was removed by opium, and for a week she had a distaste for food, but no other symptom of consequence.**

* Dr. Sigmond in Lancet, 1837-38, i. 228, from Turner's Treatise on Diseases of the Skin.
† Ibidem, p. 227.
‡ I. 240.　　　　　　　　§ Opera Omnia, p. 729.
‖ Arch. Gén. de Médecine, xix. 330.
¶ Sur l'usage et les Abus des Caustiques. Paris, 1817. Quoted by Wibmer Smith found two drachms kill a dog when swallowed, and half a drachm proved fatal in two dogs when applied to a wound.
** Lancet, 1836-37, i. 401.

Mr. Brett has described a case, in which the symptoms were occasional vomiting, stupor, languid pulse, cold clamminess of the skin, afterwards severe cramps of the legs, tenderness of the abdomen, dysuria, and some purging, and on the third day ptyalism ; but the patient recovered.* M. Devergie has given a case somewhat similar, but without any ptyalism having followed the irritant effects of the poison.† In 1840 I was consulted on the part of the Crown in the case of a girl, who, there was every reason to suppose, had been killed in twelve hours by red-precipitate. The symptoms towards the close were pain in the throat, inability to swallow, vomiting, and excessive prostration ; extensive red patches were found on the villous coat of the stomach after death ; and I detected mercury in the solid contents and likewise in the inner coat of the stomach. The case did not go to trial, because, although a man by whom she was pregnant came under some suspicion, it rather appeared that the deceased had herself swallowed the poison with the view of inducing miscarriage. Dr. Sobernheim has given the particulars of the case of a young man who died from swallowing an ounce of red-precipitate. He suffered for some hours from vomiting, diarrhœa, pain in the stomach, tenderness of the belly, and colic ; next day he had no pain, but coldness, lividity, stiffness, and an imperceptible pulse; and he expired in thirty-three hours. The poison was found abundantly in the stomach and duodenum after death, and some grains of it rested upon little ulcers.‡ As to Turbith-mineral, two scruples will kill a cat in four hours and a half; and several instances of violent and even fatal poisoning with it are mentioned by the older modern authors.§

The white precipitate or chloride of mercury and ammonia is probably also irritant, though inferior in power to the preparations just mentioned. Two scruples given to a dog occasion vomiting, pain, and some diarrhœa; and cases are recorded of death in the human subject from less doses.‖ But there are no recent facts as to the activity of this compound, and the older cases, which would assign to it very great energy, are open to the objection that this preparation was in former times often impure.

The bichloride or corrosive sublimate is a powerful corrosive or irritant, according to the dose and state of concentration ; and it also excites mercurial erethysm in a violent degree. The nitrates too are corrosive, and not inferior in activity to the bichloride, as may be inferred from Dr. Bigsby's case, noticed at page 314.

The bicyanide or prussiate of mercury, from the researches of Ollivier, and an interesting case he has published of poisoning with it in the human subject, appears to resemble corrosive sublimate closely in all its effects, except that it does not corrode chemically. Twenty-three grains and a half proved fatal in nine days.¶ M. Thibert has described a case in which ten grains caused death in the same

* London Medical Gazette, xiii. 117.   † Cours de Médecine-Légale.
‡ Handbuch der Toxicologie, 1838, p. 250.
§ Wibmer. Die Wirkung der Arzneimittel und Gifte, iii. 66.
‖ Ibidem, iii. 647.
¶ Arch. Gén. ix. 102.

period of time.* The symptoms in both instances were those of severe irritation of the stomach, extensive inflammation of the organs in the mouth, and suppression of urine ; and in Thibert's case a small quantity of albuminous fluid was discharged from the bladder instead of urine.

The protochloride or calomel, and probably also the protoxide, are the most manageable of the preparations of mercury for inducing ptyalism. Calomel is also an irritant ; that is, it causes irritation and inflammation in the alimentary canal when swallowed. This part of its properties as a poison will require a word or two of explanation.

Calomel is universally employed as a laxative, but to secure this effect being produced it is commonly combined with other purgatives. When given alone a few grains will in some constitutions induce a violent hypercatharsis ; and larger, but still moderate, doses have with most people such a tendency to cause severe griping and diarrhœa as to have led to the practice of combining it with opium when the object is to salivate. These considerations clearly establish that calomel, in a moderate dose of five or ten grains, is an irritant.

It farther appears that in larger doses it is said to have occasionally produced very violent effects, nay, even death itself, by its irritant operation. Hoffmann has mentioned two instances where fifteen grains of calomel proved fatal to boys between the ages of twelve and fifteen. One of them had vomiting, tremors of the hands and feet, restlessness and anxiety, and died on the sixth day. The other, he merely mentions, died after suffering from extreme anxiety and black vomiting.† Another fatal case has been related by Ledelius in the German Ephemerides, which was caused by a dose of half an ounce taken accidentally. Vomiting soon ensued, and a sense of acridity in the throat; then profuse diarrhœa to the extent of twenty evacuations in the day ; next excessive prostration of strength and torpor of the external senses ; and death followed in little more than twenty-four hours.‡ Wibmer quotes Vigetius, an author of the beginning of last century, for a similar case, likewise fatal, which was occasioned by half an ounce, — also Hellweg, a writer of the previous century, for the case of a physician, who took an ordinary medicinal dose by way of experiment, and died in five hours under all the symptoms of violent irritant poisoning.§

These observations being kept in view, what explanation will the toxicologist give of the effects which in modern times have been ascribed to large doses of calomel ? It was stated not many years ago by several East India surgeons, apparently with the universal assent of their brethren in later times, that this drug in the dose of a scruple administered even several times a day, is not only not an

* Thibert, Anatomie Pathologique, extracted in the American Journal. of Med. Science, April, 1842, p. 490.
† De Medicamentis insecuris et infidis, in Oper. Omn. vi. 314.
‡ Miscellanea Curiosa, 1692. Dec. ii. Ann. x. p. 34.
§ Die Wirkung der Arzneimittel und Gifte, iii. 72.

31*

irritant, but even on the contrary a sedative ;* and that in some diseases, for example yellow fever, it has been given in the dose of five,
ten, or twenty grains, four or six times a day, till several hundred
grains were accumulated in the body, yet without causing hypercatharsis, nay, with the effect of checking the irritation which gives
rise to black vomit in yellow fever, and to the vomiting and diarrhœa observed in the cholera of the East.   It is quite impossible for
a European physician to doubt these statements ; for all practitioners
in hot climates concur in them, and now that analogous practices have
been transferred to Britain, repeated opportunities have occurred for
establishing the fidelity of the original reporters.   Some American
physicians, advancing beyond the Hindostan treatment, have since
given calomel in bilious fever in the dose of forty grains, one drachm,
two drachms, and even three drachms, repeatedly in the course
of twenty-four hours for several days together, — and with similar
phenomena.   In one instance 840 grains were given in the course of
eight days in these enormous doses.   The largest dose was three
drachms ; and it was followed by only one copious evacuation, and
that not till after the use of an injection.†   This practice appears
not to have been altogether unknown in former times.   Ledelius,
the author formerly quoted, states, that he had been accustomed to
give doses of a scruple, and that Zwölffer even gave a drachm in one
dose.‡

It must be also added, that while the facts quoted above from
Hoffmann, Ledelius, and others assign to single large doses a
powerful and dangerous irritant action, very different results have
been occasionally observed in recent times where even so large
a quantity as one or two ounces had been taken.   Thus, in the
case of a lady mentioned by Wibmer, who took by mistake the
enormous quantity of fourteen drachms, although acute pain in
the belly ensued, together with vomiting and purging, these symptoms were speedily subdued by oleaginous demulcents ; and after
a smart salivation, she recovered entirely in six weeks.§   Another case has been related by Mr. H. P. Robarts, where an
ounce was swallowed by a young lady by mistake for magnesia,
with no other effect than nausea at first, rather severe griping
and slight tenderness of the belly afterwards, and subsequently
languor, headache and indigestion ; yet the powder was retained
two hours.‖

It is impossible in the present place to enter into the physiological
action of calomel as a remedy ; but every one must be satisfied that,
with all which has been already written, much still remains to be
done before the facts now mentioned can be explained satisfactorily.
Can the violent effects described by Hoffmann, Ledelius and Hellweg

* Johnson on Tropical Climates. pp. 45, 151, 267. — Annesley on the Diseases of
India. — Musgrave on Mercury, in Edin. Med. and Surg. Journ. xxviii. 42.
† Dr. Fletcher. American Journal of Med. and Phys. Sciences, vii. 561.
‡ Miscellanea Curiosa, l. c.
§ Die Wirkung der Arzneimittel und Gifte, iii. 72.
‖ London Medical Gazette, 1837-38, ii. 610.

have arisen from the calomel having been imperfectly prepared
and adulterated with a little corrosive sublimate? Or may they be
explained by reference to the fact, that the presence of hydrochlorates
in solution, particularly hydrochlorate of ammonia, tends to convert
calomel into corrosive sublimate.* Mr. Alfred Taylor has made
some experiments, to show that the latter explanation will not
suffice.†

Meanwhile, taking the facts as they stand, it is plain that great
caution must be used in ascribing violent irritant properties generally,
or even symptoms of irritant poisoning in a particular case, to large
doses of calomel.

With the view of illustrating the importance of the preceding
observations, it may be useful to mention here the heads of a case
already briefly alluded to for another purpose, the trial of William Paterson for murder (319).‡ His wife during the month
previous to her death had two attacks of diarrhœa, with an interval of a fortnight between them. On the second occasion it became profuse and exhausting, but without any material pain or
considerable vomiting; looseness of the teeth and salivation ensued, and she died in nine days. On examination of the body,
the anus was found excoriated, the whole intestines checkered
with dark patches, and the stomach red, ulcerated, and spotted
with black, warty excrescences; but the late Dr. Cleghorn of
Glasgow could not detect any poison by chemical analysis. It
was proved that the prisoner, besides procuring, a few months
before his wife's death, a variety of poisons, such as hydrochloric
acid, cantharides, and arsenic, had also on different occasions
during her last illness purchased in a suspicious manner four
doses of calomel varying from 30 to 60 grains each. Among
the various ways in which he was charged with having poisoned
the deceased, that which was best borne out by the general as
well as medical facts consisted in his taking advantage of an existing inflammation of the mucous membrane of the bowels, —
whether arising from a natural cause or from poison it was in
this view of the case immaterial to inquire, — and keeping up and
aggravating the inflammation by purposely administering at intervals large doses of calomel. On the trial Dr. Cleghorn and
other witnesses gave their opinion that the doses purchased by
the prisoner, if administered, would cause the symptoms and
morbid appearances observed in the case. On the other hand,
the late Dr. Gordon deposed to the effect, that all the symptoms
of the case might arise under the operation of natural disease,
and that such doses of calomel were by no means necessarily injurious; the late Mr. John Bell deposed, that it had even been
given in much larger doses without injury; and the profession

* M. Mialhe in Annales de Chimie et de Physique, Juin, 1842.
† Manual of Medical Jurisprudence, p. 178.
‡ For the documents in this trial I am indebted to my late colleague Dr. Duncan,
Junior, who was concerned in it.

are now well aware, though not at the time of this trial, that in the very malady alleged by the prisoner to have carried off the deceased, namely dysentery, the administration of calomel in repeated large doses is accounted by many a proper method of cure. The doses purchased by the prisoner were considerably larger, it is true. But there was not any evidence of his having administered his purchases in single doses as he got them; and even though there had been evidence to that effect, it would not remove altogether the difficulty of deciding the question, as to the irritating action of calomel, on which the issue of the trial in one view of the case chiefly depended.

It is probable that all the compounds formed by corrosive sublimate with animal and vegetable substances are feebly poisonous, or at least very much inferior in activity to corrosive sublimate itself. This has been shown by Orfila to be the case with the compound formed by albumen. Sixty grains of this compound, being equivalent to nearly five grains of corrosive sublimate, produced no bad effect whatever on a dog or a rabbit.* The same has been satisfactorily proved by Taddei as to the compound formed by gluten. Twelve grains of corrosive sublimate decomposed by his emulsion of gluten had no effect whatever on a dog.† It is important to remark, however, that if there be an excess of the decomposing principle, so that the precipitate is party redissolved, the irritant action of the corrosive sublimate is not so much reduced, though it is still certainly diminished. Orfila has settled this point in regard to albumen.‡ The power of producing mercurial erethysm is possessed by all mercurial compounds whatever, and among the rest by the compounds now under consideration.§

The present section may now be concluded with a few remarks on the strength of the evidence derived from the symptoms which are produced by the compounds of mercury.

If the medical jurist should meet with a case of sudden death like that of the animals experimented on by Sir B. Brodie, the symptoms alone could not constitute any evidence of poisoning with corrosive sublimate. All he could say would be that this variety of poisoning was possible, but that various natural diseases might have the same effect. This feebleness in the evidence from symptoms, however, is of little moment; because the dose must be great to cause such symptoms, and little can be vomited before death ; so that the poison will be certainly found in the stomach.

Should the patient die under symptoms of general irritation in the alimentary canal, poisoning may be suspected. But it would be impossible to derive from them more than presumptive evidence. The suspicion must become strong, however, if the ordinary signs of irritation in the alimentaay canal are attended with the discharge of blood upwards and and downwards. And the presumption will, I appre-

* Toxicol. Gén. i. 310.
† Recherches sur un Nouvel Antidote contre le sublimé corrosif, p. 34.
‡ Toxicol. Gén. p. 311.   § Taddei, Recherches, &c. p. 92.

hend, approach very near to certainty, — at least of the administration of some active irritant poison, — if, at the moment of swallowing a suspected article, and but a short time before the symptoms of irritation began in the stomach and bowels, the patient should have remarked a strong, acrid, metallic taste, and constriction or burning in the throat.

When upon all these symptoms salivation is superinduced, the evidence of poisoning with corrosive sublimate or some other soluble salt of mercury is almost unequivocal. That is, if, after something has been taken which tasted acrid, and caused an immediate sense of heat, pricking, or tightness in the throat, the characteristic signs of poisoning with the irritants make their appearance in the usual time, and are soon after accompanied or followed by true mercurial salivation, — it may be safely inferred that some soluble compound of mercury has been taken. Before drawing this inference, however, it will be necessary to determine with precision all the classes of symptoms, more particularly the nature of the salivation. It should also be remembered that salivation may accompany or follow the symptoms of inflammation in the stomach, in consequence of calomel having been used as a remedy. But if proper attention be paid to the fallacies in the way of judgment, I conceive that an opinion on the question of poisoning with corrosive sublimate may be sometimes rested on the symptoms alone. This is another exception to the rule laid down by most modern toxicologists and medical jurists respecting the validity of the evidence of poisoning from symptoms.

For a good example of the practical application of these precepts, the reader may consult the trial of Mr. Hodgson, for attempting to poison his wife. In the instance which gave rise to the trial in question, a violent burning sensation in the throat was felt during the act of swallowing some pills ; in the course of ten minutes violent vomiting ensued, afterwards severe burning pain along the whole course of the gullet down to the stomach, next morning diarrhœa, and on the third day ptyalism. There were many other points of medical evidence which left no doubt that corrosive sublimate was swallowed in the pills. But even the history of the symptoms alone would have led to that inference.[*]

SECTION III. — *Of the Morbid Appearances caused by Mercury.*

The morbid appearances observed in the bodies of persons killed by corrosive sublimate will not require many details ; since most of the remarks formerly made under the head of the pathology of the irritants generally, and of arsenic in particular, apply with equal force to the present species of poisoning. Still there are some peculiarities deserving of notice, which arise from the greater solubility or stronger irritant action of corrosive sublimate.

The mouth and throat are more frequently affected than by arsenic ;

[*] Edin. Med. and Surg. Journal, xxii. 438.

and a remarkable appearance sometimes observed, and not excited, so far as I know, by arsenic, is shrivelling of the tongue, with great enlargement of the papillæ at its root.[*]

The disorder of the alimentary canal is also usually more general, and reaches a greater height before death takes place. Sometimes the irritation and organic injury are confined to the stomach;[†] but more commonly the throat, stomach, gullet, rectum, nay, even also the colon, are affected. The black or melanotic extravasation into the mucous membrane of the stomach, which has been already several times described as a common effect of the more violent irritants, is also produced by corrosive sublimate. In Devergie's case and in that of Dr. Venables it was present in a very great degree.[‡]

The coats of the stomach, and also those of the intestines, more particularly the colon and rectum, have frequently been found destroyed. So far as I have been able to ascertain, two kinds of destruction of the coats may be met with, — corrosion and ulceration.

The first is the result of chemical decomposition of the tissues. This kind is evidently to be looked for only when the quantity has been considerable and the dose concentrated. Nay even then it is rare. For on account of the solubility of corrosive sublimate, the facility with which it is decomposed by the secretions or accidental contents of the stomach, and the violence and frequency of the vomiting, this poison is peculiarly liable to be prevented from exerting its corrosive action on the membranes. Hence it is that proper chemical corrosion of the coats of the stomach is seldom witnessed in man.

The appearance of this corrosion differs according to the rapidity of the poisoning. In very rapid cases, for example in animals which have survived only twenty-five minutes, the villous coat has a dark-gray appearance, without any sign of vital reaction.[§] But this variety has never been witnessed in man, in whom the action has been hitherto much less rapid. In the most rapid cases, such as that of Dr. Bigsby, which terminated in two hours and a half [314], or those related by Mr. Valentine, of which one ended fatally in eleven and another in twenty-four hours, the corrosion was black, like the charring of "leather with a red-hot coal, and the rest of the stomach scarlet-red or deep rose-red ;— showing that inflammation had set in." In the former of these two cases the corrosion was as big as a half-crown, in the latter three inches in diameter. In a third case, where the patient lived thirty-one hours, the stomach was perforated.[||] In the case described by Dr. Venables, and formerly alluded to, where life was prolonged for eight days, there was a patch on the under surface of the stomach as large as two crown-pieces, hard, elevated, and of a very dark olive or almost black colour, besides very general erosion of the villous coat.[¶] In all these cases the disintegrated spot was probably situated where the poison first chiefly lodged.

* As in Devergie's Case (Arch. Gén. ix 468), in which they were as big as peas.
† Ibidem.   ‡ Devergie in Arch. Gén. ix. 468.
§ Sir B. Brodie in Philos. Trans. 1812.
∥ Edin. Med. and Surg. Journ., xiv. 472, 473.
¶ London Medical Gazette, viii. 618.

The corrosion caused by mercury, if examined before the slough is thrown off, will be found to possess an important peculiarity : the disorganized tissue yields mercury by chemical analysis. Professor Taddei repeatedly obtained the metal from the membranes of animals which he had poisoned with corrosive sublimate.* It is probable that mercury may be thus detected although death may not have taken place for some time after the poison was swallowed. For the slough was found adhering in one of Mr. Valentine's cases, where life was prolonged for seventy hours ; and it was not entirely removed even in eight days in one of the cases described by Dr. Venables.

Although, however, it is sometimes possible to find the poison in the stomach, the medical jurist must not perhaps expect to find it so often in the present instance as in that of poisoning with arsenic. For on account of its greater solubility corrosive sublimate cannot adhere with such obstinacy to the villous coat, and is therefore more subject to be discharged by vomiting. Nevertheless, the insoluble compound formed by antidotes may adhere to the coats like arsenic, and so resist the tendency of vomiting to displace them. In Devergie's case, notwithstanding twenty-three hours of incessant vomiting, although no poison could be detected in the fluid contents of the stomach, it was distinctly found in small whitish masses that lay between the folds of the rugæ.†

It may be here farther observed that corrosive sublimate, as well as other salts of mercury, may undergo in the alimentary canal after death the same change which is produced in arsenic from the gradual action of hydrosulphuric acid gas. It may be converted into the sulphuret. I am not acquainted indeed with any actual instance of such conversion ; but that it may occur we can scarcely doubt, not merely from theoretical considerations, but likewise because Orfila met with an instance where calomel taken daily in a case of gastro-cephalitis was discharged by stool in the form of a black sulphuret.‡

Another important consideration is, that corrosive sublimate may be decomposed and reduced to the metallic state by the admixture of various substances either given at the same time or subsequently, and the longer the inspection is delayed, the more complete will be the decomposition which is accomplished. Iron, zinc, and other metals are the most active of these substances.§

The other forms of destruction of the coats of the alimentary canal is common ulceration, either such from the beginning, or what was originally corrosion converted into an ulcer in consequence of the disorganized spot being thrown off by sloughing.

I have seen this appearance to an enormous extent in the great intestines of a man who survived nine days. Numerous large, black, gangrenous ulcers, just like those observed in bad cases of dysentery,

* Recherches sur un Nouvel Antidote, &c. p. 61.
† Archives Gén. de Méd. ix. 470.
‡ Journal de Chim. Médicale. viii. 268.
§ Orfila, Traité de Médecine Légale, iii. 134.

were scattered over the whole colon and rectum. In this instance, which occurred to the late Dr. Shortt, the stomach was also ulcerated, but the small intestines were not.

Sometimes the ulceration seems to be a variety of softening of the mucous tissue, as in a case described by Dr. Alexander Wood of this city, which proved fatal in fourteen days, and in which the stomach, cæcum, and ascending colon presented round, softened, greenish spots about the size of a sixpence, and accompanied in the stomach with a tendency to detaching of the membrane in the form of a slough.*

The destruction of the villous coat of the stomach occasioned by corrosive sublimate and other soluble salts of mercury may be distinguished from spontaneous gelatinization by one of two characters. If the slough remains attached, mercury will be detected in it: if separation has taken place, the ulcer exposed presents surrounding redness and other signs of reaction.†

All the other effects of inflammation may be produced by corrosive sublimate, as by arsenic and other irritants. More frequently here than in the case of arsenic peritonæal inflammation is met with. In Devergie's case the external surface of the stomach along both its curvatures presented the appearance of red points on a violet ground. In Mr. Valentine's cases there was much minute vascularity, not only of the outside of the stomach but also of the whole peritonæum lining the viscera and inside of the abdomen; and there was even some serous effusion into the cavity. In Dr. Venables's case the peritonæal coat of the stomach was highly vascular and inflamed, and the omentum also injected.

The urinary organs, and particularly the kidneys, are often much inflamed by poisoning with corrosive sublimate. Dr. Henry has related a case in which this poison proved fatal on the ninth day, and where the left kidney was found to contain an abscess.‡ In all of Mr. Valentine's cases the kidneys were inflamed, and the bladder excessively contracted, so as not to exceed the size of a walnut. In Ollivier's case, caused by the cyanide of mercury, the scrotum was gorged and black, the penis erected, and the kidneys a third larger than natural. In the case described by Dr. Venables both kidneys, but especially the left, were large, flaccid, and vascular, the ureters turgid and purple, and the bladder contracted, empty, and red internally.

Orfila has observed that the internal membrane of the heart is sometimes inflamed and checkered with brownish-black spots. Some remarks have been already made on the light in which this appearance ought to be viewed by the pathologist (p. 271).

Whatever may be the real state of the fact as to the alleged power of arsenic to preserve from decay the bodies of those poisoned with it, all authors agree that corrosive sublimate possesses no such pro-

* Edin. Med. and Surg. Journal, li. 115.
† The reader may apply this statement to the trial of Mr. Angus, p. 118.
‡ Edin. Med. and Surg. Journal, vii. 151.

perty. Yet it is well known to be a good antiseptic, when applied topically. The experiments of Klanck, noticed under the head of Arsenic, prove that corrosive sublimate at all events does not retard putrefaction in the bodies of those poisoned with it ; and Augustin in his analysis of Klanck's researches infers that it even promotes decay.* I have met with one example in the human subject which seems to confirm Augustin's opinion. In the case formerly quoted from the Medical and Physical Journal, which was fatal in four days, the relater found the body forty-two hours after death so putrid, though in the month of January, that the examination of it was very unpleasant, the belly being black, and a very offensive odour being exhaled.† Little importance, however, can be attached to a solitary case ; for on the contrary Sallin relates a case where the body of a man supposed to have been poisoned with corrosive sublimate was found not decayed, but imperfectly mummified, after sixty-seven days.‡

It is unnecessary to detail the proofs to be found in the dead body of mercurial salivation having existed during life. They are of course to be looked for in the mouth, and in the adjoining organs. We must not, however, expect to see much appearance of disease in the salivary glands; for according to Cruveilhier, in persons who die of mercurial salivation these glands do not present any trace of inflammation themselves, but merely serous effusion into the cellular tissue around them.§

Professor Orfila has made some useful experiments as to the effects of corrosive sublimate on dead intestine, which it may be proper to notice in a few words. When applied in the form of powder to the rectum of an animal newly killed, the part with which it is in contact becomes wrinkled, and as it were granulated, harder than natural, and of alabaster whiteness, intermingled with rose-red streaks, apparently the ramifications of vessels. When the membrane is stretched upon the finger, the wrinkling disappears. The muscular coat is of a snow-white colour, and even the serous coat is white, opaque, and thickened. The parts not in contact with the powder retain their natural appearance, and the line of demarcation between the affected and unaffected portions is abrupt. If the powder is not applied till twenty-four hours after death, the parts it touches become thick, white, and hard ; but no red lines are visible. It is easy to draw the distinction between these appearances and the effects of corrosive sublimate during life.

Little need be said of the force of the evidence of poisoning with corrosive sublimate, derived from the morbid appearances. If the gullet, stomach, and colon be all inflamed and ulcerated, and these injuries have taken place during a short illness, the presumption in favour of some form of irritant poisoning will be strong. And the presumption of poisoning with corrosive sublimate will be strong, if

* Augustin's Repertorium, B. i. H. ii. 11. † xli. 207.
‡ Journal de Médecine, l. iii. 15, or Recueil Périodique de la Soc. de Méd. vii. 343.
§ Revue Medicale, 1830, ii.

the usual marks of salivation are also found in the mouth and throat.
But such evidence can never amount to more than a strong presumption or probability.

SECTION IV. — *Of the Treatment of Poisoning with Mercury.*

The treatment of poisoning by the compounds of mercury may be
referred to two heads, — that which is required when irritation of
the alimentary canal is the prominent disorder, and that which is
designed to remove mercurial salivation.

Irritation and inflammation of the alimentary canal are to be treated
nearly in the same way as when arsenic has been the poison swallowed. In the instance of corrosive sublimate we also possess a
convenient and effectual antidote.

Several substances may be used as antidotes; but those which
have hitherto been most employed are albumen and gluten.

It has been already hinted that albumen, in the form of white of
eggs beat up with water, impairs or destroys the corrosive properties
of bichloride of mercury, by decomposing it and producing an insoluble mercurial compound. For this discovery and the establishment of albumen as an antidote, medicine is indebted to Professor
Orfila. He has related many satisfactory experiments in proof of its
virtues. The following will serve as an example of the whole.
Twelve grains of corrosive sublimate were given to a little dog, and
allowed to act for eight minutes, so that its usual effects might fairly
begin before the antidote was administered. White of eight eggs
was then given; after several fits of vomiting the animal became
apparently free from pain; and in five days it was quite well.* According to Peschier the white of one egg is required to render four
grains of the poison innocuous.† The experiments of the Parisian
toxicologist have been repeated and confirmed by others and particularly by Schloepfer; who found that when a dose was given to a
rabbit sufficient to kill it in seven minutes if allowed to act uncon-
trolled, the administration of albumen, just as the signs of uneasiness
appeared, prevented every serious symptom.‡ Dr. Samuel Wright
has found that if the administration of albumen is followed up by
giving some astringent decoction or infusion, the beneficial effects
are more complete, because the compound formed is less soluble in
an excess of albumen.§

The virtues of albumen have also been tried in the human subject
with equally favourable results. The recovery of the patient, whose
case was quoted formerly (p. 312), from Orfila's Toxicology, seems
to have been owing in great measure to this remedy. In the Medical
Repository another case is related, in which it was also very serviceable.‖ A third very apposite example of its good effects is related

* Toxicologie Gén. i. 313.   † Corvisart's Journal de Médecine, xxxviii. 77.
‡ Dissert. Inaug. p. 36.
§ See my Dispensatory, p. 518. Dr. Wright's Thesis on certain points connected
with the action of mercury and its salts has not yet been published.
‖ London Med. Repository, xix. 408.

by Dr. Lendrick. His patient had taken about half a drachm of corrosive sublimate, and was attacked with most of the usual symptoms, except vomiting. White of eggs was administered a considerable time afterwards, the beneficial effects of which were instantaneous and well-marked ; and the patient recovered.* A few years ago Orfila's discovery was the means of saving the life of M. Thenard the chemist. While at lecture, this gentleman inadvertently swallowed, instead of water, a mouthful of a concentrated solution of corrosive sublimate ; but having immediately perceived the fatal error, he sent for white of eggs, which he was fortunate enough to procure in five minutes. Although at this time he had not vomited, he suffered no material harm. Without the prompt use of the albumen, he would almost infallibly have perished.†

Albumen is chiefly useful in the early stage of poisoning with corrosive sublimate, and is particularly called for when vomiting does not take place. But it farther appears to be an excellent demulcent in the advanced stages.

On a previous occasion, mention was made of a few of the facts brought forward by Professor Taddei to prove the virtues of the gluten of wheat as an antidote for poisoning with corrosive sublimate [297, 336], so that nothing more need be said on the subject in the present place. As it is difficult to bring the whole of a fluid containing corrosive sublimate into speedy contact with pulverized gluten, which when put into water becomes agglutinated into a mass, the discoverer of this antidote proposes to give it in the form of emulsion with soft soap. This is made by mixing, partly in a mortar and partly with the hand, five or six parts of fresh gluten with fifty parts of a solution of soft soap. And in order to have a store always at hand, this emulsion, after standing and being frequently stirred for twenty-four hours, is to be evaporated to dryness in shallow vessels, and reduced to powder. The powder may be converted into a frothy emulsion in a few minutes.‡ Taddei made use of this powder with complete success in the case of a man who had swallowed seven grains of corrosive sublimate by mistake for calomel. Violent symptoms followed the taking of the poison ; but they were immediately assuaged by the administration of the antidote ; and the person soon got quite well.§ It is probable that wheat-flour will prove an effectual antidote by reason of the gluten it contains. On agitating for a few seconds a solution of twelve grains of corrosive sublimate along with three ounces of a strong emulsion of flour, and immediately filtering, — I find that ammonia and carbonate of potass have little or no effect, that hydriodate of potass occasions a yellow precipitate, and that the acrid, astringent taste of the solution is removed ; whence it may be inferred, that the corrosive sublimate is all decomposed, that little mercury remains in solution, and that what does remain is in the form of a chloride of mercury and gluten.

* Trans. of Dublin Coll. of Phys. iii. 310.
† Journal de Chim. Méd. Mars, 1825.
‡ Recherches sur un Nouvel Antidote, &c. p. 26.
§ Giornale di Fisica, 1826, vi. 170, and Buchner's Repertorium für die Pharmacie ii. 229,

When neither albumen nor gluten is at hand, milk is a convenient antidote of the same kind.

Iron filings would appear to be also a good antidote.   MM. Milne-Edwards and Dumas have found that when they were administered in the dose of an ounce to animals after twelve or eighteen grains of corrosive sublimate had remained long enough in the stomach for the symptoms to begin, the animals recovered from the effects of the poison, and died only some days afterwards of the effects of tying the gullet, which operation was necessary to prevent them vomiting.   The iron obviously acts by reducing the corrosive sublimate to the metallic state.*

Meconic acid, the peculiar acid of opium, which will be described under the head of that poison, is also probably a good antidote. Pettenkoffer correctly remarks that this acid has a great tendency to form very insoluble salts with the metallic oxides, particularly with the deutoxides, and above all when the acid is previously in union with a base which constitutes a soluble salt.†   On this account it must be a good antidote.   Pettenkoffer adds, that the precipitating action of the meconates is the reason why " the operation of corrosive sublimate on the animal body is almost entirely prevented by opium." Opium, however, cannot be safely used in such quantity as to decompose all the corrosive sublimate in a case of poisoning ; for I find that an infusion of thirty-three grains is required to precipitate all which can be thrown down from a solution of five grains of the mercurial salt.   I am not aware of any instances on record where poisoning with corrosive sublimate has been prevented or cured by opium given so as to decompose the salt ; but a very remarkable case will be related under the head of Compound Poisoning, where the phenomena of its action were masked and altered in a singular manner. There is little doubt that the alkaline meconates must prove valuable antidotes for corrosive sublimate.   At present an effectual barrier to their employment is their rarity ; but they might be rendered more accessible, as a great quantity of meconate of lime, which is at present put to no use, is formed in the manufacture of muriate of morphia ; and meconate of potass may easily be prepared in sufficient quantity from the meconate of lime.

It has been alleged by Dr. Buckler of Baltimore, that a mixture of gold-dust and iron-filings is an effectual antidote ; but Orfila denies this statement ; and the fact if true would be unimportant, on account of the improbability of the materials being ever at hand in practice.‡

M. Mialhe suggested not long ago as an antidote the proto-sulphuret of iron prepared by decomposing sulphate of protoxide of iron by hydrosulphate of ammonia ; and Orfila found that it is a perfect chemical antidote, which altogether prevents the poisonous action of corrosive sublimate, if administered to animals either before or immediately after the poison ; but he further ascertained that the lapse

* London Medico-Chirurgical Review, v. 612.
† Buchner's Repertorium für die Pharmacie, iv. 51.
‡ Annales d'Hygiène Publique, xxviii. 427.

of ten minutes was sufficient to render it of no use.* It is difficult'
however, to perceive why in this respect it should differ from white
of egg or any other chemical antidote.

As to the old antidotes for poisoning with corrosive sublimate,
such as the alkaline carbonates, the alkaline hydrosulphates, cinchona,
mercury, charcoal, — Orfila has given them all a fair trial, and found
them all inefficacious. It would appear, however, from a case related in a late American journal, that frequent doses of charcoal powder have much effect in soothing the bowels and allaying the inflammation after the poison is evacuated.†

The treatment of mercurial salivation consists in exposure to a cool
pure air, nourishing diet, and purgatives, if the intestinal canal is not
already irritated. In some of the inflammatory affections it induces,
venesection is required ; in others it is hurtful. In some complaints
induced by mercury, as in iritis, the poison appears to be its own antidote ; for nothing checks the inflammation so soon and so certainly as
mercurial salivation.

Dr. Finlay of the United States proposed to check mercurial salivation by small doses of tartar emetic frequently repeated, so as to
act on the skin ;‡ and Mr. Daniell has recommended large doses of
the acetate of lead as an effectual antidote for the same purpose.§ I
have tried both of these plans several times with apparant success.
In one instance particularly, where a severe salivation was threatened
by the administration of six grains of calomel in three doses, and
where profuse salivation, ulceration of the tongue and swelling of
the face actually did commence with violence, the mercurial affection
after a few days rapidly receded under the use of large doses of acetate of lead. — Dr. Klose, a German physician, says he has found
iodine to possess the property of arresting the effects of mercury on
the mouth.‖ The iodide of potassium is generally acknowledged to
be one of the best remedies for eradicating the constitutional infir-
mities left in many by severe courses of mercury.

A great deal might be said on the treatment of the secondary effects of poisoning with mercury. But a thorough investigation of the
subject would lead to such details as would be inconsistent with the
other objects of this work.

CHAPTER XV.

OF POISONING WITH COPPER.

POISONING with the salts of copper was not long ago a common accident, in consequence of the metal being much used in the fabrica-

---

* Journal de Chimie Médicale, 1843, p. 10.
† Dr. Hort. American Journal of Med. Science, vi. 540.
‡ Edin Med. and Surg. Journal, xxix. 218.
§ Lond. Med. Repos. N. S. vi. 368.   ‖ Lond Med. Gazette, 1836-37, ii. 144.

32*

tion of vessels for culinary and other domestic purposes, or ignorantly resorted to by confectioners and others to impart a good colour to sweatmeats and preserves. Such accidents have been materially diminished in frequency since the poisonous qualities of the metal, and the circumstances under which it is acted on by articles of food, have become known. Nevertheless they are still frequent enough. The diffusion among the common people of the knowledge of the properties of copper has also naturally led some persons to have recourse to its preparations for the purpose of self-destruction. Poisoning with copper has seldom been caused by the wilful act of another person ; for the deep colour of its compounds and their strong disagreeable taste render it a difficult matter to administer them secretly. This, however, though difficult, is not impossible : whatever may be swallowed accidentally, may be also administered secretly. In 1795 a woman Inglis was tried at Aberdeen for administering sulphate of copper with intent to poison ; but the charge was not proved.* In 1842 an attempt was made at Béziers in France to poison a young woman by dissolving this salt in her coffee; but the first mouthful caused such a sense of constriction in the throat as to apprize her of something deleterious being present, and she escaped after suffering from soreness of the mouth, vomiting and cramps.† A case of imputed poisoning with sulphate of copper has been related at page 76.

SECTION I.— *Of the Chemical History and Tests of the Preparations of Copper.*

Metallic copper has a special red colour, to which it gives its own name. Its specific gravity is nearly 9, its hardness considerable, its tenacity great, its point of fusion about 27° W. or at a full-white heat.

It unites with oxygen in two proportions, forming a yellowish-red protoxide, and a peroxide, which, when dry, is brownish-black—when hydrated, azure-blue. It unites also with sulphur in two corresponding proportions, forming a gold-yellow proto-sulphuret, the natural copper-pyrites, and a black bisulphuret, which is formed by sulphuretted-hydrogen in all the solutions of this metal. The peroxide unites with ammonia. The acids all unite with the oxide and form blue or green salts, some of which are soluble, some insoluble. The oxide is frequently mixed with other matters to form various pigments ; but in such compounds the union is generally mechanical, not chemical. Of the substances thus formed and existing in nature and the arts the following only require notice here. 1. *Mineral green*, and other pigments formed with the hydrated oxide. 2. *Natural verdigris*, or the carbonate. 3. *Blue vitriol*, or the sulphate. 4. *Artificial verdigris*, or the mixed acetates.

1. *Mineral Green.*

The description of this substance and its chemical properties must

* Burnett on Criminal Law, 547.   † Journal de Chimie Médicale, 1842, p. 771.

be introduced with a short account of the tests for the unmixed *per-oxide*. When free of water the peroxide is a brownish-black powder or granular mass, which is usually procured by decomposing nitrate of copper at a low red heat. It is easily known by the solvent power of nitric acid, the blue colour of the filtered solution, and the beautiful deep violet tint communicated to the solution by an excess of ammonia. The last property is considered by chemists the most satisfactory proof of the presence of oxide of copper in a fluid. It is alone quite free of fallacy, and may be applied to all the soluble and also many insoluble compounds of copper, provided they are not mixed with a large proportion of vegetable or animal fluids, in which case the colour is often greenish.

In the case of the peroxide and of copper poisons generally, the process of reduction, which has been applied with such delicacy and precision to arsenical and mercurial poisons, loses all its advantages. The metal remains in the flux, and intimately diffused ; so that of its physical qualities the colour only can be estimated, and even that but inaccurately, except in the instance of one compound, verdigris.

The *hydrated peroxide of copper*, when newly formed and well prepared, has a fine azure-blue colour ; but on exposure to a gentle heat, it parts with its water, and becomes the anhydrous peroxide. It is procured by precipitating any of the soluble salts of copper by means of caustic potass. It is at once known by the action of ammonia, which immediately forms with it a deep violet blue solution.

Mineral green, as already mentioned under the head of Arsenic (p. 223), was originally an arsenical pigment introduced into the art of colour-making by Scheele, and now sometimes sold in this country by the name of emerald-green. But the mineral green of the colourist now contains no arsenic, being a hydrate of peroxide of copper intimately mixed with a little lime, which is generally carbonated. This variety of mineral-green probably varies a little in composition. Some parcels I have found to contain the lime in the state of carbonate ; in others the lime was chiefly caustic.

The best method of determining its nature is to dissolve it in diluted hydrochloric acid, which leaves only a slight cloudiness from accidental impurities; and then to transmit through the filtered solution a stream of sulphuretted hydrogen gas. The copper on boiling is all thrown down in the form of a black bisulphuret, and hydrochlorate of lime remains in solution. The lime is then to be detected by its proper tests, after the solution has been filtered and neutralized (see p. 192). In general this long process is unnecessary, as the medical jurist may be simply required to say whether the suspected substance contains copper. In that case it is only requisite to subject the substance to the action of ammonia, as if it was hydrated peroxide.

Verditer, another green pigment, the basis of which is always oxide of copper, does not appear to differ essentially in composition from mineral green. The samples I have examined consist of a large proportion of hydrated oxide of copper, and a small proportion of carbonate of lime.

2. *Natural Verdigris.*

This is a compound of no great importance in a medico-legal point of view. Nevertheless an instance has been lately published in which it was taken for the purpose of committing suicide, and was found abundantly in the stomach.* The carbonate of copper exists naturally in two states. In one form it constitutes the rust of copper, or natural verdigris, and is produced as a powdery crust on metallic copper by long exposure to moist air. It is insipid and insoluble, so that pure water left in vessels incrusted with it does not become poisonous. It dissolves with effervescence in sulphuric acid, and without effervescence in ammonia, forming the usual violet solution. In another form it exists in the mineral kingdom, constituting the chief part of a beautiful ore, malachite, and also a considerable proportion of some blue-copper ores.

3. *Blue Vitriol.*

Blue vitriol, blue copperas, blue stone, vitriol of copper, as it is variously called in common speech, is the sulphate of copper. In the solid form it constitutes large crystals of a deep blue colour, and an acrid, astringent, metallic taste, efflorescent in dry air, and very soluble in water. Under the action of heat it first loses its water of crystallization without undergoing the watery effusion; then its sulphuric acid is driven off partly unchanged, partly decomposed; and at last the brown peroxide is left behind in a state of considerable purity. If carbonaceous matter be previously mixed with the sulphate, the oxide is decomposed at a low red heat, so that the process of reduction may be performed in a glass tube. For the reasons formerly stated, this process does not constitute a convenient or characteristic test for sulphate of copper. The best mode of ascertaining its nature is to dissolve it, and then to apply the tests for the solution.

There are many excellent tests for copper in solution. But the four following are the most delicate and characteristic, — ammonia, sulphuretted hydrogen, ferro-cyanate of potass, and metallic iron.

1. *Ammonia* causes a pale azure precipitate, which is redissolved by an excess of the test, forming a deep violet-blue transparent fluid. If the solution is very diluted, there is no previous precipitation; the fluid becomes violet without its transparency being disturbed. This is a perfectly characteristic test of copper, and one of great delicacy.

2. *Sulphuretted hydrogen gas* causes a dark brownish-black precipitate, the sulphuret of copper. This test is one of very great delicacy; but it is not alone decisive of the presence of copper, since lead, bismuth, mercury, and silver, are similarly affected by it. A method, however, will be presently described, by which the precise nature of the sulphuret may be determined.

The alkaline hydrosulphates, for example the hydrosulphate of ammonia, answer equally well with sulphuretted-hydrogen. The

* Degrange, London Medical Gazette, 1842-43, i 495.

solution of the common liver of sulphur throws down, not a black, but a chestnut precipitate.

3. *Ferro-cyanate of potass* causes a fine hair-brown precipitate, the ferro-cyanide of copper. This test is also exceedingly delicate and characteristic.

4. A polished rod or plate of *metallic iron*, held in a solution of sulphate of copper, soon becomes covered with a red powdery crust, which is metallic copper ; and ere long the solution is changed in colour from blue to greenish-yellow. The action is simple ; the iron merely displaces the copper in the solution, in which a sulphate of iron is consequently formed. This test is characteristic, and even of considerable delicacy. At the same time other substances may cause a reddish encrustation on iron by simply rusting it, so that the test cannot be relied on alone.

The four preceding reagents taken together are amply sufficient to prove the existence of copper in a solution. Three other tests, however, may be here briefly alluded to.

Caustic potass in a solution not too diluted causes a fine azure-blue precipitate, the hydrated peroxide of copper.

Oxide of arsenic, with the previous addition of a few drops of ammonia, causes a fine apple-green or grass-green precipitate, the arsenite of copper. This test, which is both delicate and characteristic, has been already fully considered under the head of Arsenic.

The process by fluid reagents, as hitherto laid down, merely proves the presence of copper, but does not indicate the acid with which the oxide is combined. In order to determine whether it is sulphuric acid, the fluid must also be tested with nitrate of baryta followed by nitric acid : a heavy white precipitate is thus produced, which the excess of nitric acid does not redissolve.

4. *Artificial Verdigris.*

Artificial verdigris is a common pigment, which is met with in the form either of earth-like masses, or of a light powder of a greenish-blue colour and peculiar disagreeable smell, approaching that of vinegar. Like blue vitriol it has a strong metallic, astringent taste. The effect of heat is peculiar. Some acetic acid is in the first place distilled over ; a portion of the acid, however, is decomposed and reduces the oxide ; and a low red heat is sufficient to make the outer crust of the verdigris distinctly copper-red, when the material is contained in a glass tube.

Artificial verdigris varies somewhat in composition. Foreign verdigris contains chiefly the hydrated diacetate, with a little carbonate, oxide, and even metallic copper, along with particles of the fruit and fruit-stalks of the grape. British verdigris consists of little else than the hydrated diacetate. It is known by the following characters. Ammonia dissolves it almost entirely, forming a deep violet solution. Diluted sulphuric acid dissolves it, evolving an odour of acetic acid, and forming a solution of sulphate of copper, which may be

known by the tests for that salt. Boiling water converts it partly
into an insoluble brown powder, which is oxide of copper in union
with a small proportion of acetic acid, and partly into a greenish-
blue neutral acetate, which is dissolved, and may be known by the
four tests for sulphate of copper, and the want of action of nitrate of
baryta.

It may be right to notice shortly three other salts of copper, the
nitrate, the ammoniacal sulphate, and the muriate. The *nitrate*
forms a violet solution, which is acted on by reagents in the same
way as the dissolved acetate, but has not any odour of vinegar.
The *ammoniacal sulphate* [ammoniated copper — ammoniuret of cop-
per], has been occasionally used in medicine. It forms, when solid,
small scaly crystals, of an intense violet colour and strong ammoniacal odour ; and when dissolved it retains its peculiar colour even
though very much diluted. — The *muriate* of copper has a lively
grass-green colour, and is acted on by reagents in the same way as
the solution of verdigris.

Of the corrosion of copper by articles of food and drink. — To these
observations on the chemical history of copper a few remarks must
be added relative to the action of various articles of food or drink
upon the metal. Unpleasant accidents have often happened from
the use of copper vessels in the preparation of food ; and it is therefore necessary for the medical jurist to know the circumstances, so
far as they have been investigated, under which the poison may be
dissolved.

Dr. Falconer found, that distilled water kept several weeks on a
polished plate of copper, neither injured its lustre, nor acquired any
taste, nor become coloured with ammonia ;[*] and Drouard afterwards
observed, that distilled water, kept for a month on copper filings,
did not contain any of the metal.[†] Eller of Berlin, however, remarked, that water, if it contain a considerable quantity of common
salt, as four ounces in five pounds, or a twentieth part, will give
slight traces of copper after being boiled in a brass pan ; and that if
the pan be made of copper, a powder is procured by evaporation,
which when treated with acetic acid yields so much as 20 grains of
acetate of copper.[‡] But it is a singular circumstance, also observed
by the same experimentalist, that if beef or fish be boiled with the
usual allowance of salt, and with the addition also of various vegetable substances, the liquid does not yield any copper. This observation has been lately denied by Professor Orfila ; who says he found
copper deposited on a plate of iron in salt water in which beef had
been boiled, and that he also obtained copper from the beef itself.[§]
The quantity thus dissolved, however, must be exceedingly small, if
the copper be kept clean and free of oxide ; for copper vessels,

[*] Falconer on the Poison of Copper, p. 23.
[†] Expériences sur l'Empoisonnement par l'oxyde de Cuivre. Diss. Inaug. Paris,
1802. Quoted in Orfila's Toxicol. i. 502.
[‡] Sur l'usage prétendu dangereux de la vaisselle de cuivre dans nos cuisines. His-
toire de l'Acad. Roy. des Sciences de Berlin, 1756, p. 12.
[§] Toxicol. Gén. 1843, i. 612.

although they have often been the source of fatal accidents, if care-lessly used in the preparation of food, have appeared under careful management to be quite harmless. An excellent practical confirma-tion of this will be found in Michaelis's Commentaries. He states, that in the Orphan Hospital of Halle, the food was in his time pre-pared in large copper vessels, which were kept remarkably clean ; and that out of a population of eight or nine hundred he never heard of any one having suffered from symptoms of poisoning with copper.* Several other saline matters promote the solution of copper in water. Thus Dr. Falconer found that alum has this effect when aided by heat ; and probably nitre and Epsom salt possess the same quality.† Their mode of action is not very well known.

It is a common though erroneous idea, that milk, heated or allowed to stand in a copper vessel, becomes impregnated with the metal. Eller has shown, that, on the contrary, if the vessel be well cleaned, milk, tea, coffee, beer, and rain water, kept in a state of ebullition for two hours, do not contract the slightest impurity from copper ;‡ and the same remark has been also made by Dr. Falconer with re-spect to cabbage, potatoes, turnips, carrots, onions, rice, and barley.§

But Eller farther remarked, that, if the vessel is not thoroughly clean, then all acid substances dissolve the carbonate that encrusts it, especially if left in it for some time. Nay, it appears that some acid matters, though they do not dissolve clean copper by being merely boiled in it a few minutes, nevertheless, if allowed to cool and stand some time in it, will acquire a sensible impregnation.‖ Dr. Falconer also observed that syrup of lemons, boiled fifteen minutes in copper or brass pans, did not acquire a sensible impreg-nation ; but if it was allowed to cool and remain in the pans for twenty-four hours, the impregnation was perceptible even to the taste, and was discovered by the test of metallic iron.¶ This fact has been farther confirmed by the researches of Proust,** who states, that, in preparing food or preserves in copper, it is not till the fluid ceases to cover the metal, and is reduced in temperature, that so-lution of the metal begins. Inattention to this difference has been the cause of fatal accidents, of which the following case from Wild-berg's Practical Manual will serve as a good example. A servant left some sour-krout for only a couple of hours in a copper pan which had lost the tinning. Her mistress and a daughter, who took the cabbage to dinner, died after twelve hours illness ; and Wildberg found the cabbage so strongly impregnated with copper, that it was detected by the test of metallic iron.††

Some wines have the same power, by reason of the acid they contain. Hence Eller found twenty-one grains of the acetate in five pounds of French white wine, after being boiled in a copper vessel. An epidemic disease, mentioned by Fabricius, which broke out in

* Beck's Medical Jurisprudence, 460.   † Falconer, &c. pp. 48, 98, 110.
‡ Sur l'usage, &c. p. 12.   § Falconer, &c. p. 63.
‖ Histoire de l'Acad de Berlin, 1756, p. 16.
¶ Falconer, &c. p. 79.   ** Annales de Chimie, lvii. 79, 81.
†† Practisches Handb. für Physiker, iii. 312, Case 49.

1592 among the senators of Bern, and a number of their guests who had been invited to a great entertainment, was supposed to have arisen from a poisonous impregnation of this kind. The wine used at the feast had been kept cool in copper vessels immersed in a very cold well. Many of the company were attacked with dysenteric symptoms, and some died.*

Vinegar also dissolves metallic copper. Dupuytren observed that the vinegar sold by hawkers in the streets of Paris generally contained copper from the action of the acetic acid on the stop-cocks of the little vessels used in retailing it.† Others in like manner have found copper in vinegar pickles prepared in copper vessels. Thus Dr. Percival found a strong impregnation of copper in pickled samphire, of which a young lady ate one morning two breakfast platefuls, and which proved fatal to her in nine days.‡ And Dr. Falconer once detected so large a quantity in some pickled cucumbers bought at a great London grocer's, that it was deposited on a plate of iron, and imparted its peculiar taste and smell to the pickles.§ It seems indeed to have been at one time the custom to make a point of adulterating pickles with copper; for in many old cookery-books the cook is told to make her pickles in a copper pan, or to put some halfpence among the pickles to give them a fine green colour.||

The action of the vegetable acids, and more particularly of vinegar on copper, depends on the co-operation of the atmospheric air held in solution by the fluid, and in contact with its surface. Without such co-operation the copper cannot be oxidated. This fact, which was determined experimentally by Proust,¶ will explain the observations of Eller and Falconer, — that it is not dangerous to boil acidulous liquids in copper vessels, while it is very unsafe to keep these fluids cold in the same vessels. In the latter instance the liquid is impregnated with atmospheric air, while in the former the usual aëriform contents are driven off by the heat. I must observe, however, in limitation of Proust's statement, that strong vinegar, such as the pyroligneous acetic acid, will become impregnated to a certain extent if boiled in copper vessels. The action which takes place is the same as that remarked by him in the case of cold vinegar:¶ the copper where it is always covered remains quite bright; but at the edge of the fluid it becomes oxidated, and the oxide is dissolved by the occasional bubbling up of the acid.

In the last place, the property of oxidating and uniting with copper is likewise possessed by fatty matters and oils. According to Falconer, fatty substances do not act on metallic copper unless they are rancid.** But Proust is probably more correct when he states, that they will act, though fresh, provided they are aided by the co-operation of atmospheric air.†† I have found, that, if a plate of cop-

---

* Fabricii Hildani Opera omnia. Genevæ, 1682. De Dysenteria, p. 669.
† Orfila, Toxicol. Générale, i. 507.
‡ Trans. London College of Physicians, iii. 80.
§ On the Poison of Copper, 86.
|| On the Poison of Copper, 88; also Paris and Fonblanque's Medical Jurisprudence, ii. 289.   ¶ Annales de Chimie, lvii. 80.
** On the Poison of Copper, p. 18.   †† Annales, &c. p. 80.

per be thrust into a mass of fresh butter, its surface becomes dark in twenty-four hours, and the butter becomes green wherever it is in contact both with the copper and the air, but not where it covers the metal closely. In fresh hog's lard, however,' I have found that the whole lard in contact with the copper becomes blue even at a depth to which the air can scarcely reach. The action of oils is similar. It is even probable that they act when hot ; for Mr. Travis found that hot oil became green when kept for only four or five minutes in a copper vessel.* Dr. Falconer mentions that the property of acting on copper is possessed in an eminent degree by volatile oils, and especially by oil of cloves and oil of cinnamon.†

The general result of the preceding observations is, that there is hardly any article of food or drink which may not become impregnated with copper if kept in copper vessels, as there are few articles which do not contain either an acid or some fatty matter ; and it farther appears, that the impregnation will scarcely ever take place during the boiling of such articles, but only during the preservation of them in a cold state. It must also be considered, that, independently of these chemical impregnations, articles of food may be mixed mechanically with copper, in consequence of the vessels being allowed, through the carelessness of the cook, to become covered with rust or carbonate, which is subsequently removed by the friction of the solid parts of any article that is boiled in them.

In order to prevent accidental impregnations, copper vessels are usually tinned. The tinning consists of an alloy of tin and lead, which is much less easily attacked than the copper, and the safety of which is farther insured by the circumstance, that the substances endowed with the property of dissolving lead, cannot attack that metal before the whole tin of the alloy is oxidated.‡ The tinning of copper, however, has been found to be but a partial protection, as the tinning is apt to be worn away without attracting the attention of servants. Hence the use of copper in the fabrication of kitchen utensils is becoming every day more and more limited, especially since the manufacture of cast-iron vessels was brought to perfection in this country.

Many instances might be adduced of the ignorance and carelessness which prevailed, even not far back in the last century, as to the employment of copper vessels for culinary purposes. In addition to the instances already quoted, the following are well deserving of notice. Gmelin was consulted by the abbot of a monastery, on account of a violent disease which prevailed throughout the whole brotherhood of monks. The symptoms were obstinate and severe colic, retching and bilious vomiting, costiveness, flatus, burning pain in the pit of the stomach, under the sternum, in the kidneys and extremities, and paralytic weakness in the arms. On inquiring into the cause of this singular combination of symptoms, Gmelin found that every vessel in the kitchen, the pots and pans, and even the

* Medical Observations and Inquiries, ii. 11. † On the Poison of Copper, 106.
‡ Proust, Annales de Chimie, lvii. 83.

milk pails and butter dishes for storing the butter, were made of copper.* In 1781 an establishment of Jacobin monks at Paris were all violently affected from a similar error. The cook on a Friday and the subsequent Saturday, after boiling fish for the dinner of the monks in a copper pan, and drawing off the water, poured vinegar over the fish, and left it thus in the pan for a considerable time. On the evening of Friday several of them were taken severely ill with headache, acute pain in the stomach and bowels, precordial anxiety, purging, great feebleness, and cramps in the legs. The rest of them, to the number of twenty-one in all, were similarly attacked next morning; and the symptoms continued in most of them for five or six days.†

A singular variety of adulteration with copper was brought not long ago into public notice on the continent, — namely, the impregnation of bread with the sulphate of copper, which was used in small quantity for promoting the fermentation of the dough. This practice was first detected in some of the towns of Flanders, but was afterwards found to prevail in France.‡ Some chemists of reputation have indeed doubted altogether the existence of the practice; and M. Barruel in particular, who was consulted on the subject by the Prefecture of Paris, publicly declared his disbelief, because he remarked that, instead of favouring the panary fermentation, a very small proportion of sulphate of copper actually impeded it, and besides gave the bread a greenish colour of such depth that no customer would take it for a wholesome article.§ Subsequent inquiries, however, have shown that Barruel must have allowed himself to be misled, probably by using too much of the sulphate of copper. For the bakers of St. Omer admitted that they practised this ulceration for the sake of saving their yeast, the proportion required being an ounce of the salt in two pints of water, for every hundred weight (*quintal*) of dough, or about an 1800th part.‖ And it appears from an interesting set of experiments by M. Meylink, a chemist of Deventer, that, contrary to the statements of Barruel, sulphate of copper not only possesses the property of promoting the panary fermentation, but likewise constitutes in several important respects a source of adulteration, which ought to be prohibited and strictly looked after. He found that when he added to half a Flemish pound of dough from one grain to eight grains of sulphate of copper, fermentation took place more quickly than in the same dough without such addition, and nearly in proportion to the quantity of the salt used; — that the adulterated loaves when taken out of the oven were much better raised, and the loaf with only one grain of the salt likewise much whiter, than those which were not adulterated; — that a slight increase, however, in the proportion rendered the loaf greenish, and gave it a peculiar taste; but especially that the employment of the salt of copper even

* Geschichte der Mineralischen Gifte, p. 77.
† Lond. Med. Journal, ii. 411, from Journ. de Méd.
‡ Archives Gén. de Méd. xix. 471.
§ Annales d'Hygiène Publ. et de Méd. Légale, iii. 342.
‖ Archives Gén. de Méd. xxi. 145.

in the small proportion of one grain had the singular effect of bringing about the complete fermentation of the dough with considerably less loss of weight than occurs in the common process of baking, the loss in the sound and in the adulterated loaves being in the proportion of 116 to 100.* It certainly seems fully proved, then, that the adulteration of bread with sulphate of copper is an important fraud in more ways than one. Some doubt may be entertained whether any injury can result to the human body from even the habitual use of so small a quantity as that employed by the bakers; and at all events, we may be satisfied that if any bad effects do result, this can only happen from the continual use of the adulterated bread for a great length of time. But there can be no doubt that the practice is a fraud on the public, by enabling the baker to make his loaves of the standard weight with a less allowance of nutritive material.

Another important adulteration also indicated by foreign chemists, is that of syrup made with the coarsest kinds of sugar, and decolorized by means of sulphate of copper. The colour is removed by adding a solution of the sulphate to the syrup boiling hot, and decomposing the salt by lime; but a portion of the salt is often left behind, and in consequence accidents have arisen from such syrups being used in making various medicinal preparations.†

Of the detection of copper in organic mixtures. — As in the instance of arsenic and mercury, so in that of copper the presence of vegetable and animal principles interposes material obstacles in the application of the ordinary tests and methods of analysis. Some substances, such as albumen, milk, tea, coffee, and the like, decompose the solutions of the salts of copper, throwing down the oxide of copper in union with various proximate principles. Others, such as red wine, bile, vomited matter, and the tissues composing the stomach, although they do not decompose the soluble copper salts, alter materially the action of reagents on them. These facts were established long ago by Professor Orfila;‡ and various processes were suggested by him, by myself in former editions of this work, and by various other authors, with the view of overcoming the difficulties in question.

More lately a fresh difficulty has been started, which has been thought to render every prior process fallacious, including that which I have proposed. For it is alleged that copper exists naturally as a constituent part of many vegetable and animal substances, and more especially in the organs of the human body. This statement is so important as to deserve attentive consideration before fixing on a method of analysis for medico-legal cases.

Some time ago Meissner pointed out the existence of a trace of copper in some vegetable substances;§ and more recently M. Sarzeau alleged that a minute quantity of this metal, sometimes not above a

* Buchner's Repertorium für die Pharmacie, xxxiii. 236.
† Pignant in Journ. de Chim. Méd. viii. 339.
‡ Toxicologie Gén. 1826, i. 510.
§ Schweigger's Journal der Chemie, xvi. 340, 436.

1,500,000th and never exceeding a 120,000th part, may be detected not only in all vegetable substances, but likewise in the blood, as well as other fluids and solids of the animal body.   Among vegetable substances he examined with great care cinchona-bark, madder, coffee, wheat and flour ; and he succeeded in separating metallic copper from them all.*

The accuracy of these researches was called in question. By some chemists the discoveries of Meissner and Sarzeau were confirmed so far as they relate to vegetable substances. By others the confirmation was extended to the animal body, and more especially to the human organs and secretions. Thus M. Devergie says, that, having been struck with the singular circumstance of two cases occurring to him in a single year, where analysis indicated copper in the tissues of the alimentary canal of persons suspected of having died of poison, he was led to inquire, along with M. O. Henry, whether the metal was contained naturally in the textures of the human body ; and that in the course of many experiments, although unable to detect any in a solution made by means of weak acetic acid, he could always find it by the process of incineration.† Orfila has also repeatedly detected traces of copper in the bodies of animals not poisoned with the preparations of that metal.‡

By other experimentalists opposite results have been obtained, more especially in regard to animal solids and fluids.   In the course of an inquiry relative to the question, whether poisons pass into the blood, I failed to detect copper in the blood, muscles, or spinal marrow of animals, although the method of analysis must have enabled me to discover extremely minute quantities of that metal.   Afterwards M. Chevreul was unable to detect the slightest trace of copper in beef, veal, or mutton ; nor was he more successful in the case of wheat, provided care was taken to keep the sample clean.§   And more recently MM. Flandin and Danger have denied that there is any copper ever found naturally in the body.‖

These discrepant results appear to be in a great measure reconciled in an extensive inquiry into the subject by M. Boutigny ; who found that wheat, wine, cider, and some other substances of a vegetable nature, do frequently present minute traces of copper, but only when copper is contained in the manure used in raising the grain, apples, and the like ; that manure from the streets of great towns always contains copper, and introduces it into vegetable articles grown where such manure is used ; and that the occasional presence of the same metal in animal substances may be traced either to copper vessels having been employed in preparing or preserving them, or to the animals producing them having been fed on vegetables presenting from the causes mentioned above a faint cupreous im-

* Journal de Pharmacie, xvi. 505.
† Bulletins de la Société Roy. de Méd. 1838-39, p. 113.
‡ Journal de Chimie Médicale, 1840, p. 475.
§ Ibid. viii. 442, 573.
‖ L'Experience, Avril 27, 1843.

pregnation.* — Another fallacy, which may account for the alleged invariable success of some chemists, has been pointed out by M. Hiers-Reynaert of Bruges. Having once obtained copper in a specimen of suspected bread, when he used paper for a filter, but none when he used linen, he was led to examine various filtering papers, and found that some kinds contain an appreciable trace of copper.† This important fact must be attended to in all medico-legal investigations.

On the whole, whatever may be thought of the physiological question, whether copper forms a constituent of the textures and fluids of vegetables and animals, it seems well established that this metal is often present there in minute proportion ; and consequently its possible presence must not be overlooked in medico-legal researches. Fortunately methods of analysis are known which this source of fallacy does not affect.

Process. The following method emrbraces all possible cases ; and it is exempt, so far as yet appears, from every source of error.

1. Should the subject of analysis not be a liquid, render it such by dividing it into small fragments, and boiling it gently for an hour in distilled water acidulated with acetic acid, which must previously be ascertained not to contain any copper. If the liquid be not viscid, filter it at once ; but if it be too viscid for filtration, pass it through a muslin sieve, add two volumes of rectified spirit to it when cool, and then filter it. Transmit through a small portion of it a stream of hydrosulphuric acid gas ; and if a brownish-black precipitate or cloud form, subject the whole liquid to the gas. A brown precipitate, which is sulphuret of copper, will separate either immediately, or after ebullition and repose for an hour. Collect the precipitate, if abundant, by filtration, if scanty, by repeated subsidence and affusion. Dry it, subject it to a low red heat, and then heat it with a little strong nitric acid, which will convert the sulphuret into the sulphate of copper. This salt, dissolved out by boiling distilled water, may be subjected to the tests described above, and especially to ammonia.

2. If the copper be extremely minute in quantity, sulphuretted hydrogen will not act upon it in a fluid much charged with organic matter. To meet this possible case, which may occur when the subject of analysis is an organ of the human body into which the poison has been conveyed by absorption, — let the liquid be evaporated to dryness, and charred in the following manner. Heat in a porcelain basin a quantity of nitric acid equal in weight to the residuum, together with a fifteenth of chlorate of potash. Add the dry residuum in successive portions of such magnitude as not to occasion too great effervescence. When it has been all added, heat the product till it become dark-red and thick. It will then, or soon afterwards, begin suddenly to char, and at length a thick vapour will arise in dense clouds ; upon which, the charring being complete, the heat must be withdrawn. Pulverise the carbonaceous mass ; boil it

* Journal de Chimie Méd. ix. 147.   † Ibidem, 1840, p. 28.

33*

with nitric acid diluted with its own volume of water; and evaporate the filtered fluid to dryness, so as to expel any excess of acid. Dissolve the saline residuum, and test the solution with the usual reagents.

The first branch of this process is nearly the same with the one adopted in the last edition of the present work. The second is derived from a process lately proposed by Orfila.*

The principles on which it is founded are these. 1. Of the numerous organic compounds formed by vegetable and animal principles with the salts of copper, all either dissolve in very weak acetic acid, or part with their oxide of copper to it. This was pointed out by me in my last edition. 2, Weak acetic acid, as already mentioned (p. 356), has been shown by M. Devergie to be incapable of dissolving that copper which is contained naturally in the tissues, at least so as to render it discoverable by the subsequent steps of the process. 3, According to Orfila, copper naturally present in organic substances, is never indicated by the second branch of the process, provided the charred product of the action of nitric acid and chlorate of potash be not heated to incineration. It does not appear why the charring process, when so conducted, should separate adventitious copper, and not that which is present naturally. But the empirical fact may be accepted in the mean time, as it rests on apparently careful experiments.

Orfila does not use acetic acid in the first branch of his process, but merely infuses the suspected matter in cold water, and if copper be not thus found, he has recourse to boiling water. But this method introduces needless complexity; and besides neither maceration, nor boiling with mere water, will dissolve out the whole oxide of copper. Acidulation with acetic acid dissolves it all; and Devergie has shown that this advantage is gained without any additional fallacy arising from the possible presence of copper as a natural ingredient of the substance under examination (p. 356).

SECTION II. — *Of the Action of Copper, and the Symptoms it excites in Man.*

The symptoms caused by copper have at least two varieties in their character. One class arises from its local action on the alimentary canal; the other from its operation on distant organs.

This double influence is proved by the experiments of Drouard on animals, published in his inaugural dissertation at Paris in 1802; and by those of Orfila in his Toxicology.

When Drouard gave twelve grains of verdigris to a strong dog fasting, he observed that it caused aversion to food, efforts to vomit, diarrhœa, listlessness, and death in twenty-two hours; and that the stomach was but little inflamed. When two grains dissolved in water were injected into the jugular vein of another dog, it caused vomiting and discharge of fæces in seven minutes, then rattling in the throat,

* Toxicologie Gén. 1843, i. 637.

and death in half an hour; and there was no particular morbid appearance in the body. — Half a grain killed another in four days; and in addition to the preceding symptoms, there was palsy of the hind legs for a day before death. Six grains of the sulphate introduced into the stomach killed a dog in half an hour, without producing any appearance of inflammation.[*]

These experiments prove that it is not by causing local irritation that this poison proves fatal. But its mode of action is more distinctly shown in the later and more accurate experiments of Orfila. He found that twelve or fifteen grains of the neutral acetate generally killed dogs within an hour; and that besides the usual symptoms of irritation in the stomach, they often had insensibility, almost always convulsions, and immediately before death rigidity, or even absolute tetanus. He likewise remarked violent convulsions and insensibility when a grain of this salt was injected into the veins; and death was then seldom delayed beyond ten minutes. In no case was there any particular morbid appearance, except loss of contractility in the voluntary muscles.[†] More recently results nearly the same have been obtained by Mitscherlich; and when doses of two drachms of sulphate of copper were given, he observed after death pale blueness of the villous coat of the stomach, mingled with brownness, — the apparent effect of chemical action.[‡]

Allied to these results are those obtained by my late colleague, Dr. Duncan, and by Mitscherlich, when the sulphate was applied to a wound. Dr. Duncan observed that death took place in twenty-two hours, and the body was every where in a healthy state. Mitscherlich found that a drachm of either sulphate or acetate proved fatal in four hours, with symptoms of extreme prostration. The experiments of M. Smith, repeated by Orfila, are at variance with these; for one or two drachms of the acetate applied to a wound in the thigh of a dog caused only local inflammation, and no constitutional symptoms.[§]

It follows from the researches now detailed, that the salts of copper act in whatever way they are introduced into the system, and the more energetically, the more directly they enter the blood. The inquiries of Mr. Blake farther show, that when injected into the blood-vessels, they act with peculiar force in exhausting muscular irritability, and occasion death by paralysing the heart if they are injected into a vein. Six grains of the sulphate injected into the jugular vein of a dog reduced the force of the heart's contractions, and fifteen grains arrested them in twelve seconds, leaving in the dead body distension of the heart, loss of contractility, and florid blood in the left cavities. Ten grains injected into the aorta through the axillary artery caused no sign of obstruction in the capillary system; and small doses of three or four grains occasioned vomiting, dyspnœa, and

[*] Orfila. Toxic. Gén. i. 511.
[†] Ibid. Toxic. i. 513.
[‡] Buchner's Repertorium für die Pharmacie, lxxvi. 352.
[§] Toxicol. Générale, i. 515.

stiffness of the limbs; and immediately after death the muscles had lost their irritability.[*]

Copper has been sought for, with variable success, in the blood of animals poisoned with its salts. Drouard was unable to detect it in the blood. But this need not excite surprise, because the same physiologist could not detect it, even when he had injected it into a vein. — Lebküchner, who published a thesis at Tübingen in 1819, on the permeability of the living membranes, succeeded in discovering it. He introduced four grains of the ammoniacal sulphate into the bronchial tubes of a cat, and five minutes afterwards, when the animal was under the action of the poison, he drew some blood from the carotid artery and jugular vein; and he detected copper in the serum of the former, but not in the latter, by sulphuretted-hydrogen and hydrosulphate of ammonia.[†] — Afterwards Dr. Wibmer of Munich also succeeded in discovering it. In a dog which had taken from four to twenty grains of the neutral acetate daily for several weeks, he found the metal in the subtance of the liver, but not anywhere else. In the charcoally matter left by incinerating the liver, nitric acid formed a solution, which when neutralized gave the characteristic action of the salts of copper with sulphuretted-hydrogen, ferrocyanate of potash, and ammonia.[‡] Fischer also found copper in the blood of a dog which in forty-three days had got gradually-increasing doses of acetate of copper, till at length twelve grains were taken daily.[§] Orfila has recently often detected copper in the liver, spleen, heart, kidneys, and lungs of animals poisoned with its salts.[||] These facts are not all invalidated by the late discovery of the presence of copper in the animal tissues of men and animals not poisoned with its preparations. For in the experiments of Wibmer and of Orfila the quantity found in cases of poisoning was much larger than in the ordinary state of things; and the poison was accumulated in particular organs, especially the liver. The absorption of copper may therefore be considered as fully substantiated; and it is equally important whether it be regarded as a physiological or medico-legal fact.

Dr. Duncan's experiment on its effect when applied to a wound shows that it may prove fatal when applied externally. Yet in small quantities, the sulphate is daily used with safety for dressing ulcers.

As to the preparations of copper which are poisonous, it is pretty certain that, like all other metals, it is not deleterious unless oxidated, and that its soluble salts are by far the most energetic. Portal, indeed, has related the case of a woman who, while taking from a half a grain to four grains of copper filings daily, was seized with symptoms of poisoning.[¶] But it is probable the filings were oxidated;

* Edinburgh Med. and Surg. Journal, lvi 110

† Utrum per viventium adhuc anim. membr. et arter. pariet. mat. ponderab. permeare queant, 13.

‡ Ueber die Wirkung des Kupfers auf den thierischen Organismus, in Buchner's Repertorium für die Pharmacie, xxxii. 337, 1829.

§ Ibidem, lxxii. 56. || Journal de Chimie Médicale, 1840, p 475.

¶ Observations sur les effets des vapeurs méphitiques, 437.

for Drouard gave an ounce to dogs without injuring them at all,[*] and Lefortier more lately observed that two drachms had no effect.[†] The same explanation must be given of the injury sustained by those artisans who prepare and use what is called "bronze dust" in printing and paper-staining. If the substance employed be nothing else than an alloy of copper and zinc, as is alleged, the injurious effects to be mentioned presently can only be explained on the supposition that the copper becomes oxidated either before or after coming in contact with the body. It deserves to be added, that many persons have swallowed copper coins and retained them for weeks without having any symptoms of poisoning.

The sulphuret is equally innocuous with the metal if pure; but it appears probable that it becomes oxidated by long exposure to the air, and passes into the state of sulphate. Orfila found that an ounce of recently prepared sulphuret had no effect on a dog; but half an ounce of a parcel which had been long kept caused vomiting, and yielded a little sulphate to water.[‡] The power of the oxides has not been ascertained. They are certainly poisonous; and Lefortier found that both the red ditoxide and black protoxide undergo solution in no long time in the stomachs of dogs.[§] The hydrated protoxide is probably more active. From some experiments made at the hospital of St. Louis in Paris, it appears that twelve grains will cause nausea, pain in the stomach and bowels, vomiting and diarrhœa.[‖] There is no doubt that the carbonate or natural verdigris, the phosphate, and even the subphosphate, though quite insoluble in water, are capable of acting as poisons, because Lefortier found that they are soon dissolved in the stomachs of dogs, and in small doses cause severe vomiting in the course of fifteen minutes.[¶] But it is chiefly in the soluble salts that we are to look for the full development of the action of this poison. A very small quantity of the sulphate will prove fatal; for, as already noticed, Drouard found that six grains killed a dog in half an hour.

The symptoms caused by the soluble salts of copper in man are, in a general point of view, the same with those caused by arsenic and corrosive sublimate. But there are likewise some peculiarities. According to the cases related by Orfila in his Toxicology, the first symptom is violent headache, then vomiting and cutting pains in the bowels, and afterwards cramps in the legs and pains in the thighs. Sometimes throughout the whole course of the symptoms there is a peculiar coppery taste in the mouth, and a singular aversion to the smell of copper. Drouard notices this in his thesis; and says, that, having himself been once poisoned with verdigris, the smell of copper used to excite nausea for a long time after.[**] Another symptom, which occasionally occurs in this kind of poisoning, and never, so far as I know, in poisoning with arsenic or corrosive sublimate, is

* Orfila, Toxicol. Gén. i. 500.
† Annales d'Hygiène Publique, 1840, xxiv. 100.
‡ Arch. Gén. de Médecine, xix. 329.   § *Ut supra*, 103, 106.
‖ Corvisar.'s Journal de Medecine, xviii. 54.
¶ Ut supra, 108, 110, 113.   ** Ut supra, xviii. 56.

jaundice. It likewise appears that, when the case ends fatally, convulsions and insensibility generally precede death.

A set of cases illustrating the slighter forms of poisoning with copper has been published by M. Bonjean of Chambery. The cause was the preparation of an acid confection in a copper vessel. Two women suffered from severe headache, constriction of the throat, nausea, colic, and extreme weakness. Two young men, who had eaten the confection more freely, had for some hours excruciating colic, severe pain in the mouth and throat, impeded breathing, and hurried irregular pulse; and for twenty-four hours they suffered severely from headache and prostration of strength.*

The following case communicated to Professor Orfila by one of his friends will convey a good idea of the symptoms in severe cases, which do not prove fatal. A jeweller's workman swallowed intentionally half an ounce of verdigris, suspended in water. In fifteen minutes he was attacked with colic pains and profuse vomiting and purging. When seen by the physician eight hours afterwards there was not much vomiting, but frequent eructation of a matter containing verdigris, some salivation, a small pulse, and blueness about the eyes. In sixteen hours jaundice began to appear. In the course of the night he was a good deal relieved from the colic pains by three alvine discharges; and next morning he had ceased to vomit, and the pain had disappeared. But he complained of a taste of copper in his mouth, and the jaundice had increased. From this time he recovered rapidly, and on the fourth day convalescence was confirmed.†

When the poisoning ends fatally, convulsions, palsy, and insensibility, the signs in short of some injury done to the brain, are very generally present. This is illustrated by a good example in Pyl's Essays and Observations. It was the case of a confectioner's daughter, who took two ounces of verdigris, and died on the third day under incessant vomiting and diarrhœa, attended towards the close with convulsions, and then with palsy of the limbs. This case, however, is chiefly valuable for the dissection, which will be noticed presently.‡ But two cases of the same description are related in greater detail by Wildberg in his Practical Manual, which clearly show the action of this poison on the brain. They are the cases formerly alluded to of a lady and her daughter who were poisoned by sour-krout kept in a copper pan. Soon after dinner they were attacked first with pain in the stomach, then with nausea and anxiety, and next with eructation and vomiting of a green, bitter, sour, astringent matter. The pain afterwards shot downwards throughout the belly, and was then followed by diarrhœa; afterwards by convulsions, at first transient, then continued; and finally by insensibility. The daughter died in twelve hours, the mother an hour later.§ In these three cases, although there was not any jaundice

* Journal de Chimie Médicale, 1841, p. 309.   † Toxicol. Gén. i. 519.
‡ Aufsätze und Beobacht. aus der gericht. Arneiwiss. viii. 85.
§ Practisches Handbuch für Physiker, iii. 308.

noticed during life, the skin was very yellow after death. — In some instances it would appear that narcotic symptoms form the commencement and irritant symptoms the termination of the poisoning. This unusual relation occurs in a case of recovery related by M. Julia-Fontenelle, and also, though less remarkably, in a fatal case mentioned by Wibmer. The subject of the former was a man who intentionally took a solution of copper in vinegar, prepared by keeping several sous-pieces seven days in that fluid. In three hours he was found in a state of insensibility, with the jaws locked, the muscles rigid and frequently convulsed, the breathing interrupted, and the pulse small and slow. In half an hour he was so far roused that he could tell what he had done ; and soon after taking white of eggs the convulsions ceased : but next day the belly was hard and tender, and the repeated application of leeches was required to subdue the abdominal irritation that ensued.* In the fatal case by Wibmer, that of a girl of 18, who was poisoned by a dish of beans having been cooked in a copper vessel, sickness, pain of the belly and vomiting speedily arose, but were soon followed by convulsions and loss of consciousness. Next day there was little pain, but extraordinary paralytic weakness of the arms and legs : the abdomen afterwards became distended and painful ; and death took place in seventy-eight hours.† — A case where convulsions were produced by two drachms of blue vitriol is mentioned by Dr. Percival.‡ — In other instances it would appear that no nervous affection occurs at all, as in the case of a young lady related by Percival, who, when poisoned with pickled samphire containing copper, suffered chiefly from pains in the stomach, an eruption over the breast, general shooting pains, thirst, a frequent small pulse, vomiting, hiccup, and purging. Death occurred on the ninth day, without stupor or convulsions.§

Besides these effects when introduced in considerable doses and in the form of soluble salts, copper is said to produce other disorders when applied to the body for a long time in minute quantities and in its metallic or oxidized state. Among those artisans who work much with copper various affections are thought to be gradually engendered by merely handling the metal. Patissier in his treatise on the diseases of artisans says, that copper-workers have a peculiar appearance which distinguishes them from other tradesmen, — that they have a greenish complexion, — that the same colour tinges their eyes, tongue, and hair, their excretions, and even their clothes through the medium of the perspiration, — that they are spare, short in stature, bent, their offspring ricketty, and they themselves old and even decrepit at their fortieth or fiftieth year.‖ Mérat also asserts that they are liable to the painters' colic, that peculiar

* Journ. de Chimie Médicale, v. 413.
† Die Wirkung der Arzneimittel und Gifte, ii. 253.
‡ Trans. London Coll. Phys. iii. 88.
§ Quoted by Dr. Thomson in Lancet, 1836-37, ii. 640.
‖ Traité des Maladies des Artizans, p. 78.

disease soon to be noticed as a common effect of the long-continued
application of lead.*

But these notions must be received with some limitation. At least
the alleged effects on copper-workers are by no means invariable. For
copper-workers now-a-days in this country and elsewhere are by no
means the unhealthy persons Patissier represents them to be. As to
colica pictonum, it is very rare among them ; and possibly the cases
noticed by Mérat might have been produced by the secret introduction of lead into the body, if indeed they were not cases of common
colic.

A very singular set of cases was lately brought under notice by
Mr. Gurney Turner, where poisoning seemed to have been occasioned
by the external application or inhalation of the fine dust used for
imitating gilding by painters, paper-stainers, and porcelain-painters,
and which is said to be essentially brass in a state of fine division.
The workmen who use it, are very apt to be attacked with irritation
about the private parts, and a vesicular eruption about the hairs on
the pubes, — with loss of appetite, tendency to vomiting, and other
symptoms of irritation in the stomach, — with obstinate constipation,
— with soreness and dryness of the throat and irritation in the nose,
— and with want of sleep, and a remarkable greenness of the hair
over the whole body.†

SECTION III. — *Of the Morbid Appearances caused by Copper.*

The appearances found in the body after death by poisoning with
copper are chiefly the signs of inflammation.

Where death takes place very rapidly, however, it is probable, that
no diseased appearance whatever will be perceptible. At least this
was the case in the animals experimented on by Drouard and Orfila ;
and little doubt can therefore be entertained that the result would be
the same with man also in similar circumstances.

When death ensues more slowly, as in the only fatal cases yet
on record of its action on man, the marks of inflammation coincide
with the signs of irritation during life. The best account I have seen
of the morbid appearances under such circumstances is in the cases
related by Pyl, by Wildberg, by Wibmer, and by Dégrange.

In Pyl's case the whole skin was yellow. The intestines, particularly the lesser intestines, were of an unusual green colour, inflamed,
and here and there gangrenous. The stomach was also green ; its
inner coat was excessively inflamed ; and near the pylorus there was
a spot as big as a crown, where the villous coat was thick, hard,
and covered with firmly adhering verdigris. The lungs are likewise said to have been inflamed. The blood was firmly coagulated.

In the cases related by Wildberg, which are very like each other,
the skin on various parts, and particularly on the face, was yellow,
but on the depending parts livid. The outer coat of the stomach

* Traité de la Colique Métallique, p. 103.
† London Medical Gazette, 1838-39, i. 195, 697.

and intestines was here and there inflamed ; and the inner coat of the former was very much inflamed, and even gangrenous* near the pylorus and cardia. The duodenum and jejunum, and likewise the gullet, were in a similar state. The blood in the heart and great vessels was black and fluid.

In the case of the girl referred to by Wibmer, the skin was ochre-yellow, the stomach green, much inflamed, especially near the pylorus, the gullet and intestines also inflamed, the diaphragm red, the brain healthy, the lungs and heart " gorged with thick blood."

In the case of poisoning with carbonate of copper described by Dégrange [p. 348], in which, however, it is probable that death was accelerated by a fall, there was found congestion of the surface of the brain, arborescent redness of the gullet and a green sand over its sur-face, general greenness of the villous coat of the stomach, with vas-cularity of the fundus and points of superficial ulceration, greenness of the whole intestines, with black vascular ecchymosed spots and softening, except in the ileum, and redness of the inner surface of the heart. Copper was detected in the contents of the stomach and intestines.

The intestines have been found perforated by ulceration, and their contents thrown out into the sac of the peritonæum. Portal has re-lated one case where the small intestines were perforated, and several where the perforation was in the rectum, which portion of the intes-tines, as well as the duodenum, jejunum, and ileum, was also ex-tensively ulcerated.†

The existence of verdigris in the form of powder lining the inside of the stomach after incessant vomiting for three days, is of course an important circumstance in the inspection of the body. But too much reliance ought not to be placed on mere bluish or greenish colouring of the membranes. For Orfila‡ and Guersent§ have both observed, that the inside of the stomach as well as its contents may acquire these tints in a remarkable degree in consequence of natural disease.

SECTION IV. — Of the Treatment of Poisoning with Copper.

The treatment of poisoning with tne salts of copper has been ex-amined in relation to the antidotes by M. Drouard, M. Marcelin-Du-val, Professor Orfila, and M. Postel.

The alkaline sulphurets were at one time thought to be antidotes for the poisons of copper, but without any reason. Drouard found that fifteen grains of verdigris killed a dog in thirty hours, notwith-standing the free use of the liver of sulphur.||

Afterwards M. Marcelin-Duval was led from his experiments to

* Gangrene could not have taken place in thirteen hours. The appearance must have been black extravasation, which has often been mistaken for gangrene. See page 267.

† Portal sur les effets des vapeurs méphitiques, 436, 439.

‡ Orfila, Tox. Gén. i. 530.

§ Dict. des Sciences Médicales, vii. 564. || Orfila, Tox. Gén. i. 534.

34

infer that sugar was an antidote,* and in the first editions of his Toxicology Professor Orfila agreed with him, and related some experiments of his own, which, along with those of Duval, seemed to place the fact beyond all doubt. Later and more careful experiments, however, satisfied Orfila, that it only acts as an emollient after the poison has been removed from the stomach, and that it has no effect at all if the poison is retained by a ligature in the gullet.† Sugar being thus rejected as well as the sulphurets, he was led to try the effects of albumen ; and his experiments induced him to recommend that substance as an antidote in preference to every thing else. He found that the white of six eggs completely neutralized the activity of between 25 and 36 grains of verdigris; so that even when the mixture was retained in the stomach by a ligature on the gullet no effect ensued which could be ascribed to the poison. He infers that white of egg is the best antidote for poisoning with copper.‡ He likewise found the ferrocyanate of potass not inferior.§

Since the publication of these inquires the subject has been again examined by M. Postel, who reverts to the original proposition of Duval, that sugar is really a good antidote; and he rests this conclusion partly on direct comparative experiments, showing that it is at least equally effective with white of egg, and partly on the singular fact as certained by him, that sugar, which was believed to decompose the salts of copper only at the temperature of 212°, does actually accomplish this decomposition at the temperature of the human body, and throws down the copper in the form of oxide.‖

According to the experiments of MM. Milne-Edwards and Dumas, metallic iron is likewise a good antidote : they found that when fifteen, twenty, and even fifty grains of sulphate of copper, acetate of copper, or verdigris, were given to animals, and an ounce of iron filings administered either immediately before, or immediately afterwards, — the gullet being tied to prevent the discharge of the poison, — death did not ensue for five, six, or even eight days, and consequently proceeded from the operation on the gullet ; and that in one experiment, on the ligature being removed from the gullet, the opening healed up, and complete recovery took place.¶

Before quitting the subject of the treatment, it is necessary to caution the practitioner particularly against the employment of vinegar, — a substance often ignorantly used for this, in common with many other, species of poisoning. On account of its solvent power over the insoluble compounds formed by the salts of copper with animal and vegetable matters, it must be injurious rather than useful.

* Orfila, Tox. Gén. i. 535.   † Ibidem, i. 539.
‡ Ibidem, i. 540.   § Ibidem, 541.
‖ Journal de Pharmacie, xviii. 570.
¶ London Medico-Chirurgical Review, v. 611.

CHAPTER XVI.

OF POISONING WITH ANTIMONY.

The fourth genus of the metallic irritants includes the preparations of antimony. Poisoning with antimonial preparations is not common. They are employed extensively in medicine, however, and consequently accidents have sometimes occurred with them. One of them is also often foolishly used, in the way of amusement, to cause sickness and purging, and likewise to detect servants who are suspected of making free with their mistress's tea-box or whisky-bottle ; and in both of these ways alarming effects have sometimes been produced. In 1837 a woman was tried in England for attempting to poison a child with tartar-emetic ; but the poison appeared to have been given through ignorance.* In large doses some of the antimonial compounds may cause death ; and one of them, the chloride of antimony, now very little used in this country, is a violent corrosive.

Section I. — *Of the Chemical History and Tests for the preparations of Antimony.*

Metallic antimony has a bluish-white colour, not liable to tarnish. Its specific gravity is 6·7. It is easily fused, but is not very volatile. In certain circumstances, however, it easily undergoes a spurious sublimation, by being carried along with gases disengaged while it is in the act of being reduced.

A great number of preparations of antimony were at one time to be found in the shop of the apothecary ; but they are now reduced to a few. Those which require notice here are the oxide, chloride, and tartar-emetic.

The *oxide* [sesquioxide] is a white heavy powder, which is best known by its solubility in tartaric acid, and the effects of the tests for tartar-emetic on the solution.

The *chloride* [sesquichloride], as usually seen, is a yellow or reddish liquid, but when pure is colourless. It is highly corrosive. It is readily known by the effect of water in decomposing it, — an insoluble white subchloride being thrown down, and hydrochloric acid remaining in solution. The latter is detected by nitrate of silver ; and the precipitate is known by being soluble in a solution of tartaric acid, and then presenting the reactions of tartar-emetic.

Tartar-Emetic.

In its solid state tartar-emetic forms regular tetraedral or more generally octaedral crystals, which are colourless when pure, efflorescent, and of a slightly metallic taste. As commonly seen in the shops it is in the form of a white, or pale yellowish-white powder.

* Taylor's Medical Jurisprudence, 1844, p. 206.

When heated it decrepitates and then chars ; and if the heat be increased the oxide of antimony is reduced by the carbonaceous matter, and little globules appear, like those of quicksilver in point of colour.   The best way of reducing tartar-emetic is to char it in a porcelain vessel or watch-glass, and then to increase the heat till the charred mass takes fire.   Or the charred mass may be introduced into a tube and heated strongly with the blowpipe, after which glo-bules of antimony will be found lining the bottom of the glass where the material has been.   None of it is ever sublimed.   It is not easy to procure distinct globules by heating tartar-emetic at once in a small tube.

According to Dr. Duncan, tartar-emetic is soluble in three parts of boiling and fifteen of temperate water.   The solution presents the following characters with reagents.

1. *Caustic potass* precipitates a white sesquioxide, but only if the solution is tolerably concentrated.   The first portions of the test have no effect.   The precipitate is redissolved by an excess of potass.

2. *Nitric acid* throws down a white precipitate, and takes it up again when added in excess.

3. The *Infusion of Galls* causes a dirty, yellowish-white precipi-tate ; but it will not act on a solution which contains much less than two grains per ounce.

4. The best liquid reagent is *Hydrosulphuric acid*.   In a solution containing only an eighth part of a grain per ounce, it strikes an orange-red colour, which, when the excess of gas is expelled by heat, becomes an orange-red precipitate ; and if the proportion of salt is greater, the precipitate is thrown down at once. — The colour of the precipitate is so peculiar as to distinguish it from every other sulphu-ret ; but if any doubt regarding its nature should occur, it may be known by collecting it, dissolving it with the aid of gentle heat in hydro-chloric acid, and adding water to the solution ; which will then yield a white precipitate, the sesquioxide of antimony in union with a little chlorine.

5. When the solution is put into Marsh's apparatus for detecting arsenic [p. 211], the flame yields a dark brownish-black, obscurely shining crust on a surface of porcelain held across it, and a white crystalline powder if the porcelain be held just above the flame.   The dark crust is antimony, the white one its oxide.   The former has only a distant resemblance to the brilliant stain of arsenic, notwith-standing all that has been said of their similarity.   It is well, however, to use some other test for distinguishing the two metals besides their appearance ; and the most convenient is a solution of chloride of lime, which instantly makes an arsenical crust disappear, but does not affect an antimonial one.

Tartar-emetic, like the soluble salts of mercury and copper, is decomposed by various organic principles.   All vegetable sub-stances that contain a considerable quantity of tannin have this effect ; of which an example has been already mentioned in the action of infusion of galls.   Decoctions of cinchona bark decompose it still more effectually. The animal principles do not act on tartar-emetic, with the exception of milk, which is slightly coagulated by a concentrated solution. Many vegetable and animal substances, though they do not decompose it, alter the operation of the fluid tests. Thus tea, though it does not effect any distinct decomposition of the salt, will prevent the action of gall-infusion; and French wine gives a violet tint to the precipitates with that test and with acids.* Hydrosulphuric acid, however, acts under all circumstances, and always characteristically, whatever the colour of the fluid may be. Dr. Turner found that when transmitted through a diluted solution in tea, porter, broth, and milk, with certain precautions to be mentioned presently, he procured a precipitate which either showed its proper colour at once, or did so at the margin of the filter on which it was collected.†

The circumstances now referred to render it necessary to resort to other means, besides the simple application of liquid reagents, for the purpose of detecting tartar-emetic in complex organic mixtures. This subject has been ably investigated, first by Dr. Turner,‡ and afterterwards by Professor Orfila.§ The result of the researches of both seems to me to be that the most convenient method yet proposed is the following.

Process for Tartar-emetic in Organic Mixtures. — If the subject of analysis be not already liquid enough, add distilled water. Then acidulate with a little hydrochloric and tartaric acids; the former of which throws down some animal principles, while the latter dissolves readily all precipitates formed with tartar-emetic by reagents or organic principles except the sulphuret. Filter the product.

1. Subject a small portion of the liquid to a stream of hydrosulphuric acid gas, and if it be perceptibly coloured orange-red, treat the whole liquid in the same way; boil to expel the excess of gas, collect the precipitate, dry it, and reduce it by hydrogen gas in the following manner. Put the sulphuret in a little horizontal tube, transmit hydrogen through the tube by means of the apparatus reprsented in Figure 9, and when all the air of the apparatus is expelled, apply heat to the sulphuret with a spirit-lamp. Hydrosulphuric acid gas is evolved, and metallic antimony is left, if the current of hydrogen be gentle, or it is sublimed if the current be rapid. — When there is much animal or vegetable matter present in the sulphuret, the metal is not always distinctly visible. In that case, dissolve the antimony by the action of nitric acid on the mixed material and broken fragments of the tube, and throw down the orange sulphuret again from the neutralized solution by hydrosulphuric acid.

2. If hydrosulphuric acid do not distinctly affect the liquid, or if no precipitate be separated after boiling, or so small a quantity as

---

* Orfila, Toxicol. Générale, i. 466.
† Edinburgh Med. and Surg. Journal, **xxviii. 71.**
‡ Ibid. xxviii. 71.
§ Journal de Chimie Médicale, 1840.

34*

cannot well be collected, — evaporate the liquid to dryness, char it by means of nitric acid and chlorate of potash, as directed for copper (p. 357), boil the carbonaceous mass for half an hour in a mixture of eight parts of hydrochloric acid and one of nitric acid, and introduce the filtered solution into the modification of Marsh's apparatus for detecting arsenic described in page 204, but without the tube *e h*. Kindle the gas at *e*, and try whether a black, dull stain, not removable by solution of chloride of lime, be produced on a surface of porcelain held across the flame. If no stain be produced, there was no antimony in the liquid under examination. If the porcelain be stained, apply the heat of a spirit-lamp flame to the tube *d e*. Antimony will de deposited within the tube where the heat is applied. In order to ascertain its nature, break the tube, heat the portion containing the crust with nitro-hydrochloric acid, evaporate to dryness, dissolve the residue in hydrochloric acid, decompose a part of this solution with water, and subject the rest to a stream of hydrosulphuric acid gas, which will produce the usual orange sulphuret of antimony.

3. If antimony be not indicated in either of these ways in the fluid part of the subject of analysis, the solid portion may next be subjected to the second process ; but success will very seldom attend the search when the previous steps have failed.

The first branch of this process,—a slight modification of Dr. Turner's,—is a very delicate and satisfactory method of detecting antimony in organic mixtures. Some practice is required to transmit the hydrogen gas with the proper rapidity. The gas ought to be allowed to pass for some time before the spirit-lamp flame is applied, otherwise the oxygen remaining in the apparatus may cause an explosion, or will oxidate the metallic antimony, formed by the reduction of the sulphuret. As soon as the reduction of the sulphuret begins, the tube is blackened on account of the action of the sulphuretted-hydrogen on the lead contained in the glass. This obscures the operations within the tube ; but on subsequently breaking it, a metallic button or a sublimate will be easily seen. When the sulphuret is considerable in quantity and the gaseous current slow, the metal remains where the sulphuret was ; but if the mass of sulphuret is small and the current rapid, then the metal is sublimed and condensed in minute scaly brilliant crystals.

The second branch of the process is a modification of the method lately employed by Professor Orfila for detecting antimony in the textures and secretions of animals poisoned with tartar-emetic. It is probably more delicate than the other, but not more satisfactory.

The method of analysis here recommended, as well as every other yet proposed for organic mixtures, merely detects the presence of antimony. It does not indicate the state in which the metal was combined. It is a process in short for antimony in every state of combination.

It is almost unnecessary to observe that when the contents of the stomach or vomited matters are the subject of analysis, care must be taken to ascertain that tartar-emetic was not administered as a remedy.

SECTION II. — *Of the Action of Tartar-Emetic, and the Symptoms it excites in Man.*

There is little peculiarity in what is hitherto known of the symptoms of poisoning with tartar-emetic in man. Cases in which it has been taken to the requisite extent are rarely met with; and it has seldom remained long enough in the stomach to act deleteriously. But its action on animals would appear from the experiments of Magendie to be in some respects peculiar.

He found that dogs, like man, may take a large dose with impunity, for example half an ounce, if they are allowed to vomit; but that if the gullet is tied, from four to eight grains will kill them in a few hours. His subsequent experiments go to prove that death is owing to the poison exciting inflammation in the lungs. When six or eight grains dissolved in water were injected into a vein, the animal was attacked with vomiting and purging, and death ensued commonly within an hour. In the dead body he found not only redness of the whole villous coat of the stomach and intestines, but also that the lungs were of an orange-red or violet colour throughout, destitute of crepitation, gorged with blood, dense like the spleen, and here and there even hepatized. A larger quantity caused death more rapidly without affecting the alimentary canal; a smaller quantity caused intense inflammation there and death in twenty-four hours; but the lungs were always more or less affected.*

It is a fact, too, worthy of notice, that in whatever way this poison enters the body its effects are nearly the same. This is shown not only by the researches of Magendie already mentioned, but likewise by the experiments of Schloepfer, who found that a scruple dissolved in twelve parts of water and injected into the windpipe, caused violent vomiting, difficult breathing, and death in three days; and in the dead body the lungs and stomach were much inflamed, particularly the former.† It farther appears from an experiment related by Dr. Campbell, that, when applied to a wound, it acts with almost equal energy as when injected into a vein. Five grains killed a cat in this way in three hours, causing inflammation of the wound, and vivid redness of the stomach.‡ He did not find the lungs inflamed.

Magendie infers from his own researches that tartar-emetic occasions death when swallowed, not by inflaming the stomach, but through means of a general inflammatory state of the whole system subsequent to its absorption, — of which disorder the affection of the stomach and intestines and even that of the lungs are merely parts or symptoms. The later experiments of Rayer tend in some measure to confirm these views, by showing that death may occur without inflammation being excited any where. In animals killed in twenty-five

* Memoire sur l'Emétique, or Orfila, Toxicol. Gen. i. 469.
† De Effectibus liquidorum, &c. p. 32.
‡ Diss. Inaug. de Venenis Mineral. Edin. 1813. P. 23.

minutes by tartar-emetic applied to a wound, he, like Dr. Campbell, could see no trace of inflammation in any organ of the great cavities.*

Orfila has proved by analysis the important fact that tartar-emetic is absorbed in the course of its action, and may be detected in the animal tissues and secretions. He found that, when it is applied to the cellular tissue of small dogs, two grains disappear before death : That antimony may be detected by his process given above throughout the soft textures generally, but especially in the liver and kidneys : but that it is quickly discharged from these quarters through the medium of the urine. Hence in an animal that died in four hours he found it abundantly in the liver and still more in the urine ; in one that survived seventeen hours, the liver presented mere traces of the poison, but the urine contained it in abundance ; and in one that lived thirty-six hours, there was a large quantity in the urine, but none at all in the liver. He also ascertained that antimony is generally to be found in the urine of persons who are taking tartar-emetic continuously in large doses for pneumonia according to Rasori's mode of administering it.†   These results have been confirmed by the conjoined researches of Panizza and Kramer, who found antimony in the urine and blood of a man during a course of tartar-emetic.‡   And Flandin and Danger also satisfied themselves that in animals it may be generally detected in the liver.§

Effects on Man. — When tartar-emetic is swallowed by man, it generally causes vomiting very soon and is all discharged ; and then no other effect follows. But if it remains long in the stomach before it excites vomiting, or if the dose be large, more permanent symptoms are sometimes induced. The vomiting recurs frequently, and is attended with burning pain in the pit of the stomach, and followed by purging and colic pains. There is sometimes a sense of tightness in the throat, which may be so great as to prevent swallowing. The patient is likewise tormented with violent cramps. Among the cases hitherto recorded no notice is taken of pulmonary symptoms ; which might be expected to occur if Magendie's experiments are free of fallacy.

The late introduction of large doses of tartar-emetic into medical practice having excited some doubt as to its poisonous properties, it becomes a matter of some moment to possess positive facts on the subject. The following cases may therefore be quoted, which will satisfy every one that this substance is sometimes an active irritant.

The first is particularly interesting from its close resemblance to cholera. It occurred in consequence of an apothecary having sold tartar-emetic by mistake for cream of tartar. The quantity taken was about a scruple. A few moments afterwards the patient com-

* Diction. de Méd. et de Chir. Pratiques, Art. Antimoine, iii. 69.
† Journal de Chim. Médicale, 1840, p. 291, and Orfila, Toxicologie Générale, 1843, i. 475.
‡ Annales d'Hygiène-Publique, xxix. 427.
§ Buchner's Repertorium für die Pharmacie, lxxviii. 107, from Comptes Rendus de l'Institut.

plained of pain in the stomach, then of a tendency to faint, and at last he was seized with violent bilious vomiting. Soon after that he felt colic pains extending throughout the whole bowels, and accompanied ere long with profuse and unceasing diarrhœa. The pulse at the same time was small and contracted, and his strength failed completely ; but the symptom which distressed him most was frequent rending cramp in the legs. He remained in this state for about six hours, and then recovered gradually under the use of cinchona and opium ; but for some time afterwards he was liable to weakness of digestion.[*]

The next case to be mentioned, where the dose was forty grains, proved fatal, although the person vomited soon after taking it. The symptoms illustrate well the compound narcotico-acrid action often observed in animals. The poison was taken voluntarily. Before the person was seen by M. Récamier, who relates the case, he had been nearly two days ill with vomiting, excessive purging, and convulsions. On the third day he had great pain and tension in the region of the stomach, and appeared like a man in a state of intoxication. In the course of the day the whole belly became swelled, and at night delirium supervened. Next day all the symptoms were aggravated ; towards evening the delirium became furious ; convulsions followed ; and he died during the night, not quite five days after taking the poison.[†]

Severe effects have also been caused by so small a dose as six grains. A woman, who swallowed this quantity, wrapped in paper, was seized in half an hour with violent vomiting, which soon became bloody. In two hours the decoction of cinchona was administered with much relief. But she had severe colic, diarrhœa, pain in the stomach, and some fever ; of which symptoms she was not completely cured for five days.[‡] A case has been published, where a dose of only four grains caused pain in the belly, vomiting, and purging, followed by convulsions, failure of the pulse, and loss of speech ; and recovery took place very slowly.[§] Under the head of the treatment another case will be noticed where half a drachm excited severe symptoms, and was probably prevented from proving fatal only by the timely use of antidotes.

While these examples prove that tartar-emetic is occasionally an active irritant in the dose of a scruple or less, it must at the same time be admitted to be uncertain in its action as a poison. This appears from the late employment of it in large doses as a remedy for inflammation of the lungs. The administration of tartar-emetic in large doses was a common enough practice so early as the seventeenth century, and was also occasionally resorted to by physicians between that and the present time. But it is only in late years that, by the recommendations of Professor Rasori of Milan,[||] and M.

* Orfila, Toxicol. i. 74.   † Ibid. i. 478.
‡ Bulletins des Sciences Médicales, xvii. 243.
§ Taylor's Medical Jurisprudence, 205, from Casper's Wochenschrift.
|| Edin. Med. and Surg. Journal, xxii. 227.

Laennec of Paris, it has again become a general method of treatment. According to this method, tartar-emetic is given to the extent of twelve, twenty, or even thirty grains a-day in divided doses ;
and not only without producing any dangerous irritation of the alimentary canal, but even also not unfrequently without any physiological effect whatever. Doubts were at one time entertained of the
accuracy of the statements to this effect published by foreign physicians ; but these doubts are now dissipated, as the same practice has
been tried, with the same results, by many in Britain. Rasori
ascribes the power the body possesses of enduring large doses of
tartar-emetic without injury, to a peculiar diathesis which accompanies the disease and ceases along with it. And it is said, that the
same patients, who, while the disorder continues, may take large
doses with impunity, are affected in the usual manner, if the doses
are not rapidly lessened after the disease has begun to give way.
The testimony of Laennec on the subject is impartial and decisive.
He observes he has given as much as two grains and a half every
two hours till twenty grains were taken daily, and once gave forty
grains in twenty-four hours by mistake ; that he never saw any harm
result ; and that vomiting or diarrhœa was seldom produced, and
never after the first day. The power of endurance he found to diminish, but not, as Rasori alleges, to cease altogether, when the fever
ceases ; for some of his patients took six, twelve, or eighteen grains
daily when in full convalescence.* My own observations correspond with Laennec's, except as to the effects of large doses during
convalescence, of which effects I have had no experience. I have
seen from six to twenty grains, given daily in several doses of one
or two grains, check bad cases of pneumonia and bronchitis, without
causing vomiting or diarrhœa after the first day, and also without increasing the perspiration. At the same time I have twice seen the
first two or three doses excite so violent a purging and pain in the
stomach and whole bowels, that I was deterred from persevering with
the remedy. In continued fever too I have repeatedly found that the
doses mentioned above did not cause any symptoms of irritation in
the stomach or intestines.

The large quantities now mentioned have even been sometimes
given in a single dose with nearly the same results. Dr. Christie
mentions in his Treatise on Cholera that he sometimes gave a scruple
in one dose with the effect of exciting merely some vomiting and
several watery stools. But he admits that in one instance symptoms
were induced like those of a case of violent cholera.†

The same large doses have been given by some in delirium tremens without any poisonous effect being produced. A correspondent
of the Lancet has even mentioned that on one occasion, after gradually increasing the dose, he at last wound up the treatment, successfully as regarded the disease, and without any injury to the patient,

* Laennec, Auscultation Médiate, i. 493.
† On the Nature and Treatment of Cholera, p. 24.

by giving four doses of twenty grains each, in the course of twenty minutes.*

These facts are sufficiently perplexing, when viewed along with what were previously quoted in support of the poisonous effects of tartar-emetic. On a full consideration of the whole circumstances, however, I conceive the conclusion which will be drawn is, that this substance is not so active a poison as was till lately supposed ; — that in the dose of four, six, or ten grains, it may cause severe symptoms, but is uncertain in its action, — and that although there appears to be some uncertainty in the effects of even much larger doses, such as a scruple, yet in general violent irritation will then be induced, and sometimes death itself.

An instance is related in the Journal Universel of a man who, while in a state of health, swallowed seventeen grains, and then tried to suffocate himself with the fumes of burning charcoal. He recovered, though not without suffering severely from the charcoal fumes; but he could hardly be said to have been affected at all by the tartar-emetic.[†] Here the inactivity of the poison was probably owing to the narcotic effects of the fumes.

The effects of tartar-emetic on the skin are worthy of notice ; but they have not yet been carefully studied. Some facts tend to show that even its constitutional action may be developed through the sound skin. Mr. Sherwen attempted to prove by experiments on himself and two pupils, that five or seven grains in solution will, when rubbed on the palms, produce in a few hours nausea and copious perspiration.[‡] His observations have been confirmed by Mr. Hutchinson.[§] But Savary, a French physician, on repeating these experiments, could remark nothing more than a faint flat taste and slight salivation ;[||] and Mr. Gaitskell could not remark any constitutional effect at all.[¶] Sometimes it has appeared to cause severe symptoms of irritant poisoning when used in the form of ointment to excite a pustular eruption. An instance of this has been described in a late French Journal.[**] Nay, in the Medical Repository there is a case, in which the external use of tartar-emetic ointment is supposed to have been the cause of death. The subject was an infant, two years old, who, soon after having the spine rubbed with this ointment, was seized with great sickness and frequent fainting, which in forty-eight hours proved fatal.[††] Considering the numerous opportunities which medical men have had of witnessing the effects of tartar-emetic applied in the same manner, and that these are solitary cases, doubts may be entertained whether the irritant symptoms in the one case, or the child's death in the other, were occasioned in the way supposed.

Although the constitutional action of tartar-emetic is not easily developed through the sound skin, its local effects are severe and unequivocal. When applied to the skin it does not corrode, but

* Mr. Greenwood, Lancet, 1835-36, ii. 142.
    Renauld in Journ. Univ. des Sciences Médicales, xvii. 120.
‡ Mem. of Lond. Med. Soc. ii. 386.   § Ibidem, v. 81.
|| Corvisart's Journ. de Med. xxvi. 221.   ¶ Mem. of Lond. Med. Soc. iv. 79.
** Journal de Chimie Médicale, iv.   †† Lond. Med. Repos. xvi. 357.

excites inflammation, on which account it is much used instead of cantharides. It does not blister; but after being a few days applied, it brings out a number of painful pustules ; if it be persevered in, the skin ulcerates ; and if it be applied to an ulcerated surface it causes profuse suppuration, or sometimes even sloughing.

Tartar-emetic is one of the substances which appear to possess the property of acting on the infant through the medium of its nurse's milk. I do not know, indeed, what may be the general experience on this point ; but a French physician, M. Minaret, has published a clear case of the kind, in the instance of a young woman who was taking tartar-emetic for pleurisy, and whose infant was attacked with a fit of vomiting immediately after every attempt to suck the breast.*

There is some reason to suppose, that the vapours of antimony may prove injurious when inhaled. Four persons, constantly exposed in preparing antimonial compounds to the vapour of antimonious acid and chloride of antimony, were attacked with headache, difficult breathing, stitches in the back and sides, difficult expectoration of viscid mucus, want of sleep and appetite, mucous discharge from the urethra, loss of sexual propensity, atrophy of the testicles, and a pustular eruption on various parts, but especially on the scrotum. They all recovered.†

SECTION III.—*Of the Morbid Appearances produced by Tartar-emetic.*

The morbid appearances caused by tartar-emetic have not been often witnessed in man.

In M. Récamier's case there were some equivocal signs of reaction in the brain. The organs in the chest were healthy. The villous coat of the stomach, except near the gullet, where it was healthy, was everywhere red, thickened, and covered with tough mucus. The whole intestines were completely empty. The duodenum was in the same state as the stomach ; but the other intestines were in their natural condition.

M. Jules-Cloquet observed in the body of a man who died of apoplexy, and who in the course of five days had taken forty grains of tartar-emetic, without vomiting or purging, — that the villous coat of the stomach had a deep reddish-violet colour, with cherry-red spots interspersed; and that the whole small intestines were of a rose-red tint spotted with cherry-red.‡

The only other dissection I have seen noticed is one by Hoffmann. He says that in a woman poisoned by tartar-emetic he found the stomach gangrenous, and the lungs, diaphragm, and spleen as it were in a state of putrefaction.§ Little credit can be given to this description.

In animals Schloepfer found the blood always fluid.‖

* London Medical Gazette, xii. 496.
† Lohmerer in Journal de Chimie Médicale, 1840, p. 629.
‡ Orfila, Toxicol. Générale, i. 480.
§ De Medicamentis Venenorum vim habentibus. Opera Omnia, T. 1. p. ii. 213.
‖ Diss. Inaug. de Effectibus liquidorum, &c. p. 32.

SECTION IV. — *Of the Treatment of Poisoning with Antimony.*

The treatment of poisoning with tartar-emetic is simple. If the poison be not already discharged, large draughts of warm water should be given and the throat tickled, to bring on vomiting. At the same time some vegetable decoction should be prepared, which possesses the power of decomposing the poison ; and none is better or more likely to be at hand than a decoction of cinchona-bark, particularly yellow-bark. The tincture is also a good form for giving this antidote. The administration of bark has been found useful even after vomiting had continued for some length of time, probably because a part of the poison nevertheless remained undischarged. Before the decoction is ready, it is useful to administer the bark in powder. It is alleged, however, by M. Toulmouche that decoction of cinchona is not nearly so serviceable as infusion of galls, and that powder of galls is better still.* When there is reason to believe that the patient has vomited enough, and that a sufficient quantity of the antidote has been taken, opium is evidently indicated and has been found useful ; but venesection may be previously necessary if the signs of inflammation in the stomach are obstinate.

The following case related by M. Serres was probably cured by cinchona. At all events, the effect of the antidote was striking. A man purchased half a drachm in divided doses at different shops, and swallowed the whole in a cup of coffee. Very soon afterwards he was attacked with burning pain in the stomach, convulsive tremors, and impaired sensibility, — afterwards with cold clamminess of the skin, hiccup, and some swelling of the epigastrium, but not with vomiting. Decoction of cinchona was given freely. From the first moment almost of its administration he felt relief, and began to sweat and purge. Next morning, however, he vomited, and for some days there were evident signs of slight inflammation in the stomach ; nay, for a month afterwards he had occasional pricking pains in that region ; but he eventually recovered.† Another and more pointed case has been related by Dr. Sauveton of Lyons. A lady swallowed by mistake for whey a solution of sixty grains of tartar emetic. In ten minutes she was seen by her physician, and at this time vomiting had not commenced. Tincture of bark was immediately given in large doses. No unpleasnnt symptom occurred except nausea and slight colic.‡

Orfila considers that the diuretic plan of treatment recommended by him for arsenic [p. 288] is equally applicable in the case of antimony. Having ascertained that a grain and a half of tartar-emetic applied to a wound constantly killed dogs in a period varying from seventeen to thirty-six hours, if no treatment was employed, — he administered to them in this way a dose varying from a grain and a

* Archives Générales de Médecine, xlvii. 364.
† Orfila, Toxicol. Générale, i. 475.
‡ Bulletins des Sciences Médicales, vi. 259.

half to three grains, and by then giving diuretics effected a cure in four out of five instances.*

Chloride of Antimony.

The chloride of antimony [sesquichloride, muriate, or butter of antimony] being now put to little use and seldom seen except as an intermediate product obtained in the preparation of other compounds of antimony, it is rarely met with as the cause of poisoning, and therefore scarcely deserves notice here, were it not that its effects differ widely from those of tartar-emetic and other antimonials.

It is easily known by the characters mentioned above. It has not yet been made the subject of investigation by experiments on the lower animals. Mr. Taylor has collected three cases of poisoning with it, which show that it is a powerful corrosive and irritant, and that its effects, as hitherto witnessed, seem to depend entirely on this action. In one instance, that of a boy, twelve years old, who swallowed four or five drachms of the solution by mistake for ginger beer, the symptoms were vomiting in half an hour, then faintness and extreme feebleness, and next day heat in the mouth and throat, difficulty in swallowing, slight abrasions of the lining membrane of the mouth, and general fever ; but he got quite well in eight days. In the case of another boy, ten years old, who got about the same quantity by mistake for antimonial wine, there was an immediate sense of choking and inability to speak, then vomiting and pain in the throat, next a general state of collapse, with dilated pupils and a tendency to stupor, and on the subsequent day bright scarlet patches on the throat, with difficulty of swallowing. This patient also recovered completely in a few days. The third was the case of a surgeon who took intentionally between two and three fluid ounces, and was found in an hour by his medical attendant in a state of great prostration, and affected with severe efforts to vomit, violent griping, and urgent tenesmus. Reaction soon ensued, the pain abated, and the pulse rose to 120 ; a strong tendency to doze succeeded ; and in ten hours and a half he expired. The whole inside of the alimentary canal, from the mouth to the jejunum, was black as if charred ; the mucous membrane seemed to have been removed along the whole of this extent of the canal ; and the submucous and peritoneal coats were so soft as to be easily torn with the finger.†

CHAPTER XVII.

OF POISONING WITH TIN, SILVER, GOLD, BISMUTH, CHROME, ZINC, AND IRON.

SEVERAL other metallic compounds produce effects analogous to

* Bulletins de l'Acad. Roy. de Médecine, 1840, vi. 140.
† Manual of Medical Jurisprudence, 1844, p. 209.

those of the preparations of arsenic, copper, mercury, and antimony. But they may be passed over shortly; because they are little known as poisons, and it is therefore only necessary that their leading properties be mentioned. They are the compounds of tin, silver, gold, bismuth, chrome, zinc, and iron.

Of Poisoning with Tin.

The chlorides of *tin* are used in the arts of colour-making and dyeing, and the oxide of tin forms part of the putty-powder used for staining glass and polishing silver plate.

There are two chlorides, the protochloride and bichloride. They both form acicular crystals, which are very soluble. It is needless to notice their tests or chemical history; but in order that the following account of their effects on man and animals may be understood, it is necessary to mention, that they are decomposed by almost all vegetable infusions and animal fluids.

Orfila found, that a solution of six grains of the protochloride injected into the jugular vein of a dog killed it in one minute, — that two grains caused death by tetanus in fifteen minutes, — and that so small a quantity as half a grain caused death in twelve hours, the only symptoms being somnolency and catalepsy or fixedness of position.

To these dreadful effects when introduced into the blood, its effects when swallowed are not nearly proportionate. From eighteen to forty-four grains killed dogs in one, two, or three days, efforts to vomit and great depression being the only symptoms; and after death the stomach was found excessively inflamed, and sometimes ulcerated. Its effects when applied externally are still less violent. Two drachms applied to a wound merely caused violent inflammation and sloughing of the part, and death in twelve days, without any internal symptom during life or appearance after death.*

These phenomena, considered along with the violent symptoms excited when the poison is injected into the veins, show that, when swallowed or applied outwardly, it acts only as a local irritant.

Tin is absorbed in the course of its action, and may be detected in the liver, spleen, and urine, by boiling them in water acidulated with hydrochloric acid, evaporating the decoction to dryness, charring the residue by means of nitric acid as directed for copper, treating the carbonaceous mass with a mixture of twenty parts of hydrochloric acid and one of nitric acid, evaporating the solution to dryness so as to expel any excess of acid, dissolving what is left in hydrochloric acid diluted with twice its volume of water, and then transmitting hydrosulphuric acid gas. If the precipitated sulphuret of tin has not a fine yellow colour, it must be heated with a little strong nitric acid; after which, if the residuum be again dissolved in diluted hydrochloric acid, a characteristic yellow bisulphuret will be thrown down

* Toxicologie Générale, i. 555.

by hydrosulphuric acid gas.   This process may be applied to all organic mixtures containing tin.*

The oxide of tin, according to Schubarth, is quite inactive; for he gave an entire drachm to a dog without being able to observe any effect from it whatever.† This is what would be expected from its extreme insolubility.   Yet Orfila has stated in the early editions of his Toxicology, and repeats in that of 1843, but without noticing the contradictory observations of Schubarth, that one or two drachms of the oxide occasion in dogs all the phenomena of irritant poisoning, and prove invariably fatal.‡

The metal has been proved by Bayen and Charlard to be inactive.§ It has been given expressly to dogs without any effect being observed; and it is given in large doses to man for worms, without detriment.   No importance therefore can be attached to some alleged cases of poisoning with this metal. ‖

Cases of poisoning with the preparations of tin are rare.   Orfila briefly notices a set of cases which occurred to M. Guersent.   Several persons in a family took the protochloride, in consequence of the cook having mistaken a packet of it for salt and dressed their dinner with it.   They had all colic, some of them diarrhœa; none vomited; and all recovered in a few days.¶   A case is related in the Medical Times of death apparently caused by so small a quantity as half a tea-spoonful of a solution of protochloride.   The effects were vomiting, acute pain in the stomach, anxiety, restlessness, thirst, and a frequent, hard, small pulse.   These symptoms increased next day; and on the third day death took place, preceded by delirium :** As this was a case of suicide, it is probable that some other poison, or a larger dose of the chloride of tin was taken.

Little need be said of the morbid appearances.   Besides the signs of violent irritation caused by the poisons of tin in common with other irritants, Orfila always found in dogs a peculiar tanned appearance of the villous coat of the stomach.   In the case from the Medical Times the gullet was red, the stomach inflamed externally, and internally thickened, vascular, and pulpy.

Of Poisoning with Silver.

Of the preparations of *silver*, the only one which requires notice is the nitrate or lunar caustic.

It exists in two forms, — crystallized in broad, transparent, colourless tables, — and fused into cylindrical, crystalline, grayish pencils.   Both forms are essentially the same in chemical nature. — The most convenient tests are, 1, *Hydrochloric acid*, or any hydrochlorate, which even in a state of extreme dilution causes with it a dense

---

* Orfila. Journal de Chimie Médicale, 1842, p. 346.
† Horn's Archiv für Medizinische Erfahrung, 1823, ii. 415.
‡ Toxicol. Gén. 1843, ii. 10.
§ Recherches Chimiques sur l'Etain, Paris, 1781.
‖ See Wibmer, die Wirkung der Arzneimittel und Gifte, v. 168.
¶ Toxicologie Gén. 1843, ii. 5.   ** Medical Times, Oct. 9, 1841.

white precipitate, passing, under exposure to light, into dark brown; and 2, *Ammonia*, followed by the solution of oxide of arsenic; if the nitrate of silver is not too much diluted it gives a dark brown precipitate with ammonia, soluble, however, in an excess of that alkali; and when the solution has thus been restored, arsenic throws down a lively yellow precipitate, passing rapidly to brown, if left exposed to the light.

Most organic substances, but in particular all animal fluids, with the exception of gelatin, decompose nitrate of silver.

It appears from the experiments of Orfila, that, like the chlorides of tin, the nitrate of silver is a deadly poison when introduced into the veins; but that, by reason of its facility of decomposition, it cannot enter the blood through ordinary channels in a quantity sufficient to develope any remote action. When two grains in solution were injected into the jugular vein of a dog it died in six minutes, difficult respiration being the chief symptom; the third part of a grain caused death in four hours and a half, violent tetanus having preceded death; and in both animals the blood in the heart was found very black and the lungs gorged, or vivid red. According to Mr. Blake, the salts of silver when directly introduced into the blood, do not act on the heart, but operate by causing obstruction of the capillary system. If they are injected into the aorta, the systemic capillaries are obstructed, the nervous system is consequently oppressed, respiration is arrested through the medium of this nervous oppression, and death takes place by asphyxia, the heart continuing to beat vigorously. If again they are injected into a great vein, immediate obstruction of the pulmonary capillaries takes place, so that the blood ceases to be transmitted to the left side of the heart.[*]

To the violent action exerted by nitrate of silver when directly admitted into the blood, its effects through the medium of the stomach bear no proportion or resemblance. Thus, when twelve grains of the salt were introduced into the stomach in the solid state, its effects were so slight as not to be distinguishable from those of the ligature on the gullet practised to prevent its discharge by vomiting. When introduced in a state of solution, however, and in a larger dose, in the dose of 36 grains, for example, it is more energetic. Death ensued in thirty-six hours, but without any particular symptoms; and in the dead body the villous coat of the stomach was found generally softened, and corroded near the pylorus by little grayish eschars like those formed by this poison on the skin.[†]

Hence it appears that nitrate of silver does not act remotely, but simply as a local irritant and corrosive: The corrosion it produces is incompatible with its absorption in large quantity. This inference is confirmed by the experiments of Schloepfer, on its effects when introduced into the trachea. He found that it caused inflammation of the windpipe, and pneumonia passing on to hepatization of the lungs, but no symptom referrible to a remote action.[‡] Its pure cor-

[*] Edinburgh Med. and Surg. Journal, lvi. 119.   [†] Toxicol. Gén. i. 581.
[‡] De Effect. Liquid. ad vias aëriferas applic. Tübingæ, 1816, p. 33.

35*

rosive properties have long pointed it out to the surgeon as the most convenient of all escharotics.

Nitrate of silver is absorbed, however, in the course of its action. It would seem to be absorbed when it is taken medicinally in frequent small doses. It is not easy to account otherwise for the singular blueness of the skin, sometimes observed after the protracted use of lunar caustic as a remedy for epilepsy and other diseases.* The effects of the poison on the constitution in such cases are not very well known. It appears, however, that considerable doses may be taken for a great length of time without injury, and that the first and only unpleasant effects produced by its too free administration are such as indicate simply an injury of the stomach. The only exception to this general statement I have met with is a case by Wedemeyer, where, after the remedy had been taken for six months on account of epilepsy, that disease disappeared, and dropsy, with diseased liver at the same time commenced, and soon proved fatal. It is probable, however, that the nitrate of silver had no share in the ultimate event. In this instance the whole internal organs were more or less blue; and metallic silver, it is said, was found in the pancreas, and in the choroid plexus of the brain.† Silver has been found in the urine of persons who were taking it medicinally. A young man who had used the nitrate for some time observed that his urine became muddy soon after being passed, and that the sediment became black if exposed to the light; and when the sediment was digested in ammonia, chloride of silver was detached by neutralizing the ammoniacal liquor.‡

But it also appears that some nitrate of silver is absorbed when it is given in a single large dose. For in animals poisoned with it Orfila found that silver may be detected in the liver and spleen by charring these organs with nitric acid as in the instance of poisoning with copper, and then treating the residue with boiling diluted nitric acid, and adding hydrochloric acid to the solution. He also found silver in the urine by charring the extract with heat, acting on the charcoal with ammonia, and saturating the filtered ammoniacal solution, — chloride of silver being then detached.§ These results have been confirmed by the experiments of Drs. Panizza and Kramer of Milan,‖ who found silver in the blood after the administration both of the nitrate and chloride.

Boerhaave has noticed a case of poisoning with this substance, but in very brief terms. He says it caused gangrene. Schloepfer in his thesis notices a case by Dr. Albers of Bremen in which croup was brought on by a bit of lunar caustic dropping into the windpipe. M. Poumarede has related an instance of poisoning with an ounce of nitrate of silver in solution. A few hours afterwards the individual

* London Medico-Chirurgical Transactions, vii. 2. Journal der Practischen Heilkunde, Juli, 1824.

† Wibmer. Die Wirkung, &c. i. 212, from Rust und Casper's Kritische Repertorium, xix. 454.

‡ Journal de Chimie Médicale, 1842, p. 351.

§ Ibid. 1843, p. 348.

‖ Annales d'Hygiène Publique, xxix. 430.

was found insensible, with the eyes turned up, the pupils dilated, the jaws locked, and the arms and face agitated with convulsions. A solution of common salt was immediately given as an antidote. In two hours there was some return of consciousness, and abatement of the convulsions, but still complete insensibility of the limbs, with redness of the features, and pain in the stomach. In eleven hours he could articulate. For thirty-six hours he continued subject to fits of protracted coma; but he eventually recovered. Sixteen hours after taking the poison he vomited a large quantity of chloride of silver.*

The treatment of poisoning with the nitrate of silver is obvious. The muriate of soda by decomposing it will act as an antidote; and any signs of irritation left will be subdued by opium.

Of Poisoning with Gold.

Gold in various states of combination was at one time much used in medicine, and an attempt has been lately made to revive its employment.

Its poisonous properties are powerful, and closely allied to those of the chlorides of tin and nitrate of silver. In the state of chloride it occasions death in three or four minutes when injected into the veins, even in very minute doses; and the lungs are found after death so turgid as to sink in water. But if swallowed, corrosion takes place; the salt is so rapidly decomposed, that none is taken up by the absorbents; and death ensues simply from the local injury.†　It has been of late used in medicine in France as an antisyphilitic; but even doses so small as a tenth of a grain have been known to produce an unpleasant degree of irritation in the stomach.‡

In the state of fulminating gold, this metal has given rise to alarming poisoning in former times, when it was used medicinally. Plenck in his Toxicologia says it excites griping, diarrhœa, vomiting, convulsions, fainting, salivation; and sometimes has proved fatal.§ Hoffmann likewise repeatedly saw it prove fatal, and the most remarkable symptoms were vomiting, great anxiety and fainting. In one of his cases the dose was only six grains.‖ These compounds are now so little met with that they need not be noticed in greater detail.

Of Poisoning with Bismuth.

Bismuth, in its saline combinations, is also an active poison. One of its compounds, the trisnitrate, white bismuth, or magistery of bismuth, is a good deal used in medicine and the arts; and pearl white, one of the paints used in the cosmetic art, is the tartrate of this metal.

The former substance is an active poison. It is got by dissolving bismuth in nitric acid, and pouring hot water over the crystals; a

---

* Journal de Chimie Médicale, 1839, p. 434.
† Orfila, Toxicol. Générale, i. 593.
‡ Magendie, Formulaire pour les nouveaux Médicamens.　　　§ Toxicol. 241.
‖ Medicina Rationalis Syst. ii. c. 8. Sect. 12.

supernitrate being left in solution, and the trisnitrate thrown down in the form of a white powder.

Orfila found that the soluble part of fifteen grains of the nitrate, when injected into the jugular vein of a dog, caused immediate giddiness and staggering, and death in eight minutes. He also remarked that forty grains mixed with water and introduced into the stomach, caused all the customary signs of irritation, and death in twenty-four hours; and that a great part of the villous coat of the stomach was reduced to a pulpy mass, and likewise exhibited several ulcers.[*]

Similar effects were produced by the trisnitrate; but a larger dose was required. Two drachms and a half killed a dog in twenty-four hours; and redness and eroded spots were found in the stomach.

In some more recent researches Orfila found that the poison is absorbed, and may be detected, like other metallic poisons, in the liver, spleen, and urine. The process for this purpose, applicable also to all organic mixtures, consists in boiling the solids in water acidulated with a twentieth of nitric acid, evaporating the solution to dryness, charring the residue with nitric acid, as directed for copper, boiling the charcoal in diluted nitric acid, and thus obtaining an acid solution of nitrate of bismuth, which may be known by the effects of water and of hydrosulphuric acid.[†]

Orfila remarks, that Camerarius of Tübingen once detected the adulteration of wine with the oxide of bismuth, and that the bakers in some parts of England used to render their bread white and heavy by mixing the trisnitrate with flour; but he has not stated his authority for this accusation. It may be discovered in any such mixture by calcining the suspected substance in a crucible, and then separating the metallic bismuth by means of nitric acid. But the adulteration of bread with bismuth is very questionable, as there are many cheaper methods for effecting the purpose, without adding any thing positively deleterious.

The following is the only case with which I am acquainted of poisoning with the preparations of bismuth in the human subject. A man subject to water-brash took two drachms of the trisnitrate with a little cream of tartar by mistake for a mixture of chalk and magnesia. He was immediately attacked with burning in the throat, brown vomiting, watery purging, cramps, and coldness of the limbs, and intermitting pulse, and then with inflammation of the throat, difficult swallowing, dryness of the membrane of the nose, and a constant nauseous metallic taste. On the third day he had hiccup, laborious breathing, and swelling of the hands and face; and suppression of urine was then discovered to have existed from the first. On the fourth day swelling and tension of the belly were added to the pre-existing symptoms, on the fifth day salivation, on the sixth delirium, on the seventh, swelling of the tongue and enormous enlargement of the belly; and on the ninth he expired. The urine continued suppressed till the eighth day. — On inspection of the body it was found that from the back of the mouth to the rectum there were but few points

[*] Toxicol. Gén. i. 501.   [†] Journal de Chimie Médicale, 1842, p. 344.

of the alimentary canal free of disease. The tonsils, uvula, pharynx, and epiglottis, were gangrenous, the larynx spotted black, the gullet livid, the stomach very red, with numerous purple pimples, the whole intestinal canal red, and here and there gangrenous, especially at the rectum. The inner surface of the heart was bright red. The kidneys and brain were healthy.*

Of Poisoning with Chrome.

The next metal whose properties deserve notice is *chrome*. As it is now extensively used in the art of dyeing it is necessary to mention its effects, more especially as they are singular. They have been ascertained experimentally with great care by Professor Gmelin of Tübingen. He found that in the dose of a grain the *chromate of potass* had no effect when injected into the jugular vein of a dog, — that four grains produced constant vomiting, and death in six days without any other striking symptom, — and that ten grains caused instant death by paralysing the heart. Its effects, when introduced under the skin, are still more remarkable. It seems to cause general inflammation of the lining membrane of the air passages. When a drachm was thrust in the state of powder under the skin of the neck of a dog, the first symptoms were weariness and a disinclination to eat. But on the second day the animal vomited, and a purulent matter was discharged from the eyes. On the third day it became palsied in the hind legs ; on the fourth it could not breathe or swallow but with great difficulty ; and on the sixth it died. The wound was not much inflamed ; but the larynx, bronchi, and minute ramifications of the air tubes contained fragments of fibrinous effusion, the nostrils were full of similar matter, and the conjunctiva of the eyes was covered with mucus. In another dog, an eruption appeared on the back, and the hair fell off.†

The effects of the salts of chrome on man have not been well ascertained, but seem to be peculiar. Dr. Schindler of Greifenberg relates the following case of fatal poisoning with bichromate of potash. A colourman having swallowed a solution of it, vomiting was brought on by warm water, soap and oil, and kept up until the discharges ceased to be yellow. The man got apparently well and passed a quiet night ; but next morning he felt excessively weary, had stitches in his back and kidneys, passed no urine, and was affected with purging. A restless night followed. On the subsequent morning, he lay motionless and like one fatigued to the extremest degree ; in which state he died, fifty-four hours after swallowing the poison. The stomach was healthy, the intestines reddish, the kidneys gorged with blood and marbled internally with dark-red patches, and the bladder empty.‡ — Mr. Wilson of Leeds has described the case of an elderly man who took the poison in the evening, and was found

* Bulletins des Sciences Méd. xx. 188. From the Heidelberg Klinische Annalen, also Wibmer, Die Wirkung der Arzneimitiel und Gifte, i. 416.

† Versuche über die Wirkungen des Baryts, Strontians, Chrom, &c. auf den thierischen Organismus. 1824.

‡ Buchner's Repertorium für die Pharmacie, lxix. 387.

dead about twelve hours afterwards, without any sign of vomiting, purging, or convulsions; and no morbid appearance was found but redness of the villous coat of the stomach, and an inky-like fluid in it, containing a large quantity of bichromate of potash.*

To these facts may be added another not less singular, which my late colleague Dr. Duncan informed me has been observed by the workmen in Glasgow, who use the bi-chromate of potass in dyeing. When this salt was first introduced into the art of dyeing, the workmen who had their hands often immersed in its solution were attacked with troublesome sores on the parts touched by it; and the sores gradually extended deeper and deeper, without spreading, till they sometimes actually made their way through the arm or hand altogether.†

Of Poisoning with Zinc.

The compounds of zinc, which have been long used in considerable doses in medicine, have sometimes occasioned serious and even fatal effects. Partly on this account, and partly because one of them, the sulphate of zinc, being the emetic most commonly used in the treatment of poisoning, is apt to complicate various medico-legal analyses, it will be proper to notice both its physiological properties and the mode of detecting it by chemical means.

The only important compound of this metal is the sulphate or white vitriol. As usually sold in the shops, it forms small, prismatic crystals, transparent, colourless, of a very styptic metallic taste, and exceedingly soluble in water. That which is kept by the apothecary is tolerably pure; but there is a salt sometimes met with in commerce which contains an admixture of sulphate of iron, and with which the natural action of the tests for zinc is materially modified.

The solution of the pure salt is precipitated white by the caustic alkalis, an oxide being thrown down, which is soluble in an excess of ammonia. The alkaline carbonates also precipitate it white, the carbonate of ammonia being the most delicate of these reagents. The precipitate is soluble in an excess of carbonate of ammonia, and is not thrown down again by boiling. The precipitate produced both by the alkalis and by their carbonates becomes yellow, when heated nearly to redness; and on cooling it becomes again white. This is a characteristic property, by which the oxide of zinc may be known from most white powders. But oxide of antimony is similarly affected. The ferro-cyanate of potass also causes a white precipitate. A stream of sulphuretted-hydrogen likewise causes a white precipitate, the sulphuret of zinc, the colour of which distinguishes the present genus of poisons from all those previously mentioned, as well as from the poisons of lead. The precipitate is apt to be suspended till the excess of gas is expelled by ebullition. The action of this test will not distinguish sulphate of zinc from the salts of peroxide of iron, by which white sulphur is disengaged from the gas in consequence of

* London Medical Gazette 1843-44, ii.
† Ed. Med. and Surg. Journ. xxvi. 133.

the peroxide of iron being reduced to the state of protoxide. The same decomposition takes place wherever there is free chlorine, as in impure samples of muriatic or nitric acid.

When the sulphate of zinc contains iron, the alkalis throw down a greenish-white precipitate, the alkaline carbonates a grayish or reddish-white, the ferro-cyanate of potass a light-blue, but sulphuretted-hydrogen the usual white precipitate. Tincture of galls, which merely renders the pure salt hazy, causes a deep violet coagulum if there is any ferruginous impurity.

The sulphate of zinc is acted on by albumen and milk precisely in the same manner as the sulphate of copper. The salt is decomposed, and the metallic oxide forms an insoluble compound with the animal matter.

When the sulphate of zinc has been mixed with vegetable and animal substances, the action of the tests mentioned above is modified. In such circumstances I have found the following process convenient.

The mixture being strained through gauze, it is to be acidulated with acetic acid, and filtered through paper. The acetic acid dissolves any oxide of zinc that may have been thrown down in union with animal matter. The filtered fluid is then to be evaporated to a convenient extent, and treated when cool with sulphuretted-hydrogen gas, — upon which a grayish or white milkiness or precipitate will be formed. The excess of gas must now be expelled by boiling, and the precipitate washed by the process of subsidence and affusion, and collected on a filter. It is then to be dried and heated to redness in a tube. When it has cooled, it is to be acted on by strong nitric acid, which dissolves the zinc and leaves the sulphur. The nitrous solution should next be diluted, and neutralized with carbonate of ammonia ; after which the liquid tests formerly mentioned will act characteristically. The effect of carbonate of ammonia, and that of heat on the carbonate of zinc which is thrown down, ought to be particularly relied on.

I have tried this process with the matter vomited after the administration of sulphate of zinc, in a case of pretended poisoning, and found it to answer exceedingly well.

Orfila has lately suggested the following method. Boil the suspected substance in water, evaporate the filtered decoction to dryness, char the residuum with nitric acid as directed for copper in similar circumstances, digest the charcoal in diluted muriatic acid, and subject the filtered solution to hydrosulphuric acid. If the sulphuret be not white, but yellowish from iron, heat it with strong nitric acid, dry the product, and heat it to redness; dissolve it in weak nitric acid ; throw down the oxide of iron by an excess of ammonia, which retains the oxide of zinc ; and then having filtered the fluid, separate the oxide of zinc by neutralizing the ammonia.[*]

Orfila has furnished the only accurate information hitherto possessed regarding the effects of sulphate of zinc on the animal system.[†] He

* Journal de Chimie Médicale, 1842, p. 353.   † Toxicologie Gén. i. 569.

found that dogs might be made to swallow 7½ drachms without any permanent harm being sustained, provided they were allowed to vomit; for in a few seconds the whole poison was invariably discharged, and the animals, after appearing to suffer for four or five hours, gradually recovered their usual liveliness. But the result is different if the gullet be tied: violent efforts to vomit ensue, and death follows in three days, the intermediate phenomena being those of local irritation chiefly, and the appearances in the dead body those of incipient inflammation of the stomach, without corrosion. — When injected into the veins, the effect of sulphate of zinc is much more violent, in an inferior dose. Forty-eight grains occasioned almost instant death; and half the quantity proved fatal in three minutes. Orfila does not appear to have ascertained the cause of death in the last two experiments. But Mr. Blake found that when this salt is injected into the veins in the dose of three grains, it causes some depression of the heart; that thirty grains arrest the action of the heart in eight seconds, leaving that organ exhausted of irritability and full of florid blood in its left cavities; and that when injected into the arterial system in the dose of sixteen grains, it seemed not to cause any obstruction of the capillaries, but to act on the nervous system, producing extreme prostration, without insensibility or convulsions.* These experiments, when taken together, show that sulphate of zinc, though a moderately active irritant, is more indebted for its activity to a remote operation on some vital organ.

Sulphate of zinc is absorbed in the course of its action ; for Orfila has lately found it by his process for complex mixtures in the spleen, liver, and urine of animals.†

The effects of the preparations of zinc on man in large doses have not been particularly studied. In the dose of a scruple or a drachm, the sulphate is the most immediate emetic known; and it is to be inferred, that if larger doses are rejected, as is the fact, with equal rapidity, they will in general cause no more harm than the medicinal dose.

Nevertheless, some people have suffered severely from over-doses of sulphate of zinc, and a few have even perished. Instead of presenting here a general view of the symptoms, it will be preferable to relate the heads of such cases as have been published.

The first to be mentioned is related by Foderé, who, in consequence of the violent symptoms produced, assigns to the present poison very active properties. " A patient of mine," says he, " a custom-house officer, having got from a druggist six grains of sulphate of zinc to cure a gonorrhœa, was attacked with inflammation in the lower belly, attended by retraction of the navel and severe colic, which yielded only to repeated blood-letting, general as well as local, oleaginous emollients, opiates, and the warm-bath."‡ This case is noticed here chiefly to prevent any one from being misled by it, as it

* Edinburgh Med. and Surg. Journal, lvi. 110.
† Journal de Chimie Médicale, 1842, p. 353.
‡ Médecine Légale, iv. 165.

has been quoted by other medico-legal authors. For assuredly some other cause must have co-operated before such symptoms could arise; since I have in many cases given the same dose thrice daily for several days, without ever observing more than slight sickness; and Dr. Babington once gave thirty-six grains thrice a day for some weeks with as little effect.[*]

Parmentier, the chemist, met with an instance, in which about two ounces of white vitriol in solution were swallowed by mistake. The countenance became immediately pale, the extremities cold, the eyes dull, and the pulse fluttering. The patient, a young lady, then complained of a burning pain in the stomach, and vomited violently. But potass being now administered in syrup, the pain ceased, the vomiting gradually abated, and the lady soon recovered completely.[†]

In the Journal de Médecine, another instance is related by M. Schueler, in which a very large dose did not produce material injury. The symptoms were pain in the stomach and bowels, with vomiting and diarrhœa. They were dispelled in a few hours by the administration of cream, butter, and chalk.[‡]

The following is a fatal case recorded by Metzger, but it is not a pure example of poisoning with zinc, though accounted such by the relater; for a small quantity of sulphate of copper was mixed with the sulphate of zinc. Three persons in a family took this mixture, which had been given them by a grocer in mistake for pounded sugar. They were all seized with violent vomiting; and a boy twelve years of age died in less than twelve hours.[§]

Another and an unequivocal case has been lately recorded in Horn's Archiv from Mertzdorff's experience. No part of the history of the symptoms is mentioned, except that there had been vomiting. But Mertzdorff has described carefully the morbid appearances, which are interesting; and he detected the poison in the stomach by a satisfactory analysis.[‖]

Two other cases, which are presumed to have arisen from the commercial sulphate of zinc, and which proved fatal, have been recently published by Dr. Sartorius of Aachen; but they do not appear to me to have been satisfactorily traced to this poison, and it is therefore unnecessary to quote them.[¶]

Dr. Werres of Cologne has related the particulars of three cases of poisoning with some preparation of zinc in milk-porridge. One of the persons, a child four years old, was seized with vomiting in three minutes, and, after frequent violent returns of it, died in convulsions within eight hours. The others also suffered severely from vomiting, but recovered.[**]

It does not appear that workmen who are exposed to the fumes of zinc ever suffer materially. But there is a case in Rust's Magazin,

* Guy's Hospital Reports, vi. 17.
† Orfila, Tox. i. 573.　　　　　‡ Journal Gén. de Médecine, lvi. 22.
§ Materialien für die Staatsarzneikunde, i. 122.
‖ Horn's Archiv, 1824, ii. 259.
¶ Buchner's Repertorium für die Pharmacie, xxvii. 317, and xxxiii. 104.
** Henke's Zeitschrift für die Staatsarzneikunde, xxiii. 164.

which shows that these fumes are not quite harmless.   An apothecary's assistant, while preparing philosopher's wool, incautiously filled
the whole laboratory with it.   The same day he was seized with
tightness in the chest, headache and giddiness ; next morning with
violent cough, vomiting, and stiffness of the limbs ; on the third day
with a coppery taste in the mouth, some salivation, gripes, and such
an increase of giddiness that he could not stand.   He was then freely
purged, after which a fever set in, ending in perspiration ; and he
got well in three weeks.*

From these cases, and the experimental researches of Orfila, it is
clear that the preparations of zinc, though not very active poisons,
are nevertheless far from being innocuous.   We are not acquainted
with their effects when long and habitually introduced into the body
in small quantities.   About the time when physicians began to study
with care the dangerous consequences of employing lead and copper
in the manufacture of culinary vessels, it was conceived by some that
zinc might prove a safe substitute.   It was farther imagined by some
military economists in France, that zinc might be profitably used instead of tinned iron in the manufacture of canteens and other articles
of camp equipage, because the worn and damaged vessels would
sell as old metal at little short of their original price, while tinned
iron as old metal bears no value at all.   But from the experiments of
Deyeux and Vauquelin it subsequently appeared, that in the course
of many culinary operations zinc is more liable to be attacked than
either copper or lead ; — that water left for some time in zinc vessels
oxidates them, and acquires a metallic taste ;— that if water acidulated with vinegar or lemon-juice is boiled in zinc, a solution is
formed, in which the metal may be detected by its tests ; — and that
sea-salt, sal-ammoniac, and even butter, have the power of dissolving
it also.†   Some singular inquiries were afterwards prosecuted by
Devaux and Dejaer among the Spanish prisoners at Liége, with the
view of proving, that frequent small quantities of zinc dissolved in
the manner mentioned, and habitually taken with the food, have no
injurious tendency ; that even in large doses it can hardly be accounted poisonous, as it merely gives rise to vomiting and slight diarrhœa ; and that an adulteration to such an amount would always
betray itself by its strong disagreeable taste.‡   These are certainly
valuable facts, though not quite satisfactory.   But it is unnecessary
to inquire minutely into their validity ; for, independently of all
other considerations, vessels constructed of zinc are too brittle for
domestic purposes.   With regard to the effects of frequent small doses
of sulphate of zinc, the only positive information I can communicate
is, that I have often given medicinally from three to six grains thrice
a day for two or three weeks, without observing any particular effect
except in some persons sickness when the largest doses were taken ;
and others have frequently made the same observation.§   On the

* Magazin für die gesammte Heilkunde, xxi. 563.
† Annales de Chimie, lxxxvi. 59.
‡ Orfila's Toxicologie, i. 567, from the Procès-verbal of the public meeting of the
Society of Liége in 1813.
§ See Dr. Babington's Paper in Guy's Hospital Reports, vi. 16.

other hand, Dr. Nasse of Berlin says a patient of his, who had taken twenty grains of oxide of zinc daily till 3247 grains were swallowed, was attacked with paleness, emaciation, weakness of intellect, obstinate constipation, coldness and œdema of the limbs, extreme dryness of the skin, and a thready scarcely perceptible pulse. But he quickly recovered under the use of laxatives and tonics.[*]

Sulphate of zinc is said to have proved fatal when applied externally. In Pyl's memoirs there is a case of this nature, which was attributed to sulphate of zinc having been used as a lotion for a scabby eruption on the head. The subject was a child, six years old, and otherwise healthy. The wash, which was a vinous solution, had not been long applied before the child complained of acute burning pain of the head, which was followed by vomiting, purging, convulsions, and death in five hours. The cause of these symptoms, though the particulars of the case were ascertained judicially by an able medical jurist, Dr. Opitz of Minden, is nevertheless very doubtful, as daily use is made of the salt for similar purposes without any such effect. Appearances of congestive apoplexy were found within the skull; and the reporter ascribes death to the wash having produced repulsion of the cutaneous disease, and determination of blood to the head.[†]

The only opportunities which have occurred of observing the morbid appearances after poisoning with sulphate of zinc taken internally, are the cases by Metzger, Mertzdorff, and Werres.

In the first, which was a mixed case, the only appearances of note were slight inflammation in the stomach, and excessive gorging of the lungs with fluid blood; from which Metzger oddly enough concludes that the child was suffocated by the vomiting. In the second case, Mertzdorff found the stomach and intestines, but particularly the latter, contracted, — their outer surface healthy — the inner membrane of the stomach grayish-green, with several spots of effused blood, and greenish, fluid contents, — the inner membrane of the small intestines similarly spotted, — the rest of the body quite natural. It has been already mentioned that Mertzdorff detected the poison in the body. He found it not only in the contents, but likewise in the coats of the stomach and intestines. In the third, Werres found a reddish-brown patch and some vascularity in the stomach.

Of Poisoning with Iron.

In previous editions of this work the preparations of iron were arranged among those substances which are not usually considered poisonous, but which may nevertheless prove injurious when taken in large quantity. But the soluble salts of iron, although not very active, seem sufficiently so to entitle them to a regular place among poisons; and one of them, the sulphate, has actually been used, as will presently appear, for the purpose of committing murder.

[*] Journal de Chimie Médicale, 1839, p. 389, from Casper's Wochenschrift.
[†] Aufsätze und Beob. ii. 12.

There are many soluble salts of iron which in all probability may prove hurtful ; but the only ones which have been brought under notice in medico-legal researches are the sulphate of the protoxide, and the mixed chlorides.

The sulphate of the protoxide of iron, commonly called green-vitriol or copperas, occurs in commerce in crystals or crystalline masses of various shades of bluish-green. It is easily known by its colour and its strong styptic inky taste. When in solution, the iron may be detected by ferrocyanate of potash, sulphuretted-hydrogen, and tincture of galls. Ferrocyanate of potash causes a blue pre-cipitate, at first pale, but gradually passing to deep Prussian blue. Sulphuretted-hydrogen has no effect, but if an alkali, such as ammonia, be added to disengage the oxide of iron, a black precipitate of sul-phuret of iron is immediately produced. Tincture of galls occasions a deep purplish-black precipitate, the tannate of iron, and it acts with greater delicacy in very diluted solutions, if the oxide of iron be disengaged by carbonate of soda. These tests prove the presence of iron in solution. A white precipitate under the action of nitrate of baryta will indicate that the oxide is dissolved by sulphuric acid.

The most familiar form of chloride of iron is the tincture of the chloride, which sometimes contains only the sesquichloride, some-times consists of a mixture of this with the protochloride. It is known by the three tests for oxide of iron described above, and by nitrate of silver occasioning a heavy white precipitate, insoluble in nitric acid.

For detecting iron in organic mixtures, where the liquid reagents do not act satisfactorily, the simplest process is to digest the mix-ture, if there be any solid matter, in water acidulated with acetic acid, to evaporate the filtered liquid to dryness, to incinerate the extract in a porcelain crucible, to act on the product with diluted sul-phuric acid, and then to treat the solution with the three liquid reagents.

Professor Gmelin found that sulphate of iron merely caused vo-miting in dogs who were made to swallow two drachms of it, that rabbits might take forty grains without any apparent injury, and that twenty grains in a state of solution might even be injected into the veins of a dog without producing any particular symptom.[*] From these and some other facts of the like kind it was generally held, that sulphate of iron is not a poison. But Smith ascertained that a dose of two drachms will prove fatal to dogs in little more than twenty-four hours, when it is introduced into the stomach, and in half that time if applied to a wound ; and that it occasions some redness of the alimentary mucous membrane, and the effusion of a thick layer of tough mucus. It is remarkable, however, that, like Gmelin, he found no effect to flow from the transfusion of a solution of seven grains into the veins, except transient vomiting and expressions of pain.[†]

The effects which have been observed in the human subject are conformable with those witnessed in experiments on the lower ani-

* Versuche über die Wirkung des Baryts, &c.   † Toxicologie Gén. 1843, ii. 44.

mals, the symptoms being those of pure irritant poisoning. Few illustrative cases, however, have as yet been made public. In Rust's Journal there is the case of a girl, who took as an emmenagogue, an ounce of green vitriol dissolved in beer, and suffered in consequence from colic pains, constant vomiting and purging for seven hours, but eventually recovered under the use of mucilaginous and oily drinks.* A fatal case of poisoning with this substance occurs in the Parliamentary Returns of death from poison in England during the years 1837–38 [see p. 90]. — Dr. Combe of Leith has communicated to me an instructive case of fatal poisoning with the tincture of the chloride of iron, which was taken to the extent of an ounce and a half by a gardener accidentally instead of whisky. Violent pain in the throat and stomach, tension and contraction of the epigastrium, and nausea immediately ensued; afterwards coldness of the skin and feebleness of the pulse were remarked; and then vomiting of an inky fluid, with subsequently profuse vomiting of mucus and blood, and also bloody stools under the use of laxatives. He remained for some days in a very precarious state, but then began to rally, and in three weeks resumed his occupation. But in two weeks more Dr. Combe found him emaciated, cadaverous in appearance, and affected with pains in the stomach, costiveness, and thirst; in which state he lingered for five days more, and then died. In the dead body there was found great thickening towards the pylorus, a cicatrized patch there three inches long and two inches broad, and another large patch of inflammatory redness surrounded by a white border. The preparation taken in this instance contained a third of its volume of hydrochloric acid and a tenth of its weight of oxide of iron; and consequently some of the acid was free.

The following remarkable case, in which I was lately consulted on the part of the Crown, will show that sulphate of iron is a more important poison than has been commonly thought. Suspicions having arisen in December, 1840, respecting the death of a child in the county of Fife about four months before, an investigation was made by the law authorities; and the body was disinterred and inspected by Mr. Dewar and Dr. James Dewar of Dunfermline. It was ascertained that the child, a girl four years of age, and previously in good health, was attacked with violent vomiting and purging immediately after breakfasting on porridge, and died in the course of the afternoon of the same day. A boy two years older, having seen a blue solution put into the porridge, and observing that the porridge had a bad taste, took only three spoonfuls of it, but became for a time very sick. The girl, being fed by a woman in the house, was made to take all her share; and in the course of the day the same person was seen by two children of the family to give a blue solution to the sick girl for drink. The woman was proved to have purchased sulphate of copper, and admitted having bought about this time both that salt and sulphate of iron, for the alleged purpose of dyeing some clothes. Poisoning with sulphate of copper was therefore suspected.

* Magazin für die gesammte Heilkunde, xxi. 247.

36*

On examining the body, which had been buried four months, the Messrs. Dewar found the external parts considerably decayed, — the stomach soft, gelatinous, and of a uniform intense black colour through the whole thickness of its parietes, — the gullet and duodenum similarly affected, but not so deeply on their outer surface, — the spleen, kidneys, and lower parts of the liver similarly stained with a black pulp, which could be wiped off, — and the whole alimentary canal lined with a thick layer of jet-black mucus, from the pharynx down to the very anus. Inferring that the cause of this extraordinary blackness was decomposition of sulphate of copper by hydrosulphuric acid gas disengaged during the decay of the body, they proceeded to search for that metal in the form of sulphuret both in the contents and texture of the stomach, but without success: there was not a trace of copper to be found. Being then led from some circumstances in the analysis to suspect that the black matter might be sulphuret of iron, they proceeded to search for that substance, and ascertained that a large quantity existed both in the textures of the stomach and in the black mucus which lined it. They further ascertained that there was no iron in a state capable of being dissolved by water, but that a much larger quantity of sulphuric acid was associated with the black matter than could have proceeded from the sulphates naturally contained in the animal textures or in the mucous secretions. They had also an opportunity of examining several large buff-coloured stains on various articles of dress, worn by the child and by the woman at the time the poisoning was supposed to have happened; and they detected a large quantity of oxide of iron in all of them. The whole case was subsequently submitted to me for my opinion, together with a portion of the stomach, the entire intestines, and several stained articles of dress. The results of the analysis of the tissues of the stomach, the black intestinal mucus, and the stains on the cloth were the same in my hands. — It is not easy to see how any other conclusion could be drawn from the whole circumstances, than that a soluble preparation of iron had been administered a short time before death, and that it had been entirely decomposed and converted into sulphuret of iron by the evolution of hydrosulphate of ammonia during the decay of the body. In consequence of important defects in the evidence criminating a particular individual, and especially because all the essential facts depended on the testimony of children, who, after the lapse of some time, did not adhere to their original statement, it was judged improper to bring this case to a trial.

A few years afterwards another case somewhat similar was submitted by the law authorities to the same gentlemen, to whom I am indebted for the particulars. A woman far advanced in pregnancy, and enjoying excellent health, was suddenly seized about midnight with vomiting and purging, and died in fourteen hours. Various circumstances having raised suspicions as to the cause of death, the body was disinterred a few days after burial, and carefully examined by Mr. Dewar and Dr. Dewar. The organs were in general healthy.

There were some dark red patches on the villous coat of the stomach, and a general blush pervaded the whole alimentary canal, which was empty of every thing but a reddish-brown mucus. The intestines were in several places irregularly contracted and hard. The stomach, small intestines, and rectum contained iron in large quantity, dissolved either by sulphuric or hydrochloric acid. Sulphate of iron was found in the house. — No trial took place in this instance either, because there was a want of evidence to attach guilt to any particular individual, although it was highly improbable that the woman had taken the poison herself.*

A short notice may here be added of the toxicological effects of the rarer metals, which have been examined chiefly by Professor Gmelin of Tübingen.† — Oxide of *osmium* is nearly as active as arsenic, for a grain and a half will kill a dog in a few hours by the stomach, and in one hour through a vein. Twelve grains of hydrochlorate of *platinum* will kill a dog within a day through the stomach, with symptoms of pure irritation; and so will half that quantity through a vein. — The hydrochlorates of *iridium* and *rhodium* are rather less active. — The hydrochlorate of *palladium* is equally powerful when introduced into the stomach, and much more so through a vein, for two-thirds of a grain will kill dogs in a minute.

The salts of other metals appear less active. — *Molybdenum*, in the form of molybdate of ammonia, seems a feeble poison; thirty grains killed a rabbit in two hours, but produced in dogs merely some vomiting and purging; and ten grains injected into the jugular vein did not prove fatal. — *Manganese*, according to Gmelin, is likewise a feeble poison, but has peculiar effects. A drachm of the sulphate killed a rabbit in an hour. Thirty grains swallowed by a dog had no effect. Two drachms thrust into the cellular tissue had no effect. Twelve grains injected into a vein occasioned death in five days: and in the dead body, the stomach, duodenum, and liver were found much inflamed. Manganesic acid, according to Professor Hünefeld, appears also to act on the liver, but is a feeble poison. A rabbit received two drachms in three days in doses of ten or fifteen grains, without presenting any symptom except increased flow of urine. Being then killed, the liver was found soft, at one part bright-red, elsewhere dark-brownish-red, and it yielded manganese by incineration.‡ Some singular observations have been lately published by Dr. Couper of Glasgow, the purport of which is, that manganese belongs to the class of insidious, cumulative poisons, and that it has the property of slowly bringing on, in those who breathe or handle the oxide, a paraplegic affection which is incurable unless taken under treatment early. Five cases of the kind occurred subsequently to 1828, in the great chemical manufactory of Tennant and Company, among the workmen employed in grinding the black oxide of man-

* I shall take an early opportunity, with the permission of Messrs Dewar, of publishing some of the details of these two cases, which are most interesting in various respects.
† Versuche über die Wirkung des Baryts, &c. Heidelberg, 1824.
‡ Horn' Archiv für Medizinische Erfahrung, 1830, ii.

ganese.* On the other hand, Dr. Thomson of Glasgow has recently stated that an ounce of sulphate of manganese is an effectual and safe laxative.† *Uranium* is an active poison when injected into a vein, for three grains of the muriate proves fatal instantly ; but dogs may swallow fifteen, or from that to sixty grains without any other effect except slight vomiting [Gmelin]. *Cobalt* is more active. Thirty grains of the oxide occasion death in a few hours through the stomach. Twenty-four grains of the muriate applied to the cellular tissue excite vomiting. Three grains of sulphate injected into a vein prove fatal in four days. — *Tungsten, cerium, cadmium, nickel,* and *titanium* can scarcely be considered poisons. *Tungstate* of ammonia in the dose of a drachm had no effect when swallowed by a dog; forty grains of tungstate of soda, which is more soluble, operated as an emetic ; but this dose will prove fatal to rabbits in a few hours. A drachm of the muriate of *cerium* had little or no effect on a dog, and half that dose had no effect on a rabbit. The oxide of *cadmium* in the dose of twenty grains, made a dog vomit ; and ten grains had no effect at all.‡ Twenty grains of sulphate of *nickel* made a dog vomit ; forty grains applied to the cellular tissue had no effect at all on the general constitution ; but ten grains injected into the jugular vein occasioned immediate death [Gmelin]. A drachm of *titanic* acid had no effect on a dog.

CHAPTER XVIII.

OF POISONING WITH LEAD.

POISONING with lead is a subject of great consequence in Medical Police, as well as Medical Jurisprudence. Its preparations have been used for the purpose of intentional poisoning. At the Taunton Assizes in March, 1827, a servant-girl was tried for attempting to administer sugar of lead to her mistress in an arrow-root pudding : and although the charge was not made out, it appeared from the prisoner's confession that she really had made the attempt. Sugar of lead has also been often taken by accident.

In relation to medical police lead is a subject of great importance. This metal is used in so many forms, and in so many of the arts, and its effects when gradually introduced into the body are so slow and insidious, that instances of its deleterious operation are frequently met with. Such accidents, indeed, are less common now, than they used to be before the late improvements in chemistry. But they are still sufficiently frequent to render it necessary for the toxicologist to investigate the properties of lead attentively.

SECTION I. — *Of the Chemical History and Tests for the Preparations of Lead.*

The physical characters of lead in its metallic state are familiar to

---

* British Annals of Medicine, i. 41.   † Ibidem, i. 52.
‡ Schubarth, Journal der Praktischen Heilkunde, lii. 101.

every one. It is easily known by the dull bluish-gray colour it assumes when exposed some time to the air, by the brilliant bluish-gray colour of a fresh surface, and by the facility with which it may be cut. The compounds which require particular notice are four in number, litharge, red lead, white lead, sugar of lead, and Goulard's extract. The first three are very much used by house-painters and glaziers, the last two are extensively employed in surgery, and the sugar of lead is also used in many of the arts.

2. Of Litharge and Red Lead.

Litharge is the protoxide of lead in a state of semivitrification. *Red lead* is a compound of two equivalents of protoxide and one of deutoxide. The former is generally in the form of a grayish-red heavy powder, sometimes partly crystalline ; the latter in the form of a bright red powder approaching in colour to vermilion. They may be known by their colour ; — by their becoming black when suspended in water and treated with a stream of sulphuretted-hydrogen gas ; — and by litharge being entirely, and red lead partly, soluble in nitric acid, and forming a solution which possesses the properties to be mentioned presently for solutions of the acetate. The chemical actions concerned in these changes are obvious, except in the instance of nitric acid on red lead. Here the acid dissolves the protoxide only, and the deutoxide, which seems to act the part of an acid in the pigment, is separated in the form of a brown powder.

2. Of White Lead.

White lead, which is the carbonate of the metal, is in the form of a heavy snow-white powder, or in white chalk-like masses. It consists of variable proportions of the hydrated oxide and neutral carbonate ; those specimens are the whitest which contain most carbonate ; and the best English white lead I find to contain four equivalents of carbonate and one of hydrated protoxide. The grayer variety, formed by the action of distilled water on metallic lead, consists of only two of the former to one of the latter.[*] It may be known by its being blackened like the two former compounds by sulphuretted-hydrogen,—by being soluble with effervescence in nitric acid, — and by becoming permanently yellow when heated to redness, in consequence of the expulsion of its carbonic acid, and its conversion into protoxide. These tests, however, apply with exactness only to the pure carbonate, in which state white lead is not often met with in the shops. It is generally adulterated with sulphates, in consequence of which it is only partially acted on by nitric acid, and does not become distinctly yellow under a strong red heat. Dutch white-lead contains no less than between 78·5 and 25 per cent. of impurities insoluble in nitric acid, Venetian white-lead from 11 to 14·5 per cent., Munich white-lead between 1 and 7·5 per cent.[†] I have met, however, with perfectly pure specimens in the shops of this city.

[*] See a paper by myself in Edinburgh Royal Society Trans., 1842, xv. 276, 274.
[†] Buchner's Repertorium für die Pharmacie, xxxviii. 125.

3. *Of Sugar of Lead.*

Sugar of lead is the acetate of this metal. It is sold in the form either of a white heavy powder, or of aggregated masses of long four-sided prismatic crystals. It has a sweetish astringent taste, and a slight acetous odour. It is very soluble.

When in the solid state, it may be known by its solubility in water, and by the effects of heat. It first undergoes the aqueous fusion, then abandons a part of its acid empyreumatized, as may be perceived by the smell, next becomes charred, and finally presents globules of lead reduced by the charcoal of the acid. The best way of effecting its reduction on the small scale is to char it, and then direct on the mass the point of a blowpipe-flame: in an instant globules are developed. It is not easily reduced in a tube; at least I have never been able to succeed in that way.

In the fluid state the acetate of lead, as well as all its soluble salts, may be detected by the following system of reagents, — hydrosulphuric acid, bichromate of potass, hydriodate of potass, and metallic zinc, — which are the best of the numerous reagents yet proposed.

1. *Hydrosulphuric acid* causes a black precipitate, the sulphuret of lead. This is a test of extreme delicacy; and it acts in whatever state of combination the lead exists, whether fluid or solid.

It is preferable to the hydrosulphate of ammonia as a medico-legal test; for, as Fourcroy observed, the hydrosulphate of ammonia acts on many sound wines as if they contained lead,[*] while hydrosulphuric acid never causes with them a black precipitate, unless they contain either lead or some other metallic impregnation. It must be remembered that many other metallic solutions, such as those of mercury, copper, silver and bismuth, yield a black precipitate with this test.

2. *Chromate of potass*, both in the state of proto-chromate and bichromate, causes a fine gamboge-yellow precipitate, the chromate of lead. For the characteristic action of this reagent, it is desirable that the suspected liquid be neutral. It forms with solutions of the sulphate of copper a precipitate nearly of the same colour as the chromate of lead.

3. *Hydriodate of potass* causes also a lively gamboge-yellow precipitate, the iodide of lead. The action of this test is impaired in delicacy by a considerable excess of nitric acid, or acetic acid. These acids cause a yellow coloration with the test, though no lead be present.

4. *A rod of zinc* held for some time in the solution displaces the lead, taking its place, and throwing down the lead in the form of a crystalline arborescence. This is a very characteristic test; and also one of much delicacy; for I have found a small thread of zinc will very easily detect a twentieth part of a grain of lead dissolved in the form of acetate in 20,000 parts of water. It acts also on the nitrate of lead. Its action is impaired or prevented by an excess of acetic or nitric acid.

* Mem. de l'Acad. des Sc. 1787, 281, sur les vins lithargyriés.

These tests are amply sufficient for determining the presence of lead in a solution, provided they act characteristically. Others have been also used, however; and it is therefore right to notice them cursorily.

The *alkaline carbonates* throw down a white precipitate in a very diluted solution of lead. This test is ineligible, because the alkaline carbonates cause a white precipitate with many other salts. It might be rendered decisive, however, by washing the precipitate thoroughly, suspending it in pure water and transmitting sulphuretted-hydrogen, which blackens it. No other white carbonate is similarly altered except those of bismuth and silver, which are rare.

The *soluble sulphates* likewise cause with solutions of lead a white precipitate, the sulphate of lead. To this test the same objections apply as to the carbonates of the alkalis.

The *ferrocyanate of potash* causes a white precipitate, the ferrocyanate of lead. This is an objectionable test, as many other substances besides lead are similarly acted on by it.

4. *Goulard's Extract.*

Goulard's extract, the diacetate of lead, is easily distinguished from the acetate or sugar of lead by the effect of a stream of carbonic acid, which throws down a copious precipitate of carbonate of lead. The proper method of analyzing it is to transmit this gas till it ceases to act any longer, and then to subject the precipitate and solution to the tests for carbonate of lead, and acetate of lead. Solutions of the common acetate usually give a scanty white precipitate with carbonic acid, in consequence of containing a faint excess of oxide.

The presence of vegetable or animal matters may either decompose the salts of lead, or materially alter the action of the preceding reagents.

It appears from the experiments of Orfila, that most vegetable infusions possess the power of decomposing them more or less. The acetate furnishes, for example, an abundant precipitate with infusion of galls, or with infusion of tea. Almost all animal fluids, with the exception of gelatin, possess the same property; albumen, milk, bile, beef-tea, all give with it a copious precipitate. In fluids which do not decompose it altogether, the colour of the precipitate formed by the tests is so materially altered, that they cannot be relied on for the detection of lead. The test, however, which undergoes least alteration is hydrosulphuric acid.

Before proceeding to the detection of lead in complex organic mixtures, some remarks will be required on its relations to medical police. Here the various ways in which it is apt to be insidiously introduced into the body, chiefly by the action of chemical agents on metallic lead itself, will come under consideration.

Of the Action of Air and Pure Water on Lead.

When lead is exposed to the air it becomes tarnished. This

arises from a thin crust of carbonate of lead being formed ; for the
crust dissolves with brisk effervescence in acetic acid.   The formation of carbonate is accelerated by moisture and probably by the
presence of an unusual proportion of carbonic acid in the air.

The action of water on lead, which is of much greater consequence, has been made the subject of observation by the curious for
many ages.   The Roman architect, Vitruvius, who, it is believed,
flourished in the time of Cæsar and Augustus, forbids the use of this
metal for conducting water, because cerusse, he says, is formed on it,
which is hurtful to the human body.*   Galen also condemns the use
of lead pipes, because he was aware, that water transmitted through
them contracted a muddiness from the lead, and those who drank
such water were subject to dysentery.†   If we trace the sciences of
architecture, chemistry, and medicine downwards from these periods,
nothing more will be found than a repetition of the statements of Vitruvius and Galen, with but a few particular facts in support of them,
till we arrive at the close of the last and beginning of the present
century.

The first person that examined the subject minutely, was Dr.
Lambe of Warwick ; who inferred from his researches, that most, if
not all, spring waters possess the power of corroding and dissolving
lead to such an extent as to be rendered unfit for the use of man,
and that this solvent power is imparted to them by some of their
saline ingredients.‡   The inquiry was afterwards undertaken more
scientifically by Guyton-Morveau ; who, in opposition to Dr. Lambe,
arrived at the conclusion, that distilled water, the purest of all
waters, acts rapidly on lead by converting it into a hydrated oxide,
and that some natural waters, which hardly attack lead at all, are prevented doing so by the salts they hold in solution.§   A few years
later Dr. Thomson of Glasgow also examined the subject, and, as-
senting to Dr. Lambe's proposition, that most spring waters attack
lead, maintains nevertheless that the lead is only held in suspension,
not in solution ; and that the quantity suspended in such waters, after they have passed through lead pipes, pumps, and cisterns, is too
minute to prove injurious to those who make habitual use of them.‖
In the first edition of this work an extended account was given of
an investigation I made into the whole subject of the action of different waters on lead.¶   Additional observations were afterwards
published on the same point by Captain Yorke,** and by Mr. Taylor.††
And I have added some new facts in a late paper.‡‡

* Vitruv. de Architectura, L. viii. c. 7, Quot modis ducantur aquæ.   Editio Dan.
Barbari, 1567, pp. 262, 265.
  † De Medic. secundum locos, lvii.
  ‡ Researches into the Properties of Spring Waters, 1803, p. 193.
  § Annales de Chim. lxxi. 197, l'an 1809.
  ‖ Experiments in Scudamore's analysis of Tunbridge Water, 1816.
  ¶ A Treatise on Poisons, &c.   First Edition, 1829.
  ** Philosophical Magazine.   Third Series, v. 81, 1834.
  †† Guy's-Hospital Reports, 1838, iii. 60.
  ‡‡ Transactions of the Royal Society of Edinburgh, 1842, xv. 265.

The inquiry is of so great practical consequence, that I need not offer any apology for reproducing it here in detail, with such additions as ulterior experience and the researches of others enable me to make. Professor Orfila takes no notice of this important subfect, except in a few lines containing several inaccurate statements.[*]

Distilled water, deprived of its gases by ebullition, and excluded from contact with the air, has no action whatever on lead. If the water contains the customary gases in solution, the surface of the metal, freshly polished, becomes quickly dull and white. But if the surface of the water be not at the same time exposed to the air, the action soon comes to a close. — When the air, on the other hand, is allowed free access to the water, a white powder appears in a few minutes on and around the lead ; and this goes on increasing till in the course of a few days there is formed a large quantity of white matter which partly floats in the water or adheres to the lead, but is chiefly deposited on the bottom of the vessel. If this experiment be made with atmospheric air deprived of carbonic acid, the white substance puts on the form of a fine powder, which I find to be a hydrated oxide ; for when dried at 180° F. it gives off water on being heated to redness, and dissolves without effervescence in weak nitric acid. — But if the surface of the water be exposed to the open air, the substance formed consists of minute brilliant pearly scales, which with the aid of a powerful microscope are seen to be thin equilateral triangular tables, often grouped into hexaedral tables, or worn at the edges into the form of rosettes. This substance, which has a pale grayish hue when dried, I have ascertained to be a carbonate of lead, consisting of two equivalents of neutral carbonate and one of hydrated protoxide.[†] The formation of carbonate takes place with considerable rapidity. In twelve ounces of distilled water, contained in a shallow glass basin loosely covered to exclude the dust, twelve brightly polished lead rods weighing 340 grains, will lose two grains and a half in eight days ; and the lead will then show evident marks of corrosion. The process of corrosion goes on so long as atmospheric air is allowed to play freely on the surface of the water. In twenty months I have obtained 120 grains from an ounce of lead rods kept in 24 ounces of distilled water.

During these changes, a minute quantity of lead is dissolved. This is best proved by carefully filtering the water, then acidulating with a drop or two of nitric acid, and evaporating to dryness. I have never failed to detect lead in the residue by expelling the excess of nitric acid by heat, dissolving it in distilled water, and applying hydrosulphuric acid, hydriodate of potass, and chromate of potass to the solution. The lead is first dissolved in the form of hydrated oxide. For, if the air admitted to the water be deprived of carbonic acid, a clear liquid is obtained by filtration, and this is turned brown by hydrosulphuric acid. But a great part of the hydrate is speedily separated in the form of carbonate. For the filtered liquid speedily

* Toxicologie Gén. 1843, i. 657.
† Transactions of the Royal Society of Edinburgh, xv. 265.
37

becomes turbid if exposed to the air; and on evaporating it, the residuum dissolves in weak nitric acid with brisk effervescence. Captain Yorke estimates the quantity dissolved when the water is saturated at a 10,000th part.*

By far the greatest part of the lead, however, which disappears, will be found in the white pearly crystals. This crystalline powder is not, — as alleged by Guyton-Morveau, and after him by some systematic writers, a hydrated oxide of lead, but, as stated above, a particular variety of carbonate, containing more hydrated oxide than exists in common white lead. At first I thought it was neutral carbonate. Captain Yorke was led to suppose it hydrated oxide. In 1842 I found that, if it be exposed for some time to the action of aërated water after the lead has been removed, it invariably consists of two equivalents of neutral carbonate and one of hydrated oxide.

It will be inferred from the preceding facts, that distilled water for economical use should never be preserved in leaden vessels or otherwise in contact with lead. Even the distilled water of aromatic plants should not be so preserved, because the essential oil which communicates to them their fragrance does not take away the power which pure distilled water possesses of acting on lead. This fact was first announced in the second edition of the present work. A druggist in Edinburgh requested me to examine a reddish-gray crystalline, pearly sediment formed copiously in a sample of orange-flower water. I found this to be carbonate of lead coloured by the colouring matter of the water, and obviously produced by the action of the water on lead solder used instead of tin solder, and coarsely and liberally applied to the seams of the copper vessel in which the water had been imported from France. The filtered fluid did not contain a particle of lead. The same observation has been since made by a French pharmaceutic chemist, M. Barateau, who seems at a loss, however, to account for the formation of the carbonate of lead.† It appears from an inquiry of MM. Labarraque and Pelletier, conducted at the request of the Prefecture of Paris, that the orange-flower water, which is extensively used there, is often adulterated with lead in solution. They impute this to careless distillation; for then some of the decoction is driven over with the distilled liquid, and consequently produces a fluid which becomes acetous by keeping and dissolves the lead solder of the *estagnons* or copper vessels. Pure orange-flower water does not acidify by keeping.‡ M. Chevallier in a more recent investigation arrived at the same results, and found that few specimens of the orange-flower water of Paris were altogether free of lead.§ In none of these inquiries have the authors adverted to the action of pure water in forming carbonate of lead.

* The statement here given of these phenomena is somewhat different from what is contained in the last edition of this work. The present account is derived from ulterior experiments, partly published in my paper in the Edinburgh Transactions. The discrepancies formerly prevailing between my own researches and those of Captain Yorke are now completely reconciled.

† Journal de Chim. Méd. ix. 714.

‡ Annales d'Hyg. Publ. et de Méd. Lég. iv. 55. 1830.

§ Journal de Chim. Médicale, ix. 716. This adulteration has likewise since then attracted attention in London. See British Annals of Medicine, 1837, i. 15.

Of the Action of Solutions of Neutral Salts on Lead.

The property which pure aërated water possesses of corroding lead is variously affected by foreign ingredients which it may hold in solution.

Of these modifying substances none are more remarkable in their action than the neutral salts, which all impair the corrosive power of the water. Important practical consequences flow from that action ; for it involves no less than the possibility of employing lead for most of the economical purposes to which the ingenuity of man has applied that useful metal. The first experimentalist who made it an object of attention was Guyton-Morveau ; whose experiments are imperfect and in some respects erroneous. Having found that distilled water corrodes lead, he proceeded to inquire why no change of the kind takes place in some natural waters ; and being aware that most spring and river waters differ from that which has been distilled, chiefly in containing sulphate of lime and muriate of soda, he tried a solution of each of these salts, and discovered that the addition of a certain quantity of either to distilled water takes away from it the power of attacking lead, — that this preservative power is possessed by so small a proportion as a 500th part of sulphate of lime in the water, — and that the nitrates are also probably endowed with the same singular property.* Here his researches terminated.

Extending Guyton-Morveau's inquiries to other proportions of the same salts, and likewise to many other neutral salts, I was led to the conclusion, that all of them without exception possess the power of impairing the action of distilled water on lead. At least I found this power to exist in the case of sulphates, muriates, carbonates, hydriodates, phosphates, nitrates, acetates, tartrates, and arseniates.

The degree of this preservative power differs much in different salts. The acetate of soda is but an imperfect preventive when dissolved in the proportion of a hundredth part of the water : white crystals are formed, and the lead loses about a fourth of what is lost in distilled water in the same time. On the contrary, arseniate of soda is a complete preservative when dissolved in the proportion of a 12,000th ; and phosphate of soda and hydriodate of potass are almost effectual preservatives in the proportion of a 30,000th part only of the water.†
Muriate of soda and sulphate of lime hold a middle place between these extremes, and are both of them much more powerful than Guyton-Morveau imagined : the former preserves in the proportion of a 2000th to the water, the latter in the proportion of nearly a 4000th. Nitrate of potass is little superior to the acetate of soda : in the pro-

* Annales de Chimie, lxxi. 197.

† In distilled water containing a 12,000th of anhydrous *arseniate of soda* three lead rods weighing 71·235 grains became in thirty-three days 71·240 ; in a solution of a 15,000th the lead, though slightly whitened, retained its weight exactly, weighing at the end, as at the beginning, of the experiment 62·622 grains. In distilled water containing a 35,000th of anhydrous *phosphate of soda,* three lead rods, which weighed together 73·949 grains, became in thirty-two days 73·946 ; and in a comparative experiment with a solution containing a 27,000th they gained 0·015.

portion of a hundredth it prevents the action of the water almost entirely; but if the proportion be diminished to a 160th, the loss sustained by the lead is fully a third of the loss in distilled water.

When lead has been exposed for a few weeks to a solution of a protecting salt and has acquired a thin film over its surface, it not only is not acted on by the solution, but is even also rendered incapable of being acted on by distilled water.

The preservative power depends on the acid, not on the base of the salt. The acetate, muriate, arseniate, and phosphate of soda differ exceedingly in power. On the other hand, the sulphates of soda, magnesia, and lime, as well as the triple sulphate of alumina and potass, preserve as nearly as can be determined in the same proportion.

When we attempt to ascertain the relative preserving power of the neutral salts, it will appear that those whose acid forms with the lead a soluble salt of lead are the least energetic ; while those whose acid forms an insoluble salt of lead are most energetic. The protecting powers of acetate of soda, nitrate of potass, muriate of soda, sulphate of lime, arseniate of soda, and phosphate of soda, are inversely as the solubility of the acetate, nitrate, muriate, sulphate, arseniate, and phosphate of lead. The existence of this ratio might naturally lead to the inference that the protecting power depends simply on the salt in solution being decomposed, so that there is formed on the surface of the lead a thin crust consisting of the oxide of the metal in union with the acid of the decomposed salt, and constituting an insoluble film which is impermeable to aërated water: for example, that phosphate of soda acts in the small proportion of a 30,000th part by forming on the surface of the metal an impermeable film of phosphate of lead, which is known to be one of the most insoluble of all the neutral salts. But this is not altogether a correct statement of the fact.

When the protection afforded is complete, as for example by a 27,000th of phosphate of soda, a 12,000th of arseniate of soda, or a 4000th of sulphate of soda, the lead undergoes no change in appearance or in weight for several hours, or even days. At length the surface becomes dull, then white, and gradually a uniform film is formed over it. This film, examined at an early period, is found to consist of carbonate of lead, — being entirely soluble in diluted acetic acid, although the salts in solution is a sulphate or phosphate. But after a few weeks the carbonate is mixed with a salt of lead, containing the acid of a part of the neutral salt dissolved in the water : if, after five or six weeks' immersion in a preservative solution of phosphate or sulphate of soda, the film on the lead be scraped off and immersed in diluted acetic acid, effervescence and solution take place, but a part of the powder remains undissolved ; and if the protecting salt has been the muriate of soda, the whole powder is dissolved, but muriatic acid will be found in solution by its proper test, the nitrate of silver. — In all such protecting solutions the lead gains weight for some weeks; but at length it ceases to undergo farther change, and is not acted on even if removed into distilled water.

The crust, when formed thus slowly, adheres with great firmness. The most careful analysis cannot detect any lead, either dissolved in the water, or floating in it, or united with the insoluble matter left on the side of the glass by evaporation. In short, the preservation of the lead from corrosion, and of the water from impregnation with lead, is complete.[*]

When the protection afforded is not quite complete, — for example in distilled water containing a 4000th of muriate of soda, a 6000th of sulphate of soda, a 15,000th of arseniate of soda, or a 35,000th of phosphate of soda, — besides a powdery crust, small crystals, with several facettes, are sometimes formed on the lead, while, at the same time, a minute white film will very slowly appear on the bottom of the glass, on its side where it is left dry by the evaporation of the water, and likewise on the surface of the water itself. These detached films are composed of carbonate of lead, with a little of the muriate, sulphate, arseniate, or phosphate of lead, according to the nature of the acid in the alkaline salt which is dissolved in the water. In the course of the changes now described, the lead in general no longer gains, but loses weight. The loss, however, is exceedingly small. — No lead can be discovered in solution, if the water before evaporation is carefully filtered.

On progressively trying solutions of weaker and weaker preservative power, it will be remarked, that the quantity of the detached powder, and the proportion of carbonate in it, progressively increase ; and likewise, that what is formed on the lead adheres more and more loosely. In distilled water and weak solutions of acetate of soda, or nitrate of potass, the lead never becomes so firmly encrusted, but that gentle agitation of the water will shake off the powder.

It is worthy of notice that, although a small quantity of lead is dissolved by distilled water after it has remained some time in contact with the metal, yet not a trace is found in solution where a protecting salt is present. In solutions even weakly preservative I never could detect any lead dissolved. Thus, in distilled water containing a 4000th of muriate of soda, or a 160th of nitre, the lead lost weight, and loose crystals of carbonate were formed ; yet even after thirty days no lead could be found in solution by the process with which I have always detected it in pure distilled water. Free exposure to the air is probably in part the cause of this. For it will be seen afterwards that some natural waters in passing through a long course of lead pipes, within which the action goes on without direct access of the atmosphere, contract an impregnation, which is invisible when the water is newly drawn, but after a few hours' exposure to the air shows itself in the form of a white film and milkiness.

The general result of these experiments appears to be, that neutral salts in various, and for the most part minute, proportions, retard

[*] Sometimes, however, a minute trace of white powder is attached to the bottom of the glass wherever the lead touches it. This is carbonate of lead at first, and afterwards a mixture like that described in the text.

37*

or prevent the corrosive action of water on lead, — allowing the carbonate to deposit itself slowly, and to adhere with such firmness to the lead as not to be afterwards removable by moderate agitation, adding subsequently to this crust other insoluble salts of lead, the acids of which are derived from the neutral salts in solution, — and thus at length forming a permanent impermeable skreen, through which the action of the water cannot any longer be carried on.

An important subject of inquiry regards the natural causes by which the preservative power of the neutral salts is impaired. This topic I have not hitherto been able to examine with all the care which is desirable.

From the effect of the water of Edinburgh when highly charged with carbonic acid, I was led to infer in former editions of this work that an unusual quantity of carbonic acid is a counteracting agent. For if Edinburgh water charged with it be corked up with some lead rods in a phial half-filled with water, and half with atmospheric air, the lead, which in common Edinburgh water, as will presently be mentioned, hardly loses any of its brilliancy for six or seven days, becomes quite white in twelve or sixteen hours. Subsequent experiments by Captain Yorke seemed to him to render this conclusion doubtful; nor do I attach much consequence to the observation just quoted. On the other hand it is said Professor Daniell has found all waters dissolve lead, if they contain an excess of carbonic acid.* The point would be best settled by the effect of a natural carbonated water passing through a long lead pipe.

On the Action of Natural Waters on Lead.

The preceding observations on the action of water on lead may be resorted to for explaining many interesting facts, and correcting some erroneous statements, which have been published by authors as to the corrosion of lead by natural processes.

Rain and Snow-Water. — It has been stated by Dr. Lambe that rain-water does not corrode lead, that " its effect is so slight as not to be discernible within a moderate compass of time."† But this observation is far from being correct. Rain or snow-water, collected in the country at a distance from houses, and before it touches the earth, being nearly as pure as distilled water, ought to act with equal rapidity on lead. I have accordingly found by a comparative experiment with that mentioned in p. 401, that in twelve ounces of snow-water, collected ten miles west from Edinburgh, and at some distance from any house, twelve lead rods weighing 340 grains lost two grains in eight days, and the usual crystals began to form in less than an hour. But when collected in a great city, rain or snow-water is much impaired in activity. Thus in an experiment made with eaves'-droppings collected from the roof of my house in Edinburgh, after half an hour of gentle rain from the south-east, — the first rain which had fallen for several weeks, — there was no action at all. Yet even

* Mr. Morson in Pharmaceutic Journal, ii. 355.   † On Spring Waters, p. 23.

when collected in a great city, and in circumstances which at first sight would appear not very favourable to its action, — for example from eaves'-droppings a few hours after the beginning of a shower, — it retains a little of its corroding property; and when collected in like manner after twelve or twenty-four hours' rain, it corrodes almost as rapidly as distilled water. Thus with four ounces of eaves'-droppings collected after the shower last alluded to had continued four hours, the crystalline powder began to cover the bottom of the glass in five hours, and in nine days three lead rods weighing fifty-seven grains lost a fifth of a grain. And in another experiment made with eaves'-droppings after a day's steady rain from the north-east, the powder began to form in half an hour, and the loss sustained by the lead in thirty-three days was a grain and a third, being very nearly what is lost in distilled water during the same time.

We must obviously be prepared to look for an explanation of these differences in the relative purity of the different waters. Accordingly, in the eaves'-droppings at the beginning of the shower the nitrates of baryta and silver caused, the former a distinct, the latter a faint precipitation, which, as oxalate of ammonia had no effect, arose from the presence of alkaline sulphates and muriates: but after a four hours' shower nitrate of baryta alone acted, and caused merely a faint haze: and after a twenty-four hours' shower, as well as in snow-water from the country, none of the three tests had any effect whatever.

Hence, perhaps even in a town, but at all events certainly in the country, it would be wrong to use for culinary purposes rain or snow-water which has run from lead roofs or spouts recently erected. When the roof or spout has been exposed for some time to the weather the danger is of course much lessened, if not entirely removed; because exposure to the weather encrusts it with a firmly adhering coat of carbonate, through which, as already observed, even distilled water will not act. But I believe it would be right to condemn the turning even old leaden roofs to the purpose of collecting water for the kitchen. Although the purest rain-water cannot act on them when it is once fairly at repose, we do not know what may be the effect of the impetus of the falling rain on the crust of carbonate; and if the crust should happen to be thus worn considerably, or detached by more obvious accidents, the corrosion would then go on with rapidity as long as the shower lasted. Acid emanations too disengaged in the neighbourhood, and other more obscure causes may enable rain-water actually to dissolve even the crust of carbonate.

These remarks on the effect of rain-water on lead are pointedly illustrated by what Tronchin has recorded of the circumstances connected with the spreading of the lead colic at Amsterdam, about the time he wrote his valuable essay on that disease. Till that period lead colic was seldom met with in the Dutch capital. But soon after the citizens began to substitute lead for tiles on the roofs of their dwelling-houses, the disease broke out with violence and committed great ravages. Tronchin very properly ascribed its increase to lead entering the body insidiously along with the water, which for culinary purposes was chiefly collected from the roofs during rain. He farther attempts to account for the rain-water having acquired the power of corroding the lead, by supposing that it was rendered acid in consequence of the roofs having been covered with decaying leaves from trees which abounded in the city ; and without a doubt this explanation accords with the season at which the lead colic was observed to be most frequent, — namely, the autumn. But he does not seem to have been aware that rain-water itself possesses the corroding property, independently of any extrinsic ingredient except the gases it receives in its passage through the atmosphere.* — Mérat has referred to a Dutch author, Wanstroostwyk, for an account of a similar incident which happened at Haarlem.†

The co-operating effect of acid emanations in the atmosphere is well exemplified by an interesting incident which occurred this year in Manchester, as detailed in some documents put into my hands by Dr. Hibbert Ware. A gentleman being seized with symptoms, which in the opinion of his medical adviser were owing to the insidious introduction of lead into the body, it was found by Mr. Davies that the rain-water from a leaden roof, which had been used in the family for nine years, contained a considerable impregnation of lead. At first this excited some surprise, because the roof was an old one. But on farther inquiry it was found, that the rain in descending contracted an impregnation of hydrochloric acid from the vapours which escaped from an adjoining manufactory. A portion of the water which was sent to me contained so much lead dissolved that it became dark-brown on the addition of hydrosulphuric acid, and a considerable black precipitate was slowly deposited.

Spring-Water. — Most spring-waters, unlike rain or snow-water, have little or no action on lead, because they generally contain a considerable proportion of muriates and sulphates.

As an example of a spring water which does not act on lead at all, the mineral water of Airthrey, near Stirling, may be mentioned. In four ounces of water from the strongest spring at Airthrey, I kept for thirty-five days three bright rods of lead weighing 47·007 grains ; and at the end of that period the rods were very nearly as brilliant as when they were first put in, and weighed 47·004 grains. This result is easily explained on considering the nature of the water. It contains no less than a seventy-seventh part of its weight of saline matters, which are chiefly muriates, and partly sulphates.

Another good illustration occurred to me lately, which contrasts well with some instances of an opposite description to be mentioned presently. The house of Phantassie in East-Lothian was supplied with water by a lead pipe from a distance of a mile. About a year afterwards, when I had an opportunity of examining into the circum-

* Tronchin de Col. Pict. 66. — 1757.

† De la Colique Métallique, 99, from Wanstroostwyk de l'Electricité Médicale, p. 224.

stances, I found the cistern singularly clean and free of incrustation, and the water quite free of lead. The composition of the water explained these facts. It contains a 4,900th of salts, a large proportion of which consists of carbonates of lime and magnesia.

The water of Edinburgh is another example of spring water nearly destitute of action on lead. But it is not so completely inactive as the water of Airthrey. In four ounces of water three bright rods weighing fifty-seven grains lost in seven days a 250th of a grain, in twenty-one days a 100th, in thirty-five days a 66th, and in sixty-three days a 59th of a grain. In seven days the lead was hardly tarnished at all, and not a speck of powder could be seen in the water, or on the glass. In twenty-one days, but still more in thirty-five or sixty-three days, the lead was uniformly dull; and on the surface of the water, as well as on the bottom of the glass, and on the side where left dry by the evaporation of the water, there were many white, filmy specks, which became black with the hydrosulphate of ammonia. In another experiment 145 grains of lead kept for six months in six ounces of Edinburgh water, which was filled up as it evaporated, lost a fifteenth of a grain ; and the white incrustation on the bottom and sides of the glass gave a large proportion of black precipitate when scraped together and treated with hydrosulphate of ammonia. These experiments are of some practical importance. For they show that the impregnation which the water of Edinburgh can receive in a few days from being kept in lead is so small as to be barely perceptible by the nicest analysis; but that the impregnation may be material if the same portion of water is kept in lead for a considerable length of time. Hence the perfect safety of the leaden cisterns and service-pipes used in this city. The same portion of water rarely remains in them above a single day. and therefore cannot become impregnated in a degree that is appreciable by the nicest examination. Dr. Thomson of Glasgow, in an interesting inquiry made in 1815 into the purity of the water which supplies Tunbridge, has stated that, when he lived in Edinburgh some years before, he could always detect a minute trace of lead suspended in the water, which at that time was brought six miles in leaden pipes.* I presume it is owing to the main pipes being now made of iron that this impregnation no longer exists. For I have found that the residue of two gallons of water, very carefully collected by gentle evaporation of successive portions in a small vessel, did not furnish the slightest trace of lead, when strongly heated with black flux and then acted on by nitric acid.† The feeble action of the Edinburgh water on lead arises from the salts it holds in solution. It contains about a 12,000th part of its weight of solid matter, of which about two-thirds are carbonate of lime, and one-third consists of the sulphates and muriates of soda, lime, and magnesia.

* Appendix to Dr. Scudamore's Analysis of the Mineral Water of Tunbridge, p. 51.

† Some effect may perhaps be also owing to a difference between the proportion of saline matter contained in the water of the Crawley spring, which has been introduced into the city since Dr. Thomson resided here, and the proportion in the water with which the city was at that time supplied. I am not aware, however, of the difference between them, or that any material difference does exist.

Many instances might be quoted of spring waters which act with inconvenient or dangerous rapidity on lead. But it is hardly worth while mentioning more than one or two of these, because the nature of the waters has been seldom described.

A striking example was related by Dr. Wall of Worcester. A family in that town, consisting of the parents and twenty-one children, were constantly liable to stomach and bowel complaints; and eight of the children and both parents died in consequence. Their house being sold after their death, the purchaser found it necessary to repair the pump; because the cylinder and cistern were riddled with holes and as thin as a sieve. The plumber who renewed it informed Dr. Wall that he had repaired it several times before, and in particular had done so not four years before the former occupant died.* The nature of the water was not determined. Most of the water around Worcester is very hard; but this will not account for its operation in the instance now described.

Another incident of the same kind, but hardly so unequivocal in its circumstances, was related in 1823 by Dr. Yeats of Tunbridge. A plumber undertook to supply that town with water for domestic purposes, and in 1814 laid a course of leaden pipes for a quarter of a mile. In the subsequent year many cases of lead colic occurred among the inhabitants who were supplied by those pipes; and one lady particularly, who was a great water-drinker, lost the use of her limbs for some months. The inhabitants naturally became alarmed; iron pipes were substituted; and no case of colic appeared afterwards. Mr. Brande analyzed the water which had passed through the pipes and detected lead in it, while at the same time none could be detected at the source.† Some uncertainty was supposed to have been thrown over these statements by the analytic researches of Drs. Thomson, Scudamore, and Prout, and Mr. Children.‡ But water like that in question can scarce fail to act powerfully on lead in favourable circumstances; for according to the analysis of Dr. Thomson it is extremely pure, as it contains only a 38,000th part of saline matter, three-fourths of which are a feebly protecting salt, the muriate of soda.§ I am satisfied, therefore, from my experiments, and the facts which follow, that no such water could be safely conveyed through new lead pipes; and that it would be dangerous even to keep it long in a lead cistern. It is difficult to account for the failure of the gentlemen above-mentioned to find lead in the water, except by supposing that they had analyzed what had been exposed for some time to the air, and deposited its oxide of lead in the form of carbonate.

Since my attention was first turned to this subject, the three following incidents have occurred to me, which show the danger of conveying very pure water in long lead pipes. 1. A gentleman in Dumfries-shire resolved to bring to his house in leaden pipes the

* Trans. of London College of Physicians, ii. 400.
† Hints on a mode of procuring Soft Water at Tunbridge — Journal of Science, xiv. 352.
‡ Scudamore's Pamphlet — Appendix — *passim*.   § Ibidem, p. 47.

water of a fine spring on his estate, from a distance of three-quarters of a mile. As I happened to visit him at the time, I took the opportunity of examining the action of a tumbler of the water on fresh cut lead, and could not remark any perceptible effect in fourteen days. It appeared to me, therefore, that the water might be safely conveyed in lead pipes ; and they were laid accordingly. No sooner, however, did the water come into use in the family, than it was observed to present a general white haze, and the glass decanters in daily use acquired a manifest white, pearly incrustation. On examining the cistern, the surface of the water, as well as that of the cistern itself, where in contact with it, was found completely white, as if coated with paint ; and the water taken directly from the pipe, though transparent at first, became hazy and white when heated or left some hours exposed to the air. On afterwards analyzing the water direct from the spring, I found it of very unusual purity ; as it contained scarcely a 22,000th of solid ingredients, which were sulphates, muriates, and carbonates. The reader can be at no loss to perceive why the experiment with a few sticks of lead in a tumbler was not a correct representation of what was subsequently to go on in the pipes : in fact, as the pipes were 4000 feet long, and three-fourths of an inch in diameter, each portion of water may be considered as passing successively over no less than 784 square feet of lead before being discharged. The remedy employed in this case will be mentioned presently [p. 415]. 2. A gentleman in Banff-shire introduced a fine spring into his house from a distance of three-quarters of a mile by means of a lead pipe. Two years and a half afterwards he was attacked with stomach complaints, obstinate constipation, and severe colic, for which he was under medical treatment for three months, with only partial and temporary relief. At last on leaving home and repairing to Edinburgh, he soon got quite well. Two other members of his family were similarly, but more slightly affected. On returning home some time afterwards, the same symptoms began to show themselves ; but he had not been many weeks there, when his attention was accidentally drawn to a notice of my experiments, and of the last case, in Chambers's Journal. He then saw that a white film lined the inside of the water-bottle in his dressing-room ; and the water was declared by a chemist to contain lead. I lately had an opportunity of analyzing the water, and found it to contain only a 16,500th of solid matter, the principal salt being chloride of sodium, and the others being sulphates of magnesia and lime, with very little carbonate. This, therefore, was exactly a case in which action upon lead might have been anticipated, as the principal proportion of the very small quantity of saline matter present was a feebly protective salt. 3. The third instance occurred at a country residence of Lord Aberdeen. Mr. Johnston, surgeon at Peterhead, being called to visit the housekeeper, found her affected with vomiting, constipation, acute pain at the pit of the stomach, retraction of the navel, and great feebleness. Little improvement was effected in three days, when Mr. Johnston, astonished at this,

and reflecting on the cause, suddenly was attracted by the appearance
of a silvery film on the inside of his patient's water-bottle, and recol-
lected at the same time my narrative of the Dumfries-shire case.   He
then perceived that the disease was lead-colic, treated it accordingly,
and slowly accomplished a cure.   The housekeeper's niece, a young
girl who had resided only a few weeks with her, and who was the
only other individual that had lived in the house above a few days
together for more than a year before, had begun also to suffer from
the premonitory symptoms.   About twelve months before this incident happened, a spring of water, which had been analyzed and pro-
nounced extremely pure, was brought to the house in a lead pipe ;
and the housekeeper had used this water for eight months before she
took ill. Mr. Johnston found that the water issued from the pipe was
quite clear, but that a white silvery film formed on its surface under
exposure to the air ; and he ascertained that the first-drawn water
contained lead in solution, and that the film was carbonate of lead.
I had an opportunity of analyzing the water, which proved to be by
no means very pure, as it contained a 4460th of solids.   But as the
solid matter consisted almost entirely of chlorides, namely, in a great
measure of chloride of sodium and a very little of the chlorides of
magnesium and calcium, as there was no carbonate present, and the
sulphates constituted only a 32,000th of the water, — it is plain from
the principles formerly laid down that the action which took place
was to be anticipated from the nature of the spring.*

For other instances of the corrosive action of spring water on lead
the reader may refer to Dr. Lambe's treatise.   Dr. Lambe was led
by his researches to imagine that no spring water whatever was destitute of this property in a dangerous degree.   This wide conclusion
is not supported by valid facts.   Yet his work contains several ac-
curative and instructive examples of the action in question.   Thus
among other instances he mentions that he had found the water of
Warwick to act on lead with great rapidity, and once saw holes and
furrows in a cistern there, which was the second that had been used
in the course of ten years.†   Sir G. Baker, in a letter to Dr. Heberden,
has related another striking instance of the same kind.   Lord Ash-
burnham's house in Sussex was supplied from some distance with
water, which was conveyed in leaden pipes.   The servants being
often affected with colic, which had even proved fatal to some of
them, the water was carefully examined, and found to contain lead.
The solvent power of the water was ascribed to its containing an
unusual quantity of carbonic acid gas.‡   This may be doubted.

In the course of the preceding remarks, allusion has been made to
the danger of keeping the same portion of water for a length of
time in leaden cisterns, if it has the power of acting on lead even in
a trifling degree.   The following illustrations deserve particular
notice.

It was mentioned in p. 409, as the result of experiments on the

* Edinburgh Royal Society Transactions, xv. 265.
† On Spring Waters, p. 14.   ‡ Ibidem, 116.

small scale, that although the water of Edinburgh does not contract a sensible impregnation of lead on remaining a few days in contact with it, yet a sufficient action ensues in the course of a few months, to show that it might be dangerous to keep that water long in a lead cistern. After coming to this conclusion, I had an opportunity of verifying it on a large scale. A cistern in my laboratory in the University having been left undisturbed for four or five months with about six inches of water in it, I found so large a quantity of pearly crystals lying loose on the cistern and diffused through the water, that when the whole was shaken up and transferred to a glass vessel, the water appeared quite opaque. Mérat observes that at the laboratory of the Medical Faculty of Paris there was procured by evaporating six loads, or probably about 1000 pounds of water, which had been kept two months in a leaden pneumatic trough, no less than two ounces of finely crystallized carbonate of lead.* Water in such circumstances has proved eminently poisonous. Thus, the crew of an East-India packet having been put on short allowance of water, in consequence of being delayed by contrary winds, the men got their share each in a bottle ; but the officers united their shares and kept it all in a lead cistern. In three weeks all the officers began to suffer from stomach and bowel complaints, and had the lead colic for six weeks ; while the men continued to enjoy good health. The surgeon detected lead in a tumbler of water without the process of concentration, by adding to it the sulphuret of potass.† A similar accident has been briefly alluded to by Van Swieten. He mentions, that he was acquainted with a family who were all attacked with colica pictonum in consequence of using for culinary purposes water collected in a large leaden cistern and kept there for a long time.‡ The composition of the water has not been mentioned in any of these instances ; but the water of Paris is so strongly impregnated with calcareous salts, that in ordinary circumstances its action on lead must be trifling.

It was probably from confounding the consequences of keeping the same water long in a lead cistern with the action in ordinary circumstances, that Dr. Lambe was led into the error of supposing that all spring waters whatever act on lead so powerfully, as to render it in his opinion advisable to abandon the use of this metal in the fabrication of pipes and cisterns. It must be admitted, however, that in all likelihood many waters will contain a trace of lead, without being kept more than the usual time in the pipe or cistern. For Dr. Lambe's results correspond to a certain extent with the more recent and accurate researches of Dr. Thomson, who mentions many instances where a faint trace of lead was found in the residue of the evaporation of a large quantity of spring water by himself, as well as by Dr. Dalton, Dr. Wollaston, and Mr. Children.§ But, as Dr. Thomson properly

* De la Colique Métallique, p. 98.
† Dr. Duncan's Medical Commentaries, xix. 313.
‡ Comment. ad Boerhaav. § 1060, T. iii. 347. Edit. Lugd. Batav. 1753.
§ Scudamore on the Analysis of Tunbridge Water, Appendix, 51, 53.

38

adds, when the quantity does not exceed a 600,000th or a millionth part of the water, as in these instances, it is ridiculous to imagine that any harm can result to man from the constant use of it for domestic purposes.

Another fact of some practical consequence, which flows from the experimental conclusions stated above is, that although it may be perfectly safe to keep some waters in leaden cisterns, it may be very unsafe to use covers of this metal, because the water which condenses on the covers must be considered as pure as distilled water. It has been found that white lead forms in much larger quantity on the inside of the covers of cisterns than on the cisterns themselves, where both are constructed of lead. A remarkable illustration of this is mentioned in a paper read before the Academy of Sciences at Paris in 1788 by the Comte de Milly. About a year after getting two leaden cisterns erected in his house, to keep the water of the Seine for general domestic purposes, he was attacked with severe and obstinate colic; which led him to examine his cisterns. He found that the sides, where they were occasionally left exposed by the subsidence of the water, and more especially the leaden cover, were lined with a white liquid, which was constantly dropping from the lid into the cistern, like the drops in caverns where stalactites are formed. The water was in consequence so strongly impregnated with lead as to give a dark precipitate with liver of sulphur.* The reason of this occurrence is, that the water in the cistern is a solution of preventive salts, but what reaches the lid is in a manner distilled. In Edinburgh the lids of the cisterns are invariably made of wood, whether on account of its superior cheapness merely, or because a leaden cover had been found perishable, I have not been able to discover.

It may be well to conclude these remarks on the action of spring waters on lead with a general summary of the chief circumstances to be adverted to in using lead for keeping or conveying water; to which may be added a few hints for preventing action where it is found to have taken place.

The general results of the preceding inquiries are that rain or snow-water for culinary use should not be collected from leaden roofs, nor preserved nor conveyed in lead; — that the same rule applies to spring waters of unusual purity, where for example the saline impregnation does not exceed a 15,000th of the water; — that spring water which contains a 10,000th or 12,000th of salts may be safely conveyed in lead pipes, if the salts in the water be chiefly carbonates and sulphates; — that lead pipes cannot be safely used, even where the water contains a 4000th of saline matter, if this consist chiefly of muriates; — that spring water, even though it contain a large proportion of salts, should not be kept for a long period in contact with lead; — and that cisterns should not be covered with lids of this metal.

Where action is observed to take place in the instance of particu-

* Rozier. Observations sur la Physique, xiii 145.

lar waters, it may in some cases be impossible to prevent it by any attainable means. But the inquiries detailed above suggest two modes by which a remedy may be generally found. It appears that, where a crust of carbonate is allowed to form slowly and quietly on the surface of lead, even distilled water ceases to have any material action ; and that the action is reduced almost to nothing if a crust be thus formed in a solution containing a minute quantity of some powerfully protecting salt, such as phosphate of soda. It appears to me then that a remedy may be often found in the instance of unusually pure spring waters — either by leaving the new pipes filled with the water for a few months, care being taken not draw any water from them in the interval, — or perhaps even more effectually by filling the pipes for a similar period with a solution containing about a 25,000th of phosphate of soda. I had determined to try the latter plan with the pipes in the Dumfries-shire case mentioned above, but recommended that in the first instance the pipes should be left for a few months full of the water of the spring, and the stopcocks kept carefully shut ; and on this being done for three or four months, it was found that the water afterwards passed with scarcely any impregnation of lead, and what little was contracted at first gradually diminished in the course of time. — Probably neither of these methods will be of more than temporary use, when the chief or only salt present is chloride of sodium, even though the proportion be considerable. Both plans seemed to answer for a time in the instance which occurred at Lord Aberdeen's (p. 411); but after a while the action recommenced, probably owing to the deposited carbonate being slowly dissolved. At the time of publication of my paper in the Transactions of the Royal Society of Edinburgh, the cure appeared complete, and was there represented to be so.

I should add that an effectual remedy has been lately introduced by a patent invention for covering lead pipes both externally and internally with a thin coating of tin.

In the remarks now made on the action of water on lead no account has been taken of the effect of the galvanic fluid in promoting it. This, however, is a most important co-operating agent, or rather perhaps it ought to be considered a distinct power ; for it acts with energy where water alone acts least, namely, when there is saline matter in solution, because then a galvanic current of greater force is excited. In general it is necessary that two different metals be present in the water before galvanic action be excited ; but a very slight difference may be sufficient. For example, it seems enough that the lead contain here and there impurities, constituting alloys slightly different from the general mass of the pipe or cistern. It is probable that galvanic action may be thus excited by the joinings being soldered with the usual mixture of lead and the more fusible metals. At least I have seen pipes deeply corroded externally, when made of sheets of lead rolled and soldered ; and the action was deepest on each side of the solder, which had itself entirely escaped corrosion. Even inequalities in the composition of the

lead may have the same effect. Sheet lead long exposed to air or
water is sometimes observed to be corroded in particular spots;
and these will always be found in the neighbourhood of parts of
the metal differing in colour, hardness or texture from the general
mass. I have not analyzed such spots; but I conceive the supposition now made is exceedingly probable, and supplies a ready explanation of the corrosion. Similar effects may arise simply from
fragments of other metals lying long in contact with the lead.
They may also arise from portions of mortar being allowed to lie on
the lead; but the action here is not galvanic.

I have no doubt that many of the instances of unusually rapid corrosion of lead by water, such as that mentioned by Dr. Wall [p. 410]
are really owing, not to the simple action of water, but to an action
excited obscurely in one or other of the ways now mentioned.

Of the Action of Acidulous Fluids on Lead and its Oxide.

Water acidulated with various acids acts on lead with different
degrees of rapidity.

The effect of acidulation with *carbonic acid* has not yet been accurately ascertained. The effect of *sulphuric acid* is peculiar. Distilled water feebly acidulated with that acid acts much less rapidly
on lead than when quite pure. Thus I have found that, if it contained a 4000th or even only a 7000th of sulphuric acid, fifty grains
of lead kept in it for thirty-two days gained a seventh or a twelfth of
a grain in weight, and were covered with beautiful crystals of sulphate of lead. A minute trace of lead could be detected in the
water. *Hydrochloric acid* is somewhat more active as a solvent.
Distilled water containing a 3000th of that acid acquired in thirty-
two days a sweetish taste, and yielded by evaporation a considerable
quantity of muriate of lead, while the lead rods lost weight, and
were covered with acicular crystals of the same salt.

It is much more important, however, to consider the effects of the
vegetable acids on lead and its oxide, because their solvent power
is a fruitful source of the accidental as well as intentional adulteration
of many articles of food and drink.

Acetic acid in the form of common vinegar, even when much diluted, attacks and dissolves metallic lead, if by exposing the surface
of the fluid to the air, a constant supply of oxygen be maintained to
produce oxidation. The *citric acid* will attack it under the same
circumstances, but acts more slowly. In a solution of five grains of
citric acid in twenty-four parts or two drachms of water, three lead
rods lost two grains in weight in nine weeks. The greater part of
the citrate of lead separated slowly in white powdery crystals; but a
small portion was dissolved by the excess of acid, and imparted to
the fluid a pleasant sweetness. *Tartaric acid* acts much less energetically. In a comparative experiment with the last, the lead
gained nearly half a grain in weight by acquiring a crystalline coat
of tartrate of lead. But I could not detect any lead in solution; and

there was no loose powder. The tartrate of lead is very sparingly soluble in an excess of its acid, so that a sweet taste cannot be communicated by it to a fluid acidulated with tartaric acid. *Malic acid*, according to MM. Chevallier and Ollivier, acts so quickly as a solvent, that if a solution be kept in a lead vessel for three hours, the metal may be detected in the fluid by any of its ordinary tests.[*]

The acids act with greater rapidity on the protoxide of lead than on the metal; and the presence of air is of course not required to enable them to effect its solution.

The solvent power of the acids is liable to be counteracted by various substances; the operation of which, however, has not been well ascertained. It appears that substances containing gallic acid or tannin throw down the lead; and on this account various adulterations which would otherwise take place are either prevented or corrected. It has been also ascertained by Proust, that the vegetable acids do not attack lead when it is alloyed with tin. For as the latter metal has a stronger attraction than the former for acids, no lead can be oxidated before the tin undergoes that change.[†]

From what has been said of the action of the vegetable acids, it follows that the preparation or preservation of articles of food and drink in leaden vessels is fraught with danger. For, if they contain a vegetable acid, more particularly the acetic, as many of them do, and if they are allowed to remain in the vessel for a moderate length of time, they will be apt to be impregnated with the metal. In this way lead has been often insidiously introduced into the food of man.

Thus milk has been poisoned by being kept in leaden troughs. An instance of the kind has been related by Dr. Darwin. A farmer's daughter used to wipe the cream from the edge of the milk which was kept in leaden cisterns, and being fond of cream, had a habit of licking it from her finger. She was seized in consequence with the symptoms of lead colic, afterwards with paralytic weakness of the hands, and she died of general exhaustion.[‡] The circumstances under which the lead is acted on have not been carefully examined. It appears to be sometimes used with safety. It will of course be dissolved, if the milk should become sour.

Rum has been also supposed to be sometimes adulterated with lead by being left in contact with the metal. The dry belly-ache of the West Indies, which appears to be the same disease with the lead colic, has been ascribed by some to the same cause. But on this subject precise information is still wanted. Dr. J. Hunter has stated, that an epidemic colic, which attacked three of our regiments in Jamaica during the years 1781 and 1782, and which seized almost every man of them, was traced by him to the presence of lead in the rum; and he endeavours to show that the spirit might dissolve the lead in passing through the leaden worms of the distilling apparatus.[§] He adds in another work, that, according to information communi-

* Annales d'Hygiène Publique, 1842, xxvii. 111.
† Ann. de Chim. lvii. 82.   ‡ Zoonomia, ii. 130.
§ Trans. of London College of Physicians, iii. 227.
38*

cated by Dr. Franklin, the legislature of Massachusetts passed an act in 1723, prohibiting the use of leaden still-heads and worms in the distillation of spirituous liquors.* It is certain that rum has been often impregnated with lead; but it is by no means clear that Dr. Hunter has successfully accounted for the mode in which the adulteration is effected.

Wine has been accidentally impregnated in like manner, in consequence of the bottles having been rinsed with shot, and some of the shot left behind. An interesting example of this has been related in the Philosophical Magazine. Severe abdominal symptoms were caused by a bottle of wine; and the cause was discovered to be the action of the wine on some shot in the bottom of the bottle. The shot had been so completely dissolved, that it crumbled when squeezed between the fingers.† The illness in this instance must have been owing to the arsenic contained in the shot, because the quantity of lead was hardly sufficient to excite violent symptoms. — At one time home-made British wines must have been frequently adulterated with lead, from the makers being ignorant of the dangerous nature of the adulteration. Sir G. Baker quotes the following receipt in a popular cookery book of his time: " *To hinder wine from turning.* — Put a pound of melted lead in fair water into your cask, pretty warm, and stop it close."‡

But by far the most remarkable adulteration of the kind now under review is that of cider. At one time a disease in every respect the same as the lead colic used to prevail in some of the southwest counties of England at the cider season; and it was generally ascribed, in consequence apparently of the opinion of Huxham, to the working people indulging too freely in their favourite beverage during the season of plenty. The subject, however, was carefully investigated in 1767 by Sir George Baker, who succeeded in proving, that the disease arose from the cider being impregnated with lead, sometimes designedly for the purpose of correcting its acescency when spoiled, but chiefly by accident, in consequence of the metal being used for various purposes in the construction of the cider-house apparatus. The substance of his researches is, — that a disease in all respects the same with the lead colic was in his time so prevalent in Devonshire as to have supplied 289 cases to the Exeter Hospital in five years, and 80 to the Bath Infirmary in a single season (1766); while, on the contrary, it was little, if at all, known in the adjoining counties of Gloucester, Worcester, and Hereford, although cider is there an equally common drink among all ranks: — that in the latter counties lead was seldom or never used in constructing the apparatus of the cider-houses, while in Devonshire it was used sometimes for lining the presses, but more commonly for fastening the iron cramps, and filling up the stone joinings of the grinding troughs, and for conveying the liquor from vessel to vessel: — that lead did not exist in the

* On the Diseases of the Army in Jamaica, p. 269.
† Philosophical Magazine, liv. 229.
‡ Trans. of London College of Physicians, i. 216.

cider of Herefordshire, but might be detected both in the ripe cider, and more especially in the must, of Devonshire : — that from eighteen bottles of cider, a year in bottle, $4\frac{1}{2}$ grains of metallic lead were procured.* The accuracy of these facts, and the soundness of the conclusions which Sir George Baker drew from them have been universally admitted ; and lead is now, I believe, completely excluded from the cider apparatus.

Notwithstanding the notoriety of these facts, accidents from adulterated cider seem still to occur occasionally in France. So recently as 1841 a set of cases which presented the incipient symptoms of lead colic were traced by MM. Chevallier and Ollivier to cider having been adulterated with lead to the amount of nearly two grains and a half per quart, in consequence of a publican having kept his cider for two days in a vessel lined with lead.[†]

If lead is previously oxidated, the presence of vegetable acids in articles kept in contact with it is still more likely to give rise to a poisonous impregnation, than in the case of lead itself.

Of accidental adulterations of this kind the most important is that which arises from the action of vegetable acids on the glazing of earthenware. This glaze is well known to contain generally a considerable quantity of oxide of lead, and in consequence is more or less easily dissolved by vegetable acids. A good example has been noticed by Dr. Beck.[‡] A family in Massachusetts, consisting of eight persons, were all seized with spasmodic colic, obstinate costiveness, and vomiting ; and the disease was satisfactorily traced to a store of stewed apples, which had been kept some months in an earthenware vessel and had corroded the lead glazing. Another interesting example has been described by Dr. Hohnbaum of Hildburghausen. A family of five persons were all violently affected for a long time with spasmodic colic, and some with partial palsy. After examining many articles of food, Dr. Hohnbaum at last found that the vinegar for dressing their salads was kept in a large earthenware vessel capable of holding eight or ten quarts, and glazed with lead ; that an ounce of vinegar remaining in the vessel contained no less than nine grains of lead ; and that the whole glazing of the vessel was completely dissolved.[§] Accidents like this appear from the statements of the same author to have been common in Germany not long ago. Luzuriaga attributes the great prevalence of colic in Madrid and the neighbourhood to the general use in the kitchen of earthenware glazed with lead.[‖] Jacob imputes it to the same cause.[¶] But others have doubted the accuracy of this explanation.

The effect of acids on lead glazing appears to be variable. Some-

* On the Cause of the Endemical Colic of Devonshire. Transactions of the London Coll. of Phys. i. ii. and iii.

† Annales d'Hygiène-Publique, 1842, xxvii. 104.

‡ Elements of Medical Jurisprudence, ii. 319.

§ Zeitschrift für die Staatsarzneikunde, 1827, xiii. 151.

‖ Mérat de la Colique Métallique.

¶ Diss. Inaug. sur la Collique de Madrid. Analyzed in Corvisart's Journal de Médecine, xxxiv. 208.

times they hardly act on it at all.* The difference probably depends on differences in the composition of the glaze. Gmelin says, that if there is little oxide of lead present, acids and fat do not corrode it; but that potters often use too much, to render the glaze more fusible; and that then it is easily corroded.† Westrumb states, that, if the lead glaze is thoroughly vitrified and not cracked, the strongest acids do not attack it.‡ Farther experiments are still required to elucidate this subject.

It is not, however, by accident only that the food or drink of man is subject to be poisoned with lead. Many articles are adulterated with it designedly for a variety of purposes. These adulterations it is necessary for the medical jurist to study.

No kind of adulteration with lead is more common than that of wine; which, when too acid and harsh from the first, or rendered acescent by decay, may be materially improved in taste by the addition of litharge.

The practice of correcting unsound wines in this way seems to have been well known at an early period. Betwixt the years 1498 and 1577, various decrees were passed against it by the German emperors; and in some provinces the crime was even punished capitally.§ For some time afterwards the dangerous effects of the practice appear to have been lost sight of in Germany. But towards the close of the seventeenth century, the attention of physicians and legislators in that country was pointedly directed to the subject by various writers in the *Acta Germanica*.‖ The same practice has been long prevalent in France. The famous endemic colic of Poitou, which appeared in 1572, and raged for sixty or seventy years, has been with justice ascribed in modern times to the adulteration of wine with lead, and has given to the lead colic its scientific name of *colica pictonum*. More recently, the practice became exceedingly prevalent in Paris. About the year 1750, the farmers-general found that for some years before that, 30,000 hogsheads of sour wine were annually brought into Paris for the alleged purpose of making vinegar, while the previous yearly imports did not exceed 1200. An inquiry was accordingly set on foot; which led to the discovery, that the vinegar merchants corrected the sour wines with litharge, and thus made them marketable.¶ Notwithstanding the active system of medical police in the French capital, the crime is not yet eradicated. Indeed the small tart wines used so abundantly there by all ranks, hold out great encouragement and facilities to its perpetration.

The process employed for correcting the acescency of wine is not precisely known. Some wines are easily corrected; Mérat found that a bottle of harsh wine, which had a sharp, bitterish, rather acrid

---

* Hohnbaum, &c. p. 157.   † Geschichte der Mineralischen Gifte, 194.

‡ Note in an Essay by his Son, — Ueber Vergiftung durch Käse. Horn's Archiv, 1828, i. 83.

§ Gmelin's Geschichte der Mineralischen Gifte, 216.

‖ Cockelius, Acta, &c. Dec. i. An. iv. Obs. 30. Brunnerus, Ibidem, Obs. 92. Vicarius, Ibidem, Obs. 100. Riselius, Ibidem, Dec. i. An. v. Obs. 251.

¶ Paris and Fonblanque's Med. Jurisprudence, ii. 347.

taste, took up in forty-eight hours twelve grains of litharge, and became palatable.* With other wines this simple method will not answer, because the colour is destroyed, and a taste is substituted which has no resemblance to that of the genuine wine. Thus Orfila remarked, that Burgundy, neutralized with litharge, acquired a saccharine taste and became pale-red, because the insoluble salts of lead which were formed, combined with and removed the colouring matter.† On the whole, it is probable that the adulteration of wine with lead can only be practised with success on the common tart kinds, such as those used by the lower orders on the continent.

Some excellent observations have been published on this subject by Fourcroy. In order to render what he has said intelligible, it is necessary to premise. that in the course of the fermentation of wine, the bitartrate of potass, which accelerates the conversion of the sugar of the fruit into alcohol, is itself partly converted into malic acid ; that in sound wine, therefore, there is a mixture of tartaric and malic acids ; but that if the malic acid originally existed in the fruit in too great abundance, the fermentation of the sugar is imperfect, and the wine is consequently both too acid and too weak ; and lastly, that all wines, if neglected, are apt to ferment too much, in consequence of which they pass the vinous stage of fermentation, and become impregnated with acetic acid.‡

Now Fourcroy found that the oxide and other preparations of lead correct acescency and harshness in wines, not so much by throwing down the acids, as by combining with them in solution, and imparting to the liquor the peculiar sweetness of lead. Hence tart wines, which owe their acidity to too great a proportion of tartaric acid or bitartrate of potass, cannot be improved by adulteration with oxide of lead. For the bitartrate of potass cannot act at all as a solvent on the oxides or carbonate of lead, and even pure tartaric acid takes up so little, that wine containing it, could not acquire the sweet taste which is the purpose of the adulteration. This statement I have confirmed. But the case is very different when the wine contains acetic acid, the presence of which is the general cause of spoiling or acidity. For Fourcroy remarked, that acetic acid dissolves not only oxide and carbonate of lead, but likewise the tartrate, notwithstanding its great insolubility in water or in its own acid. Hence the presence of tartaric acid in a wine spoiled by co-existence of the acetic, will not prevent the liquor from taking up oxide of lead in sufficient quantity to acquire an improved taste and flavour. Nay, an obvious mode of correcting excessive acidity, produced by too much tartaric acid, is to add tartaric acid, and then to treat the mixture with oxide of lead. Fourcroy farther thinks, that the malic acid possesses the same solvent power as the acetic over tartrate of lead, and that its presence may therefore be the reason why some tart wines, which do not contain the acetic acid, becomes nevertheless impregnated with the poison. The solvent power of acetic acid is increased by the

* De la Colique Métallique, 212.   † Toxicologie Gén. i. 616.
‡ Dr. Macculloch on the Art of Wine-making, in Edin. Horticultural Mem. i. 134.

presence of other vegetable principles in the wine.* I may add, that I have found the citric acid to possess the same property with the acetic and malic acids. It dissolves so much of the tartrate of lead as to acquire a pleasant sweetness, unmixed with metallic astringency.

The practice of adulterating wine with lead does not seem to have been ever pursued to any material extent in Britain. Home-made wines may be adulterated in this way, as may be inferrred from the receipt formerly quoted for preventing acescency. But I have never heard that any such adulteration has been suspected in the foreign wines usually drunk in this country. Considering, indeed, the nature of these wines, and the class of people who alone make use of them, it is not likely that adulteration with lead could be practised with success. If the foreign wines used in Britain should become acescent, lead could hardly restore their taste so thoroughly as to impose on the consumer.

Sometimes spirituous liquors and preserves have been adulterated with lead, in consequence of sugar of lead having been used to clarify them, or to render them colourless. Cadet de Gassicourt says it is a common practice in France to clarify honey and sugar of grapes, and to make brandy pale in this way ; and M. Boudet has detected lead in many samples of these articles in Paris.† Hollands has likewise been poisoned in the same manner. Dr. Shearman mentions his having detected an extensive adulteration of smuggled Geneva by an excise officer, which had been sold and dispersed over an extensive tract of country, and which committed great ravages among the inhabitants.‡

The adulterations hitherto noticed take place through means of the chemical action of the adulterated articles on lead or its oxide. Some other substances are occasionally contaminated by its compounds being merely mechanically mixed with them. There is no end to the number and variety of adulterations of this kind. But the following will serve as examples. Gaubius once detected an adulteration of butter with white lead at a time when it was very scarce in Flanders, owing to a dreadful mortality among cattle.§ An instance of poisoning with lead, in consequence of cheese having been mixed with red lead, is mentioned in the Repertory of Arts.‖ This variety deserves to be remembered. Red lead was at one time a good deal used to communicate the peculiar reddish-yellow colour, which is supposed to characterize the finer qualities of certain kinds of English cheese. In the Transactions of the Medical Society of London, a singular instance has been related by Mr. Deering, of lead colic attacking a whole family, and proving fatal to two of them, in consequence of the insidious introduction of white lead into the body. Although the nature of the symptoms in the several cases left no doubt that

* Sur les Vins lithargyriés Mém. de l'Académie, 1787, p. 280.
† Journal Gén. de Médecine, xliv. 321.
‡ Edin. Medical and Surgical Journal, viii. 213.
§ Dehaen, Ratio Medendi, P. x. c. viii. § 1.
‖ Repertory of Arts, First Series, viii. 262.

lead was the cause of them, it was long before the source of the poison was discovered. Every vessel and article used in the kitchen was in vain examined; when at length it was discovered that the sugar used by the family had been taken from a barrel which had formerly contained white lead, and that, as the sugar from the centre of the barrel had been dug out, and given away to various friends, the outer part of it next the white lead was chiefly used by the family themselves.*

Process for detecting Lead in Organic Mixtures.

In the first place, a little nitric acid should be added to the suspected matter before filtration; for nitric acid redissolves any insoluble compound formed by the salts of lead with albumen and other animal principles, as well as some of those formed with vegetable principles; and consequently renders it more probable, that the poison will be detected in the first part of the analysis, if present at all.† This being done, sulphuretted-hydrogen gas is to be transmitted through the fluid part of the mixture; and if a dark-coloured precipitate is formed, the whole is to be boiled and filtered to collect the precipitate.

In order to ascertain that the precipitate positively contains lead, those who are accustomed to use the blowpipe may put the sulphuret into a little hole in a bit of charcoal, and reduce it by the fine point of a blowpipe-flame; when a single globule is procured, which is easily distinguished by its lustre and softness. A better process, for those not accustomed to the blowpipe, and perhaps a better test of the existence of lead in all circumstances, is to heat the sulphuret to redness in a tube, and to treat it with strong nitric acid, without heat or with the aid of a gentle heat only. The lead is thus dissolved without the sulphur being acted on. The solution is then to be diluted with water, filtered, evaporated to dryness, and gently heated to expel the excess of nitric acid. If the residue be dissolved in water, it will present the usual characters of a lead solution when subjected to the proper liquid tests. Of these the hydriodate of potass is to be preferred when the quantity is too small for trying more of them. But for this purpose care must be taken to expel all the excess of nitric acid, because an excess will strike a yellow colour with the test though lead be not present.

If the preceding process should not detect lead in the filtered part of the mixed fluid, then the insoluble matter left on the filter is to be incinerated, and the residuum dissolved in nitric acid, and tested as above. This branch, however, will be rarely required, if lead be present, because the precaution of adding nitric acid, previous to filtration, dissolves the lead from most of its compounds which are insoluble in water. The process of incineration in medico-legal ana-

* Trans. of Lond. Med. Society, i., or Edin. Med. and Surg. Journal, viii. 211.

† The precipitate formed by the acetate of lead with albumen is dissolved by nitric acid. From that formed with milk the acid removes the oxide of lead entirely, leaving the casein.

lysis generally should be avoided if possible, as it is not easily ma-
naged by unpractised persons. — The present branch of the process
of analysis will be particularly required for the contents of the stomach or vomited matter, when any sulphate or phosphate has been
given as an antidote.

A process different from the preceding, and analogous to those for
detecting copper and antimony in complex organic mixtures, has
lately been proposed by Professor Orfila, especially for those cases in
which lead is to be sought for in the textures of the body, where
death is supposed to have been occasioned by it. The subject of
analysis, such as the liver, spleen, or kidneys, being cut into small
pieces, and boiled in distilled water, and the filtered decoction being
evaporated to dryness, the extract is to be carbonized with nitric acid
as directed under the head of copper (p. 357); and care must be
taken that the heat be not raised to redness, so as to inflame the
mass. The residuum is then to be boiled with nitric acid ; the solution being evaporated to dryness to expel the excess of acid, the saline matter left is to be re-dissolved and acted on by hydrosulphuric
acid gas; and the sulphuret thus formed may be recognized by the
means mentioned above.*

A question has been recently started, whether all the processes for
detecting lead in the tissues of the human body are not rendered fallacious by the alleged existence of lead in the healthy animal textures.
In the first place, however, it is doubtful, as will be seen presently,
whether lead ever exists naturally in the animal organs. But besides,
the fallacy, if a real one, is obviated by the process of Orfila ; who
states that lead, naturally combined in the animal tissues, cannot be
indicated by his method, if the animal matter be charred by nitric
acid without deflagration. And farther, in regard to the tissues of
the stomach in cases of acute poisoning with the preparations of lead,
it appears that in most instances there may be seen on the villous coat
little white points, which are blackened by hydrosulphuric acid, a
phenomenon never occasioned by lead naturally contained in the substance of the membrane. [See p. 439.]

SECTION II. — *Of the Action of Lead and the Symptoms it excites
in Man.*

The effects of the preparations of lead on the body are very
striking. They differ according to the rapidity with which it enters
the system. Large doses of its soluble salts cause symptoms of irritant poisoning. The gradual introduction of any of its oxidated preparations in minute quantities brings on a peculiar and now well-
known variety of colic, which is often followed by partial palsy, and
in violent cases by apoplexy.

The physiological effects and mode of action of the soluble salts
in irritating doses have been examined experimentally by Professor
Orfila, M. Gaspard, Dr. Schloepfer, and Dr. Campbell. Their expe-

* Journal de Chimie Médicale, 1842, 339.

riments agree in showing that these poisons have a direct irritating action, and a remote operation of an unknown kind; but the results obtained by different experimentalists differ as to some of the details. The acetate may be taken as a type of the whole genus.

Orfila found that it was hardly possible to bring dogs under the action of the acetate if swallowed in solution, because they speedily discharged it all by vomiting. But if the salt was given in powder in the dose of half an ounce, or if the solution was retained in the stomach by a ligature on the gullet, the symptoms produced were those of violent irritation in the first instance, succeeded by extreme weakness and death, sometimes in nine hours, more generally not till the second day or later. The appearances in the body were unnatural whiteness of the villous coat when death was rapid, and vascular redness when death was slower. The whiteness in the former case Orfila ascribes to chemical action. But as neither this appearance nor the redness in the latter case was considerable, while at the same time the symptoms were not those of continuous irritation, he was led to doubt whether the poison causes death in consequence of its irritant properties. And the phenomena observed by him when acetate of lead was injected into the jugular vein prove that death is owing to certain remote effects. Introduced through this channel thirteen grains killed a dog almost immediately, death being preceded by no other symptom except convulsive respiration; five grains killed another in five days, and the leading symptoms were weariness, languor, staggering, and slight convulsions, none of which symptoms appeared till the third day; and it is remarkable that in neither animal could he find any morbid appearance on dissection.* Mr. Blake states that large doses, such as a drachm, suddenly arrest the heart's action; but that small doses of three grains, injected into the jugular vein, cause diminished action of that organ, and afterwards gorging and hepatization of the lungs; and that when injected backwards into the aorta from the axillary artery, this salt occasions obstruction of the capillary circulation, indicated by increased arterial pressure,—and then an action on the nervous system, producing insensibility, violent movements of the tail, and at last arrestment of the respiration. It may be inferred from Mr. Blake's researches that lead obstructs both the systemic and pulmonary capillaries, that it acts powerfully on the nervous centre, and that it likewise depresses the heart's action when the dose is large.†

The experiments of Gaspard coincide with those of Orfila in assigning considerable activity to the acetate of lead when it is directly introduced into the blood, — the quantity of two or four grains generally causing death in three or five days.‡ The experiments of Campbell farther show that death may be induced by applying it to a wound, and that the symptoms antecedent to death resemble those remarked by Orfila when it is injected into a vein.§ But the two

* Toxicologie Générale, i. 630.
† Edin. Med. and Surg. Journal, lvii. 117.
‡ Journal de Physiologie, i. 284.   § Diss. Inaug. p. 27.
39

last experimentalists differ from Orfila in assigning to sugar of lead a property like that possessed by arsenic, of acting on the alimentary canal, even when applied to a wound, or directly introduced into the blood. For Campbell found the stomach corrugated and red, and the small intestines also vascular; while Gaspard not only observed analogous appearances after death, but even also witnessed all the symptoms of violent dysentery during life. In farther proof of the local irritating power of this poison, it may be added, that when sugar of lead was injected into the rectum Campbell found it to cause purging, tenesmus, itching of the anus, and great debility.

I have found that the nitrate of lead is powerfully irritant and corrosive in the dose of 400 grains. This quantity dissolved in four ounces of water killed a strong dog in sixteen hours, producing violent efforts to vomit and diarrhœa. And after death the whole inner membrane of the gullet and stomach, and the villi of the upper half of the small intestines, were uniformly white, brittle, and evidently disintegrated ; and the mucous coat of the great intestines was bright red in parallel lines.

The only inquiries I have hitherto met with, which assign to lead in continued small doses the power of producing in animals the peculiar colic and palsy often produced by it in man are those of Schloepfer, related in his thesis on the effects of poisons when injected into the windpipe. He found that the acetate, introduced through this channel in successive doses of ten grains, brought on all the symptoms of *colica pictonum*, preceded by oppressed breathing, and ending fatally with palsy and convulsions in the course of three weeks.[*] More recently Dr. Wibmer, in the course of some experiments on the long-continued use of acetate and carbonate of lead, remarked weakness and stiffness of the limbs in dogs ; and in the rabbit I have observed in the like circumstances gradually increasing weakness, ending in complete palsy of the fore legs.

The compounds of lead seem to produce their effects on the animal body through the medium of absorption. At all events they are absorbed in the course of their action, and are diffused throughout the animal textures. Lead was long sought for with variable and dubious success in the fluids and solids of men and animals killed by it or labouring under its effects. But the late improvements in physiological science and chemical analysis have demonstrated, that it may always be detected in favourable circumstances in the liver and kidneys, often in the spleen and in the urine, and sometimes even in the muscles. Wibmer was the first who satisfactorily proved its presence. In dogs poisoned slowly by the acetate or carbonate of lead in frequent small doses, and dying with symptoms of lead-colic and palsy, he found the metal distinctly in the liver, muscles, and spinal cord, and more obscurely in the blood, by drying and deflagrating the animal matter with nitre, acting on the residue with nitric acid, neutralizing the solution, and testing it with hydrosul-

[*] De Effectibus liquidorum in vias aëriferas, &c. p. 43.

phuric acid, carbonate of potash, and iodide of potassium.* On repeating these experiments, I succeeded in detecting lead in very minute quantity in the lumbar and dorsal muscles of rabbits, but not any where else.† Professor Orfila has since frequently found lead, by means of his method of analysis described at page 424, in the kidneys, liver, and urine of animals which had taken large doses of acetate of lead, and once in the urine of a girl who had swallowed above an ounce of the acetate twenty-five hours before the urine was passed.‡ About the same time M. Ausset, under the directions of Lassaigne, detected lead largely in the blood and urine of a horse during life, and in the liver and kidneys after death.§ Mr. Alfred Taylor found traces of it in the milk of a cow accidentally poisoned by carbonate of lead.‖ M. Tanquerel Desplanches says it has been detected by M. Devergie and himself in the palsied parts of persons who had died of colica pictonum ;¶ and Dr. Budd observes, that Mr. Miller found lead in abundance in the paralysed extensors of the hand in a man who died in a London Hospital of the epileptic form of the effects of this poison.**

These facts seem to outweigh the negative results obtained by others. Nor are they invalidated by the alleged existence of lead in the healthy animal textures. For in the first place, — although M. Devergie says he has always found traces of lead in the substance of the stomach and intestines of men and women, who had not used preparations of lead or been in any way exposed to it,†† and Professor Orfila confirmed these observations by also finding traces of lead in the alimentary canal under similar circumstances,‡‡ — the conclusion flowing from their researches is after all doubtful ; for in a later inquiry MM. Danger and Flandin could not find any lead, unless it had been purposely introduced into the body.§§ And secondly, — Devergie adds to his remarks, that the quantity of lead he found in the textures and secretions of those who had died of lead-colic was far greater than in those who had not been exposed to lead preparations before death ; and Orfila ascertained that the process by which he detects adventitious lead is incapable of indicating that which may be present naturally in the body.‖‖

It is probable that all the preparations of lead are poisonous except the metal, and perhaps also the sulphuret. The experimentalists at the Veterinary School of Lyons found that nearly four ounces of the metal might be given to a dog without even vomiting being excited ; and Orfila remarked that an ounce of carefully prepared sul-

* De effectu plumbi in organismo animali sano, &c. auctore Carol. Wibmer. Monachii, 1829, p. 29.

† Treatise on Poisons, Edition 1836, p. 509.

‡ Bulletin de l'Académie Roy. de Méd. 1840, vi. 283, and Toxicologie Gén. 1843, i 668, 684.

§ Journal de Chim. Med. 1842, 344. ‖ Guy's Hospital Reports, 1841, vi. 175.

¶ Archives Gén. de Médecine, liv. 106.

** London Med. Chir. Trans., 1842, xxv. 115.

†† Annales d'Hygiène Publique, xx. 463, xxiv. 180. ‡‡ Ibidem, xxi. 164.

§§ L'Experience, Avril 27, 1843.

‖‖ Toxicologie Gén. 1843, i. 670.

phuret had as little effect.* The effects, which have been occasionally ascribed to lead-shot, and which will be mentioned by and by [see p. 435], seem at variance with these experiments, but cannot outweigh such precise negative results. It is probable that irritant poisoning can be produced only by those compounds which are soluble, such as the acetate, subacetate, and nitrate. It appears indeed from the experiments of Orfila with the acetate and my own with the nitrate, that these compounds are true corrosives, and of no mean energy when given in large doses moderately diluted.

The insoluble compounds, such as the carbonate, red oxide and protoxide, possess little irritant power. The experimentalists of Lyons found litharge to be irritant in large doses of half an ounce.† Orfila gave dogs large doses of the red oxide and carbonate without observing any signs of irritation in the stomach. A case has been published of a young woman who swallowed accidentally an ounce and a half of the carbonate without any bad effect whatever either at the time or afterwards ;‡ and Dr. Ogston of Aberdeen has informed me he met with a similar case, that of a girl who took an ounce with the view of destroying herself, but without sustaining any harm whatever. In a remarkable case, published by Mr. Cross of London, in which six drachms were taken accidentally by a pregnant female instead of magnesia, vomiting and violent colic were produced, and afterwards fainting, paralysis of the extensor muscles, and contraction of the flexors; all of which symptoms, however, after enduring without abatement till eight hours after the poison was swallowed, gradually disappeared under antidotes and laxatives. But such a case bears no great resemblance either to the acute or chronic form of poisoning with lead, and was probably hysterical.§ Orfila has found that an ounce and a quarter of sulphate of lead had no effect whatever on a dog.‖ Mr. Taylor mentions a case where the chloride of lead caused vomiting, but no other ill consequence.¶ Dr. Cogswell found that three drachms of iodide of lead caused in a dog merely depression and weakness for a few days ; but forty grains killed a rabbit in twelve days, with symptoms of exhaustion and constipation ; and doses frequently repeated, to the amount of eleven drachms in eighteen days, killed a dog under symptoms nearly the same.**

It may be presumed that all the compounds of lead which are soluble in water or in the animal fluids may produce in favourable circumstances the lead colic and palsy. Dr. A. T. Thomson, indeed,†† has endeavoured to show by some experiments, that the carbonate is the only compound of lead which possesses this singular power; and that if the acetate of lead produces similar effects, it is only because that salt usually contains an excess of oxide which becomes

* Arch. Gén. de Médecine, xix. 328.   † Corvisart's Journal de Médecine.
‡ Krüger in Rust's Magazin für die gesammte Heilkunde, xi. 535.
§ Lancet, 1838, i. 786.   ‖ Toxicologie Gén. i. 690.
¶ Manual of Medical Jurisprudence, 189.
** Experimental Inquiry on Iodine, p. 140.
†† London Medical Gazette, v. 538.

carbonate from the action of free carbonic acid in the stomach and other parts of animals, or because the salt is decomposed by double decomposition from the accidental presence of alkaline carbonates. It does not appear to me, however, that the researches of Dr. Thomson, taken along with the prior inquiries of other physiologists, will bear out this conclusion. The experiments of Wibmer in particular would seem to show that the carbonate is at least not more active than the acetate ; nor does it appear probable that the small doses of acetate given by him, seldom exceeding two or three grains at a time, could yield any carbonate in the alimentary canal of a dog, where there is commonly much free muriatic acid. Farther, in many of the instances of lead colic related above as produced by cider, wine, and other acid substances acting on lead or its oxide, the acid must have been so greatly in excess, that it was scarcely possible that carbonate of lead could have been formed afterwards by any ordinary accident. And even supposing the carbonate to be more active than other compounds in occasioning colic and palsy, as Dr. Thomson's inquiries would tend to show, the fact may be admitted without necessarily leading to the inference, that it is the only active compound of lead, or that other preparations must be converted into the carbonate before they can act as slow poisons. For the superior activity of the carbonate may be owing to the great obstinacy with which its impalpable powder adheres to moist membranous surfaces, and the consequent greater certainty of its ultimate absorption. It certainly appears at least but consistent with a general law, to which hitherto no undoubted exception has been found, that the carbonate must be dissolved before it can act constitutionally.

The symptoms observed in man from the preparations of lead are of three kinds. One class of symptoms indicate inflammation of the alimentary canal : another spasm of its muscles : and a third injury of the nervous system, sometimes apoplexy, more commonly palsy, and that almost always partial and incomplete. Each of these classes of symptoms may exist independently of the other two ; but the last two are more commonly combined.

The irritant effects of large doses of the soluble salts of lead come first under consideration. Of these the acetate, or sugar of lead may be taken as an example.

Here it will, in the first instance, be observed that, according to the experiments mentioned above, the acetate of lead, though certainly an irritant poison, is not very energetic, — being much less so than the vulgar generally believe, and far inferior to most of the metallic poisons hitherto treated of. This farther appears from the experience of physicians as to its effects in medicinal doses. The acetate has been often given in pretty large doses in medical practice ; and although it has sometimes excited colic when continued too long, ordinary irritation of the stomach seems to have been rarely observed. Mr. Daniell, in a paper on its effects as a remedy for mercurial salivation, states that he gave it in doses of ten grains three times a day, and that he never observed it to excite any other un-

39*

pleasant symptom except slight colic, which seldom came on till after the fourth dose.* I have often given it in divided doses to the amount of eighteen grains daily for eight or ten days, without remarking any unpleasant symptom whatever, except once or twice slight colic. Van Swieten even mentions a case in which it was given to the amount of a drachm daily for ten days before it caused any material symptom.†

Yet facts are not wanting to prove that acetate of lead in an improper dose will produce violent and immediate effects. The symptoms are then either those of simple irritation, or more commonly those of inflammation united with the peculiar spasmodic colic of lead, and sometimes followed by convulsions and coma, or by local palsy.

In one of Sir George Baker's essays there is an instance of immediate and violent symptoms having been caused by a drachm taken twice with a short interval between the doses. The subject was a soldier who took it in milk to cure a diarrhœa. Five hours after the first dose he was seized with pain in the bowels and a feeling of distension round the navel. After the second these symptoms became much more acute ; and he was soon after seized with bilious vomiting, loss of speech, delirium, and profuse sweating, while the pulse fell down to 40. He recovered, however, with the aid of diluents and cathartics.‡

A case which proved rapidly fatal has been related in a French journal. A drummer in a French regiment, who was much given to drinking, stole some Goulard's extract, and drank it for wine. Neither the first symptoms nor the dose could be ascertained. On the second day he was affected with loss of appetite, paleness, costiveness, and excessive debility ; on the third day he had severe and excessive colic, drawing in of the belly, loss of voice, cold sweats, locked jaw, and violent convulsions ; and he expired before the evening of the same day. The morbid appearances will be mentioned in their proper place. Sugar of lead was detected in the stomach.§

In both these instances the disorder excited partook very much of the character of the spasmodic colic which is caused by the gradual introduction of lead into the body ; and in the last the whole course of the man's illness was very like that of the worst or most acute form of *colica pictonum.* But in another example which came under my own notice, the symptoms were more nearly those of ordinary irritation,—namely, vomiting, burning, and pricking pain in the throat, gullet, and stomach, with trifling colic subsequently ; but the patient recovered in two or three days. The quantity taken was supposed to exceed a quarter of an ounce. So, too, in a case which occurred to M. Villeneuve of Paris, the symptoms were chiefly vomiting and purging, with faintness and some convulsions. His patient swallowed intentionally above an ounce of acetate of lead in solution.

* Lond. Med. Repos. N. S. vi. 368.
† Comment. 1060, T. iii. p 347. Editio Dan Barbari.
‡ Trans. Coll. Phys. London, iii. 426.   § Journal Universel, xx. 351.

Sulphate of soda and sulphate of magnesia were given promptly as antidotes; in an hour the symptoms had abated materially; and next day she was well.[*] This was the case in which Orfila found lead in the urine. Of the same nature, also, are two cases briefly alluded to by Mr. Taylor, as having been caused in London in 1840 by Goulard's extract. The subjects, who were children, were seized with vomiting, purging, and other symptoms like those of Asiatic cholera; and both died within thirty-six hours.[†]

In another instance, related by Mr. Iliff of London, where an ounce of the acetate was accidentally swallowed in solution, the symptoms were at first colic pains and vomiting, in the course of a few hours vomiting and tenderness, and, after these symptoms receded, a peculiar state of rigidity and numbness, which was not entirely removed for several days. In this case no remedies were used for three hours; and even two hours later, when the stomach-pump was resorted to on account of the slightness of the vomiting, lead was found in the first fluid withdrawn, — a new proof of the feeble action of acetate of lead, compared with some other metallic poisons.[‡]

So much for the operation of the acetate of lead in large doses. Physicians, however, are much better acquainted with the effects of lead when introduced in the body continuously and insidiously in minute quantities. For all tradesmen who work much with its preparations are apt to suffer in this way, and many other persons have been brought under its action in consequence of articles of food and drink being impregnated with it. The disease which is thus induced may be divided into two distinct stages.

The first stage is an affection of the alimentary canal, the leading feature of which is violent and obstinate colic. This symptom at times begins abruptly during a state of sound health; but much more commonly it is ushered in by a deranged state of the stomach, not unlike common dyspepsia, seldom so severe as to excite alarm, and commonly imputed at first to a wrong cause. There is general uneasiness and depression, a dingy yellowish complexion, weakness and numbness in the limbs, a sweetish styptic taste and fetid breath, a slaty tint of the teeth and gums, with a blue line along the margin of the gums where they touch the teeth, a slow hard pulse, great emaciation, loss of appetite and tendency to indigestion. This state, which was first well characterized by Mr. Wilson[§] of Leadhills, and has lately been more fully described by M. Tanquerel,[||] is of great moment as apprizing the workman of the necessity of taking active measures for preventing the more formidable effects, which otherwise are sure to follow. Of the warning symptoms none is so invariable or so characteristic as the blue line along the edge of the gums, an appearance which was first noticed by Dr. Burton of St. George's,

* Bulletin de la Soc. Roy. de Méd. 1840, vi. 283.
† Manual of Medical Jurisprudence, p. 186.
‡ London Medical Repository, 1824, N. S. iii. 37.
§ Edinburgh, Phys. and Lit. Essays, i.
|| Traité des Maladies de Plomb. 1843.

London,* and has been since observed in every case of lead colic, whether impending or present. — If alarm be not taken in time, the obscure complaints hitherto mentioned become attended by and by with uneasy sensations in the stomach, stretching ere long throughout the whole belly. At the same time the stomach becomes irritable, and the food is rejected by vomiting. Cramps in the pit of the stomach then arise, and extend to the rest of the belly, till at length the complete colic paroxysm is formed. The pain is sometimes pretty constant; sometimes it ceases at intervals altogether; but much more commonly there are remissions rather than intermissions; and it is remarked that both the remissions and exacerbations are much longer than those of common colic. The pain is very generally, yet not invariably, relieved by pressure; even strong pressure seldom causes any uneasiness, provided it be not made on the epigastrium; nay, some patients have been known to bear, with relief to the paroxysms, the weight of two or three people standing on the belly.† The belly is almost always hard, the abdominal muscles being contracted: sometimes it is rather full, more commonly the reverse, and the navel is often drawn in so as almost to touch the spine. The bowels all the while are obstinately costive. Either there is no discharge from them at all; or scanty, knotty fæces are passed with much straining and pain. This state, long supposed to depend on spasm, is now known to arise on the contrary from paralysis, of the intestinal muscular coat. In a few instances diarrhœa takes the place of the opposite affection. The urine is commonly diminished. The saliva has been described as greater than natural in quantity and bluish in colour; but Dr. Burton says he did not observe a single instance of this in forty cases which he carefully examined. From the beginning, or more generally after a few hours or days, the limbs are racked with diffuse cutting pains; which, according to Tanquerel, affect chiefly the limbs, especially near the joints, are worst at night, are often attended with cramps, and are relieved by pressure. The aspect of the countenance is dull, anxious, and gloomy: in advanced cases the expression of gloomy anxiety exceeds that of almost all other diseases. It appears from the latest works on this disease published in France, and particularly from the able treatise of Mérat, that the pulse is rarely accelerated, but on the contrary often retarded.‡ This does not accord with the experience of some earlier writers;§ and in the few cases I have seen in this city the pulse has been always frequent. It cannot be questioned, however, that, as Mérat states, fever is not essential. The skin has a dull, dirty, cadaverous appearance, is often, though not always hot, and in either case is bedewed with irregular, clammy, cold perspiration.

This, the first stage of colica pictonum, may end in three ways. In the first place, the patient may recover at once from it as from an

* London Medical Gazette, 1839-40, 1, 687.
† Mérat de la Colique Métallique, 51.
‡ Ibid., p. 55.
§ Tronchin de Colica Pictonum. Genevæ, 1757.

ordinary colic ; and it is consolatory to know, that a first attack, taken under timely management, is for the most part easily made to terminate in that favourable manner. In such circumstances it rarely endures beyond eight days. But it is exceedingly apt to recur, if, for example, the patient expose himself to what in ordinary circumstances would cause merely a common colic or diarrhœa ; and if he returns to a trade which exposes him again to the poison of lead, the disease is sure to recur sooner or later, and repeatedly, unless he observes the greatest precautions. In one or other of these returns, sometimes even in the first attack, the colic is not succeeded by complete recovery, but gives place to another more obstinate and more alarming disease. This secondary affection is of two sorts. One, which occurs chiefly in fatal cases, is a species of apoplexy. The other, which does not of itself prove fatal, is partial palsy.

In violent and neglected cases of colica pictonum, the colic becomes attended in a few days with giddiness, great debility, torpor, and sometimes delirium ; as the torpor advances the pains in the belly and limbs abate ; at length the patient becomes convulsed and comatose, from which state very few recover. Tanquerel, who is unnecessarily minute in subdividing the various affections produced by the poison of lead, distinguishes four kinds of affections of the head, coma, epilepsy, delirium, and a combination of all these.* A very rare termination allied to that now described is sudden death during the colic stage, without any symptom which would lead one to suspect its approach. A case of this kind has been related by M. Louis. His patient, five minutes after talking to the attendant of his ward, was found at his bedside in the agony of death ; and no cause for so sudden a death could be found on dissection.† Somewhat similar was a case which occurred in 1838 at the hospital of La Charité at Paris. A man labouring for three days severely under the colic stage of the disease, began to breathe stertorously soon after straining at stool, and died in three hours.‡ In a case which occurred to Dr. Elliotson death was owing to concomitant perforation of the stomach, a concurrence which was probably accidental, but which was also once observed by Dr. Copland.§

In cases, on the other hand, which have not been neglected, and particularly when the attack is not the first, the departure of the colic often leaves the patient in a state of extreme debility, which by and by is found to be a true partial palsy, more or less complete. This affection is sometimes present before the colic departs, but is apt to escape notice till the pain abates. Occasionally it supervenes on a sudden, but more generally it is preceded by a sense of weariness, numbness and tremor of the parts. The palsy is of a peculiar kind. It affects chiefly the upper exremities, and is attended with excessive muscular emaciation. The loss of power and substance is most re-

* Archives Gén. de Médecine, liv. 111.   † Louis, Recherches Pathologiques
‡ London Medical Gazette, 1837-38, ii. 158.
§ British Annals of Medicine, i. 145.

markable in the muscles which supply the thumb and fingers ; and in every case which I have seen the extensors suffered more than the flexors. The paralysis is hardly ever complete, except perhaps in the extensors of the fingers. When it is considerable, the position of the hands is almost characteristic of the disease. The hands are constantly bent, except when the arms hang straight down by the side ; they dangle loosely when the patient moves ; he cannot extend them, and raises one arm with the aid of the other. The palsy is attended, according to Tanquerel, with diminished heat in the parts, and feeble pulsation in the arteries which supply them. There is seldom any loss of sensation in the affected parts. But the paralysis sometimes affects the nerves of the other senses. Thus two cases of paralysis of the nerves of vision have been related by Dr. Alderson of Hull ;* and Tanquèrel says this affection is not uncommon in Paris, and is attended with dilated and immovable pupils. The latter author also once met with deafness in the same circumstances. — Patients affected with lead palsy usually complain of racking pains in the limbs and arms, digestion is feeble, and trivial causes renew the colic. From this deplorable condition it is still possible to restore the sufferer to health, chiefly by rigorous attention to regimen. But he too often dies in consequence of a fresh attack of colic as soon as he returns to his fatal trade.

The lead palsy, however, does not always come on in this regular manner. Sometimes the primary stage of colic is wanting, so that the wasting of the muscles and loss of power are the first symptoms. I have seen a characteristic example of the kind in a sailor who had been employed for a month in painting a vessel. He had great weakness and wasting of the arms and hands, particularly of the ball of the thumb ; but except a tendency to indigestion, costiveness, and transient slight pain of the belly, he had suffered no previous disorder of the intestines. I have seen the paralytic affection confined to the extensors of one hand in a compositor, and Dr. Chowne met with a similar affection of both hands in a gas-fitter.† Dr. Bright observed palsy without colic in the case of a painter three times in the course of seven years.‡ — In like manner, according to Tanquerel, the neuralgic affection may occur severely without any precursory colic ; and the same author has witnessed both coma and convulsions in the same circumstances.

Colica pictonum, with the collateral disorders specified above, is the only disease which has been distinctly traced to the operation of lead insidiously introduced into the body. But many other disorders have been ascribed to its agency. Boerhaave seems to have imagined that consumption might be so induced ; and Dr. Lambe thought that to this cause may be traced the increased prevalence of " scrofula, phthisis, dropsy, chronic rheumatism, stomach complaints, hypochondriasis, and the host of nervous complaints which infest modern life."§ These conjectures are wholly destitute of foundation in fact.

* London Med.-Chir. Transactions, xxii. 82.
† Lancet, 1838-39, i. 65.   ‡ Reports of Medical Cases, p. 394.
§ Lambe on Spring Waters, p. 71.

In whatever form lead is habitually applied to the body, it is apt to bring on the train of symptoms mentioned above ;— the inhalation of its fumes, the habitual contact of any of its compounds with the skin, the prolonged use of them internally as medicines, or externally as unguents and lotions, and the accidental introduction of them for a length of time with the food, may sooner or later equally induce colica pictonum.

Instances have occurred of colic being produced by the prolonged employment of the compounds of lead inwardly in medical practice. Such cases are so uncommon that it is evident some strong constitutional tendency must co-operate. But it is in vain to deny, as some do, that the medicinal employment of preparations of lead internally is unattended with any risk whatever of slow poisoning. Dr. Billing of Mulhausen relates a case of death, apparently from the comatose affection succeeding the colic stage of poisoning with lead, in the instance of a boy of fifteen, to whom he gave acetate of lead in gradually increasing doses for six weeks, till he took two grains daily.[*] Tanquerel met with a case of colic produced by 130 grains taken in fourteen days, and another occasioned by 149 grains in sixteen days.[†] Sir George Baker has mentioned similar instances.[‡] It would even appear that metallic lead may have the same effect when taken inwardly. Thus Dr. Ruva of Cilavegno has related the case of a man who was violently attacked with the colic form of the effects of lead after taking six ounces of shot by direction of a quack for the cure of dyspepsia, and was seized again with the same symptoms six days afterwards on taking four ounces more. On the second occasion he had violent colic, great feebleness of the limbs, constant vomiting of any thing he swallowed, severe headache, and other analogous symptoms, of which he was not effectually cured for seven weeks.[§] A case somewhat similar, but less severe, has been described by Dr. Bruce.[∥] — With regard to lead colic being excited by unguents and lotions applied to the surface of the body, Sir George Baker mentions a case of violent colic brought on by litharge ointment applied to the vagina ; he adds that children have been thrown into convulsions by the same substance sprinkled on sores : and he quotes Zeller for a case where symptoms of poisoning were occasioned by sprinkling the axilla with it, as a cure for redness of the face.[¶] Dr. Wall, in a letter to the preceding author, mentions his having seen the bowels affected by Goulard's extract applied to ulcers ; in another paper he has given two unequivocal cases, in one of which colic was brought on by saturnine lotions applied to a pustular disease, and in the other by immersing the legs twice a day for ten days in a bath of the solution of acetate of lead :[**] and lately Dr. Taufflieb of Barr observed lead colic to arise from

* Hufeland's Journal der Praktischen Heilkunde, Mars, 1839.
† Archives Gén. de Médecine, liv. 106.
‡ Transactions of London Coll. of Phys. i. 236, 301, 304.
§ Annali Universali di Medicina, 1837, iv. 426.
∥ Lancet, Dec. 31, 1842.
¶ Trans. of Lond. Coll. Phys. i. 311.   ** Ibid. iii. 435.

the continued use of diachylon plaster during eleven weeks for dressing an extensive ulcer.* Such accidents are exceedingly rare, and some auxiliary cause must have favoured the operation of the poison in the cases now noticed; for every one knows that free use is made of lead unguents and lotions, yet we seldom hear of any bad consequences. — These cases, however, will probably remove the doubts which some entertain of the possibility of lead colic being induced by the application of the compounds of lead to the sound skin in those trades which compel the workmen to be constantly handling them. At the same time it must be admitted, that in all these trades there exists a more obvious and ready channel for the introduction of the poison; because the workmen are either exposed to breathe its fumes, or are apt to transfer its particles from the fingers into the stomach with their food. — Of all exposures none is more rapid and certain than breathing the vapours or dust of the preparations of lead. But for that very reason workmen who are so exposed seldom suffer; because the greatness of the risk has led to the discovery of means to avert it, and the openness of the danger renders it easy for the workmen to apply them. Tanquerel mentions a singular case of a woman who was attacked in consequence of the fine dust of white lead ascending through chinks in the floor from a room below, where a perfumer was in the practice of grinding and sifting that substance.† — It may be added that Dr. Otto of Copenhagen has published an extraordinary instance of fatal lead-colic, originating in the habitual use of Macuba snuff adulterated with twenty per cent. of red lead.‡

To these observations on the various ways in which lead insidiously enters the system a few remarks may be added on the trades which expose workmen to its influence. The most accurate information on this subject is contained in the work of Mérat.

He places foremost in the list miners of lead. In this country miners are now rarely affected, because the frequency of colica pictonum among them formerly led their masters to study the subject, and to employ proper precautions for removing the danger. It has been stated by Dr. Percival, and is generally thought, that the whole workmen in lead mines are apt to be attacked with the colic, — those who dig the sulphuret as well as those who roast the ore.§ If this idea were correct, it would be in contradiction with the general principle in toxicology, that the metals are not poisonous unless oxidated. But the opinion is in all probability founded on error; for, according to information communicated to me by Mr. Braid, and confirmed since by personal investigation, the workmen at Leadhills who dig and pulverize the ore, although liable to various diseases connected with their profession, and particularly to pectoral complaints, never have lead colic till they also work at the smelting furnaces.

* Archives Gén. de Médecine, 1838, i. 353.
† Ibid., liv. 106.
‡ London Medical Gazette, April, 1843.   § On the Poison of Lead, p. 22.

Next to miners may be ranked manufacturers of litharge, red-lead and white-lead. The workmen at these manufactories are exposed to inhale the fumes from the furnaces or the dust from the pulverizing mills. It has been chiefly among the workmen of a former white-lead manufactory in the neighbourhood of Edinburgh that I have had an opportunity of witnessing the lead colic. By a simple change the proprietor made in the process, and which will be mentioned presently, the disease was almost extirpated some years before the manufactory was given up.

Next in order, perhaps in the same class with colour-makers, are house-painters. The causes of their liability is the great quantity of the preparations of lead contained in the paints they use. It would appear that lead colic is most frequent among people of that trade in cities of the largest size. In Geneva, as I am informed by my friend Dr. C. Coindet of that place, colica pictonum is now almost unknown and never occurs among painters. In Edinburgh it is also little known among painters. A journeyman painter, a patient of mine in the Infirmary, had been seventeen years in the trade, and yet did not know what the painters' colic or lead palsy meant. In London, according to the Dispensary reports, and in Paris, according to the tables of Mérat, many workmen of that trade suffer. I have been informed by an intelligent workman, once a patient of mine, who had been a journeyman painter both in London and Edinburgh, that the number of his acquaintances who had been affected with colic in the metropolis was incomparably greater than here. This man ascribed the difference to the working hours being more in the former place, so that the men had not leisure enough to make it worth their while to clean themselves carefully in the intervals. This appears a rational explanation. I do not not know how the great prevalence of colic among painters in Paris is to be accounted for.

Plumbers, sheet-lead manufacturers, and lead-pipe makers, are also for obvious reasons apt to suffer; but as they are not necessarily exposed to the vapours of lead, and suffer only in consequence of handling it in the metallic form, it ought to be an easy matter to protect them. They themselves conceive that a very hazardous part of their occupation is the removing the melted lead from the melting pot, to make the sheets or pipes; but this operation cannot be dangerous if the melting pots are properly constructed.

A few cases of lead colic occur among glass-blowers, glaziers, and potters, who use the oxide of lead in their respective trades.

There are a few also among lapidaries and others, who use it for grinding and polishing, and among grocers and colourmen who sell its various preparations. Printers seldom suffer from the colic, but are generally thought liable to partial palsy of the hands, which is ascribed to frequent handling of the types. I have met with one case apparently of this nature.

Lead is not the only metal to which the power of inducing colica pictonum has been ascribed. Mérat has mentioned several instances
40

of the disease occurring among brass-founders and other artizans who work with copper.* Tronchin quotes Scheuchzer for a set of well-marked cases in a convent of monks, where the malady was supposed to have been traced to all the utensils for preparing and keeping their food having been made of untinned copper.† The same author mentions two cases, one of which came under his immediate notice, where the apparent cause was the long-continued use of antimonial preparations internally.‡ Mérat likewise found a few iron-smiths and white-iron-smiths in the lists kept at one of the Parisian hospitals.§ Chevallier alleges that colic occurs at times among money-changers at Paris, and others who constantly handle silver.‖ Cases have even been noticed by Mérat among varnishers, plasterers, quarrymen, stone-hewers, marble-workers, statuaries, saltpetre-makers;¶ and Tronchin enumerates among its causes the immoderate use of acid wine or of cider, checked perspiration, sea-scurvy, and melancholy. But the only substance besides lead, whose operation in producing colica pictonum has been traced with any degree of probability, is copper; and even among artizans who work with copper the disease is very rare. As to the other tradesmen mentioned by Mérat, it is so very uncommon among them, that we may safely impute it, when it does occur, to some other agent besides what the trade of the individual exposes him to; and in general the secret introduction of lead into the body may be presumed to be the real cause. Still, however, the connection of colica pictonum with other causes besides the poison of lead is upheld by so many facts, and is believed by so many authorities, that this disease cannot be safely assumed, even in its most characteristic form, as supplying undoubted evidence of the introduction of lead into the system. Dr. Burton thinks it will when the blue line at the edge of the gums is seen.

The work of Mérat contains some interesting numerical documents, illustrative of the trades which expose artisans to colica pictonum. They are derived from the lists kept at the hospital of La Charité in Paris, during the years 1776 and 1811. The total number of cases of colica pictonum in both years was 279. Of these, 241 were artisans whose trades exposed them to the poison of lead, namely, 148 painters, 28 plumbers, 16 potters, 15 porcelain-makers, 12 lapidaries, 9 colour-grinders, 3 glass-blowers, 2 glaziers, 2 toy-men, 2 shoemakers, a printer, a lead-miner, a leaf-beater, a shot-manufacturer. Of the remainder, 17 belonged to trades in which they were exposed to copper, namely, 7 button-makers, 5 brass-founders, 4 braziers, and a copper-turner. The remaining twenty-one were tradesmen, who worked little, or not at all with either metal, namely, 4 varnishers, 2 gilders, 2 locksmiths, a hatter, a saltpetre-maker, a winegrocer, a vine-dresser, a labourer, a distiller, a stone-cutter, a calciner,** a soldier, a house-servant, a waiter, and an attorney's clerk. — Age or youth seems not to afford any protection against the poison. Of the 279 cases, 24

* De la Colique Métallique.   † De Colica Pictonum, p. 56.   ‡ Ibid. p. 65.
§ De la Colique Métallique, p. 23.
‖ Journal de Chim. Médicale, 1840, 328.   ¶ Ibid. *passim.*
** Calcineur, — a calciner of gypsum, I believe.

were under twenty, and among these were several painter-boys not above fifteen years old; 113 were between nineteen and thirty; 66 between twenty-nine and forty; 38 between thirty-nine and fifty; 28 between forty-nine and sixty; and 10 older than sixty. These proportions correspond pretty nearly with the relative number of workmen of similar ages. — Among the 279 cases fifteen died, or 5·4 per cent.

There seems to have lately been little or no diminution in the frequency of the disease in Paris. In 1833-4-5-6, there were treated in the hospitals 1541 cases, or 385 annually; of whom one in 39½ died. And in 1839-40-41 there were 761 cases, or 252 annually; of whom one in 24½ died. Of 302 cases in 1841 no fewer then 266 were from white-lead manufactories.*

SECTION III. — *Of the Morbid Appearances caused by Lead.*

The morbid appearances caused by poisoning with lead are in some respects peculiar.

In acute poisoning, from the irritant action of its soluble salts, as in the case of the drummer poisoned by Goulard's extract, the lower end of the gullet, the whole stomach and duodenum, part of the jejunum, and the ascending and transverse colon, have been found much inflamed, and the villous coat of the stomach as if macerated. In Mr. Taylor's two cases Dr. Bird found the villous coat of the stomach gray, but otherwise natural; and the intestines were much contracted.

The stomach in the first of these cases contained a reddish-brown, sweetish, styptic fluid, in which lead was detected by chemical analysis,† — an important medico-legal fact, since the man survived nearly three days. Some valuable observations have been made by Professor Orfila as to the presence of lead in the textures of the stomach in such instances. When small doses of acetate or nitrate of lead were administered to dogs and allowed to act for two hours only, the villous coat presented numerous streaks of white points, which contained lead, as hydrosulphuric acid blackened them. These points, though less distinct, were still visible, when the animals were allowed to live four days after the excess of salt had been removed; and even after seventeen days, although no such appearance remained, lead could still be detected in the tissues of the stomach.‡

The blood in animals is sometimes altered. Dr. Campbell found it fluid. In a dog poisoned with litharge, the experimentalists of the Veterinary School at Lyons found it of a vermilion colour in the veins, and brighter than usual in the arteries.§ Mitscherlich also found it unusually red and firmly coagulated.‖

The appearances in the bodies of those who have died of the various forms of lead colic are different, and wholly unconnected with inflammation.

* Annales d'Hygiène Publique, xix. 23, xxv. 543, xxviii. 226.
† Journal Universel, xx. 353.   ‡ Annales d'Hygiène Publique, xxi. 149.
§ Corvisart's Journ. de Médecine.   ‖ British Annals of Medicine, i. 205.

The valuable work of Mérat contains four inspections after death from the acute or comatose form of colica pictonum. The bodies were plump, muscular and fat. The alimentary canal was quite empty, and the colon much contracted, — in one to an extraordinary degree. The mucous coat of the alimentary canal was everywhere healthy. He therefore infers that the disease is an affection of the muscular coat only. It is a striking circumstance, and conformable with what will be afterwards established in regard to the true narcotics, that although both of the men died convulsed and comatose, no morbid appearance was visible within the head.[*] Another case, which confirms the foregoing facts, has been described by Mr. Deering. It was that of a lady who died convulsed after suffering in the usual manner, and in whose body no trace of disease could be detected any where.[†] Senac informed Tronchin that he had dissected above fifty cases of colica pictonum, and found no morbid appearances.[‡] Schloepfer's observations on animals are to the same effect. In rabbits which died of colica pictonum the great intestines were excessively contracted, but all the other organs of the body were healthy except the liver, which was dark and brittle.[§] Mitscherlich observed in his animals extravasation of blood into the intestines, also sometimes into the cavities of the pleura and peritoneum, and occasionally under the peritoneal covering of the kidneys.[||] The only instance I have met with where morbid appearances were found within the head, was in a case mentioned by Sir G. Baker, of a gentleman who died apoplectic after many attacks of colica pictonum, and in whom the brain was found unusually soft, and blood extravasated on its surface to the amount of an ounce.[¶]

The appearances in those who have been long affected with the paralytic form of colica pictonum have been rarely observed in modern times. I am indebted to my late colleague, Dr. Duncan, Junior, for an account of the appearances in the intestinal canal of a plumber, who had been long and frequently afflicted with colica pictonum and its sequelæ. The intestines were dark, tender, and far advanced in putrefaction. The cardiac orifice of the stomach was so narrow that it would admit a goose-quill. The mesenteric glands were enlarged and hardened. The thoracic duct was surrounded by many large bodies like diseased glands, exactly of the colour of lead, and composed of organized cysts containing apparently an inorganic matter. The analysis of this matter was unfortunately neglected. The muscles in similar circumstances are much diseased. When the paralysis is not of long standing, it appears from the experiments of Schloepfer (whose animals survived about three weeks), that the whole muscular system becomes pale, bloodless, and flaccid. When the palsy is of long standing, this change increases so much, that the muscles in some parts, as in the arms and thumbs, acquire the

* De la Colique Métallique, p. 213.
† Trans. of Lond. Med. Society, 1810, or Edin. Med. and Surg. Jour. viii. 211.
‡ Tronchin de Colica Pict. p. 117.
§ De effectibus liquidorum ad vias aërif. applic. p. 43.
|| British Annals of Medicine, i. 205.
¶ Trans. of Lond. Coll. of Physicians, i. 469.

colour and general aspect of white fibrous tissue. Some observations on the nature of these changes will be found in the essays of Sir G. Baker.* The facts are communicated by Mr. John Hunter. On examining the muscles of the arm and hand of a house-painter who was killed by an accident, Mr. Hunter found them all of a cream colour, and very opaque, their fibres distinct, and their texture unusually dry and tough. These alterations he at first imagined might have been the result merely of the palsy and consequent inactivity of the muscles, but on finding the same alterations produced by the direct action of sugar of lead on muscle, he inferred that the poison gradually effected a change either on the muscles directly, or on the blood which supplied them.

In a late elaborate inquiry into the pathology of lead-colic, M. Tanquerel has arrived at the conclusion, that "the pathological phenomena are not caused by anatomical changes cognisable by the senses," and that such appearances as may be found are the effects, not the cause, of the disease.†

SECTION IV. — *Of the Treatment of Poisoning with Lead.*

The treatment of poisoning with lead, and the mode of protecting workmen from its influence, will now require a few remarks.

For the irritant form of poisoning, a safe and effectual antidote exists in any of the soluble alkaline or earthy sulphates. If none of these be at hand, then the alkaline carbonates may be given, particularly the bicarbonates, which are not so irritating as the carbonates. The phosphate of soda is also an excellent antidote. If the patient does not vomit, it will be right also to give an emetic of the sulphate of zinc. In other respects, the treatment does not differ from that of poisoning with the irritants generally.

Colica pictonum is usually treated in this country with great success by a practice much followed here in colic and diarrhœa of all kinds, — the conjunction of purgatives with anodynes. A full dose of a neutral laxative salt is given, and an hour afterwards a full dose of opium. Sometimes alvine discharges take place before the opium acts, more commonly not till its action is past, and occasionally not for a considerable time afterwards. But the pain and vomiting subside, the restlessness and irritability pass away, and the bowels return nearly or entirely to their natural condition. Sometimes it is necessary to repeat the practice. It is almost always successful. I have seldom seen the second dose fail to remove the colic, leaving the bowels at worst in a state of constipation. Dr. Alderson of Hull, who has had many opportunities of treating the workmen of a white-lead manufactory there, says powerful purgatives, such as croton-oil, are highly serviceable in severe cases, and are borne well notwithstanding the extreme debility often present.‡ M. Tanquerel says he has found this treatment more effectual in Paris than any

* Trans. of Lond. Coll. Phys. i. 317.   † Annales d'Hygiène-Publique, **xxviii**. 234.
‡ London Med. Chir. Transactions, 1839, xxii. 87.

40*

other means.* When the pulse is full and strong, I have seen venesection premised with apparent advantage ; in some instances it
appeared to me to be called for by the flushing of the face and the
violence of the spasms ; and I have never seen it otherwise than a
safe remedy, notwithstanding the fears expressed by Dr. Warren and
others.†

The hospital of La Charité in Paris has long enjoyed a high reputation for the treatment of this disease. In the first place a decoction
is given of half an ounce of senna in a pound of water, mixed with
half an ounce of sulphate of magnesia and four ounces of the wine of
antimony. Next day an ounce of sulphate of magnesia and three
grains of tartar-emetic are administered in two pounds of infusion of
cassia, to keep up the operation of the first laxative. In the evening
a clyster is given, containing twelve ounces of wine and half as much
oil. After this the patient is made to vomit with tartar-emetic, then
drenched with *ptisanes* for several days, and the treatment is wound
up with another dose of the first purgative succeeded by gentle anodynes. I am not aware of any particular advantage possessed by
this complicated and tormenting method of cure, which is not equally
possessed by the simpler plan pursued in Britain.

In 1831 M. Gendrin announced to the French Institute that he had
found sulphuric acid to be at once the most effectual remedy, and the
most certain preventive, for the injurious effects of lead ; and he has
subsequently spoken in strong terms of the utility of this treatment.‡
But the experience of others does not bear out his conclusions.§

Among the many other methods of cure that have been proposed
for the primary stage of this disease, salivation by mercury deserves
to be particularized. It appears to have been often used with success, the colic yielding as soon as ptyalism sets in.‖ If the case,
however, is severe, there is no time to lose in waiting for the action
of the mercury to commence.

The treatment in the advanced period of the disease, when palsy
is the chief symptom remaining, depends almost entirely on regimen.
The patient must for a time at least quit altogether his unlucky trade.
He should be allowed the most generous food he can digest. He
ought to take frequent gentle exercise in the open air, but never to
fatigue. The hands being the most severely injured of the affected
parts, and at the same time the most important to the workman, the
practitioner's attention should be directed peculiarly to the restoration
of their muscular power. This appears to be most easily brought
about by frictions, electricity, and regulated exercise, the hands
being also supported in the intervals by splints extending from the

* Traite des Maladies de Plomb, 1839, and Annales d'Hygiène Publique, 1842,
xxviii. 232.

† Trans. of London Coll. of Phys., ii. 83.

‡ Transactions Médicales, 1832, or, Annales d'Hygiène, 1841, xxv. 463, and xxvi.
543.

§ Annales d'Hygiène, xxv. 466.

‖ Clark, in Edin. Med. Comment. xi. 102. Berger, in Horn's Archiv für Mediz.
Erfahrung, xi. 344. London Med. and Phys. Journ. xxvi. 46.

elbows to the fingers. The dragging of the emaciated muscles by the weight of the dangling hands certainly seems to retard recovery. — Strychnia has also been repeatedly found of service in restoring muscular action. Tanquerel states that electricity and strychnia, but especially the latter, have appeared to him by far the most efficacious remedies both for muscular paralysis and for amaurosis. — In the head affections the best treatment consists in relying on nature and merely combating symptoms ; and blood-letting is of no use, however much it may seem to be indicated by the coma and convulsions.

When a person has been once attacked with colica pictonum, he is more easily attacked again. Hence if he is young enough, he should, if possible, change his profession for one in which he is not brought into proximity with lead. Few, however, have it in their power to do so. The prophylaxis, therefore, or mode of preventing the influence of the poison, becomes a subject of great importance ; and more particularly when we consider the vast number of workmen in different trades, whose safety it is intended to secure.

On this subject many useful instructions are laid down in the work of Mérat. He very properly sets out with insisting on the utmost regard being paid to cleanliness, — a point too much neglected by most artizans, and particularly by those to whom it is most necessary, the artizans who work with the metals. In proof of the importance of this rule, he observes he knew a potter, who contracted the lead colic early in life when he was accustomed to go about very dirty, but for thirty years after had not any return of it, in consequence simply of a scrupulous attention to cleanliness. In order to secure due cleanliness three points should be attended to. In the first place, the face and hands should be washed once a day at least, the mouth well rinsed, and the hair occasionally combed. Secondly, frequent bathing is of great consequence, both with a view to cleanliness and as a general tonic ; so that masters should provide their workmen with sufficient means and opportunities for practising it. Lastly, the working clothes should be made, not of woollen, but of strong, compact linen, should be changed and washed at least once and still better twice a week, and should be worn as little as possible out of the workshop. While at work a cap of some light impervious material should always be worn.

Next to cleanliness, the most important article of the prophylaxis relates to the means for preventing the food being impregnated with lead. For this end it is essential that the workmen never take their meals in the workshop, and that before eating they wash their lips and hands with soap and water, and brush out all particles of dirt from the nails. It is also of moment that they breakfast before going to work in the morning.

Derangements of the digestive organs should be watched with great care. If they appear to arise from the poison of lead, the individual should leave off work with the very first symptom, and take a laxative. Habitual constipation should be provided against.

The nature of the diet of the workmen is of some consequence. It should be as far as possible of a nutritive and digestible kind. Mérat condemns in strong terms the small tart wines generally used by the lower ranks of his countrymen. They constitute a very poor drink for all artizans; and are peculiarly ill adapted for those who work with lead, because, besides being at times themselves adulterated with that poison, they are also apt to disorder the bowels by their acidity. Beer is infinitely preferable. Various articles of diet have been recommended as tending to impede the operation of the poison. Hoffmann recommends brandy, the efficacy of which few workmen will dispute. There is some reason for believing that the free use of fat and fatty articles of food is a preservative. Dehaën was informed by the proprietor and the physician of a lead mine in Styria, that the work-people were once very liable to colic and palsy, but that, after being told by a quack doctor to eat a good deal of fat, especially at breakfast, they were exempt for three years.* Another fact of the kind was communicated to Sir George Baker by a physician at Osterhoüt, near Breda. The village contained a great number of potters, among whom he did not witness a single case of lead colic in the course of fifteen years; and he attributes their immunity to their having lived much on cheese, butter, bacon, and other fatty kinds of food.† Mr. Wilson says, in his account of the colic at Leadhills in Lanarkshire, that English workmen, who live much on fat meat, suffer less than Scotchmen, who do not.‡

Professor Liebig says that lead colic is unknown in all white-lead manufactories, where the workmen use as a beverage lemonade or sugar-water acidulated with sulphuric acid; and it was stated above that the same announcement has been made by Mr. Gendrin. This, however, is doubtful. The prophylactic effects of sulphuric acid have been denied in France by M. Tanquerel,§ and M. Grisolle;‖ the latter of whom in particular says that no advantage whatever was derived from it at the white-lead manufactory of Clichy near Paris.

Some have likewise proposed as an additional preservative, that the exposed parts of the body should be anointed with oily or fatty matters. But Mérat maintains with some reason, that the lead will be thereby enabled to penetrate the cuticle more easily by friction and pressure.

The observance of the preceding rules will depend of course in a great measure on the intelligence and docility of the workmen. It would appear that particular care should be taken in hot weather, statistical facts having shown that three times as many workmen are attacked in Paris during the month of January as in July.¶

Some other objects of much consequence are to be attained by the humanity and skill of the masters.

The workshop should be spacious, and both thoroughly and sys-

* Ratio Medendi, P. I. c. ix. de Variis.
† Trans. of London Coll. of Phys. ii. 457.
‡ Ed. Phys. and Lit. Ess. i. 521.
§ Annales d'Hygiène Publique, xxv. 466.
‖ Archives Gén de Médecine, xli. 136.
¶ Annales d'Hygiène Publique, xv. 22.

tematically ventilated, the external air being freely admitted when the weather will allow, and particular currents being established, by which floating particles are carried away in certain invariable and known courses. Miners and others who work at furnaces in which lead is smelted, fused, or oxidated, should be protected by a strong draught through the furnaces. According to Mr. Braid, wherever furnaces of such a construction were built at Leadhills, the colic disappeared ; while it continued to recur where the furnaces were of the old, low-chimneyed form. Manufacturers of litharge and red-lead used formerly to suffer much in consequence of the furnaces being so constructed as to compel them to inhale the fine dust of the oxides. In drawing the furnaces the hot material is raked out upon the floor, which is two or three feet below the aperture in the furnace ; and the finer particles are therefore driven up and diffused through the apartment. But this obvious danger is now completely averted by a subsidiary chimney, which rises in front of the drawing aperture, and through which a strong current of air is attracted from the apartment, the hot material on the ground performing the part of a fire.

In white-lead manufactories a very important and simple improvement has been effected of late in some places by abandoning the practice of dry-grinding. In all manufactories of the kind, the ultimate pulverizing of the white lead has been long performed under water. But in general the preparatory process of rolling, by which the carbonate is separated from the sheets of lead on which it is formed, continues to be executed dry. This is a very dangerous operation, because the workmen must inhale a great deal of the fine dust of the carbonate. In a white-lead manufactory which formerly existed at Portobello, the process was entirely performed under water or with damping ; and to this precaution in a great measure was imputed the improvement effected by the proprietor in the health of the workmen, and their superior immunity from disease over those of Hull and other places, where the same precaution was not taken at that time. The only operation latterly considered dangerous at the Portobello works was the emptying of the drying stove, and the packing of the white lead in barrels ; and the dust diffused in that process was kept down as much as possible by the floor being maintained constantly damp. By these precautions, by making the workmen wash their hands and faces before leaving the works for their meals, and by administering a brisk dose of castor oil on the first appearance of any complaint of the stomach or bowels, the manufacturer succeeded in extirpating colica pictonum entirely for several years. — This trade continues to be a very pernicious one in France ; for no fewer than 266 cases of colic were admitted into the Parisian hospitals in 1841 from the white-lead manufactories in and near the capital. Yet facts are not wanting there to prove that with proper care the disease may be all but extirpated. A French manufacturer, whose workmen at one time suffered severely, had no case of colic among them for nine years after breaking them in to the observance of due precautions.[*] Another says, from his

* Annales d'Hygiène Publique, xv. 36.

own experience and information obtained at other works, he is satisfied the risk is very much greater among the intemperate than among
sober workmen.*

CHAPTER XIX.

OF POISONING WITH BARYTA.

BARYTA and its salts, the last genus of the metallic irritants which
requires particular notice, are commonly arranged among earthy substances, but on account of their chemical and physiological properties, may be correctly considered in the present place. These poisons
are worthy of notice, because they are not only energetic, but likewise easily procured, so that they may be more extensively used,
when more generally known.

SECTION I. — *Of the Chemical Tests for the preparations of Baryta.*

Three compounds of this substance may be mentioned, the pure
earth or oxide, the muriate, or chloride of barium, and the carbonate. The pure earth, however, is so little seen, that it is unnecessary
to describe its chemical or physiological properties.

The *Carbonate of Baryta* is met with in two states. Sometimes it
is native, and then commonly occurs in radiated crystalline masses,
of different degrees of coarseness of fibre, nearly colourless, very
heavy, and effervescing with diluted muriatic acid. It is also sold
in the shops in the form of a fine powder of a white colour, prepared
artificially by precipitating a soluble salt of baryta with an alkaline
carbonate. It is best known by its colour, insolubility in water,
solubility with effervescence in muriatic acid, and the properties of
the resulting muriate of baryta.

The *Muriate of Baryta,* or chloride of barium, is the most common of the compounds of this earth, having been for some time used
in medicine for scrofulous and other constitutional disorders. It is
procured either by evaporating the solution of the carbonate in hydrochloric acid, or by decomposing a more common mineral, the sulphate, by means of charcoal aided by heat, dissolving in boiling
water the sulphuret so formed, and decomposing this sulphuret by
hydrochloric acid.

It is commonly met with in the shops irregularly crystallized in
tables. It has an acrid, irritating taste, is permanent in the air, and
dissolves in two parts and a half of temperate water.

The solution is distinguished from other substances by the following
chemical characters. From all other metallic poisons hitherto mentioned, it is easily distinguished by means of hydro-sulphuric acid,
which does not cause any change in barytic solutions. From the
alkaline and magnesian salts it is distinguished by the effects of the

* Annales d'Hygiène Publique, xix. 14.

alkaline sulphates, which have no visible action except on the barytic solution, and cause in it a heavy white precipitate, insoluble in nitric acid. From the chlorides of calcium and strontium, it is to be distinguished by evaporating the solution till it crystallizes. The crystals are known not to be chloride of calcium, because they are not deliquescent. The chloride of strontium (which resembles that of barium in many properties, but which must be carefully distinguished, as it is not poisonous), differs in the form of the crystals, which are delicate six-sided prisms, while those of the barytic salt are four-sided tables, often truncated on two opposite angles, sometimes on all four,— by its solubility in alcohol, which does not take up the chloride of barium,—and by its effect on the flame of alcohol, which it colours rose-red, while the barytic salts colour it yellow. The chloride of barium is known from other soluble barytic salts, by the action of nitrate of silver, which throws down a white precipitate.

Vegetable and animal fluids do not decompose the solution of chloride of barium, except by reason of the sulphates and carbonates which most of them contain in small quantities. But the action of its tests may be distinguished, although the salt has not undergone decomposition. In that case the most convenient method of analysis is to add a little nitric acid, which will dissolve any carbonate of baryta that may have been formed, — to filter and then throw down the whole baryta in the form of sulphate, by means of the sulphate of soda, — and to collect the precipitate, and calcine it with charcoal for half an hour in a platinum spoon or earthen crucible, according to the quantity. A sulphuret of baryta will thus be procured, which is to be dissolved out by boiling water, and decomposed after filtration by muriatic acid. A pure solution is thus easily obtained. Orfila has lately proposed a process more complex in its details, but the same in principle.*

Section II. — *Of the Action of the Salts of Baryta, and the Symptoms they excite in Man.*

The action of the barytic salts on the body is energetic. Like most metallic poisons, they seem to possess a twofold action, — one local and irritating, the other remote and indicated by narcotic symptoms. This narcotic action is more decided and invariable than in the instance of any of the metallic poisons hitherto noticed. Such at least is the result of the experiments of Sir B. Brodie,[†] which have since been amply confirmed by Professor Orfila[‡] and Professor Gmelin.[§] Orfila found that when the chloride was injected into the veins of a dog in the dose of five grains only, death ensued in six minutes, and was preceded by convulsions, at first partial, but afterwards affecting the whole body. Sir B. Brodie found the same effects follow in twenty minutes, when ten grains were applied to a

* Annales d'Hygiène-Publique. 1842, xxviii. 217.
† Philosophical Transactions, 1812, p. 218.   ‡ Toxicologie Gén. i. 208.
§ Versuche über die Wirkungen, &c.

wound in the back of a rabbit, — the convulsions being preceded by palsy, and ending in coma. Half an ounce when injected into the stomach excited the same symptoms in a cat, and proved fatal in sixty-five minutes, though the animal vomited. Schloepfer observed, that when a scruple, dissolved in two drachms of water, was injected into the windpipe of a rabbit, it fell down immediately, threw back its head, was convulsed in the fore-legs, and died in twelve minutes.* Gmelin observed in his experiments that it caused slight inflammation of the stomach, and strong symptoms of an action on the brain, spine, and voluntary muscles. He found the voluntary muscles destitute of contractility immediately after death; yet the heart continued to contract vigorously for some time, even without the application of any stimulus. From some experiments made on horses by Huzard and Biron, by order of the Société de Santé of Paris, it appears that the hydrochlorate, when given to these animals in the dose of two drachms daily, produced sudden death about the fifteenth day, without previous symptoms of any consequence.†   In the experiments now related, very little appearance of inflammation was found in the parts to which the poison was directly applied.   It is also worthy of remark that the heart does not seem to have been particularly affected ; and yet according to the recent researches of Mr. Blake, the barytic salts are the most powerful of all inorganic poisons in their action on the heart, when they are injected into the veins.   A quarter of a grain of the chloride appreciably depresses arterial action ; two grains completely arrest the heart's contractions in twelve seconds ; and when it is injected back into the aorta from the axillary artery, it causes at first some obstruction to the capillary circulation, but soon arrests the action of the heart, as when it is introduced into the veins.‡

The pure earth appears to produce nearly the same effects in an inferior dose.   When swallowed, the symptoms of local irritation are more violent ; but death ensues in a very short space of time, and is preceded by convulsions and insensibility.   The stomach after death is found of a reddish-black colour, and frequently with spots of extravasated blood in its villous coat.

The carbonate in a state of minute division is scarcely less active than the hydrochlorate, since it is dissolved by the acid juices of the stomach.   A drachm killed a dog in six hours ; vomiting, expressions of pain, and an approach to insensibility preceded death ; and marks of inflammation were found in the stomach.§   Pelletier made many experiments on the poisonous properties of the carbonate. Fifteen grains of the native carbonate killed one dog in eight hours, and another in fifteen.‖   Dr. Campbell found it to be a dangerous poison, even when applied externally.   Twelve grains introduced into a wound in the neck of a cat, excited on the third day languor, slow respiration, and feeble pulse ; towards evening the animal became affected with convulsions of the hind-legs and with dilated

* Diss. Inaug. de effectibus liquidorum ad vias aërif. applic. p. 30,
† Nicholson's Journal, First Series, i. 529.
‡ Ed. Med. and Surg. Journ., lvi. 114.
§ Orfila, Toxicol. Gén. i. 213.
‖ Observations sur la Strontiane.   Ann. de Chimie, xxi. 119.

pupils; and death followed not long afterwards.* This substance, before its real nature was known, used at one time to be employed in some parts of England as a variety of arsenic for poisoning rats.

The salts of baryta are absorbed in the course of their action. The chloride has been detected by Dr. Kramer both in the blood and urine by incineration with carbonate of potash, washing the ashes with weak solution of carbonate of potash, dissolving the residue in diluted nitric acid, and testing the solution for baryta.† Orfila has also obtained baryta, by his process alluded to above, in the liver, kidneys, and spleen of animals killed by the chloride.‡

The symptoms produced by the salts of baryta in man have seldom been particularly described. An instance is shortly noticed in the Journal of Science, where an ounce of the hydrochlorate was taken by mistake for Glauber's salt, and proved fatal. The patient immediately after swallowing it felt a sense of burning in the stomach ; vomiting, convulsions, headache, and deafness ensued ; and death took place within an hour.§ A similar case, fatal in two hours, has been related by Dr. Wach of Merseburg. A middle-aged woman who, though generally in good health, had suffered for a day or two from pains in the stomach, took one morning a solution of half an ounce of chloride of barium by mistake for sulphate of soda. She was soon seized with sickness, retching, convulsive twitches of the hands and feet, vomiting of clear mucus, great anxiety, restlessness, and loss of voice ; and she died under constant efforts to vomit, and violent convulsive movements, but with her faculties entire.‖

Unpleasant effects have been observed from too large doses of the chloride administered medicinally. A case is mentioned in the Medical Commentaries of a gentleman who was directed to take a solution as a stomachic, but swallowed one evening by accident so much as seventy or eighty drops. He had soon after profuse purging without tormina, then vomiting, and half an hour after swallowing the salt excessive muscular debility, amounting to absolute paraplegia of the limbs. This state lasted about twenty-four hours, and then gradually went off.¶ I have known violent vomiting, gripes, and diarrhœa produced in like manner by a quantity not much exceeding the usual medicinal doses.

Dr. Wilson of London has lately described a distinct case of poisoning with the carbonate. The quantity taken was half a tea-cupful ; but emetics were given, and operated before any symptoms showed themselves. In two hours the patient complained of dimness of sight, double vision, headache, tinnitus, and a sense of distension in the stomach, and subsequently of pains in the knees and cramps of the legs, with occasional vomiting and purging next day ; for some days afterwards the head symptoms continued, though more mildly,

* Diss. Inaug. de venenis Mineralibus, p. 31.
† Annales d'Hygiène Publique, 1842, xxix. 425.
‡ Ibidem, xxviii. 216. § Journal of Science, iv. 382.
‖ Henke's Zeitschrift für die Staatsarzneikunde, 1835, xxx. 1.
¶ Medical Commentaries, xix. 267.

and she was much subject to severe palpitations ; but she was in the way of recovery when the account of her case was published.* Mr. Parkes mentions that, according to information communicated to him by the proprietor of an estate in Lancashire, where carbonate of baryta abounds, many domestic animals on his estate died in consequence of licking the dust of the carbonate, and that it once proved fatal to two persons, a woman and her child, who took each about a drachm.† Dr. Johnstone says he once swallowed ten grains of this compound, without experiencing any bad effect.‡

Section III. — *Of the Morbid Appearances caused by the Salts of Baryta.*

In animals the mucous membrane of the stomach is usually found of a deep-red colour, unless death take place with great rapidity, in which case the alimentary canal is healthy. In all the animals, which in Dr. Campbell's experiments were killed by the application of the muriate to wounds, the brain and its membranes were much injected with blood ; and in one of them the appearances were precisely those of congestive apoplexy.

In Wach's case the stomach was dark brownish-red externally, and the small intestines brighter red. Internally the stomach presented uniform deep redness, with clots of blood, and bloody mucus scattered over it; and near the cardiac end there was a perforation, above half an inch in diameter within, and half as wide at the outside, and surrounded with swollen edges and extensive thickening of the villous coat. The small intestines were internally very red and lined with red mucus interspersed with clots of blood. The great intestines were extremely contracted. The lungs were gorged, the heart full of dark liquid blood, and the cerebral vessels distended. Chloride of barium was detected in the stomach and intestines. The perforation in this case was evidently an accidental concurrence.

Section IV. — *Of the Treatment.*

The treatment of this variety of poisoning consists chiefly in the speedy administration of some alkaline or earthy sulphate, such as the sulphate of soda or sulphate of magnesia. The poison is thus immediately converted into the insoluble sulphate of baryta, which is quite inert. Two drachms of muriate of baryta were injected by Orfila into the stomach of a dog, and eight minutes afterwards two drachms of sulphate of soda. The gullet was then secured by a ligature. At first efforts were made to vomit, and in an hour sulphate of baryta was discharged with the alvine evacuations. There was neither insensibility nor convulsions ; and the next morning the animal evidently suffered only from the ligature on the gullet. This fact not only proves the efficacy of the sulphate, but likewise shows

* London Medical Gazette, 1833-34, ii. 487.
† Parkes's Chemical Essays, ii. 219.   ‡ Essay on Poisons, p. 143.

that in the kinds of poisoning where diarrhœa occurs, the poison is very soon discharged, and ought therefore to be looked for in the evacuations from the bowels.*

A few observations may be here added on the effects of the salts of *strontia* on the animal frame.   These compounds bear a close resemblance to the salts of baryta, and the two earths were consequently long confounded together till Dr. Hope pointed out their distinctions.   One of the most striking differences is, that the salts of the strontia are very feebly poisonous.   Some experiments of this purport were made by M. Pelletier of Paris,† and by Blumenbach; but the most accurate researches are those of Professor Gmelin.   He found that ten grains of the chloride in solution had no effect when injected into the jugular vein of a dog, — that two drachms had no effect when introduced into the stomach of a rabbit, — that half an ounce was required to cause death in that way, — that two drachms of the carbonate had no effect, — and that two drachms of the nitrate, dissolved in six parts of water and given to a rabbit, merely caused increase of the frequency and hardness of the pulse and a brisk diarrhœa.‡   Mr. Blake also found that small doses of the salts of strontia have little effect when injected into the veins; but that forty grains arrest the action of the heart in fifteen seconds.§

CHAPTER XX.

The fourth order of the irritant poisons contains a great number of genera derived from the vegetable kingdom, and at one time commonly arranged in a class by themselves under the title of Acrid Poisons.   The order includes many plants of the natural families *Ranunculaceæ*, *Cucurbitaceæ*, and *Euphorbiaceæ*, and other plants scattered throughout the botanical system.   It likewise comprehends a second group consisting of some acrid poisons from the animal kingdom, namely, cantharides, poisonous fishes, poisonous serpents, and animal matters become poisonous by disease or putrefaction.

OF POISONING WITH THE VEGETABLE ACRIDS.

The vegetable acrids are the most characteristic poisons of this order.   They will not require many details, as they are seldom resorted to for criminal purposes, and their mode of action, their symptoms, and their morbid appearances are nearly the same in all.

We are chiefly indebted to Professor Orfila for our knowledge of their *mode of action*.   He has subjected them to two sets of experiments.   In the first place, he introduced the poison in various doses

---

* Toxicologie Gén. i. 216.
† Observations sur la Strontiane, Annales de Chimie, xxi. 119.
‡ Versuche über die Wirkungen, &c.   § Edin. Med. and Surg. Jour. lvi. 113.

into the stomach, sometimes tying the gullet, sometimes not : and, secondly, he applied the poison to the subcutaneous cellular tissue by thrusting it into a recent wound.

In the former way he found that, unless the gullet was tied, the animal soon discharged the poison by vomiting, and generally recovered ; but that, if the gullet was tied, death might be caused in no long time by moderate doses. The symptoms were seldom remarkable. Commonly efforts were made to vomit ; frequently diarrhœa followed ; then languor and listlessness ; sometimes, though not always, expressions of pain ; very rarely convulsions ; and death generally took place during the first day, often within three, six, or eight hours. The appearances in the dead body were redness over the whole mucous coat of the stomach, at times remarkably vivid, often barely perceptible, and occasionally attended with ulcers ; very often a similar state of the whole intestines, more especially of the rectum ; and in some instances a slight increase of density, with diminished crepitation, in patches of the lungs.

When the poison, on the other hand, was applied to a recent wound of the leg, the animal commonly whined more or less ; great languor soon followed ; and death took place on the first or second day, without convulsions or any other symptom of note. It was seldom that any morbid appearance could then be discovered in the bowels. But in every instance active inflammation was found in the wound, extending to the limb above it and even upwards on the trunk. Every part affected was gorged with blood and serum ; and an eschar was never formed. The appearances in short were precisely those of diffuse inflammation of the cellular tissue, when it proves fatal in its early stage.[*]

Since these poisons do not appear to act more energetically through a wound than through the stomach, it has been generally inferred that they do not enter the blood, and consequently that the local impression they produce is conveyed to distant organs through the nerves. This inference is correct in regard to such species of the vegetable acrids as act in small doses. But the validity of the conclusion may be questioned when the poison acts only in large doses, as in the case with many of those now under consideration. For they cannot be applied to a wound over a surface equal to that of the stomach, and may therefore be more slowly absorbed in the former than in the latter situation. And, in point of fact, a few plants of the present order have been found to act through the medium of absorption, as soon as chemistry discovered their active principles, and thus enabled the physiologist to get rid of fallacy by using the poison in small quantity. This principle has been proved to be in some plants a peculiar resin, in others a peculiar extractive matter, in others an oil, in others an alkaloid, and in others a neutral crystalline matter. But in all there exists some principle or other in which are concentrated the poisonous properties of the plant. Some of these principles appear to act through the medium of the blood.

* Toxicol. Gén. i. *passim.*

There is no doubt, however, but many plants of the present order, as well as their active principles, have a totally different and very peculiar action. They produce violent spreading inflammation of the subcutaneous cellular tissue, and acute inflammation of the stomach and intestines, without entering the blood; and death is the consequence of a sympathy of remote organs with the parts directly injured.

As to their forming a natural order of poisons, it is evident, that if a general view be taken of their properties, they are distinguished by obvious phenomena from the three orders hitherto noticed. But if their effects on man be alone taken into account, when of course their influence on the external surface of the body must be left out of view, nothing will be discovered to distinguish them from several of the metallic irritants.

The *symptoms* occasioned in man by the irritant poisons of the vegetable kingdom, are chiefly those indicating inflammation of the villous coat of the stomach and intestines. When taken in large doses, they excite vomiting soon after they are swallowed; by which means the patient's life is often saved. But sometimes, like the mineral poisons that possess emetic properties, the vegetable acrids present a singular uncertainty in this respect: they may be retained without much inconvenience for some length of time. If this should happen, or if the dose be less, in which case vomiting may not be produced at all, or if only part of a large dose be discharged at an early period by vomiting, — the other phenomena they give rise to are sometimes fully developed. The most conspicuous symptom then is diarrhœa, more or less profuse. The diarrhœa and vomiting are commonly attended by twisting pain of the belly, at first remittent, but gradually more constant, as the inflammation becomes more and more strongly marked. Tension, fulness and tenderness of the belly, are then not unfrequent. The stools may assume all the characters of the discharges in natural inflammation of the intestinal mucous membrane, but an additional character worthy of notice is the appearance of fragments of leaves or flowers belonging to the plant which has been swallowed. At the same time there is generally excessive weakness. Sometimes, too, giddiness and a tendency to delirium have been observed. But the latter symptoms are rare: if they occurred frequently, it would be necessary to transfer any poison which produced them to the class of narcotico-acrids.

The properties now mentioned have long ago attracted the attention of physicians, and led them to introduce many vegetable irritants into the materia medica. In fact they comprehended a great number of the most active, or, as they are technically called, drastic purgatives. Among others, elaterium, euphorbium, gamboge, colocynth, scammony, croton, jalap, savin, stavesacre, are of this description. The effect of most of them, however, is so violent and uncertain, that few are now much used except when combined with other milder laxatives.

The *morbid appearances* they leave in the dead body are the same with those noticed under the head of their mode of action, — more or less redness of the stomach, ulceration of its villous coat, redness of the intestines, and especially of the rectum and colon, which are often inflamed when the small intestines are not visibly affected.

In the following account of the particular poisons of this order, a very cursory view will be taken of their physical and chemical properties. A knowledge of these properties will be best acquired from any author on the materia medica ; and an account of them would be misplaced in a work which professes to describe only the leading objects of the medical jurist's attention.

A great number of genera might be arranged under the present head. But the following list comprehends all which require mention. *Euphorbia*, or spurge, the *ricinus*, or castor-oil tree, the *jatropha*, or cassava-plant, croton oil, *elaterium*, or squirting-cucumber, *colocynth*, or bitter-apple, *bryony*, or wild cucumber, *ranunculus*, or buttercup, *anemone*, *stavesacre*, *celandine*, *marsh-marigold*, *mezereon*, *spurgelaurel*, *savine*, *daffodil*, *jalap*, *manchineel*, *cuckow-pint*.

The first plants to be noticed belong to the natural order *Euphorbiaceæ*, namely, the euphorbia, ricinus, jatropha, and croton.

Of Poisoning with Euphorbium.

Euphorbium is the inspissated juice of various plants of the genus euphorbia or spurge, but is principally procured from the *E. officinarum*, a species that abounds in Northern Africa. It contains a variety of principles ; but its chief ingredient is a resin, in which its active properties reside. It has been analysed by Braconnot, Pelletier, Brandes,* and Drs. Buchner and Herberger. According to Brandes the resin forms above 44 per cent. of the crude drug, and is so very acrid, that the eyelid is inflamed by rubbing it with the finger which has touched the resin, even although it be subsequently washed with an alkali.† According to the most recent analysis, that of Drs. Buchner and Herberger, this resin is a compound substance, which consists of two resinous principles, one possessing in some degree the properties of an acid, and the other the properties of a base. The latter, which they have called euphorbin, is considered by them the true active principle of euphorbium.‡ It will be mentioned under the head of Jalap, that they have taken the same view of the nature of other resinous poisons.

Orfila found that a large dog was killed in twenty-six hours and a half by half an ounce of powder of euphorbium introduced into the stomach, and retained there by a ligature on the gullet.

The whole coats of the stomach, but especially the villous membrane, were of a deep-red or almost black colour ; the colon, and still more the rectum, were of a lively red internally, and their inner membrane was checkered with little ulcers. Two drachms of the powder thrust into a wound in the thigh, and secured by covering it

* Supplement to Dr. Duncan's Dispensatory, p. 53.
† Buchner's Repertorium für die Pharmacie, vi. 175.
‡ Ibidem, xxxvii. 203.

with the flaps of the incision, killed a dog in twenty-seven hours ; and death was preceded by no remarkable symptom except great languor. The wounded limb was found after death highly inflamed, and the redness and sanguinolent infiltration, which were alluded to in the general observations on the vegetable acrids, extended from the knee as high up the trunk as the fifth rib, — a striking proof of the rapidity with which this variety of inflammation diffuses itself.[*] Mr. Blake concludes from his experiments, that euphorbium, when injected in a state of solution in the jugular vein, acts by obstructing both the pulmonary and systemic capillaries, and so preventing the passage of the blood into the left side of the heart ; but that the heart is not primarily acted on.[†]

The most common symptoms occasioned in man by euphorbium are violent griping and purging, and excessive exhaustion ; but it appears probable that narcotic symptoms are also at times induced. A case of irritant poisoning with it has been related in the Philosophical Transactions ; but it is not a pure one, as a large quantity of camphor was taken at the same time. Much irritation was produced in the alimentary canal ; but by the prompt excitement of vomiting and the subsequent use of opium the patient soon recovered.[‡] Mr. Furnival has related a fatal case which arose from a farrier having given a man a teaspoonful by mistake for rhubarb. Burning heat in the throat and then in the stomach, vomiting, irregular hurried pulse, and cold perspiration were the leading symptoms ; and the person died in three days. Several gangrenous spots were found in the stomach, and its coats tore with the slightest touch.[§] The operation of this substance is so violent and uncertain, that it has long ceased to be employed inwardly in the regular practice of medicine, and has been even excluded from some modern Pharmacopœias. It is still used by farriers as an external application ; and in the Infirmary of this city I met with a fatal case of poisoning in the human subject, which was supposed to have been produced by a mixture containing it, and intended to cure horses of the grease. Pyl has related the proceedings in a prosecution against a man for putting powder of euphorbium into his maidservant's bed ; and from this narrative it appears, that, when applied to the sound skin, it causes violent heat, itching and smarting, succeeded by inflammation and blisters.[‖] Dr. Veitch denies that the powder has any such power ;[¶] but the effects described by Pyl correspond with popular belief.

Probably all the species of euphorbium possess the same properties as *E. officinarum*. Orfila found that the juice of the leaves of E. *cyparissias* and *lathyris* produces precisely the effects described above. Sproegel applied the juice of the latter to his face, and was attacked in consequence with an eruption like nettle-rash ; and he found that it caused warts and hair to drop out.[**] Vicat mentions analogous

---

[*] Toxicologie Gén. i. 710.   [†] Edin Med. and Surg. Journal, li. 341.
[‡] Phil. Trans. 1760, li. 662.   [§] Journal of Science, iii. 51.
[‖] Aufsätze und Beobachtungen, i. 79.
[¶] Edin. Med. and Surg Journal, xlix. 488.
[**] Toxicol. Gén. i. 712.

facts, and Lamotte notices the case of a patient who died in conse-quence of a clyster having been prepared with this species instead of the mercurialis.* The seeds and root of the *E. lathyris* or caper-spurge are used by the inhabitants of the northern Alps in the dose of fifteen grains as an emetic ; and very lately the oil of the seeds has been em-ployed in Italy as an active purgative, which in the dose of two or eight grains is said to possess all the efficacy of croton oil.† MM. Chevallier and Aubergier have also found the seeds of the E. *hybeua* and their expressed oil to be very energetic. The seeds yield 44 per cent. of oil, which in the dose of ten drops produces copious watery evacuations without pain, and resembles closely croton-oil in its effects.‡ The *E. esula* appears to be a very active species. Scopoli says that a woman who took thirty grains of the root died in half an hour, and that he once knew it cause fatal gangrene when imprudently applied to the skin of the belly.§ Withering observes that all the in-digenous species blister and ulcerate the skin, and that many of them are used by country people for these purposes.‖

I have no where seen any notice taken by authors of narcotic symp-toms as the effect of poisoning with euphorbium ; and indeed this substance has always been considered a pure irritant. I am in-formed, however, by the Messrs. Herring, wholesale druggists in London, that their workmen are subject to headache, giddiness and stupor, if they do not carefully avoid the dust thrown up while it is ground in the mill ; and that the men themselves are familiarly ac-quainted with this risk. An analogous fact has likewise been com-municated to me by Dr. Hood of this city, relative to the effects of the seeds of the *E. lathyris*. A child two years of age ate some of the seeds, and soon after vomited severely, which is the usual effect. Drowsiness, however, succeeded ; and after a few returns of vomit-ing, which were promoted by an emetic, deep sleep gradually came on, broken by convulsions, stertorous breathing and sighs. Sensi-bility was somewhat restored by blood-letting and the warm bath ; after which the tendency to sleep was interrupted by frequent agita-tion and exercise in the open air. The vomiting then recurred for a time ; but the child eventually got well.

Of Poisoning with the Seeds of the Castor-Oil Tree.

Castor-oil at present so extensively used as a mild and effectual laxative, is nevertheless derived from a plant hardly inferior in ac-tivity as a poison to that just considered. It is the expressed oil of the seeds of the *Ricinus communis* or Palma Christi. Much discus-sion has taken place as to the source of the acrid properties of this seed, some supposing that they reside in the embryo, others in the peri-sperm, others in the cotyledon, others in a principle formed from the oil

---

* Toxicol. Gén. i. 713.
† Archives Gén. de Méd. viii. 615.　　　‡ Journal de Chim. Méd. viii. 671.
§ Orfila, Toxicol. Gén. 714.
‖ Botanical Arrangement, ii. 501. Stokes's Edition.

by heat ; and the question is scarcely yet settled. It is certain, however, that, although castor oil owes its occasional acridity to changes effected by the heat to which it is sometimes exposed in the process of separation, nevertheless the cotyledons are in themselves acrid.*

Two or three of the seeds will operate as a violent cathartic. Bergius, as quoted by Orfila, says he knew a stout man who was attacked with profuse vomiting and purging after having masticated a single seed. Lanzoni met with an instance where three grains of the fresh seeds, taken by a young woman, caused so violent vomiting, hiccup, pain in the stomach, and faintness, that for some time her life was considered in great danger.† Mr. Alfred Taylor met with three cases of poisoning with castor-oil seeds. Two sisters, who took each from two to four seeds, suffered severely ; and a third, who took twenty, died in five days, with symptoms like those of malignant cholera.‡ Climate probably affects their activity ; for I have known a person eat without any effect several seeds ripened in the open air in this neighbourhood. Dogs vomit so easily that they may take thirty seeds without material inconvenience, if the gullet is not tied. But if the gullet is secured, a much less quantity will occasion death in six hours. They produce violent inflammation when applied to a wound.§

Of Poisoning with the Physic-nut.

The plants of the genus *Jatropha*, belonging to the same natural family, have all of them the same acrid properties as the castor-oil tree. The seeds of the *J. curcas*, the physic-nut of the West Indies, when applied in the form of powder to a wound, produce violent spreading inflammation of the subcutaneous cellular tissue ; and when introduced into the stomach they inflame that organ and the intestines.‖ Four seeds will act on man as a powerful cathartic.¶ I have known violent vomiting and purging occasioned by a few grains of the cake, left after expression of the fixed oil from the bruised seeds; and in some experiments performed a few years ago, I found that twelve or fifteen drops of the oil produced exactly the same effects as an ounce of castor-oil, though not with such certainty. In the last edition of this work some observations were made, on the authority of MM. Pelletier and Caventou, respecting the properties of a pure oil and a volatile acid, supposed by them to exist in the physic-nut ; but they analyzed the croton-seed by mistake for it.

Two other species have been also examined, but not with care, namely, the *Jatropha multifida*, and the *Jatropha* or *Janipha manihot*. It is probable that the seeds of both are acrid, and also the oil which may be extracted from them by pressure. But a much more interest-

* See on this subject Deyeux in Ann. de Chim. lxxiii. 106. Boutron-Charlard et Henri, in Journal de Pharmacie, x. 466. Bussy et Lecanu, ibid. xii. 481.

† Tractatus de Venenis in Opp. I. i. 308, quoted by Marx, die Lehre von den Giften, i. 128.

‡ Manual of Medical Jurisprudence, 224.

§ Toxicol. Gén. i. 706.   ‖ Ibidem, i. 715.

¶ Mr. Bennet in London Medical Gazette, ix. 7.

ing part of the latter species in a toxicological point of view is the root; the juice of which is a most energetic poison. The *Janipha manihot*, or cassava-plant, has two varieties, one of which produces a small, spindle-shaped, bland root, called, in the West Indies, sweet cassava, while the other has a much larger, bitter, poisonous root, called bitter cassava, and in universal use for obtaining the well-known amylaceous substance, tapioca. The juice of the bitter variety is watery, and so poisonous that, according to Dr. Clark of Dominica, negroes have been killed in an hour by drinking half a pint of it.* It has been commonly, but erroneously, arranged among acrid poisons. It really belongs to the narcotic class, for it occasions coma and convulsions. And we now know the cause of this extraordinary anomaly in the natural family to which the species belongs; because MM. Henry and Boutron ascertained that the juice imported into France, as well as what they expressed from fresh roots sent from the West Indies, contains hydrocyanic acid, produces in animals all the usual effects of that poison, and is rendered inert by such means as will remove the acid, — for example, by the addition of nitrate of silver.† I confirmed this singular discovery in 1838 by examination of some well-preserved juice from Demerara. It is easy to see how tapioca, which is obtained from the poisonous root by careful elutriation, becomes quite bland during the process.

Of Poisoning with Manchineel.

The *manchineel* [*Hippomane mancinella*], another plant of the same natural family, contains a milky juice, which is possessed of very acrid properties. Orfila and Ollivier have made some careful experiments with it on animals,‡ and M. Ricord has since added some observations on its effects on man.§ From the former it appears that two drachms of the juice applied to a wound in a dog will cause death in twenty-eight hours, by exciting diffuse cellular inflammation; and that half that quantity will prove fatal in nine hours when introduced into the stomach. From the observations of M. Ricord it follows that inflammation is excited wherever the juice is applied, even in the sound skin; but he denies the generally received notion, that similar effects ensue from sleeping under the branches of the tree, or receiving drops of moisture from the leaves. This notion, however, it is right to add, has been adopted by other recent authors. Descourtils, for example, states that it is dangerous to sleep under the tree; that drops of rain from the leaves will blister any part of the skin on which they fall; and that on these accounts the police of St. Domingo were in the practice of destroying the trees wherever they grew.‖ Other species of Hippomane are equally poisonous. The *H. biglandulosa* and *H. spinosa* are peculiarly so, especially the latter

* Med. Facts and Observations, vii. 293.
† Journal de Pharmacie, xxii. 118.
‡ Journ. de Chim. Méd. i. 343.   § Ibidem, i. 483.
‖ Flora Médicale des Antilles, iii. 14.

which is known to the negroes of St. Domingo by the name of Zombi apple, and is familiarly used by them as a potent poison.*

Of Poisoning with Croton.

The oil of the *Croton Tiglium* has been familiarly known for some years as a very powerful hydragogue cathartic in the dose of a few drops ; and therefore little doubt could exist that both the oil and the seed which yields it must be active irritant poisons in moderate doses. Accordingly it has been lately found by experiments in Germany that forty seeds will kill a horse in the course of seven hours ;† and Rumphius mentions that it was a common poison in his time at Amboyna among the natives. I have known most violent watery purging and great prostration caused by four drops of the expressed oil. A fatal case of poisoning with it occurred not long ago in France. A young man who swallowed two drachms and a half of the oil by mistake, instead of using it as an embrocation, was soon seized with tenderness of the belly, violent efforts to vomit, cold sweating, laborious respiration, blueness of the lips and fingers, and an almost imperceptible pulse, — then with profuse, involuntary discharges by stool, burning along the throat and gullet, and insensibility of the skin ; — and in four hours he expired. The villous coat of the stomach was soft, but not otherwise injured.‡

The activity of the seed and oil seems to depend on a peculiar volatile acid, which was discovered by MM. Pelletier and Caventou when they analysed the croton seed by mistake as the seed of the *Jatropha curcas*, or physic-nut. When the oil was saponified by potash and then freed of the acid by distillation, it became inert. On the other hand, the acid was found by them to excite inflammation of the stomach, and spreading inflammation of the cellular tissue, according as it was administered internally or applied to a wound.§

The next natural family in which plants are to be found that possess the properties of the acrid poisons, is the *Cucurbitaceæ*, or gourds. This family, it should be remarked, does not in general possess poisonous properties. On the contrary, they are, with a few exceptions, remarkably mild ; and many of them supply articles of luxury for the table. The melon, gourd, and cucumber belong to the order. The only poisons of the order which have been examined with any care are elaterium, bryony, and colocynth.

Of Poisoning with Bryony.

The roots of the *Bryonia alba* and *Dioica* possesses properties essentially the same with those of euphorbium. The *B. dioica* is a native of Britain, where it grows among hedges, and is usually known by

* Flore Médicale des Antilles, ñi. 27.

† Landsberg. Therapeutische und Toxikologische Würdigung der Grana Tiglii. Horn's Archiv für Medizinische Erfahrung, 1831, 565.

‡ Journal de Chim. Médicale, 1839, 509.

§ Journal de Pharmacie, iv. 289.

the name of wild vine, or bryony.   The flowers are greenish, and are succeeded by small, red berries.   The root, which is the most active part of the plant, is spindle-shaped, and varies in size from that of a man's thigh to that of a radish.

Orfila found that half an ounce of the root introduced into the stomach of a dog, killed it in twenty-four hours, when the gullet was tied ; and that two drachms and a half applied to a wound brought on violent inflammation and suppuration of the part, ending fatally in sixty hours.*

Bryony root owes its power to an extractive matter discovered in it by Brandes and Firnhaber, to which the name of Bryonine has been given.   According to the experiments of Collard de Martigny, bryonine acts on the stomach and on a wound exactly as the root itself, but more energetically.   When introduced into the cavity of the pleura it causes rapid death by true pleurisy, ending in the effusion of fibrin.†

Before bryony-root was expelled from medical practice, it was often known to produce violent vomiting, tormina, profuse watery evacuations, and fainting.   Pyl mentions a fatal case of poisoning with it, which happened at Cambray in France.   The subject was a man who took two glasses of an infusion of the root to cure ague, and was soon after seized with violent tormina and purging, which nothing could arrest, and which soon terminated fatally.‡   Orfila quotes a similar case from the Gazette de Santé, which proved fatal within four hours, in consequence of a strong decoction of an ounce of the root having been administered, partly by the mouth and partly in a clyster, to repel the secretion of milk.§

Of Poisoning with Colocynth.

Colocynth, or bitter-apple, is another very active and more common acrid derived from a plant of the same family, the Cucumis colocynthis.   It is imported into this country in the form of a roundish, dry, light fruit, as big as an orange, of a yellowish-white colour, and excessively bitter taste.   Its active principle is probably a resinoid matter discovered by Vauquelin, which is very soluble in alcohol and sparingly so in water, but which imparts even to the latter an intensely bitter taste.‖   It is termed Colocynthin.

According to the experiments of Orfila, colocynth powder or its decoction produces the usual effects of the acrid vegetables on the stomach and on the subcutaneous cellular tissue.   Three drachms proved fatal in fifteen hours to a dog through the former channel when the gullet was tied, and two drachms killed another when applied to a wound.¶

A considerable number of severe cases of poisoning with this sub-

* Toxicol. Gén. i. 679.   † Nouv. Bibliothèque Medicale, Mai, 1827, p. 221.
‡ Neues Magazin, i. 3, p. 557.   § Toxicol. Gén. i. 680.
‖ Journal de Pharmacie, x. 416.   ¶ Toxicol. Gén. i. 691.

stance have occurred in the human subject; and a few have proved fatal. Tulpius notices the case of a man who was nearly carried off by profuse, bloody diarrhœa, in consequence of taking a decoction of three colocynth apples.* Orfila relates that of a rag-picker, who, attempting to cure himself of a gonorrhœa by taking three ounces of colocynth, was seized with vomiting, acute pain in the stomach, profuse diarrhœa, dimness of sight, and slight delirium ; but he recovered under the use of diluents and local blood-letting.† In 1823 a coroner's inquest was held at London on the body of a woman who died in twenty-four hours, with incessant vomiting and purging, in consequence of having swallowed by mistake a teaspoonful and a half of colocynth powder.‡ M. Carron d'Annecy has communicated to Orfila the details of an instructive case, which also proved fatal. The subject was a locksmith, who took from a quack two glasses of decoction of colocynth to cure hemorrhoids, and was soon after attacked with colic, purging, heat in the belly, and dryness of the throat. Afterwards the belly became tense and excessively tender, and the stools were suppressed altogether. Next morning he nad also retention of urine, retraction of the testicles and priapism. On the third day the retention ceased, but the other symptoms continued, and the skin became covered with clammy sweat, which preceded his death only a few hours. The intestines were red, studded with black spots, and matted together by fibrinous matter; the usual fluid of peritonitis was effused into the belly; the villous coat of the stomach was here and there ulcerated ; and the liver, kidneys, and bladder also exhibited traces of inflammation.§

Of Poisoning with Elaterium.

Elaterium, which is procured from a third plant of the cucurbitaceæ, the *Momordica elaterium* or squirting cucumber, possesses precisely the same properties with the two preceding substances. It appears, however, to be more active ; for a single grain has been known to act violently on man. There can be no doubt that small doses will prove fatal ; but its strength and consequently its effects are uncertain. British elaterium, which is the feculence that subsides in the juice of the fruit, is the most powerful ; French elaterium, which is the extract of the same juice, is much weaker ; and a still weaker preparation sometimes made is an extract of the juice of the whole plant. The plant itself is probably poisonous. But the only case in point with which I am acquainted is a singular instance of poisoning, apparently produced in consequence of the plant having been carried for some time betwixt the hat and head. A medical gentleman in Paris, after carrying a specimen to his lodgings in his hat, was seized in half an hour with acute pain and sense of tightness in the head, succeeded by colic pains, fixed pain in the stomach,

* Observat. Medicinales, iv. c. 27, p. 218.
† Toxicol. Gén. i. 695.   ‡ London Courier, Sept. 9, 1823.
§ Toxicol. Gén. i. 695.

42

frequent watery purging, bilious vomiting, and some fever. These symptoms continued upwards of twelve hours.*

The active properties of this substance reside in a peculiar crystalline principle, discovered by Mr. Morries-Stirling, and named by him *Elaterine.* It is procured by evaporating the alcoholic infusion of elaterium to the consistence of thin oil, and throwing it into boiling distilled water ; upon which a white crystalline precipitate is formed, and more falls down as the water cools. This precipitate when purified by a second solution in alcohol and precipitation by water, is pure elaterine. In mass it has a silky appearance. The crystals are microscopic rhombic prisms, striated on the sides. It is intensely bitter. It does not dissolve in the alkalis, or in water, is sparingly soluble in diluted acids, but easily soluble in alcohol, ether, and fixed oil. It has not any alkaline reaction on litmus.—It is a poison of very great activity. A tenth of a grain, as I have myself witnessed, will sometimes cause purging in man ; and a fifth of a grain in two doses, administered at an interval of twenty-four hours to a rabbit, killed it seventeen hours after the second dose. The best British elaterium contains 26 per cent. of it, the worst 15 per cent.; but French elaterium does not contain above 5 or 6 per cent.† These facts account for the great irregularity in the effects of this drug as a cathartic. The principle discovered by Mr. Morries-Stirling was also discovered about the same time by Mr. Hennell‡ of London.

Of Poisoning with the Ranunculaceæ.

The natural family of the Ranunculaceæ abounds in acrid poisons. Indeed few of the genera included in it are without more or less acrid property.

The genus *Ranunculus* is of some interest to the British toxicologist, because many species grow in this country, and unpleasant accidents have been occasioned by them. The most common are the *R. bulbosus, acris, sceleratus, Flammula, Lingua, aquatilis, repens, Ficaria,* which are all abundant in the neighbourhood of this city. The *Ranunculus acris* is the only species that has been particularly examined. Five ounces of juice, extracted by triturating the leaves with two ounces of water, killed a stout dog in twelve hours when taken internally. Two drachms of the aqueous extract applied to a wound killed another in twelve hours by inducing the usual inflammation.‡

Krapf, as quoted in Orfila's Toxicology, found by experiments on himself, that two drops of the expressed juice of the *Ranunculus acris* produced burning pain and spasms in the gullet and griping in the lower belly. A single flower had the same effect. When he chewed the thickest and most succulent of the leaves, the salivary glands were strongly stimulated, his tongue was excoriated and

* Annales d'Hygiène Publique et de Méd. Lég. viii. 333.
† Edin. Med. and Surg. Journal, xxxv. 339.
‡ Journal of the Royal Institution, i. 532.   § Toxicol. Gén. i. 754.

cracked, his teeth smarted, and his gums became tender and bloody.[*]
Dr. Withering alleges that it will blister the skin. A man at Bevay
in the north of France, after swallowing by mistake a glassful of the
juice which had been kept for some time as a remedy for vermin on
the head, was seized in four hours with violent vomiting and colic,
and expired in two days.[†] The acridity of the genus ranunculus is
entirely lost by drying, either with or without artificial heat. The *R.
acris*, however, is far from being the most active species of the genus.
The taste of the leaves of *R. bulbosus, alpestris, gramineus*, and
Flammula. and also of the unripe germens of *R. sceleratus*, is much
more pungent. The *R. repens, Ficaria, auricomus, aquatilis*, and
Lingua, I have found to be bland.

The genus *Anemone* produces similar effects on the animal economy.
The most pungent species I have examined are the *A. pulsatilla, A.
hortensis*, and *A. coronaria ;* the *A. nemorosa* and *A. patens* are less
active ; and the *A. hepatica*, as well as the *A. alpestris*, are bland.
The powder of the *A. pulsatilla* causes itching of the eyes, colic and
vomiting, if in pulverizing it the operator do not avoid the fine dust
which is driven up ; and Bulliard relates the case of a man who, in
applying the bruised root to his calf for rheumatism, was attacked
with inflammation and gangrene of the whole leg.[‡] The same
author mentions an instance where violent convulsions were produced
by an infusion of the *A. nemorosa*, and the person was for some time
thought to be in great danger.[§] The acridity of the anemone is retained under desiccation even in the vapour-bath ; but is very
slowly lost under exposure to the air, not entirely, however, in two
months. The ripe fruit of the *A. hortensis* is bland. The activity
of the anemones is owing to a volatile oil, which, when left for some
time in the water with which it passes over in distillation is converted
into a neutral crystalline body called anemonine, and a peculiar acid
termed anemonic acid.[‖]

The *Caltha palustris*, or marsh marigold, a plant closely allied in
external characters to the ranunculus, is considered by toxicologists
a powerful acrid poison. Wibmer observes that it has an acrid,
burning taste,[¶]—a remark which has been also made by Haller.[**]
On the continent the flower buds are said to be sometimes pickled
and used for capers on account of their pungency. The following
set of cases which happened in 1817 near Solingen will show that in
some localities it possesses energetic and singular properties. The
poison was taken accidentally by a family of five persons, in consequence of their having been compelled by the badness of the times
to try to make food of various herbs. They were all seized half an
hour after eating with sickness, pain in the abdomen, vomiting, headache, and ringing in the ears, afterwards with dysuria and diarrhœa,
next day with œdema of the whole body, particularly of the face, and

---

[*] Toxicologie Gén. i. 754.   [†] Journal de Chimie Médicale, 1836, 273.
[‡] Histoire des Plantes Vénéneuses de la France, p. 178.   [§] Ibidem, 180.
[‖] Buchner's Repertorium für die Pharmacie, lxviii. 346.
[¶] Die Wirkung der Arzneimittel und Gifte, i. 17.
[**] Historia Stirpium Helvet.

on the third day with an eruption of pemphigous vesicles as large as almonds, which dried up in forty-eight hours. They all recovered.*

Notwithstanding these apparently pointed facts, however, I have no doubt that the marsh marigold is in some circumstances bland, and is commonly so in this country, or at least but feebly poisonous. Haller, in speaking of its acrid taste, adds that when young it is eaten with safety by goats. For my own part I have never been able to remark any distinct acridity in tasting it either before inflorescence, or in the young flower-buds, or in any part of the plant while in full flower. It produces a peculiar, disagreeable impression on the back of the tongue, when collected in dry situations; but never occasions that pungent acridity which so remarkably characterizes many species of ranunculus, anemone, and clematis.

The *stavesacre*, or *Delphinium staphysagria*, another plant of the same natural family, is interesting in a scientific point of view, because its properties have been distinctly traced to a peculiar alkaloid. The seeds, which alone have been hitherto examined, were analyzed by MM. Lassaigne and Feneulle, who, besides a number of inert principles, discovered in them an alkaloid, possessing in an eminent degree the poisonous qualities of the seeds. This alkaloid is solid, white, pulverulent but crystalline, fusible like wax, very bitter and acrid, almost insoluble in water, very soluble in ether and alcohol, and capable of forming salts with most of the acids.† It has been named *delphinia*. It was also discovered about the same time by Brandes.‡

Orfila found that six grains of it diffused through water, introduced into the stomach of a dog and retained there with a ligature on the gullet, brought on efforts to vomit, restlessness, giddiness, immobility, slight convulsions, and death in two or three hours. The same quantity, if previously dissolved in vinegar, will cause death in forty minutes. In the former case, but not in the latter, the inner coat of the stomach is found to be generally red.§

An ounce of the bruised seeds themselves killed a dog in fifty-four hours when introduced into the stomach, and two drachms applied to a wound in the thigh killed another in two days. In the former animal a part of the stomach was crimson-red; in the latter there was extensive subcutaneous inflammation reaching as high as the fourth rib.‖

Besides these four genera of the ranunculaceæ many other genera of the same natural order are equally energetic. The *Clematis vitalba* or traveller's-joy is said to be acrid, but does not taste so: the *C. flammula*, however, is pungently acrid to the taste; it reddens and blisters the skin; and when swallowed excites inflammation in the stomach. The *trollius* or globe flower is also considered acrid; and its root in appearance, smell, and taste, has been said to resemble

* Rust's Magazin für die Gesammte Heilkunde, xx. 451.
† Ann. de Chim. et de Phys xii. 358.
‡ Schweigger's Journal der Chimie, xxv. 369.
§ Toxicol. Gén. i. 739.   ‖ Ibidem, 741.

closely that of the black hellebore. The herb, however, in Scotland, has certainly none of the peculiar acrid pungency of the ranunculus, anemone, or clematis, but is on the contrary bland. Some other genera of equal power have been usually arranged with the narcotico-acrid poisons on account of their action on the nervous system ; and probably some of the present group of acrids might with equal propriety be removed to the same class.

Of plants possessing acrid properties and interspersed throughout other natural families, the only species I shall particularly notice are the mezereon, cuckow-pint, gamboge, daffodil, jalap-plant, and savine.

Of Poisoning with Mezereon.

The *mezereon* and several other species of the genus Daphne to which it belongs are powerfully acrid. They belong to the natural order Thymeleæ. The active properties of the bark of mezereon have been traced to a very acrid resin ; and those of the allied species, *Daphne alpina,* to a volatile, acrid acid.*

The experiments of Orfila have been confined to a foreign species, the *D. Gnidium* or *garou* of the French. Three drachms of the powder of its bark retained in the stomach of a dog killed it in twelve hours ; and two drachms applied to a wound killed another in two days.† The action of the other species has not been so scientifically investigated ; but fatal accidents have arisen from them when taken by the human species. Children have been tempted to eat the berries of the *D. mezereon* by their singular beauty ; and some have died in consequence. Three such cases, not fatal, have been related by Dr. Grieve of Dumfries. Two of the children had violent vomiting and purging: in the third narcotic symptoms came on in five hours, namely, great drowsiness, dilatation of the pupils, extreme slowness of the pulse, retarded respiration, and freedom from pain.‡ Vicat relates the case of a man who took the wood of it for dropsy, and was attacked with profuse diarrhœa and obstinate vomiting, the last of which symptoms recurred occasionally for six weeks.§ A fatal case, in a child about eight years of age, occurred a few years ago in this city. Linnæus in his *Flora Suecica* says that six berries will kill a wolf, and that he once saw a girl die of excessive vomiting and hæmoptysis, in consequence of taking twelve of them to check an ague.|| The *D. laureola* or spurge-laurel, a common indigenous species, abounding in low woods, is said by Withering to be very acrid, especially its root.¶

Of Poisoning with Cuckow-pint.

The *Arum maculatum,* or cuckow-pint, one of our earliest spring

* Journal de Chim. Méd. v. 567.　　　　† Toxicol. Gén. i. 703.
‡ Lancet, 1837-38, i. 44.　　§ Hist. des Plantes Venen. de la Suisse, p. 140.
|| Flora Suecica, No. 338.
¶ Withering's Arrangement, i. 403, Stokes's Edition.

42*

flowers, not uncommon in moist ground, under the shelter of woods, is one of the most violent of all acrid vegetables inhabiting this country. I have known acute burning pain of the mouth and throat, pain of the stomach and vomiting, colic and some diarrhœa, occasioned by eating two leaves. The genus possesses the same properties in other climates, the several species being everywhere among the most potent acrid poisons in their respective regions. The *Arum seguinum*, or dumb cane of the West Indies, is so active that two drachms of the juice have been known to prove fatal in a few hours.* It is not a little remarkable that the acridity of the arum is lost not merely by drying, but likewise by distillation. I have observed that when the roots are distilled with a little water, neither the distilled water nor the residuum possesses acridity. Reinsch says he has eaten powder of arum root, which, though not acrid to the taste, produced severe burning of the throat not long after it was swallowed.†

Of Poisoning with Gamboge.

The familiar pigment and purgative *gamboge* is one of the pure acrids, and possesses considerable activity. It appears from the researches of Orfila,‡ some experiments by Schubarth,§ and various earlier inquiries quoted by Wibmer,‖ that two drachms will kill a sheep; that a drachm and a half will kill a dog if retained by a ligature on the gullet, while much larger doses have little effect without this precaution, as the poison is soon vomited; that an ounce has little effect on the horse; that eighteen grains will prove fatal to the rabbit within twenty-four hours; and that the symptoms are such as chiefly indicate an irritant action. Orfila farther found that it produces intense spreading inflammation when applied to a recent wound, and in this way may occasion death as quickly and with as great certainty as when administered internally.

Gamboge in its action on man is well known to be one of the most certain and active of the drastic cathartics, from three to seven grains being sufficient to cause copious watery diarrhœa, commonly with smart colic. Larger doses will induce hypercatharsis. A drachm has proved fatal, as is exemplified by a case in the German Ephemerides where the symptoms were excessive vomiting, purging, and faintness.¶

Under this head are probably to be arranged the repeated cases, which have lately occurred in this country, of fatal poisoning with a noted quack nostrum, Morison's pills. Almost every physician in extensive practice has met with cases of violent hypercatharsis occasioned by the incautious use of these pills; and three instances are now on record where death was clearly occasioned by them.** No

* Descourtils. Flora Médicale des Antilles, iii. 57.
† Buchner's Repertorium, lxviii. 90.　　‡ Toxicologie Gén. ii.
§ Horn's Archiv für Mediz. Erfahrung, 1824, i. 65.
‖ Die Wirkung der Arzneim. und Gifte, ii. 388.
¶ Acta Curios. Nat. Dec. 1. Ann. viii. p. 139.
** Trial of Webb. Lond. Med. Gaz. xiv. 612. Inquest on Rebecca Cross. Ibidem, 759. Case by Drs. Labatt and Stokes. Dublin Journ. of Med. and Chem. Science, iv. 237.

toxicologist will feel any surprise at such results, when he learns that one sort contains, besides aloes and colocynth, half a grain of gamboge, and another three times as much, in each pill; and that ten, fifteen, or even twenty pills are sometimes taken for a dose once or oftener in the course of the day.* The symptoms in the cases alluded to were sickness, vomiting and watery purging, pain, tension, fulness, tenderness, and heat in the abdomen, with cold extremities and sinking pulse; and in the dead body the appearances were great redness of the stomach with softening of its villous coat, in the intestines softening and slate-gray coloration of the same coat, and in one instance intestinal ulceration.

Gamboge is one of the poisons whose energy seems to be irregularly modified by the co-existence of certain constitutional states in disease. Physicians in Britain cannot but be startled to hear of the practice, prevailing among the followers of Rasori in Italy, of administering this purgative in doses of a drachm and upwards in inflammatory diseases. But it is nevertheless undeniable, that it has been given to that extent in such circumstances, with no further consequence than brisk purging. Professor Linoli mentions two cases of inflammatory dropsy, in which he gave gamboge-powder in gradually increasing doses, till he reached in one instance an entire drachm, and in the other 86 grains. In the course of a month one of his patients got 1044 grains, and the other took 850 grains in twelve days. Both recovered from their dropsy, and the purging was never great.†

Of Poisoning with Daffodil.

The common *daffodil*, the *Narcissus pseudo-narcissus* of botanists, though commonly arranged with the vegetable acrids, seems not entitled to a place among them. At least the experiments of Orfila rather tend to show that it acts through absorption on the nervous system. Four drachms of the aqueous extract of this plant secured in the stomach in the usual way killed a dog in less than twenty-four hours; and one drachm applied to a wound killed another in six hours. In both cases vomiting or efforts to vomit seemed the only symptom of note; and in both the stomach was found here and there cherry-red. The wound was not much inflamed.‡

Of Poisoning with Jalap.

Jalap, the powder of the root of the *Ipomœa purga*, and a common purgative, is an active poison in large doses; and this every one should know, as severe and even dangerous effects have followed its incautious use in the hands of the practical joker. Its active properties reside in a particular resinous principle. It contains a tenth of its weight of mixed resin, which, like the resin of euphorbium, has been separated by Drs. Buchner and Herberger into two, one pos-

* Analysis by Mr. West in the first of these cases.
† Annali Universali di Medicina, 1839, iii. 41.   ‡ Toxicol. Gén. i. 744.

sessing some of the properties of acids, the other some of the properties of bases ; and the latter they consider the active principle,
and have accordingly named Jalapine.* Mr. Hume of London some
time ago procured from the crude drug a powdery substance, to which
he gave the same name, and which he conceived to be the active
principle. His analysis has not been generally relied on by chemists ;
but it is not improbable that his principle differs little from that of the
German chemists.

The action of jalap has been examined scientifically by M. Felix
Cadet de Gassicourt, who found that it produced no particular symptom when injected into the jugular vein of a dog in the dose of
twenty-four grains, or when applied to the cellular tissue in the dose
of a drachm. But when rubbed daily into the skin of the belly and
thighs it excited in a few days severe dysentery ; when introduced
into the pleura it excited pleurisy, fatal in three days ; when introduced into the peritonæum it caused peritonitis and violent dysentery, fatal in six days ; and when introduced into the stomach or the
anus, the animals died of profuse purging in four or five days, and
the stomach and intestines were then found red and sometimes ulcerated. Two drachms administered by the mouth proved fatal.[†]
Scammony, which is procured from another species of the same
family, the *Convolvulus scammonea*, has been found by Orfila to be
much less active. Four drachms given to dogs produced only
diarrhœa.[‡]

Of Poisoning with Savin.

The leaves of the *Juniperus sabina*, or savin, have been long
known to be poisonous. They have a peculiar heavy, rather disagreeable odour, and a bitter, acrid, aromatic, somewhat resinous
taste. They yield an essential oil, which possesses all their qualities
in an eminent degree.

A dog was killed by six drachms of the powdered leaves confined
in the stomach. It appeared to suffer pain, died in sixteen hours,
and exhibited on dissection only trivial redness of the stomach.
Two drachms introduced into a wound of the thigh caused death after
the manner of the other vegetable acrids in two days ; and besides
inflammation of the limb there was found redness of the rectum.[§]

Savin is a good deal used in medicine for stimulating old ulcers
and keeping open blistered surfaces ; which may be done without
danger, although it cannot be applied to a fresh wound without risk
of diffuse inflammation. Both the powder and the essential oil are
of some consequence in a medico-legal point of view, as they have
been often used with the intent of procuring abortion. The oil is
generally believed by the vulgar to possess this property in a peculiar
degree. Doubts, however, may be entertained whether any such

---

* Repertorium für die Pharmacie, xxxvii.
† Dissertation Inaugurale, quoted in Orfila, Toxicol. Gén. i. 683.
‡ Tox. Gén. i. 758. The drug must have been much adulterated, as it very generally
is ; for half a scruple is an active purgative to man.
§ Orfila, Toxicol. Gén. i. 724.

property exists independently of its operation as a violent acrid on the bowels. It has certainly been taken to a considerable amount without the intended effect ; of which Foderé has noticed an unequivocal example. The woman took daily for twenty days no less than a hundred drops of the oil, yet carried her child to the full time.* The powder has likewise been taken to a large extent without avail. A female, whose case is noticed by Foderé, took without her knowledge so much of the powder that she was attacked with vomiting, hiccup, heat in the lower belly, and fever of a fortnight's duration ; nevertheless she was not delivered till the natural time.† There is no doubt, however, that if given in such quantity as to cause violent purging, abortion may ensue ; but unless there is naturally a predisposition to miscarriage, the constitutional injury and intestinal irritation required to induce it are so great, as to be always attended with extreme danger, independent of the uterine disorder. Of this train of effects the following case, for which I am indebted to Mr. Cockson of Macclesfield, is a good illustration. A female applied to a pedlar to supply her with the means of getting rid of her pregnancy : and under his direction appears to have taken a large quantity of a strong infusion of savin-leaves on a Friday morning and again next morning. A very imperfect account was obtained of the symptoms, as no medical man witnessed them ; but it was ascertained that she had violent pain in the belly and distressing strangury. On the Sunday afternoon she miscarried ; and on the ensuing Thursday she died. Mr. Cockson, who examined the body next day, found extensive peritonæal inflammation unequivocally indicated by the effusion of fibrinous flakes, — the uterus presenting all the signs of recent delivery, — the inside of the stomach of a red tint, checkered with patches of florid extravasation, — and its contents of a greenish colour, owing evidently to the presence of a vegetable powder, as was proved by separating and examining it with the microscope. My colleague Dr. Traill has communicated to me the particulars of a similar case. A servant-girl, after being for some time in low spirits, was seized with violent colic pains, frequent vomiting, straining at stool, tenderness of the belly, dysuria and general fever ; under which symptoms she died after several days of suffering. The stomach was inflamed, in parts black, and at the lower curvature perforated. The uterus with its appendages was very red, and contained a fine *membrana decidua*, but no ovum. The lower intestines were inflamed. There was found in the stomach a greenish powder, which, when washed and dried, had the taste of savin.

A singular case is quoted by Wibmer of a woman who died from taking an infusion of the herb for the purpose of procuring miscarriage, and in whom death seems to have been occasioned by the gall-bladder bursting in consequence of the violent fits of vomiting.‡

In a charge of wilful abortion the mere possession of oil of savin would be a suspicious circumstance, because the notion that it has

* Méd. Légale, iv. 430.   † Ibid. iv. 431
‡ Die Wirkung der Arzneimittel und Gifte, iii. 191.

the power of causing miscarriage is very general among the vulgar ; while it is scarcely employed by them for any useful purpose. The leaves in the form of infusion are in some parts of England a popular remedy for worms ; and the oil is used in regular medicine as an emmenagogue.

The following list includes all the other plants which have been either ascertained experimentally to belong to the present order, or are believed on good general evidence to possess the same or analogous properties.

By careful experiment Orfila has ascertained that the Gratiola officinalis, Rhus radicans and Rhus toxicodendron, Chelidonium majus and Sedum acre, possess them ; and the following species are also generally considered acrid, namely, Rhododendron chrysanthum and ferrugineum, Pedicularis palustris, Cyclamen Europæum, Plumbago Europæa, Pastinaca sativa, Lobelia syphilitica and longiflora, Hydrocotyle vulgaris. To these may be added the common elder or Sambucus nigra, the leaves and flowers of which caused in a boy, once a patient of mine, dangerous inflammation of the mucous membrane of the bowels lasting for eight days.

CHAPTER XXI.

OF POISONING WITH CANTHARIDES.

The second group of the present Order of poisons comprehends most of those derived from the animal kingdom. In action they resemble considerably the vegetable acrids, their most characteristic effect being local inflammation ; but several of them also induce symptoms of an injury of the nervous system.

This group includes cantharides, poisonous fishes, venomous serpents, and decayed or diseased animal matter.

The first of these is familiarly known as a poison even to the common people. I am not aware that it has ever been used for the purpose of committing murder. But on account of its powerful effect on the organs of generation it has often been given by way of joke, and sometimes taken for the purpose of procuring abortion. Fatal accidents have been the consequence.

The appearance of the fly is well known. When in powder, as generally seen, it has a grayish-green colour, mingled with brilliant green points. It has a nauseous odour and a very acrid burning taste. Alcohol dissolves its active principle. This principle appears from a careful analysis by M. Robiquet to be a white, crystalline, scaly substance, insoluble in water, but soluble in alcohol as well as in oils, and termed cantharidin.*

In compound mixtures cantharides may generally be detected by the green colour and metallic brilliancy even of its finest powder, if examined in the sunshine — and sometimes by making an etherial

* Annales de Chimie, lxxvi.

extract of the suspected matter, and producing with this extract the usual effects of a blister on a tender part of the arm. By these two tests Barruel discovered cantharides in chocolate cakes, part of which had been wickedly administered to various individuals.

From the late important researches of M. Poumet* it appears, that cantharides cannot be detected by its chemical properties in the contents, or on the inner surface, of the alimentary canal of animals poisoned with it; and that in such circumstances it is seldom to be discerned even by the shining green colour of its particles, unless the matter to be examined be dried. The method he recommends for a medico-legal investigation is to detach the stomach, small intestines, and great intestines, each separately from the body, — to wash out their contents with rectified spirit, and dry the pulpy fluid on sheets of glass, — to dry the stomach and intestines by distending them, removing their mesentery, and hanging them up vertically with a weight attached to stretch them, — and then to examine both the surface of the glass, and the inside of the stomach and intestines with the aid of sunshine or a bright artificial light. In this way cantharides may be detected, by the peculiar green hue of its powder, in most cases where this poison may have proved fatal; for M. Poumet constantly found it in dogs. The same author ascertained that the green particles generally abound most in the contents of the great intestine or on its inner membrane, next in the small intestines, and least of all in the stomach; and that they may be seen in the bodies of animals at least seven months after interment. Orfila had previously ascertained, that cantharides-powder may be recognized by its brilliancy in various organic mixtures after interment for nine months.† Poumet farther states that the green particles of cantharides may be confounded with the particles of other coleopterous insects, and also somewhat resemble particles of copper and tin. But he with reason asks, what possible accident could introduce the powder of any other coleopterous insect into the alimentary canal? And as to particles of copper or tin, he ascertained, that, unlike cantharides, these substances are visible in the contents, or on the tissues, of the stomach and intestines only before desiccation, and never after it.

SECTION I. — *Of the Action of Cantharides and the Symptoms it excites in Man.*

Cantharides, either in the form of powder, tincture, or oily solution, is an active poison both to man and animals. As to its action on animals, Orfila found that a drachm and a half of a strong oleaginous solution, injected into the jugular vein of a dog, killed it in four hours with symptoms of violent tetanus; that three drachms of the tincture with eight grains of powder suspended in it caused death in twenty-four hours, if retained in the stomach by a ligature

* Annales d'Hygiène Publique, xxviii. 347.
† Revue Medicale, 1828, ii. 475.

on the gullet, — insensibility being then the chief symptom; and that forty grains of the powder killed another dog in four hours and a half, although he was allowed to vomit. In all the instances in which it was administered by the stomach, that organ was found much inflamed after death; and generally fragments of the poison were discernible if it was given in the form of powder. When applied to a wound the powder excites surrounding inflammation; and a drachm will in this way prove fatal in thirty-two hours without any particular constitutional symptom except languor.* M. Poumet has since obtained results not materially different.

These experiments do not furnish any satisfactory proof of the absorption of the poison, but rather tend to show that it does not enter the blood. Such a conclusion, however, must not be too hastily drawn; since its well-known effects on man when used in the form of a blister lead to the conclusion that it is absorbed, and that it produces its peculiar effect on the urinary system through the medium of the circulation. On account of the magnitude of the dose required to produce severe effects on animals, Orfila's experiments on the stomach and external surface of the body cannot, for reasons formerly assigned [452] be properly compared together.

The effect of cantharides, when admitted directly into the blood, seems much less than might be expected. Mr. Blake found that an infusion of two drachms injected into the jugular vein of a dog, caused some difficulty of breathing, irregularity of the pulse, and diminished arterial pressure, but apparently no great inconvenience to the animal.† The greater effect observed in Orfila's experiment was probably owing to obstruction of the pulmonary capillaries by the oil.

Orfila has examined with care not only the preparations of cantharides already mentioned, but likewise the various principles procured by M. Robiquet during his analysis; and it appears to result, that the active properties of the fly reside partly in the crystalline principle, and partly in a volatile oil, which is the source of its nauseous odour.

The symptoms produced by cantharides in man are more remarkable than those observed in animals. A great number of cases are on record; but few have been minutely related. Sometimes it has been swallowed for the purpose of self-destruction, sometimes for procuring miscarriage. But most frequently, on account of a prevalent notion that it possesses aphrodisiac properties, it has been both voluntarily swallowed and secretly administered, to excite the venereal appetite. That it has this effect in many instances cannot be doubted. But the old stories, which have been the cause of its being so frequently used for the purpose, are many of them fabulous, and all exaggerated. Often no venereal appetite is excited, sometimes even no affection of the urinary or genital organs at all; and the kidneys and bladder may be powerfully affected without the genital organs participating. It is established, too, by frequent observation, that the excitement of the genital organs can never be induced, without other violent constitutional symptoms being also brought on, to the great hazard of life.

* Toxicol. Gen. ii. 4.   † Edin. Med. and Surg. Journal, li. 344.

The following abstract of a case by M. Biett of Paris gives a rational and unexaggerated account of the symptoms as they commonly appear. A young man, in consequence of a trick of his companions, took a drachm of the powder. Soon afterwards he was seized with a sense of burning in the throat and stomach ; and in about an hour with violent pain in the lower belly. When M. Biett saw him, his voice was feeble, breathing laborious, and pulse contracted ; and he had excessive thirst, but could not swallow any liquid without unutterable anguish. He was likewise affected with priapism. The pain then became more extensive and severe, tenesmus and strangury were added to the symptoms, and after violent efforts he succeeded in passing by the anus and urethra only a few drops of blood. By the use of oily injections into the anus and bladder, together with a variety of other remedies intended to allay the general irritation of the mucous membranes, he was considerably relieved before the second day ; but even then he continued to complain of great heat along the whole course of the alimentary canal, occasionally priapism, and difficult micturition. For some months he laboured under difculty of swallowing.* — Another case very similar in its circumstances has been related by M. Rouquayrol. In addition to the symptoms observed in Biett's patient there was much salivation, and towards the close of the second day a large cylindrical mass, apparently the inner membrane of the gullet, was discharged by vomiting.†
— A case of the same kind, but less severe, is related in the Medical Gazette. A woman, who had taken an ounce of the tincture, was observed throughout the day to be apparently intoxicated. Next morning, when she for the first time told what she had done, she had excruciating pain, great tenderness and distension of the belly, a flushed anxious countenance, a dry, pale tongue, a natural pulse, and urine loaded with sediment and fibrinous matter. In the evening there was extreme weakness, cold extremities, a scarcely perceptible pulse, and retention of urine ; and at night she was delirious. After this she recovered progressively, the chief symptoms then being pain in the kidneys and inability to pass urine.‡

Among the symptoms the affection of the throat, causing difficult deglutition and even an aversion to liquids, appears to be pretty constant. The sense of irritation along the gullet and in the stomach is also generally considerable. Sometimes it is attended with bloody vomiting, as in four cases related by Dr. Graaf of Langenburg ;§ and at other times, as in the instance of poisoning with the acids, there is vomiting of membranous flakes. These have been mistaken for the lining membrane of the alimentary canal, but are really in general a morbid secretion.‖ At the same time there is reason to believe that a portion of the membrane of the gullet was discharged

* Orfila, Toxicol. Gén. ii. 28.
† Annales de la Med. Physiologique, Octobre, 1829 — extracted in Edin. Med. and Surg. Journal, xxxiv. 214.
‡ London Medical Gazette, 1841-42, i. 63.
§ Hufeland's Journal der Praktischen Heilkunde, lii. 2, 112.
‖ See an interesting case in Memorie della Soc. Med. di Genova, ii. 1, p. 29.

43

in Rouquayrol's case ; for there were ramified vessels in it, and one so large that blood issued on pricking it. A prominent symptom in general is distressing strangury, and it commonly concurs with suppression of urine and the discharge of blood.* It would appear that, when the genital organs are much affected, the inflammation may run on to gangrene of the external parts. Ambrose Paré notices a fatal instance of the kind, which was caused by a young woman seasoning comfits for her lover with cantharides.†

The preceding symptoms are occasionally united with signs of an injury of the nervous system. Headache is common, and delirium is sometimes associated with it.‡ In a case communicated to Orfila the leading symptoms at first were strangury and bloody urine ; but these were soon followed by violent convulsions and occasional loss of recollection § The quantity in that instance was only eight grains : and it was taken for the purpose of self-destruction. In one of Graaf's four cases the patient was attacked during convalescence with violent phrensy of three days' continuance.‖ An instance is also related in the Transactions of the Turin Academy, of tetanic convulsions and hydrophobia appearing three days after a small overdose of the tincture of cantharides was taken, and continuing for several days with extreme violence.¶ The cause of the symptoms, however, is here doubtful.

A rare occurrence is relapse after apparent convalescence. In a case communicated to me by Dr. Osborne of Dundee, which there was every reason to believe had arisen from cantharides administered to a girl by an unprincipled scoundrel, the usual symptoms of violent irritation in the bladder and rectum prevailed for 36 hours ; and an interval of quiet and apparent convalescence ensued for three days. But on the fifth day the urinary symptoms returned, and were attended with great prostration, a rapid feeble pulse, and severe diarrhœa for two days longer. She eventually recovered. Another girl, poisoned at the same time, had most distressing irritation in the bladder, and for some time passed nothing but drops of blood ; but she got well in two days, and had no relapse.

The following fatal cases deserve particular mention. Orfila quotes one from the *Gazette de Santé* for May, 1819, which was caused by two doses of twenty-four grains taken with the interval of a day between them, for the purpose of suicide. The ordinary symptoms of irritation in the bowels and urinary organs ensued, miscarriage then took place, and the patient died on the fourth day, with dilated pupils and convulsive motions, but with unimpaired sensibility.** Another instance related by Dr. Ives of the United States, presented two stages, like that related by Orfila, but with the remarkable difference that an interval of several days intervened between the irri-

---

* Graaf's Cases, and Rouquayrol's.
† Lib. xxi. des Venins.
‡ See the case in Memorie della Soc. Med. di Genova, ii. 1, p. 29.
§ Toxicol. Gén. ii. 23.   ‖ Hufeland's Journal, lii. 2, 114.
¶ Mem. dell' Acad. de Torino, 1802-3.
** Toxicol. Gén. ii. 30.

tant and narcotic effects. A man swallowed an ounce of the tincture and was seized in a short time with hurried breathing, flushed face, redness of the eyes and lacrymation, convulsive twitches, pain in the stomach and bladder, suppression of urine and priapism ; in the evening delirium set in, and next morning there was loss of consciousness ; but from this time under the use of bloodletting, emetics, blisters, sinapisms, and castor-oil, he got well and continued so for fourteen days. But after that interval he was suddenly attacked with headache and shivering, then with convulsions, and subsequently with coma ; which, however, was removed for a time by outward counter-irritants. Next day the coma returned at intervals, and on the subsequent day the convulsions also, which gradually increased in severity for three days more, and then proved fatal.* In this case it admits of question whether the affection which proved the immediate cause of death really arose from the cantharides, or was an independent disease. — A third case, fatal on the fourth day, occurred in April, 1830, near Uxbridge in the south of England. I have not been able to learn the particulars exactly ; but it appears to have been produced by cantharides powder, which was mixed with beer by two scoundrels at a dancing party for the purpose of exciting the venereal appetite of the females. A large party of young men and women were in consequence taken severely ill ; and one girl died, who had been prevailed on to take the powder at the bottom of the vessel, on being assured that it was ginger.

The quantity of the powder or tincture requisite to prove fatal or dangerous has not been accurately settled. Indeed practitioners differ much even as to the proper medicinal doses. The smallest dose of the powder yet known was twenty-four grains (Orfila); and the smallest fatal dose of the tincture was one ounce, which is equivalent to six grains of powder.† It is probable that this is one of the poisons whose operation is liable to be materially affected by idiosyncrasy. The medicinal dose is from half a grain to two grains of the powder, and from ten drops to two drachms of the tincture. But Dr. Beck has quoted an instance where six ounces of the tincture were taken without injury.‡ On the other hand Werlhoff has mentioned the case of a lad who used to be attacked with erection and involuntary emission on merely smelling the powder.§ This statement, though extraordinary, is not without support from the parallel effects of other substances.

The familiar effects of cantharides on the external surface of the body are not unattended with danger, if extensive, or induced in particular states of the constitution. An ordinary blistered surface often ulcerates in febrile diseases ; and in the typhoid state which characterizes certain fevers, this ulceration has been known to pass on to fatal sloughing, especially when the blister has been applied to parts on which the body rests. I have met with two such cases. On the

---

* Medizinische-Chirurgische Zeitung, 1834, iv. 298, from American Journal of Medical Science.
† Taylor's Manual of Medical Jurisprudence, 228.
‡ Medical Jurisprudence, 574, from New York Med. and Phys. Journal.
§ Mem. della Soc. Med. di Genova, ii. 1, 29.

other hand if the blistered surface be very extensive, death may take place in the primary stage of the local affection, in consequence of the great constitutional disturbance excited. Thus in 1841 a girl, affected with scabies, received cantharides ointment by mistake instead of sulphur ointment from an hospital-serjeant at Windsor Barracks; and having anointed nearly her whole body with it, was seized with violent burning pain of the integuments, followed by vesication, general fever, and the usual symptoms of the action of this poison on the urinary organs. These effects were so severe that she died in five days.[*]

Section II. — *Of the Morbid Appearances caused by Cantharides.*

The only precise account I have hitherto seen of the morbid appearances caused by cantharides is contained in the history of the case from the *Gazette de Santé.* The brain was gorged with blood. The omentum, peritonæum, gullet, stomach, intestines, kidneys, ureters, and internal parts of generation were inflamed; and the mouth and tongue were stripped of their lining membrane. — In dogs Schubarth observed, besides the usual signs of inflammation in the alimentary canal, great redness of the tubular part of the kidneys, redness and extravasated patches on the inside of the bladder, and redness of the ureters as well as of the urethra.[†] M. Poumet denies that any morbid appearance is ever found in any part of the genito-urinary organs of animals; but he sometimes found blood effused into the stomach and intestines.[‡] In Dr. Ives's case the bloodvessels of the brain and cerebellum were gorged, the cerebellum spread over with lymph, the villous coat of the stomach softened and brittle, and the kidneys inflamed and presenting blood in their pelvis.

When the case has been rapid, the remains of the powder may be found in the stomach or intestines by Poumet's process. From the researches of Orfila and Lesueur, confirmed by those of Poumet, it appears not to undergo decomposition for a long time when mixed with decaying animal matters. After nine months' interment the resplendent green points continue brilliant.[§]

Section III. — *Of the Treatment of Poisoning with Cantharides.*

The treatment of poisoning with cantharides is not well established. No antitode has yet been discovered. At one time fixed oil was believed to be an excellent remedy. But the experiments of Robiquet on the active principle of the poison, and those of Orfila on the effects of its oleaginous solution, rather prove that oil is the reverse of an antidote. The case mentioned in the Genoa Memoirs was evidently exasperated by the use of oil. When the accident is discovered early

* Report of the Coroner's Inquest in Standard Newspaper, Jan. 1841.
† Archiv. für Medizinische Erfahrung, 1834, i. 61-64.
‡ Annales d'Hygiène Publique, xxviii. 383.
§ Revue Médicale, 1828, ii. 475.

enough, and vomiting has not already begun, emetics may be given ; and if vomiting has begun, it is to be encouraged. Oleaginous and demulcent injections into the bladder generally receive the strangury. The warm bath is a useful auxiliary. Leeches and bloodletting are required, according as the degree and stage of the inflammation may seem to indicate.

Many other insects besides the *Cantharis vesicatoria* possess similar acrid properties. Two of them, however, may be briefly alluded to, because they have caused fatal poisoning. The one is the *Meloë proscarabæus*, the *Maiwurm* of the Germans, a native of most European countries. In Rust's Magazin there is an account of four persons who took the powder of this insect from a quack for spasms in the stomach. The principal symptoms were stifling and vomiting ; and two of the people died within twenty-four hours.* The other is the *Bombyx*, of which at least two species are believed to possess powerful irritant properties, the *B. pityocarpa* and *B. processionea*. The following is an instance of their effects. A child ten years old had a common blister applied to the neck and spine as a remedy for deafness ; and four days afterwards her mother dressed the abraded skin with the leaves of beet-root, from which she had previously shaken a great number of caterpillars. The child soon complained of insupportable itching and burning in the part, and endeavoured to tear off the dressings. The mother persevered, however; and her child died in two days of gangrene of the whole integuments of the back. The surgeon who saw the child on the last day of her life, ascribed the gangrene to the insects mentioned above, and states that they possess the power of exciting erysipelas when applied even to the sound skin.† It is probable that many other insects in Europe have similar properties. The *Mylabris cichorii*, which is partially used in Italy,‡ and is in common use in India and China for blistering, possesses active irritant properties. The *Cantharis ruficollis*, another species used in the Nizam's Territories in India, is also energetic. Other species known to possess activity are *Mylabris fusselini*, *Meloe majalis*, *M. trianthemum*, *Coccinella bipunctata C. septem-punctata*, and *Cantharis vittata*.

CHAPTER XXII.

OF THE DELETERIOUS EFFECTS OF POISONOUS FISH.

The species of fish which act deleteriously, either always or in particular circumstances, have also been commonly arranged in the present order of poisons.

The subject of fish-poison is one of the most singular in the whole range of toxicology, and none is at present veiled in so great obscurity. It is well ascertained that some species of fish, particu-

* Magazin für die gesammte Heilkunde, xviii. 109.
† Journal Complémentaire, xviii. 184.   ‡ Cuvier, Règne Animal, v. 63.

larly in hot climates, are always poisonous, — that some, though generally salubrious and nutritive, such as the oyster and still more the muscle, will at times acquire properties which render them hurtful to all who eat them, — and that others, such as the shell-fish now mentioned, and even the richer sorts of verbetrated fishes, though actually eaten with perfect safety by mankind in general, are nevertheless poisonous, either at all times or only occasionally to particular individuals.   But hitherto the chemist and the physiologist have in vain attempted to discover the cause of their deleterious operation.

A good account of the poisonous fishes of the tropics has been given by Dr. Chisholm[*] and by Dr. Thomas ;[†] and some farther observations on the same subject have been published by Dr. Fergusson.[‡] These essays may be consulted with advantage.   On the effects of poisonous muscles several interesting notices and essays have been written, among which may be particularized one by Dr. Burrows[§] of London, another by Dr. Combe of Leith,[||] and the observations of Professor Orfila, including some cases from the Gazette de Santé, and from the private practice of Dr. Edwards.[¶]   Of all the sources of information now mentioned, that which appears to me the most comprehensive and precise, is the essay of Dr. Combe, who has collected many facts previously known, added others equal in number and importance to all the rest put together, and weighed with impartiality the various inferences which have been or may be drawn from them. The succeeding remarks will be confined to a succinct statement of what appears well established.

In this work, however, the poisonous fishes of the West Indies and other tropical countries may be laid aside, because we are still too little acquainted with the phenomena of their action to be entitled to investigate its cause, and they are objects of much less interest to the British medical jurist than the fish-poison of his own coast.

There is little doubt that some of the inhabitants of the sea on the coast of Britain are always poisonous.   Thus it is well known that some of the molluscous species irritate and inflame the skin wherever they touch it, — a fact which is familiar to every experienced swimmer.   The fishermen of the English coast are also aware that a small fish known by the name of Weever (*Trachinus vipera*, Cuv.) possesses the power of stinging with its dorsal fin so violently as to produce immediate numbness of the arm or leg, succeeded rapidly by considerable swelling and redness ; and indeed an instance of this accident, which happened at Portobello on the Firth of Forth, has been mentioned to me by Mr. Stark, author of the Elements of Natural History, who witnessed the effects of the poison.   But our knowledge of the poisons of that class is too imperfect to require more particular notice.

* Edin. Med. and Surg. Journal, iv. 393.
† Memoirs of the London Medical Society, v. 94.
‡ Edin. Philos. Journal. i 194.   § Lond. Med. Repository, iii. 445.
| Edin. Med. and Surg. Journal, xxix. 86.   ¶ Toxicol. Gén. ii. 37.

Of fishes which are commonly nutritive, but sometimes acquire poisonous properties, by far the most remarkable is the common *Muscle.* Opportunities have often occurred for observing its effects, — so often, indeed, that its occasional poisonous qualities have become an important topic of medical police, and in some parts, as in the neighbourhood of Edinburgh and Leith, it has of late been abandoned by many people as an article of food, although generally relished, and in most circumstances undoubtedly safe. This result originated in an accident at Leith in 1827, by which no fewer than thirty people were severely affected and two killed.

Of the Symptoms and Morbid Appearances caused by Poisonous Muscles.

The effects of poisonous muscles differ in different cases. Sometimes they have produced symptoms of local irritation only. Thus Foderé mentions the case of a sailor in Marseilles, who, in consequence of eating a large dish of them, died in two days, after suffering from vomiting, nausea, pain in the stomach, tenesmus, and quick contracted pulse. The stomach and intestines were found after death red and lined with an abundant tough mucus.* One of the cases described by Dr. Combe, which, however, terminated favourably, is of the same nature. The patient had severe stomach symptoms from the commencement, attended with cramps and ending in peritonitis, which required the frequent use of the lancet.

But much more commonly the local effects have been trifling, and the prominent symptoms have been almost entirely indirect and chiefly nervous. Two affections of this kind have been noticed. One is an eruptive disease resembling nettle-rash, and accompanied with violent asthma ; the other a comatose or paralytic disorder of a peculiar description.

Of the former affection several good examples have been recorded in different numbers of the Gazette de Santé.† In these the number of muscles eaten was generally small ; in one instance ten, in another only six. Nay, in a case related with several others by Möhring in the German Ephemerides, the patient only chewed one muscle and swallowed the fluid part, having spit out the muscle itself.‡ The symptoms have usually commenced between one and two hours after eating, and rapidly attained their greatest intensity. In the patient who was affected by ten muscles the first symptoms were like those of violent coryza ; swelling and itching of the eyelids, and general nettle-rash followed ; and the eruption afterwards gave place to symptoms of urgent asthma, which were removed by ether. In other cases the symptoms of asthma preceded the eruption. In one instance the eruption did not appear at all. The swelling has not

* Medecine Légale, iv. 85.

† 1er Mars, 1812 ; 1er Octobre, 1812 ; 21 Mars, 1813 ; Avril, 1813.

‡ De Mytilorum quorundam veneno, — Acta Physico-Medica Acad. — Cæsareo-Leopoldino-Carol. &c. 1744. Appendix, p. 124.

been always confined to the eyelids, but, on the contrary, has usually extended over the whole face. All the patients were quickly relieved by ether. The eruption, though generally called nettle-rash, is sometimes papular, sometimes vesicular, but always attended with tormenting heat and itchiness. Several cases of this kind have been related by Möhring. The eruption was preceded by dyspnœa, lividity of the face, insensibility, and convulsive movements of the extremities. All recovered under the use of emetics.* This affection, however, may prove fatal. In the cases of two children related by Dr. Burrows, the symptoms began, as in Möhring's cases, with dyspnœa, nettle-rash, and swelling of the face, combined with vomiting and colic ; but afterwards the leading symptoms were delirium, convulsions, and coma ; and death took place in three days.

In these children it is worthy of remark, that none of the symptoms began till twenty-four hours after eating. In Möhring's cases, on the contrary, the symptoms began in a few minutes.

The other affection is well exemplified in the correct delineations of Dr. Combe. The following is his general summary of the cases, which, with the exception of the instance of peritonitis already alluded to, were all singularly alike in their leading features.—" None, so far as I know, complained of any thing peculiar in the smell or taste of the animals, and none suffered immediately after taking them. In general, an hour or two elapsed, sometimes more ; and then the bad effects consisted rather in uneasy feelings and debility, than in any distress referable to the stomach. Some children suffered from eating only two or three ; and it will be remembered that Robertson, a young and healthy man, only took five or six. In two or three hours they complained of a slight tension at the stomach. One or two had cardialgia, nausea, and vomiting; but these were not general or lasting symptoms. They then complained of a prickly feeling in their hands; heat and constriction of the mouth and throat ; difficulty of swallowing and speaking freely ; numbness about the mouth, gradually extending to the arms, with great debility of the limbs. The degree of muscular debility varied a good deal, but was an invariable symptom. In some it merely prevented them from walking firmly, but in most of them it amounted to perfect inability to stand. While in bed they could move their limbs with tolerable freedom ; but on being raised to the perpendicular posture, they felt their limbs sink under them. Some complained of a bad coppery taste in the mouth, but in general this was an answer to what lawyers call a leading question. There was slight pain of the abdomen, increased on pressure, particularly in the region of the bladder, which suffered variously in its functions. In some the secretion of urine was suspended, in others it was free, but passed with pain and great effort. The action of the heart was feeble ; the breathing unaffected ; the face pale, expressive of much anxiety ; the surface rather cold ; the mental faculties unimpaired. Unluckily the two fatal cases were not seen by any medical person ; and we are therefore unable to state minutely the train of symptoms.

* De Mytilorum, &c. p. 115.

We ascertained that the woman, in whose house were five sufferers, went away as in a gentle sleep ; and that a few minutes before death, she had spoken and swallowed."* She died in three hours. The other fatal case was that of a dock-yard watchman, who was found dead in his box six or seven hours after he ate the muscles.

The inspection of the bodies threw no light on the nature of these singular effects. No appearance was found which could be called decidedly morbid. The stomach contained a considerable quantity of the fish half digested.

Dr. Combe's narrative agrees with that of Vancouver, four of whose sailors were violently affected, and one killed in five hours and a half, after eating muscles which they had gathered on shore in the course of his voyage of discovery.†

In closing this account, allusion may be briefly made to a case related by Dr. Edwards, which differs from all the preceding. The symptoms were uneasiness at stomach, followed by epileptic convulsions, which did not entirely cease for a fortnight. Dr. Edwards imputed the illness to muscles ; but it must be observed that this is a solitary instance of simple convulsions arising from such a cause.‡ The case deserves particular attention, because a suspicion of intentional poison might have been excited by the circumstances in which it occurred. The individual, a young man, was attacked soon after eating in company with another, who was about to marry his mother, and with whom on that account he lived on bad terms.

Of the Source of Poison of Muscles.

Various opinions have been formed as to the cause or causes of the poisonous qualities of some muscles.

The vulgar idea that the poisonous principle is copper, with which the fish becomes impregnated from the copper bottoms of vessels, is quite untenable. Copper does not cause the symptoms described above. I analyzed some of the muscles taken from the stomach of one of Dr. Combe's patients, without being able to detect a trace of copper. Others have arrived at the same result in former cases. The only instance indeed to the contrary is a late analysis by M. Bouchardat ; who does not mention the quantity of copper he detected, or what was the source of the poisonous fish.§

The theory which ascribes their effects to changes induced by decay is equally untenable. In Dr. Burrows's two cases the muscles appear to have been decayed ; yet he very properly refuses to admit this fact as explanatory of their operation. And, indeed, it rather complicates than facilitates the explanation ; as it shows that the poison differs from animal poison generally, in not being destroyed by putrefaction. Dr. Combe's inquiries must satisfy every one, that in the Leith cases decay was out of the question, and I may add my testimony to the statement: the muscles taken from the stomach of

* Edin Med. and Surg. Journal, xxix. 88.
† Voyage of Discovery, ii. 285.   ‡ Orfila, Toxic. Gén. ii. 44.
§ Annales d'Hygiène Publique, xvii. 360.

one of his fatal cases, and likewise others obtained in the shell, and brought to me for analysis, were perfectly fresh.

By some physicians, and especially by Dr. Edwards, their poisonous effects have been referred to idiosyncrasy on the part of the persons who suffer. It can hardly be doubted that this is the cause in some instances. It was formerly mentioned that muscles, oysters, crabs, and even the richer sorts of vertebrated fishes, such as trout, salmon, turbot, holibut, herring, mackerel, are not only injurious to some people, while salutary to mankind generally, but likewise that this singular idiosyncrasy may be acquired. A relation of mine for many years could not take a few mouthfuls of salmon, trout, herring, turbot, holibut, crab, or lobster, without being attacked in a few minutes or hours with violent vomiting; yet at an early period of life, he could eat them all with impunity; and at all times he has eaten without injury cod, ling, haddock, whiting, flounder, oysters, and muscles. Among the cases which have come under Dr. Edwards's notice in Paris, there is one evidently of the same nature. In two others, the idiosyncrasy existed in regard to the muscle, and although in both of these the affection induced was slight, there is no doubt but idiosyncrasy will also account even for some instances of the severe disorders specified above. In particular, it appears sometimes to operate in the production of nettle-rash and asthma; for in the instance quoted from the Gazette de Santé, as arising from ten muscles, it happened that the father of the patient partook very freely of the same dish without sustaining any harm whatever; and in each of three distinct accidents mentioned by Möhring, it appeared that other individuals had eaten of the same dish with equal impunity.*

But idiosyncrasy will not account for all the cases of poisoning with muscles, oysters, and other fish. For, passing over other less unequivocal objections, it appears that, when the accident related above happened at Leith, every person who ate the muscles from a particular spot was more or less severely affected; and an important circumstance then observed for the first time was, that animals suffered as severely as man, a cat and a dog having been killed by the suspected article.

Another theory ascribes the poisonous quality to disease in the fish; but no one has hitherto pointed out what the disease is. The poisonous muscles at Leith were large and plump, and seemed to have been chosen on account of their size and good look. Dr. Coldstream, however, at the time a pupil of this University, and a zealous naturalist, thought the liver was larger, darker, and more brittle than in the wholesome fish, and certainly satisfied me that there was a difference of the kind. But whether this was really disease or merely a variety of natural structure, our knowledge of the natural history of the fish hardly entitles us to pronounce.

Considering the failure of all other attempts to account for the injurious properties acquired by muscles, it is extraordinary that no experiments have been hitherto made with the view of discovering in the poisonous fish a peculiar animal principle. It certainly seems

* De Mytilorum, &c. p. 117, 121, 124.

probable, that the property resides in a particular part of the fish or in a particular principle. In 1827, 1 made some experiments on those which caused the fatal accident at Leith, but without success. My attention was turned particularly to the liver; but neither there nor in the other parts of the fish could I detect any principle which did not equally exist in the wholesome muscle. This result, however, should not deter others, any more than it would myself, from a fresh investigation; for the want of a sufficient supply prevented me from making a thorough analysis; and the reader will presently find an instance related, where another singular poison, sometimes contained in sausages and in cheese, was, after repeated failures, at length traced successfully to the real cause by the hand of the analytic chemist.

M. Lamouroux, in a letter to Professor Orfila, conjectures that the poison may be a particular species of Medusa, and enters into some ingenious explanations of his opinion. But it is not supported by any material fact, and seems to be surrounded by insuperable difficulties.[*] It is not a new conjecture; for Möhring mentions in his paper formerly quoted, that several writers before him had conceived such a cause might afford an explanation of the phenomena.[†]

Little or no light is thrown on this singular subject by the nature of the localities in which the poisonous muscle has been found. Even on this point we possess little information. Both in Dr. Burrows's and Dr. Combe's cases the fish was attached to wood. At Leith they were taken from some Memel fir logs, which formed the bar of one of the wet-docks, and had lain there at least fifteen years. From the stone-walls of the dock in the immediate vicinity of this bar muscles were taken which proved quite wholesome. It is impossible, however, to attach any importance to these facts; for Dr. Coldstream informs me, that he examined muscles which were attached to the fir piles of the Newhaven Chain-pier, about a mile from Leith, and found them wholesome. In the latter animals the liver was not large, as in the poisonous muscles of Leith. Lamouroux states, but I know not on what authority, that muscles never become poisonous unless they are exposed alternately to the air and the sea in their place of attachment, and unless the sea flows in gently over them without any surf, — these conditions being considered by him requisite for the introduction of the poisonous Medusæ into the shell.

Of Poisonous Oysters.

Oysters sometimes acquire deleterious properties analogous to those acquired by muscles. But fewer facts have been collected regarding them. M. Pasquier has mentioned some cases which occurred not long ago at Havre, in consequence apparently of an artificial oyster-bed having been established near the exit of the drain of a public necessary. But I have not been able to consult his work.[‡] Another

* Toxicol. Gén. ii 45. † De Mytilorum, &c. p 134.
‡ Journal de Pharmacie, v. 25, from Essai Médical sur les huitres.

instance of their deleterious operation occurred a few years ago at Dunkirk. At least an unusual prevalence of colic, diarrhœa, and cholera was believed to have been traced to an importation of unwholesome oysters from the Normandy coast. Dr. Zandyk, the physician who was appointed to investigate the matter, found that the suspected fish contained a slimy water, and that the membranes were retracted from the shell towards the body of the animal.* Dr. Clarke believes that even wholesome oysters have a tendency to act deleteriously on women immediately after delivery. He asserts that he has repeatedly found them to induce apoplexy or convulsions; that the symptoms generally came on the day after the oysters were taken; and that two cases of the kind proved fatal.† I am not aware that these statements have been since confirmed by any other observer.

Of Poisonous Eels.

Eels have also been at times found in temperate climates to acquire poisonous properties. Virey mentions an instance where several individuals were attacked with violent tormina and diarrhœa a few hours after eating a paté made of eels from a stagnant castle-ditch near Orleans; and in alluding to similar accidents having previously happened in various parts of France, he adds that domestic animals have been killed by eating the remains of the suspected dish.‡

CHAPTER XXIII.

OF POISONING BY VENOMOUS SNAKES.

Another entire group of poisons allied to the acrid vegetables in their action, but infinitely more energetic, comprehends the poisons of the venomous serpents. If we were to trust the impressions the vulgar entertain of the effects of the bite of serpents, the poisons now mentioned would be considered true septics or putrefiants; for they were once universally believed, and are still thought by many, to cause putrefaction of the living body. This property has been assigned them probably on no other grounds, except that they are apt to bring on diffuse subcutaneous inflammation, which frequently runs on to gangrene. But there are some serpents, especially among those of hot climates, which appear also to act remotely on the centre of the nervous system, and to occasion death through means of that action.

The present group of poisons is of little consequence to the British medical jurist, as an opportunity of witnessing their effects in this country is seldom to be found. The viper is the only poisonous

* London Med. Repository, xiii. 58.   † Trans. London Coll. of Phys. v. 109.
‡ Journal de Pharmacie, v. 509.

snake known in Britain, where its poison is hardly ever so active as to occasion death.*

This serpent, like all the other poisonous species, is provided with a peculiar apparatus by which the poison is secreted, preserved, and introduced into the body of the animal it attacks. The apparatus consists of a gland behind each eye, of a membranous sac at the lateral and anterior part of the upper jaw, and of a hollow curved tooth surrounded and supported by the sac. The cavity of the tooth communicates with that of the sac, and terminates near the tip, in a small aperture, by which the poison is expelled into the wound made by the tooth.

The symptoms caused by the bite of the viper are lancinating pain, which begins between three minutes and forty minutes after the bite, and rapidly stretches up the limbs, — swelling, at first firm and pale afterwards red, livid and hard, — tendency to fainting, bilious vomiting, sometimes convulsions, more rarely jaundice, — quick, small, irregular pulse, — difficult breathing, cold perspiration, dimness of vision, and injury of the mental faculties. Death may ensue. A case is related in Rust's Magazin of a child twelve years old, who died two days after being bitten in the foot ;† another instance is briefly noticed in the French Bulletins of Medicine, of a person forty years old, dying also in two days ;‡ Dr Wagner of Schlieben mentions his having met with two instances where persons bit on the toes died before assistance could be procured ;§ and notice has been taken in Hufeland's Journal of a girl, eleven years old, having been killed in three hours at Schlawe in Prussia.‖ In the last case burning in the foot, which was the part bitten, then severe pain in the belly, inextinguishable thirst, and vomiting, preceded a fit of laborious breathing, which ushered in death. The most remarkable instance, however, of death from the bite of the European viper is one lately described by Dr. Braun, as having been occasioned in the Dutchy of Gotha by the Coluber Chersea [Kreuzotter of the Germans]. A man, who represented himself to be a snake-charmer, insisted on showing his skill before Dr. Lenz, a naturalist of Schnepfenthal ; and putting the head of a viper belonging to this gentleman's collection into his mouth, he pretended to be about to devour it. Suddenly he threw the snake from him, and it was found that he had been bitten near the root of the tongue. In a few minutes he became so faint that he could not stand, the tongue swelled a little, the eyes became dim, saliva issued from the mouth, rattling respiration succeeded, and he died within fifty minutes after being bitten.¶ A French writer observes that the common viper of France is not very deadly ; but that the bite of the red viper may occasion death in a few hours.**

* For a severe case, not fatal, occurring in Kent, see London Medical Gazette, xii. 464.
† Magazin für die gesammte Heilkunde, xx. 155.
‡ Bulletins des Sciences Medicales, x. 92.   § Ibidem, xx. 195.
‖ Journal der Praktischen Heilkunde, 1829, ii. iv. 120.
¶ Rust's Magazin für die gesammte Heilkunde, xxxii. 361.
** Robineau-Devoidy in Archives Gén. de Méd. xxi. 626.

The activity of the poison of the viper depends on a variety of circumstances. When kept long confined, the animal loses its energy ;
and after it has bitten repeatedly in rapid succession, its bite ceases
for some time to be poisonous, as the supply of poison is exhausted.
It appears also to be most active in hot and dry climates. Those
cases are always the most severe in which the symptoms begin soonest ;
and the danger increases with the number of bites. An important
observation made by Dr. Wagner is that danger need not be dreaded
except when the bite is inflicted on small organs such as the fingers
or toes, because larger parts cannot be fully included between the
animal's jaws, and fairly pierced by its fangs, but can only be scratched. The properties of the fluid contained in the reservoir do not
cease with the animal's life ; nay they continue even when the fluid
is dried and preserved for a length of time. It may be swallowed in
considerable quantity without causing any injury whatever. In the
course of some experiments lately made in Italy, a pupil of Professor
Mangili swallowed at once the whole poison of four vipers without
suffering any inconvenience ; and that of six vipers was given to a
blackbird, that of ten to a pigeon, and that of sixteen to a raven, with
no other effect beyond slight and transient stupor.*

For the most recent account of the far more terrible effects of the
cobra di capello and rattlesnake, the reader may refer to the authorities below.†

It was stated above that the poison of the viper retains its activity
when dried. I have had an opportunity of observing this in regard
to the poison of the cobra di capello, which is said to be preserved
in India by simply squeezing out the contents of the poison-bag, and
drying the liquid in a silver dish exposed to the sun. The specimen
in my possession, for which I am indebted to Mr. Wardrop of London, has the appearance of small fragments of gum-arabic. It had
been kept for fifteen years when I tried its effects on a strong rabbit.
A grain and a half dissolved in ten drops of water, having been introduced between the skin and muscles of the back, the animal in
eight minutes became very feeble and averse to stir, so that it remained still even when placed in irksome postures ; occasional slight
twitches of the limbs supervened ; at length it became extremely
torpid, and breathed slowly by means of the abdominal muscles and
diaphragm alone ; and in twenty-seven minutes it died exhausted,
without any precursory insensibility. The heart contracted readily,
when irritated nine minutes after death ; so that the poison seemed
to operate by causing muscular paralysis, and consequently arresting
the respiration.

There might also be arranged in an appendix to the present group
of poisons those *insects* whose sting is poisonous. The European
insects known to have a poisonous sting, are chiefly the scorpion,
tarantula, bee and wasp ; of which the last two only are natives of
Britain.

* Giornale di Fisica, ix. 458, and Meckel's Archiv für Anat. und Physiol. iii. 639.
† Edin. Med. and Surg. Journal, xviii. ; Phil. Trans. 1810.

The poison of these insects occasions diffuse cellular inflammation, which always ends in resolution.   It is said, however,[*] and it may be readily believed, that death has been sometimes caused in consequence of a whole hive attacking an intruder and covering his body with their stings.   In an old French journal is shortly noticed the case of a peasant who died soon after being stung over the eye by a single bee.[†]   A more probable story has been told in the Gazette de Santé of a gardener who died of inflammation of the throat, in consequence of being stung there by a wasp while he was eating an apple, in which it had been concealed.[‡]   But the same accident has often occurred without any material danger.

The treatment of poisoning by venomous serpents need not be detailed here.   The subject is introduced merely to mention that the treatment of poisoned wounds by the application of cupping-glasses has been lately resorted to with success for curing the bite of the viper.   A patient of M. Piorry, two hours after being bitten, had all the constitutional symptoms strongly developed, such as slow, very feeble pulse, nausea, vomiting, and swelling of the face.   When a cupping-glass was applied for half an hour, the general symptoms ceased and did not return.   Next day diffuse inflammation began; but it was checked by leeches.[§]   An equally successful case is related in the Calcutta Transactions by Mr. Clarke.[‖]

CHAPTER XXIV.

OF POISONING BY DISEASED AND DECAYED ANIMAL MATTER.

ANOTHER and much more important group of poisons, that may be arranged in the present order, comprehends animal matter usually harmless or even wholesome, but rendered deleterious by disease or decay.   These poisons are formed in three ways, by morbid action local or constitutional, by ordinary putrefaction, and by modified putrefaction.

Of Animal Matter rendered Poisonous by Diseased Action.

Under the first variety might be included the latent poisons by means of which natural diseases are communicated by infection, contact, and inoculation.   Such poisons, however, being usually excluded from a strict toxicological system, the only varieties requiring notice are the animal poisons engendered by disease, and which do not produce peculiar diseases, but merely inflammation.   Several species of this kind may be mentioned, comprehending the solids and fluids in various unhealthy states of the body.

[*] Wibmer, Die Wirkung der Arzneimittel und Gifte, i 200.
[†] Journal de Médecine, 1765.   [‡] Gazette de Santé, 1776.
[§] Archives Gén. de Médecine, xi. 30.
[‖] Trans. of Med. and Phys. Soc. of Calcutta, iv. 442.

One of these poisons, contained in the blood and perhaps in some of the secretions of overdriven cattle, arises under circumstances in which the body seems to deviate little from its natural condition. A good account of the effects thus induced has been given in an essay on the subject by Morand.* From the cases he describes it follows, that the flesh of such animals is wholesome enough when cooked and eaten ; but that if the blood or raw flesh be applied to a wound or scratch, nay even sometimes to the unbroken skin, a dangerous and often fatal inflammation is excited, which at times differs little from diffuse cellular inflammation, and at other times consists of a general eruption of gangrenous boils, the *pustules malignes* of the French. The deleterious effects occasionally observed to arise from offal are probably analogous in their nature and their cause. On this subject Sir B. Brodie has made some remarks which tend to show that the application of various kinds of offal to wounds, and especially pricks of the fingers with spiculæ of bone from the hare, may cause an obstinate chronic erysipelas of the hand.† I have met with a case of this nature, where the affection was erratic erythema of the hand.

Another species of poison, allied to the preceding in its effects and equally obscure in its nature, includes certain fluids of the human body after natural death, which are probably modified, if not even formed altogether, by morbid processes during life. Such poisons are the most frequent source of the dreadful cellular inflammation, often witnessed as the consequence of pricks received during dissection by the anatomist. On this interesting but obscure subject, much minute information will be found in the works quoted below.‡

It is still a matter of question among pathologists what these poisons are, and in what circumstances they spring up. By some their baneful properties have been suspected to arise from the operation of particular diseases on natural or morbid secretions ;§ and although the precise diseases inducing these properties, and the precise fluids which acquire them have by no means been satisfactorily ascertained, it appears well established that no fluid possesses them more frequently or in a higher degree than the serum effused into the cavities of the chest and belly by recent inflammation of the serous membranes of these cavities. By others the origin of the poison is suspected to be wholly independent of diseased action in the living body and to lie merely in certain changes effected in healthy se-cretions by decay. And as the accidents produced by this poison have occurred chiefly during the dissection of bodies recently dead, it is supposed to exist only for a short time at the commencement of decay, and to disappear in the farther progress of putrefaction.

But whatever may be its nature and origin, we are well enough acquainted with its effects ; which are diffuse inflammation and

* Histoire d'une Maladie très-singulière, &c. in Hist. de l'Académie des Sciences, 1766, i. 97.
† London Med. and Phys. Journal, lvii. 342.
‡ Dr. Duncan's Cases of Diffuse Inflammation of the cellular texture — in Edin. Med. Chirurg. Trans. i. 455, 470, 1824. Also,
§ Mr. Travers on Constitutional Irritation, 1826.

violent constitutional excitement, quickly passing to a state resembling typhoid fever. Sometimes the inflammation spreads steadily towards the trunk from the part to which the poison was applied ; sometimes the inflammation around the injury is trifling and limited, but a similar inflammation appears in or near the axilla, and subsequently on other parts of the body ; and the latter form of disease is always attended with the highest constitutional derangement and with the greatest danger.

Another singular poison, unequivocally the product of disease, and which acts as a local irritant, is the flesh or fluids of animals affected at the time of their death with a carbuncular disorder, denominated in Germany *Milzbrand*, and analogous to the *pustule maligne* of the French. The disease, so far as I know, has not received a vulgar name in the English language, being fortunately rare in Britain. It is a constitutional and epidemic malady, which sometimes prevails among cattle on the continent to an alarming extent, and is characterized by the eruption of large gangrenous carbuncles on various parts of the body. This distemper has the property of rendering the solids and fluids poisonous to so great a degree, that not only persons who handle the skin, entrails, blood, or other parts, but even also those who eat the flesh, are apt to suffer severely. The affection thus produced in man is sometimes ordinary inflammation of the alimentary canal, or cholera ;[*] more commonly a disorder precisely the same as the pustule maligne ;[†] but most frequently of all an eruption of one or more large carbuncles resembling those of the original disease of cattle.[‡] It is often fatal. The carbuncular form has been known to cause death in forty-eight hours.[§] It is an interesting fact, for the knowledge of which we are indebted to M. Dupuy, that the carbuncle of cattle may be caused by applying to a wound the blood or spleen of an animal killed by gangrene of the lungs.[‖]

A poison analogous to the former in its nature, which has sometimes occasioned severe and even fatal effects in man is the matter of *glanders*, a contagious disease to which the horse is peculiarly subject, and which is communicated probably by means of a morbid secretion from the nostrils. This disease has been propagated to man by infection ; at least instances have been related where grooms attending glandered horses, although they had no external injury through which inoculation could take place, were attacked with profuse fetid discharge from the nostrils, a pustular eruption on the face, and colliquative diarrhœa, which has sometimes ended fatally in a few days.[¶] In other instances inoculation of the hand with the blood of the glandered horse has produced alarming diffuse inflammation, and a carbuncular eruption.[**]

It appears probable, that some peculiar circumstances with which we are not yet acquainted must concur with the operation of the

* Rust's Magazin, xxiv. 490. Also Annali Univ. di Med. 1841, iii. 449.
† Ibidem, xxv. 108.   ‡ Kopp's Jahrbuch, v 67, and vi. 95.
§ Rust's Magazin, xxv. 105.   ‖ Revue Médicale, 1827, ii. 488.
¶ Journal der Praktischen Heilkunde, liv. iii. 62.
** Magazin der Ausländischen Literatur, iii. 460, v. 168.
44*

poisons now under review, before they can take effect. At least unequivocal facts have been published which show, that the fluids and solids, as well as the emanations of animals infected and even killed by glanders or the *pustule maligne*, may be often handled and breathed with impunity. Such is the result of a careful inquiry made under the direction of the Parisian Board of Health into the nuisance occasioned by the great Nackery of Montfaucon.* Parent-Duchatelet, the author of an elaborate report on the subject, considers it clearly established that neither the workmen nor the horses connected with the establishment, nor the tanners who are supplied with hides from it, have ever presented a single instance of disease referrible to the operation of diseased animal matter. Yet upwards of twelve thousand horses are annually flayed there, and among these it is calculated that at least three thousand six hundred are affected with carbuncle, glanders, or farcy.†

Of Animal Matter rendered Poisonous by common Putrefaction.

The second mode in which animal matters, naturally wholesome or harmless, may acquire the properties of irritant poisons, is by their undergoing ordinary putrefaction.

The tendency of putrefaction to impart deleterious qualities to animal matters originally wholesome has been long known, and is quite unequivocal. To those who are not accustomed to the use of tainted meat, the mere commencement of decay is sufficient to render meat insupportable and noxious. Game, only decayed enough to please the palate of the epicure, has caused severe cholera in persons not accustomed to eat it in that state. The power of habit, however, in reconciling the stomach to the digestion of decayed meat is inconceivable. Some epicures in civilized countries prefer a slight taint even in their beef and mutton ; and there are tribes of savages still farther advanced in the cultivation of this department of gastronomy, who eat with impunity rancid oil, putrid blubber, and stinking offal. How far putrefaction may be allowed to advance without overpowering the preservative tendency of habit, it is not easy to tell. But with the present habits of this and other civilized nations, the limit appears very confined.

* I have taken the liberty of applying this term to an establishment unique perhaps in the history of the world. The Voirie et Chantier d'"Ecarrissage of Montfaucon, which has existed close to the walls of Paris for several centuries, is an enclosure of many acres, where the contents of the necessaries of the city are collected in enormous pits, and where horses, dogs, and cats are flayed to the amount of forty or fifty thousand annually. The fat is melted for blow-pipe lamps ; the bones are in a great measure burnt on the premises for fuel ; the intestines are made into coarse gut for machinery ; the flesh, blood, and garbage are heaped to putrefy for manure ; and in summer a bed of compost is spread to breed maggots for feeding poultry. There is no drain. Description cannot convey an idea of the stench. The committee of the Board of Health, appointed to make inquiries into the best mode of abating the nuisance, in vain attempted to penetrate into the place. Yet the workmen and their families are stout, healthy, and long lived.

† Des Chantiers d'Ecarrissage. Annales d'Hyg. Publ. et de Méd. Lég. viii. 139. Sur l'enfouissement des Animaux morts de maladies contagieuses. Ibid. ix. 109.

Putrid animal matter when injected into the veins of healthy animals proves quickly fatal; and from the experiments of Gaspard and Magendie,[*] together with the more recent researches of MM. Leuret and Hamont,[†] the disease induced seems to resemble closely the typhoid fever of man.

Similar effects were observed by Magendie, when dogs were confined over vessels in which animal matter was decaying, so that they were obliged always to breathe the exhalations.[‡]   These discoveries throw some light on the question regarding the tendency of putrid effluvia to engender fever in man; and notwithstanding many well ascertained facts of an opposite import, they show that, probably in peculiar circumstances, decaying animal matter may excite epidemic fevers.   A detailed investigation of this important topic would be misplaced here, as it belongs more to medical police than to medical jurisprudence; but the two works quoted below are referred to for examples, in my opinion, of the unequivocal origin of continued fever in the cause now alluded to;[§] and other instances of the like kind will be found in the Report of the Parliamentary Commission on the Health of Towns.

Another affection sometimes brought on by putrid exhalations is violent diarrhœa or dysentery, of which a remarkable instance lately occurred in the person of a well-known French physician, M. Ollivier.   While visiting a cellar where old bones were stored, he was seized with giddiness, nausea, tendency to vomit and general uneasiness; and subsequently he suffered from violent colic with profuse diarrhœa, which put on the dysenteric character and lasted for three days.[‖]   Chevallier, in noticing this accident, mentions his having been affected somewhat in the same way when exposed to the emanations of dead bodies; and it is a familiar fact that medical men, who engage in anatomical researches after long disuse, are apt to suffer at first from smart diarrhœa.

The same remark must be applied here as at the close of the observations in the last section.   Without peculiar concurring circumstances no bad effect results.   This will follow from many facts illustrative of the innocuous nature of various trades where the workmen are perpetually exposed to the most noisome putrid effluvia.   But no facts of the kind are so remarkable as those collected in regard to the establishment at Montfaucon by Parent-Duchatelet, who makes it appear that this most abominable concentration of the worst of all possible nuisances is not merely not injurious to the health of the men and animals employed in and around it, but actually even preserves them from epidemic or epizootic diseases.[¶]

The effects of putrid animal matter when applied to wounds have

* Journal de Physiologie, ii. 1, and iii. 81.
† Journal des Progrès des Sciences Médicales, 1827, vi. 181.
‡ Journal de Physiologie, iii. 85.
§ De divers accidens graves occasionnés par les miasmes d'animaux en putréfaction. Mém. de la Soc. de Med. i. 97. — London Med. Chirurg. Review, vi. 202.
‖ Annales d'Hyg. Publique et de Med. Légale, vii. 216.
¶ Ibidem, viii. and ix. ut supra.

been investigated experimentally by Professor Orfila ; who found that putrid blood, bile, or brain, caused death in this way within twenty-four hours, — producing extensive local inflammation of the diffuse kind, and great constitutional fever. In man also several instances of diffuse cellular inflammation have been observed as the consequence of pricks received during the dissection of putrid bodies. The disease, as formerly observed, certainly arises in general from pricks received in dissecting recent bodies. At the same time, a few cases have been traced quite unequivocally to inoculation with putrid matter ;* and if any doubts existed on this point, the experiments of Orfila would remove them.

M. Lassaigne has examined chemically the putrid matter formed by keeping flesh long in close vessels, and has found it to consist of carbonate of ammonia, much caseate of ammonia, and a stinking volatile oil, — the last of which is probably the poisonous ingredient.

Of Animal Matter rendered Poisonous by Modified Putrefaction.

The third way in which animal matters naturally wholesome may become irritant poisons, is by their undergoing a modified putrefaction.

It is probable that many common articles of food occasionally become poisonous in this way ; but none are so liable to acquire injurious properties as certain articles much used in Germany, namely, a particular kind of sausage, a particular kind of cheese, and bacon. The last two species of poison have been occasionally observed in France, and probably occur in Britain also. But the first has been hitherto met with only in some districts of Germany.

The best account yet given of the *sausage-poison* is contained in two essays published by Dr. Kerner,† in a Thesis by Dr. Dann,‡ and in a prize-essay by Dr. W. Horn.§ It has at various times committed great ravages in Germany, especially in the Würtemberg territories, where 234 cases of poisoning with it occurred between the years 1793 and 1827 ; and of that number no less than 110 proved fatal.‖

The symptoms of poisoning seldom begin till twenty-four, or even forty-eight hours, after the noxious meal, and rather later than earlier, The tardiness of their approach seems owing to the great indigestibility of the fatty matter with which the active principle is mixed. The first symptoms are pain in the stomach, vomiting, purging, and dryness of the mouth and nose. The eyes, eyelids, and pupils then become fixed and motionless ; the voice is rendered hoarse, or is lost altogether; the power of swallowing is much impaired; the pulse

---

* Dr. Duncan, Edin. Med. Chirurg. Trans. i. 502 and 520.

† Neue Beobachtungen über die Vergiftungen durch dens genuss geraücherten Würste. Tübingen, 1820. — Das Fettgift, oder die Fettsäure, und ihre Wirkungen auf den thierischen Organismus. Tübingen, 1822.

‡ De Veneni Botulini viribus et natura. Diss. Inaug. Berolini, 1828.

§ De Veneno in Botulis. Commentatio in certamine lit. a gratioso Med. Ord. Berol. Præmio ornata. 1828. Analyzed by Dr. Arrowsmith in Edin. Med. and Surg. Journal, xxxiii. 28.   ‖ Horn's Archiv, 1828, i. 558.

gradually fails, frequent swoonings ensue, and the skin becomes cold and insensible. The secretions and excretions, with the exception of the urine, are then commonly suspended; but sometimes profuse diarrhœa continues throughout. The appetite is not impaired; fever is rarely present; and the mind continues to the last unclouded. Fatal cases end with convulsions and oppressed breathing between the third and eighth day. In cases of recovery the period of convalescence may be protracted to several years. The chief appearances in the dead body are signs of inflammation in the mucous membrane of the alimentary canal, — such as whiteness and dryness of the throat, thickening of the gullet, redness of the stomach and intestines; also croupy deposition in the windpipe; great flaccidity of the heart; and a tendency in the whole body to resist putrefaction. In a set of cases which occurred so lately as 1841, there was found after death abscesses in the tonsils, dark bluish redness of the membrane of the pharynx, windpipe and bronchial ramifications, gorging of the pulmonary air-tubes and condensation of the pulmonary tissue itself, dark redness of the fundus of the stomach, with circumscribed softening, a dark gray, red, or black appearance of the mucous coat of the intestines, accumulation of greenish-yellow fæces in the colon, brittleness of the liver, and enlargement of the spleen.*

The article which is apt to occasion these baneful effects is of two sorts, the white and the bloody sausage *(leberwürste, blut-würste).* Both are of large size, the material being put into swine's stomachs; and they are cured by drying and smoking them in a chimney with wood-smoke. Those which have been found to act as poisons possess an acid reaction, are soft in consistence, have a nauseous, putrid taste, and an unpleasant sweetish-sour smell, like that of purulent matter. They are met with principally about the beginning of spring, when they are liable to be often alternately frozen and thawed in the curing. Those sausages only become poisonous which have been boiled before being salted and hung up. They are poisonous only at a particular stage of decay, and cease to be so when putrefaction has advanced so far that sulphuretted-hydrogen is evolved. The central part is often poisonous when the surface is wholesome.

Various opinions have been entertained of the cause of the deleterious qualities thus contracted. In recent times the principle has been supposed to be pyroligneous acetic acid, hydrocyanic acid, or cocculus indicus. Dr. Kerner, however, has shown that none of these notions will account for the phenomena; and at first conceived he had proved the poisonous principle to be a fatty acid analogous to the sebacic acid of Thenard, and originating in a modified process of putrefaction. From the poisonous sausage he procured by double decomposition an acid similar in chemical properties to that obtained from fat by destructive distillation; and by experiments on animals he thought he observed, that the acid procured in either way produced symptoms analogous to those of poisoning with the deleterious sausage. Subsequently, however, he changed his views in some

* Röser, in London Med. Gazette, 1842-43, i. 271.

measure; and he now considers that the poison is a compound one, consisting of a fatty acid analogous to the sebacic, and of a volatile principle.* The results obtained by Dr. Dann coincide with the last opinion. Dann infers from his researches that the poisonous princi- ple does not necessarily reside in an acid, but is an acrid empy- reumatic oil, which when pure is not active, but is rendered so by uniting with various fatty acids.†

The results lately obtained by Buchner after an elaborate and careful analysis are somewhat different and probably nearer the truth. He first ascertained that the product of the distillation of fat has no analogy with the sausage-poison. He found it to consist of animal- ized acetic acid, and a fetid empyreumatic oil, the former of which has no injurious effect on animals, while the latter, though an active poison, is purely narcotic in its operation. On next examining a sausage sent to him from Würtemberg, which had violently affected four individuals and killed one of them in six days, he remarked that the poisonous principle is not soluble in water, or capable of being distilled over with it; and that cold alcohol removes a granular fatty matter, which, when purified by distilled water, has a yellowish co- lour, a peculiar nauseous smell, and a disagreeable oleaginous taste, followed by extraordinary dryness of the throat for several hours. Although it does not possess an acid reaction on litmus, it forms a soap with alkalis, and is separated again by acids unchanged; and consequently it may be considered a fatty acid, to which Buchner proposes to give the name of Botulinic acid [Würst-fett-saüre]. It concentrates in itself the poisonous properties of the crude sausage. Thirty grains of it, which formed three-fourths of the whole product of a single sausage, were given in two doses to a puppy with an in- terval of a day between them. For some hours after the second dose no apparent effect was produced. But gradually the animal became dull, lay in the same spot, wasted rapidly away notwithstanding a vigorous appetite, and died of exhaustion on the thirteenth day. Half a grain causes insupportable dryness in the throat, which does not go off for several hours.‡ With these results the contemporane- ous and unconnected researches of Dr. Schumann accord very re- markably. Alcohol boiled on the poison-sausage deposited on cool- ing a fatty matter, which, when washed with distilled water, pos- sessed all the properties specified by Buchner, as characterizing his fatty acid, and acted on animals in the same way as the sausage- poison.§

The *poison of cheese* has been for some time more generally known. Dr. Henneman has published an interesting essay on several cases which happened at Schwerin in 1823.|| Another account of a simi- lar accident which happened at Minden in 1825 has been published in Rust's Magazin.¶ But by far the best information on the subject

* Weiss. die neuste Vergift. durch Verdorbene Würste, &c. mit Vorrede und Anhang begleitet, von Dr. J. Kerner. Carlsruhe, 1821.   † Horn's Archiv, 1828, i. 596.
‡ Toxicologie, Zweite Aufl. 1829, p. 136.
§ Das Wurst-fett-gift, oder neue Untersuchung, &c. Archiv für Medizinische Erfah- rung, 1829, i. 30 and 75. || Hufeland's Journal, lvii. 2, 106.
¶ Magazin für die gesammte Heilkunde, xxi. 247.

is to be obtained from two papers in Horn's Archiv, — the one by Professor Hünefeld of Greifswald, describing the phenomena as he witnessed them in that city in 1827, and containing an elaborate chemical analysis and physiological experiments, by means of which he conceives he has discovered the deleterious principles contained in the cheese,[*] — the other by Dr. Westrumb of Hameln, who investigated the particulars of seven cases which came under his notice in 1826, and with the aid of Sertürner, the chemist, traced the properties of the poison to almost the same principles with those indicated by the researches of Hünefeld.[†] Besides the cases which have given origin to these papers, others have occurred throughout Germany in the same period; and during the third quarter of last century this kind of poisoning was so common, that several of the German states investigated the subject, and legislative enactments were passed in consequence.

For a long time the prevalent belief was that the cheese acquired an impregnation from copper vessels used in the dairies ; and accordingly the Austrian, Wirtemberg and Ratesberg States prohibited the use of copper for such purposes. This opinion, however, was proved by chemical analysis to be untenable ; and the inquiries of Hünefeld and Sertürner, have now rendered it probable that the poisonous property of the cheese resides in two animal acids, analogous, if not indentical, with the caseïc and sebacic acids.

The mode in which the formation of these acids is accounted for is as follows. According to the researches of Proust the sharp peculiar taste of old cheese is owing to the gradual conversion of the curd or caseïn into the caseate of ammonia, which in sound cheeses is always united with the excess of alkali. In the cheese in question (*barscherkäse*, *quark-käse*, *hand-käse*) the curd, before being salted, is left for some time in a heap to ferment, in consequence of which it becomes sour and afterwards ripens faster. But if the milk has been curdled with vinegar, — if the acid liquor formed while it ferments is not carefully drained off, — if the fermentation is allowed to go too far, — if too little salt is used in preserving the curd, — or if flour has been mixed with the curd, the subsequent ripening or decaying of the cheese follows a peculiar course, and a considerable excess of caseïc acid is formed, as well as some sebacic acid.

The poisonous cheeses, according to Westrumb, present no peculiarity in their appearance, taste or smell. But Hünefeld says that they are yellowish-red, soft, and tough, with harder and darker lumps interspersed, that they have a disagreeable taste, redden litmus, and becomes flesh-red instead of yellow, under the action of nitric acid.

The symptoms they cause in man appear to be nearly the same with those produced by the poisonous sausage, and usually commence, according to Hünefeld, in five or six hours, according to Westrumb in half an hour. They constitute various degrees and combinations

[*] Die Chemische Ausmittelung des Käsegifts. Horn's Archiv, 1827, i. 203.
[†] Ueber die Vergiftung durch Käse. Horn's Archiv, 1828, i. 65.

of gastro-enteric inflammation. In the most severe of Hünefeld's cases the quantity taken did not exceed four ounces, and was sometimes only an ounce.

The same author found that a drachm and a half of the caseïc acid, which he procured from the cheese, killed a cat in eight minutes, and the same quantity of the sebacic acid another in three hours. His experiments, however, are not quite conclusive of the fact that these acids are really the poisonous principles, as he has not extended his experimental researches to the caseïc and sebacic acids prepared in the ordinary way. His views will probably be altered and simplified, if future experiments should confirm the late inquiries of Braconnot, who has stated that Proust's caseïc acid is a modification of the acetic, combined with an acrid oil.* Westrumb procured analogous results with those of Hünefeld when he gave to animals the acid fat which he separated in the course of his analysis.

The poisonous cheese has been hitherto met with chiefly in some parts of Germany. From information communicated to me by Dr. Swanwick of Macclesfield, there is some reason to think that a parallel poison is occasionally met with in Cheshire, among the small hill-farms, where the limited extent of the dairies obliges the farmer to keep the curd for several days before a sufficient quantity is accumulated for the larger cheeses. — I am indebted to Mr. Wilson of Lockerby for the particulars of a set of cases, which seem to have been owing to some obscure poison in cheese. A gentleman, an hour after eating the suspected cheese, was seized with extreme weakness and severe vomiting for four hours, then with general soreness and a mercurial taste in the mouth, and afterwards with tenesmus, bloody stools, soreness of the gums, and cramps in the limbs; from which symptoms he did not recover for four weeks. Five other members of his household suffered similarly, but less severely, and also the shop-boy who ate a little while selling it. None of the ordinary mineral poisons could be detected in it. — It is hardly necessary to add, that analogous properties may be imparted to cheese by the intentional or accidental addition of other poisons of a mineral nature. This subject has been already alluded to in the section upon lead.

As connected, though indeed but remotely, with the cheese-poison, some notice may be here taken of a peculiar mode in which it has been supposed that *milk* may acquire the properties of an acrid poison. It has been several times remarked on the continent, that the milk even of the cow, but more particularly that of the ewe and goat, may act like a violent poison, although no mineral or other deleterious impregnation could be detected in it ; and these effects have been variously and vaguely ascribed to the animal having been diseased, or to its having fed on acrid vegetables, which pass into the milk without injury to its health, because though poisonous to most animals, they are not so to the Ruminantia. This singular topic cannot be thoroughly investigated, as precise facts are still wanting. But the two following examples of the accident alluded to may be

* Ann. de Chimie et de Physique, xxxvi. 159.

mentioned. One occurred at Aurillac, a village in France. Fifteen or sixteen customers of a particular dealer in goats' milk were at one and the same time attacked with all the symptoms of violent cholera ; and about twenty-four hours afterwards the goat too was taken ill with the same affection, and died in three days.* The other instance occurred at Hereford in Westphalia. Six people of a family, after partaking of goat's butter-milk, were simultaneously attacked with violent vomiting, tension of the epigastrium, and retraction of the lower belly; and several of them suffered so severely as even to have been thought by their physician, Dr. Bonorden, to be in danger.† Dr. Westrumb has alluded to similar cases in his memoir on the poison of cheese, and has proved that the ordinary explanations of them are far from satisfactory. Among other judicious observations he remarks, that the poison has been generally believed to arise sometimes from the cattle having fed on the *Euphorbia esula*, a species of spurge ; that, according to Viridet in his *Tractatus de Prima Coctione*, l. i. c. 15, certain fields in the neighbourhood of Embrim were of necessity abandoned by the shepherds, because the milk of their cows was rendered useless by the abundance of that plant among the herbage ; but that he himself has found cattle will not touch it so long as grass and other wholesome vegetables are to be found in the pasturage.‡ Professors Orfila and Marc, who were appointed by the Society of Medicine of Paris to report upon the accident at Aurillac, state, that in parallel cases which had been referred to them by the police at Paris they had been unable to detect any mineral poison ; that none of the received explanations are in their opinion satisfactory ; and that they are disposed to ascribe the poisonous alteration of the milk to new principles formed by a vital process.

Another common article of food, which has occasionally produced similar effects with the poisonous sausages and cheese, is bacon. Dr. Geiseler has related an accident which occurred in a family of eight persons, and which he traced to this cause. The symptoms were almost exactly the same with those described by Kerner, with the addition, however, of delirium and loss of recollection ; and in two they were so violent as seriously to endanger life. The father of the family alone escaped, having stewed his bacon, while the rest ate it raw.§ His escape might have arisen from the fatty acid having been decomposed, or the acrid oil expelled, by the heat. It is not improbable that other varieties of cured meat may also become poisonous. Cadet de Gassicourt mentions, that he had been frequently desired by the police to examine cured meat which had produced symptoms of poisoning at Paris,|| and Orfila makes the same remark in his Lectures on Medical Jurisprudence.¶ As the meat always came from the shops of meat-curers, and did not contain

---

* Archives Gén. xv. 460.   † Rust's Magazin, xxvii. 193.
‡ Horn's Archiv, 1828, i. 76.   § Rust's Magazin, xvi. 111.
|| London Medical and Physical Journal, xlvi. 68.
¶ Orfila, Médecine-Légale, ii. 322.

any mineral poison, it probably owed its qualities to the same ingre⁻
dient as the bacon in Geiseler's cases.   A full and interesting account
of an accident of the kind has also been given by M. Ollivier, of
which the following is an analysis.   Three members of a family at
Paris, on the day after eating a ham-pie, were seized with shivering,
cold sweats, violent pain in the stomach, frequent vomiting, burning
thirst, excessive tenderness of the belly, profuse purging, and colic ;
but they all recovered under antiphlogistic treatment.   On subsequent
inquiry it appeared that about the same period other customers of
the pastry-cook who supplied the pie had been similarly affected ;
and consequently an investigation was made into the cause under
the authority of the police.   After a very careful analysis, however,
by MM. Barruel and Ollivier, it was clearly made out, that the pie
did not contain a trace of any of the common mineral poisons ; and
therefore the only conclusion Ollivier conceived it possible to draw
was, that the ham had acquired the properties of the poisonous sausage or cheese of Germany.*   Two similar reports have been since
published, one by MM. Lecanu, Labarraque, and Delamorlière,
another by Chevallier ; and both agree in ascribing the poisonous
effects to the decay of the meat, the ordinary poisons having been
sought for in vain.   In the cases examined by Chevallier, the article
was a sort of sausage, called in Paris " Italian Cheese," and made
of scraps of various kinds of meat, especially pork.†   M. Boutigny
has published an account of a similar accident which befel a great
number of people at a festival in France.   He could not find any of
the ordinary poisons in the meat, which had been taken chiefly in
the form of sausages ; and being consequently persuaded that the
suspected articles were wholesome, he dined on stuffed turkey, sold
by the dealer who had supplied them.   But he was seized with
chilliness, contracted pulse, cold sweating, lividity of the countenance, great anxiety, and then with vomiting and purging ; after
which he slowly recovered.‡

Other articles of food have been occasionally observed to act injuriously on the health.   Thus M. Ollivier has given an account of
a whole family having been apparently poisoned with mutton under
the influence of modified decay.   Six individuals were attacked
soon after dinner with vomiting, purging, colic, tenderness of the
belly, extreme prostration, and a small hurried pulse.   Four of them
died within eight days.   General inflammatory redness, with some
extravasation under the mucous coat, was found throughout the
whole course of the small intestines.   No trace could be detected of
any of the ordinary poisons ; and Ollivier was therefore led to ascribe
the accident to some peculiar change produced in stewed mutton,
which all the individuals had partaken of at dinner.§   In 1839 a
singular accident happened at Zurich, which was ascribed to decayed
veal and *ham*.   On a fete-day 600 people, who had dined upon cold

* Archives Gén. de Méd.   † Journ. de Chim. Méd. viii. 726.
‡ Annales d'Hygiène Publique, xxi. 234.
§ Annales d'Hygiène Publique, xx. 413.

roast-veal and ham in a wooden erection, were all taken ill with shivering, giddiness, headache, burning fever, diarrhœa and vomiting; some had delirium, others a fœtid salivation and even ill-conditioned ulcers of the mouth ; and in the worst cases collapse of the countenance, involuntary stools, and extreme prostration preceded death. On dissection the alimentary mucous membrane was found softened and the intestinal follicles ulcerated. The cause was supposed to have been satisfactorily traced to incipient putrefaction of the veal and ham, which constituted the fundamental part of the repast.* Effects somewhat similar have been observed from spoiled *goose-grease*, used in dressing food. Dr. Siedler has related four cases where violent symptoms were thus induced. Two adults and two children, after eating a dish seasoned with goose-grease, were seized with giddiness, prostration of strength, anxiety, sweating, — burning pain in the lower belly, aggravated by pressure, — violent vomiting, in one case sanguinolent, — involuntary stools, and urine, and dilatation of the pupil. In one of the adults there was also complete insensibility, with imperceptible pulse for six minutes. No metallic poison could be found. The grease was acid, and of a repulsive odour ; and three ounces given to a dog acted violently and in the same manner.† Another article of food which has appeared occasionally to produce parallel effects is *smoked sprats*. An instance of their injurious operation is briefly described in the work quoted below ;‡ and Dr. O'Shaughnessey informed me some years ago, that, while in London, he met with the case of a female, advanced in pregnancy, who after eating smoked sprats, in which she remarked a disagreeable sharp taste, was attacked with severe colic, sickness, vomiting of food mixed with streaks and clots of blood, and some diarrhœa. Putrid *pickled salmon* has occasioned death in this country ;§ and I may mention that I have known most violent diarrhœa occasioned in two instances by a very small portion of the oily matter about the fins of *kipper* or smoked salmon, so that I have no doubt a moderate quantity would produce serious effects.

Although these illustrations of the effects of modified putrefaction in rendering wholesome meat noxious have been taken in a great measure from continental experience, this has been done rather because the subject has been more fully and accurately investigated there, than because similar poisons are unknown in Britain. The defective system of medical police in this country would allow such accidents as those mentioned above to pass sometimes without notice, and almost always without scientific examination; but it must not therefore be supposed that they are wholly unknown.

The following incident, which happened a few years ago on the Galloway coast, is an instance of poisoning not less alarming than any of those which have occurred in Germany. In the autumn of 1826 four adults and ten children ate at dinner a stew made with

* Journal de Chimie Med. 1842, 872.
† Journal of the Institution, ii. 414, from Hufeland Journal.
‡ Bulletins des Sciences Méd. xx. 197. § London Med. Gazette, xiv. 656.

meat taken from a dead calf, which was found by one of them on the sea shore, and of which no history could be procured. For three hours no ill effect followed. But they were then all seized with pain in the stomach, efforts to vomit, purging, and lividity of the face, succeeded by a soporose state like the stupor caused by opium, except that when roused the patient had a peculiar wild expression. One person died comatose in the course of six hours. The rest, being freely purged and made to vomit, eventually got well; but for some days they required the most powerful stimulants to counteract the exhaustion and collapse which followed the sopor. The meat, they said, looked well enough at the time it was used. Yet the remains of the fish which formed the noxious meal had a black colour and nauseous smell; and the uncooked flesh had a white, glistening appearance, and was so far decayed that its odour excited vomiting and fainting.* It is much to be regretted that this accident was not properly inquired into. The only conjecture which the facts will warrant as to the cause of the poisonous quality of the meat is, that in consequence of having lain long in the water, the flesh had begun to undergo the adipocirous putrefaction; and that in the course of the changes thus induced the meat became impregnated with some poisonous principle, like that of the German sausages, or cheese.

An accident of a similar nature, for the particulars of which I am indebted to Dr. Swanwick of Macclesfield, occurred at Stockport in the summer of 1830. A family of five persons took for dinner broth made of beef, which, owing to its black colour, the master of the family had previously said to his wife he thought bad and unfit for use. In the course of some hours two boys were attacked with sickness and vomiting, but appear to have got soon well, probably owing to the early discharge of the poison. Next morning a washerwoman who had dined with the family was seized with violent pain in the bowels, diarrhœa, racking pains and weakness in the limbs; and she did not recover for ten days. On the evening of the second day the master of the house was similarly affected, and was ill for a fortnight. And a day later his wife was also seized with a similar disorder, preceded by soreness of the throat and tongue and difficulty of swallowing, and ending fatally in fourteen days. The last person was previously in delicate health, and subject to disorder in the stomach and bowels. The investigation made by the police authorities into the circumstances of this accident was extremely imperfect: but there seems little reason to doubt that unsound meat was the cause.

I am not sure under what head to arrange the following observations, communicated to me by Dr. M'Divitt of Canterbury, and of which he has since published a detailed account.† But they may be mentioned, perhaps not inappropriately, in the present place; and at all events they deserve careful attention, as referring to a description of cases which may be mistaken for other kinds of poisoning.

It is well known that pork in all forms, but especially when fresh,

* London Med Repository, Third Series, iii. 372.
† Edin. Med. and Surg. Journal, xlvi. 293.

is apt to cause indigestion in many persons who are not accustomed to it. But Dr. M'Divitt has shown by a number of interesting cases, that even in those habituated to its use, it may, from unascertained causes, excite symptoms closely allied to those of irritant poisoning. The effects sometimes begin within three hours, the symptoms being those of an affection of the stomach, such as sudden violent pain in the epigastrium, difficult breathing, irregularity of the pulse, great prostration and alarm, coldness of the extremities and vomiting. If a longer period elapses, — and sometimes no injury accrues for many hours, or even a whole day, — the symptoms indicate an affection of the abdomen, namely, pain in the region of the duodenum, or of the sigmoid flexure of the colon, with the other symptoms just enumerated, but which ere long become attended with more pungent pain, tension and tenderness of the belly, frequency of the pulse, and ineffectual straining to evacuate the bowels. In the less urgent and slower cases of this nature there is little or no vomiting. Sometimes nettle-rash appears. Stimulants, opiates, and bloodletting are of no avail ; and the only useful remedies are emetics and cathartics, which speedily put an end to the symptoms by removing their cause. In all the cases related by the author the pork was either fresh or recently salted, fatter than usual, but not ill preserved or otherwise faulty in any appreciable respect. In every instance the individuals had eaten pork often before without injury ; and on several occasions others ate without harm the same pork which seemed deleterious.

CHAPTER XXV.

OF POISONING BY MECHANICAL IRRITANTS.

THE *fifth* order of the irritant class of poisons includes mechanical irritants.

These substances have not properly speaking any poisonous quality ; but occasion symptoms like those of poisoning, and even sometimes death itself, in consequence of their mechanical qualities only. They have therefore been excluded from every toxicological system proposed in recent times ; but in a medico-legal work on poisoning it would be wrong to pass them without notice.

The most important of the mechanical irritants are those which cause injury by reason of their roughness, sharpness, or size.

Many instances have occurred of persons having swallowed fragments of steel, copper, iron, broken glass, or entire prune-stones, cherry-stones, and the like, — who not long afterwards were attacked with signs of inflammation, or some other abdominal disease, and were carried off by it as by the administration of poison. The disorders thus induced are almost always of a chronic or lingering kind, and commonly depend on gradual perforation of the intestines by the foreign body pressing on the coats. In general the illness ends in in-

45*

flammation of the peritonæum. Sometimes the irritating substance perforates the skin and muscles as well as the intestines, and escapes outwardly; and a few individuals have even recovered under these circumstances. An excellent account of the ordinary course of such accidents is given in the London Medical and Physical Journal. The person swallowed a chocolate bean, and after experiencing many uneasy sensations throughout the belly for several days, was attacked with peritonitis and died.* Mr. Howship has related the particulars of the case of a woman, died after two years of constant suffering, in consequence of having swallowed a large quantity of cherry-stones.† Dr. Marcet has also described the case of a sailor who died in a similar way after swallowing several large clasp-knives.‡ Thus too, although it is a familiar fact, that needles and pins are in general swallowed with impunity, death nevertheless sometimes arises from this cause. Guersent mentions the case of a child who died in the course of two months of frequent vomiting caused by swallowing a pin, which was found after death pinning the stomach, as it were, to the liver.§ Dupuytren relates the case of a woman, who, after swallowing an incredible number of needles and pins, became very lean and was confined to bed by the excruciating pain excited on motion by the needles and pins escaping through the skin. There were seldom less than fifty tumours or abscesses on various parts of the body; and Dupuytren, on opening about a hundred of these, invariably found one or more needles or pins in each. She laboured under general debility, irritative fever, and marasmus, and at length died hectic. After death many hundred pins and needles were found among the muscles and viscera.‖ Many other examples might be referred to, but these will suffice for information on the ordinary effects of mechanical irritants of the kind under consideration.

From the case of Dr. Marcet and other similar facts, it appears that large and even angular bodies do not always cause serious mischief, nay, that they have been frequently swallowed without any material injury. Dr. Marcet's sailor in the course of his life had repeatedly swallowed several clasp-knives in quick succession: and nevertheless recovered perfectly after some days of slight illness. As to prune and cherry-stones, buttons, coins, needles, pins, and the like, they have been very often taken, and even sometimes in large quantities, without any harm. It is indeed extraordinary, and almost incredible, if the facts were not authenticated beyond the possibility of a doubt, how much mechanical irritation the alimentary canal has been subjected to, without sustaining any injury. Mr. Wakefield mentions that a man, who was committed to the House of Correction, swallowed seven half-crowns, to prevent the prison authorities from depriving him of them. He suffered no inconvenience for twenty months;

* London Medical and Physical Journal, xxxv. 100.
† Observations on Surgery, 276.
‡ London Medico-Chirurgical Transactions, xii. 52.
§ Annales d'Hygiène Publique, xxi. 188.
‖ Sur les Blessures par armes de guerre, i. 82. Also, Lond. Med. Gaz. 1838-39, ii. 799.

when, after an attack of sickness, slight bowel-complaint, and general tenderness of the belly, he discharged them all at one evacuation.* Many singular instances to the same effect have been related in the various medical journals of Europe. At the head of the list, however, may be placed the following, which is related by the late Professor Osiander of Göttingen, in his work on Suicide.

A young German nobleman tried to kill himself in a fit of insanity by swallowing different indigestible substances, but without success. He never suffered any particular inconvenience except a single attack of vomiting daily, though in the course of seven months after being detected he passed the following articles by stool — 150 pieces of sharp, angular glass, some ·of them two inches long — 102 brass pins — 150 iron nails — three large hair pins, and seven large chair-nails — a pair of shirt-sleeve buttons — a collar-buckle, half of a shoe-buckle, and three bridle-buckles — half a dozen sixpenny pieces — three hooks, and a lump of lead — three large fragments of a curry-comb, and fifteen bits of nameless iron articles, many of them two inches in length.†

Before such articles occasion serious harm, it is necessary that some cause coincide, by means of which the foreign bodies are detained long in the same part of the intestines ; otherwise the irritation they produce is too trivial to excite disease.

The only substance of this kind which it is necessary to particularize is *pounded glass*. A common notion prevails that pounded glass is an active poison. There is no doubt, indeed, that it does possess some irritant properties even when finely pulverized ; for it titillates and smarts the nostrils, and inflames the eyes. There is also little doubt that when swallowed in fragments of moderate size, especially if the stomach is empty, it may wound the viscera. But it is in this way only that it has any action when swallowed, and even then its effects are by no means uniformly serious. It can have no chemical action on the stomach ; it cannot act through absorption, as it is quite insolu-ble : and when finely pulverized, it cannot easily wound the villous coat of the alimentary canal, on account of the abundance and visci-dity of the lubricating mucus.

Accordingly, M. Lesauvage ascertained that $2\frac{1}{2}$ drachms of the powder may be given to a cat at once without hurting the animal, — that in the course of eight days seven ounces might be given to a dog without any bad consequence, although the period chosen for adminis-tering it was always some time before meals, — and that even when the glass was in fragments a line in length, no symptoms of irritation were induced. Relying indeed on these results he himself swal-lowed a considerable number of similar fragments ; and did not sus-tain any injury.‡ Caldani likewise, an Italian physician, after some experiments on animals, gave a boy fifteen years old several drachms of pounded glass, without observing any bad effects ; and at his request

* London Med. Gazette, 1836-37, ii. 275.
† Ueber den Selbstmord, p. 168, from Schmucker's Vermischte Chirurgische Schriften.
‡ Diss Inaug, Paris, 1810. Analyzed in Sedillot's Journal de Méd. xxxix. 331.

Mandruzzato repeated his experiments on animals, and himself swallowed on two successive days two drachms and a half each day without sustaining any injury.[*]

Similar observations have been made by others also. Dr. Turner of Spanish Town, Jamaica, has informed me, that an attempt was made there by a negro to poison a whole family by administering pounded glass ; but, although a large quantity was taken by seven persons, none of them suffered any inconvenience. Not long ago the occurrence of a similar case at Paris gave rise to a careful investigation of the whole subject by Baudelocque and Chaussier. A young man, Lavalley, married a girl who was pregnant by him ; but it was agreed that she should live with her father till her delivery was over. A month after the marriage Lavalley invited his wife and father-in-law to dinner ; and his wife ate heartily boiled pork, bloody-sausages, and roast-veal, and subsequently drank coffee with brandy in it. On returning home in the evening she became unwell, continued so all night, next morning was seized with violent pain in the stomach and vomiting, and died in convulsions. The period of her death is not mentioned in the report I have seen. A suspicion of poisoning having arisen after burial, the body was disinterred in forty-two days ; and, although it was much decayed, black points and patches could be distinguished in many parts of the bowels, together with a quantity of broken down glass. The medical inspectors accordingly declared that she had died of poisoning with pounded-glass ; and the husband was imprisoned. Baudelocque and Chaussier, who were consulted, ascribed the black patches to putrefaction or venous congestion, and declared that in whatever way the glass had got into the bowels, she had not died of poisoning with the substance, as pounded glass is not deleterious.[†] A similar opinion as to the properties of pounded glass was more lately given by Professor Marc, when consulted on a case of attempted poisoning, in which the person against whom the attempt was made felt the rough particles in his mouth while taking the second spoonful of soup in which the glass was contained.[‡]

This opinion certainly appears to be in general true. At the same time instances are not wanting to render it probable, that pounded or broken glass is occasionally hurtful. Thus, passing over the more doubtful examples recorded by the older authors, we have the two following cases related by good authorities in the most modern times. One has been published by Mr. Hebb of Worcester. A child, eleven months old, died of a few days' illness in very suspicious circumstances. On Mr. Hebb being requested by the coroner to examine the body, he found the inside of the stomach lined with a tough layer of mucus streaked with blood ; the villous coat was highly vascular,

* Saggi scient. e litter. dell' Acad. di Padova, T. iii. P. ii. p. l, quoted in Marx, die Lehre von den Giften, I. ii. 196.

† Meyan, Causes Célèbres. Edit. 2, 1808. T. ii. 324, quoted by Marx, die Lehre von den Giften, I. ii. 298.

‡ Ann. d'Hyg. Pub. et de Méd. Lég. iii. 365.

and covered with numberless particles of glass of various sizes, some
of which simply touched, while others lacerated it ; and no other
morbid appearance could be detected in the body.* The other case
is described by Portal. A man undertook for a wager to eat his
wine-glass, and actually swallowed a part of it. But he was attacked
with acute pain in the stomach, and subsequently with convulsions.
Portal made him eat a surfeit of cabbage ; and having thus enveloped the fragments, administered an emetic, which brought away
the glass and vegetables together.§ The same feat has undoubtedly
been sometimes accomplished with impunity. For example, in the
Edinburgh Medical and Surgical Journal, an instance is related of a
man who champed and swallowed three-fourths of a drinking-glass
without suffering any harm ; and the person mentioned by Osiander
swallowed many pieces of glass, and sustained no inconvenience (p.
503). But these facts will not altogether outweigh the equally pointed
narratives of Portal and Mr. Hebb. And, on the whole, the medical
jurist must come to the conclusion, that broken and pounded glass,
though generally harmless, may sometimes prove injurious or even
fatal.‡ Powdered glass, however, is probably inert.

Another variety of injury from the mechanical irritants is inflammation from hot liquids, such as *melted lead or boiling water*. These,
when swallowed, may unquestionably cause serious mischief, and
even death ; and the symptoms they induce are exactly those of the
irritant poisons properly so called.

The effects of boiling water have been investigated experimentally
by Dr. Bretonneau of Tours ; and the results illustrate forcibly the
observations which have been repeatedly made in the course of this
work, respecting the slight constitutional derangement caused by
such poisons as have merely a local irritating power. He found that
when boiling water was injected in the quantity of eight ounces
into the stomach of dogs, it excited inflammation, passing on to
gangrene, both in the villous and muscular coats. The symptoms,
however, were trifling. For a day or two the animals appeared
languid ; but in three days they generally became lively and playful,
one of them actually lined a bitch, and it was only on strangling
them and examining the bodies, that the extent of the mischief was
discovered.§

I am not aware that any such case have hitherto occurred in man.
Death from drinking boiling water, indeed, is not an uncommon accident, particularly in Ireland and some parts of England, where
children, who are in the habit of drinking cold water from the tea-
kettle, have swallowed boiling water by mistake. It appears, however, that in these instances death is not owing to inflammation of
the gullet and stomach, but to inflammation of the upper part of the
windpipe, — the water never passing lower than the pharynx. The
best information on this subject is contained in an interesting paper

* Midland Medical and Surgical Reporter, i. 47, 1828.
† Instruction sur le Traitement des Asphyxies, &c. p. 118.
‡ Med. and Surg. Journal, xxii. 233.   § Arch. Gén. de Méd. xiii. 372.

by Dr. Hall.* He has there given the particulars of four cases which came under his notice ; from which it follows that the disease induced is always *cynanche laryngea*, proving fatal by suffocation. Two of his patients died suffocated ; another, while in imminent danger, was relieved by tracheotomy, but died afterwards of exhaustion ; the fourth recovered suddenly during a fit of screaming, when apparently about to be choked ; and it was supposed that the vesicles around the glottis had been burst by the cries.

Pouring melted lead down the throat was a frequent mode of despatching criminals and prisoners in former ages. Only one authentic case is to be found on record of death from this cause in modern times. It occurred at the burning of the Eddistone light-house. A man, while gazing up at the fire with his mouth open, received a shower of melted lead from the building, and expired after twelve days of suffering. Seven ounces and a half of lead had reached the stomach ; and the stomach was severely burnt, and ulcerated.†

In concluding the Irritant Poisons, and before proceeding to the next class, the Narcotics, it is necessary to observe, that besides the substances which have been treated of, there are others not usually considered poisons, and some that are even used daily for seasoning food, which, nevertheless, when taken in large quantities, will prove injurious and even occasion all the chief symptoms of the active irritants. These substances connect the true poisons with substances which are inert in regard to the animal economy.

It is impossible to particularize all the articles of the kind now alluded to. But in illustration, I may refer in a few words to six common substances, pepper, Epsom salt, alum, cream of tartar, sulphate of potash, and common salt.

Pepper, which is daily used by all ranks with impunity, will nevertheless cause even dangerous symptoms when taken in large quantity. In Rust's Journal is noticed the case of a man affected with a tertian ague, who after taking between an ounce and a half and two ounces of pepper in brandy, was attacked with convulsions, burning in the throat and stomach, great thirst, and vomiting of every thing he swallowed. His case was treated as one of simple gastritis, and he recovered.‡

A very striking instance, which may be arranged under the present head, has also been related to me, of apparent poisoning with Epsom salt. A boy ten years old took two ounces of this laxative partly dissolved, partly mixed in a teacupful of water ; and had hardly swallowed it before he was observed to stagger and become unwell. When the surgeon saw him half an hour after, the pulse was imperceptible, the breathing slow and difficult, the whole frame in a state of extreme debility, and in ten minutes more the child died without any other symptom of note, and in particular without any vomiting.

* London Medico-Chirurgical Transactions, xii. 1.
† Philosophical Transactions, xlix. 477, 4-3.
‡ Magazin für die gesammte Heilkunde, xxi. 549.

The circumstances having been investigated judicially, it appeared that the substance taken was pure Epsom salt ; that the father, who was doatingly fond of the child, gave the laxative on account of a trifling illness which he supposed might arise from worms ; and that on the most careful inspection of the body, no morbid appearance whatever could be found in any part of it. For the particulars of this singular case, I am indebted to Dr. Dewar of Dunfermline, the medical inspector under the sheriff's warrant. It shows that in certain circumstances even the laxative neutral salts may be irritating enough to cause speedy death.

Of the same nature probably are the cases which have lately led some to ascribe poisonous properties to *sulphate of potash*, a purgative salt at one time in common use. About three years ago several instances of apparent poisoning with this substance occurred in Paris ; and one of them proved fatal. This was the case of a woman, recently delivered, who got 100 grains every fifteen minutes till she had taken six doses. Immediately after the first dose she was seized with severe pain in the stomach, nausea, vomiting, numbness, and cramps in the arms and legs, then with dyspnœa and severe purging, and in two hours she expired. The stomach and intestines were emphysematous, but otherwise healthy ; and the stomach contained sulphate of potash, but not a trace of any of the common poisons. The stock of this salt in the shop where it had been purchased was found to be perfectly pure.* — A remarkable case of the same kind lately led to a criminal trial in London. A man Haynes was charged with attempting to procure abortion by giving his wife sulphate of potash. It was proved that on two successive evenings he gave her a dose of two ounces of the salt ; that she was seized after the first dose with excessive and alarming sickness, from which, however, she soon recovered without apparent harm ; but that after the second dose she had violent vomiting and profuse purging, of which she died in five hours, without any alteration in the symptoms, except that she became insensible for five minutes before death. The whole gastro-intestinal mucous membrane was bright red, the vessels of the brain were much congested, and between two and three ounces of blood had escaped from the neighbourhood of the occipital sinus. The salt had been swallowed in a single tumbler of water, so that part of it was undissolved. Mr. Brande, who analyzed the sample which had been used, found it free of all the ordinary irritant poisons. Mr. Coward of Hoxton, to whom I owe the particulars of this singular case, was of opinion, along with other medical gentlemen concerned in it, that death arose from apoplexy brought on by the violent and unceasing vomiting.

Another cathartic, undoubtedly in general very mild in its action, the *bitartrate of potash*, has also proved fatal, when taken in immoderate quantity. Thus, a man, endeavouring to quench his thirst and cool his stomach the morning after he had been drunk, ate a quarter of a pound of this salt in lumps at once, and a good deal more

* Annales de Hygiène Publique, 1842, xxvii. 397.

throughout the day afterwards. He was in consequence attacked with incessant vomiting, frequent purging, and other signs of irritation in the alimentary canal. He died on the third day; and the stomach and bowels were found much inflamed.[*]

Even *common salt* has been known to act as a poison when taken in large quantity. A striking instance of the kind occurred in London in September, 1828. A man, who had been in the custom of exhibiting various feats of gluttony, proposed to some of his comrades one afternoon to sup a pound of *common salt* in a pint of ale, and actually finished his nauseous dish, but not without being warned of his imprudence by an attack of vomiting in the middle of it. He was soon after seized with all the symptoms of irritant poisoning, and died within twenty-four hours. The stomach and intestines were found after death excessively inflamed.[†] This remarkable case is not without its parallel. In 1839, a girl in the North of England died in consequence of taking upwards of half a pound of salt as a vermifuge.[‡] Not long ago I met with an instance of somewhat similar, but less violent effects. A student having taken upwards of two ounces of salt as an emetic, dissolved in a small quantity of water, was seized with acute burning pain in the stomach, tenderness in the epigastrium and great anxiety, without any vomiting until he drank a large quantity of warm water as a remedy. Before I saw him he had vomited freely, but still suffered severe, intermitting pain, which was removed by a large dose of muriate of morphia.

In France, though not hitherto, so far as I know, in Britain, several instances have occurred of extensive sickness in particular districts, which have been traced to the accidental adulteration of *common salt* with certain deleterious articles. In an investigation conducted by M. Guibourt, in consequence of several severe accidents having been produced apparently by salt in Paris and at Meaux, oxide of arsenic was detected;[§] and this discovery was subsequently confirmed by MM. Latour and Lefrançois, who ascertained that the proportion of arsenic was sometimes a quarter of a grain per ounce.[‖] Another singular adulteration which appears fully more frequent is with hydriodate of soda. At a meeting of the Parisian Academy of Medicine in December, 1829, a report was read by MM. Boullay and Delens, subsequent to an inquiry by M. Sérullas, into the nature of a sample of salt which appears to have occasioned very extensive ravages. In 1829, various epidemic sicknesses in certain parishes were suspected to have arisen from salt of bad quality. In the month of July no less than 150 persons in two parishes were attacked, some with pain in the stomach, nausea, slimy and even bloody purging, others with tension of the belly, puffiness of the face, inflammation of the eyes and swelling of the legs; and in several parishes in the Department of the Marne a sixth part of the population was similarly affected. The salt being suspected to be the source of the mischief,

---

[*] London Med Gazette, 1837-38, i. 177.
[†] London Courier, Oct. 1, 1828.   [‡] London Med. Gazette, 1839-40, i. 559.
[§] Journal de Chim. Méd. vi. 265.   [‖] Ibidem, vi. 458.

as it had an unusual smell which some compared to the effluvia of marshy ground, M. Sérullas analyzed it, and after him MM. Boullay and Delens; and both analyses indicated the presence of a hundredth of its weight of hydriodate of soda, besides a little free iodine.[*] Subsequently, in reference to the discovery of arsenic by other chemists in different samples of suspected salt, M. Sérullas repeated his analysis, but could detect none of that poison.[†] Still more lately the whole subject has been investigated with great care by M. Chevallier.[‡] M. Barruel states that he observed the occasional adulteration of salt with some hydriodate accidentally in 1824, while preparing experiments for Professor Orfila's lectures. He found it in two samples from different grocers' shops in Paris.[§] No satisfactory explanation has yet been given of the source of the adulteration with arsenic; but the presence of hydriodate of soda has been traced to the fraudulent use of impure salt from kelp [see p. 160].

Some difference of opinion prevails among toxicologists in regard to the alleged deleterious qualities of *alum*. On the whole it scarcely appears so active as to deserve the name of a poison; yet, like other salts, it may in large doses do serious injury. It merits particular mention among the present description of substances, partly on account of a trial at Paris, where dangerous effects were alleged to have been produced by it, and partly for the physiological inquiries made on that occasion. A druggist supplied a lady by mistake with powder of burnt alum instead of gum-arabic; and the lady, who had long laboured under chronic derangement of the stomach and bowels, took a single dose of a solution containing between ten and twenty grains of the salt. She immediately complained of acute pain in the stomach and gullet, burning in the mouth, and nausea; the symptoms of a severe attack of inflammation in the stomach and bowels ensued; and she was not considered out of danger for several days. The druggist was accordingly prosecuted, and heavy damages claimed. The attending physician ascribed the symptoms to the alum. But Marc and Orfila, who were consulted, declared that this was impossible except on the supposition that the lady had a very unusual sensibility of the stomach to irritating substances; — that it was a common thing to give three, four, and even five times the quantity in the treatment of diseases, without any such consequences resulting; — and that at the very time of the inquiry a physician in Paris was using it to the amount of six or eight drachms in a day. From an experimental inquiry conducted by Professor Orfila it appears, that large doses of calcined alum, such as one or even two ounces, excite in dogs little more than one or two attacks of vomiting, even although retained between ten and thirty minutes, — that one ounce will not excite any marked symptoms though secured in the stomach by a ligature, — but that two ounces given in the same way prove fatal in five hours, under symptoms of

---

[*] Archives Gén. de Méd. xxi. 616, or Journ. de Chim. Méd. v. 621, and vi. 63.
[†] Journal de Pharmacie, xvi. 322, or Journ. de Chim. Méd. vi. 263.
[‡] Annales d'Hyg. Publique et de Méd. Légale, viii. 25.
[§] Journal de Chim. Med. iv. 275.

46

excessive exhaustion and insensibility.* A similar inquiry was instituted about the same time by M. Devergie, who seems, however, to have remarked more activity in alum than is indicated by Orfila's experiments. He infers that two ounces may sometimes kill dogs, even though they vomit freely; that half that quantity is fatal if the gullet be tied; that calcined alum is more active than a solution of the salt; that it is a corrosive or irritant; and that probably man is more sensible to its operation than the lower animals.† Whatever may be thought of the effects of alum on the animal body when administered in large doses, it is plain from its frequent medicinal use as an internal astringent that it is not poisonous when given in small doses, like that taken by the patient in the trial alluded to. I may add that it appears very doubtful whether any injury accrues from the long-continued use of very small doses. Bakers, it is well known, are in the practice of using it in minute proportion for improving the whiteness of bread; and it has been imagined that chronic disorders of the stomach and bowels may consequently originate, by reason of its constipating tendency. These fears, however, are not borne out by facts. Either the quantity is insufficient to do harm in the way supposed; or the constitution becomes accustomed to the continual operation of the salt, and does not suffer.

CHAPTER XXIV.

CLASS SECOND.

OF NARCOTIC POISONS GENERALLY.

The term narcotism has been used by different writers with different significations, but is now generally understood to denote the effects of such poisons as bring on a state of the system like that caused by apoplexy, epilepsy, tetanus, and other disorders commonly called nervous. Narcotic poisons, therefore, are such as produce chiefly or solely symptoms of a disorder of the nervous system.

The mode in which most narcotic poisons act has been well ascertained: they act on the brain or spine or both by entering the blood-vessels. Hence they are most active when most directly introduced into the blood, that is, when injected into the veins; and when they are applied to an entire membranous surface, their energy is in the ratio of its absorbing power. Thus, when injected into the chest, they act more rapidly than when swallowed. According to the generally received opinion, they are conveyed with the blood to the brain and spine on which they act. But, according to the views of Messrs. Morgan and Addison, they produce on the inner coats of the blood-vessels a peculiar impression, which is conveyed to the centre of the nervous system along the nerves.

* Annales d'Hyg. Publique et de Med. Légale, i. 235.
† Dictionnaire de Méd. et Chirurg. Pratiques, v. 124.

The usual symptoms in man and the higher order of animals are giddiness, headache, obscurity or deprivation of the sight, stupor or perfect insensibility, palsy of the voluntary muscles or convulsions of various kinds, and towards the close complete coma. The symptoms of each poison are pretty uniform, when the dose is the same. But each has its own peculiarities, either in the individual symptoms, or in the mode in which they are combined together.

The morbid appearances they leave in the dead body are commonly insignificant. In the brain, where chiefly the physician is led from the symptoms to expect unnatural appearances, the organs are in general quite healthy. Sometimes, however, the veins are gorged with blood, and the ventricles and membranes contain serosity. The blood appears to be sometimes altered in nature ; but the alteration is by no means invariable, and sometimes none is remarked at all. Many of the statements to be found in authors on the morbid appearances caused by narcotics are far from being accurate.

Before proceeding to notice the genera of this class in their order, some remarks must be premised on the principal diseases which resemble them in the symptoms and morbid appearances. Of these the only diseases of much consequence are *apoplexy, epilepsy inflammation of the brain, hypertrophy of the brain, inflammation of the spinal cord, and syncopal asphyxia.*

Of the Distinction between Apoplexy and Narcotic Poisoning.

Of the Symptoms. — The symptoms of apoplexy are almost exactly the same as those of the narcotic poisons, namely, more or less complete abolition of sense and the power of motion, frequently combined with convulsions. This disease commonly arises from congestion or effusion of blood within the skull ; but one variety of it, the nervous apoplexy of older authors, or simple apoplexy of the moderns, is believed to be an affection of the brain, unaccompanied by any recognizable derangement of structure.

Apoplexy and narcotic poisoning may be often distinguished by the following criterions :

1. Apoplexy is sometimes preceded at considerable intervals by warning symptoms, such as giddiness, headache, ringing in the ears, depraved vision, or partial palsy. But it is an error to suppose that warning symptoms always occur ; nay, if we may trust the experience of M. Rochoux, they are by no means common : of sixty-three cases which came under his notice nine only had distinct precursory symptoms.* Poisoning with narcotics of course has not any precursory symptom except by fortuitous combination. And consequently, if warning symptoms have occurred, the presumption is, that the cause of death is a natural one.

2. Apoplexy attacks chiefly the old. It is not, however, confined to the old. On the trial of Captain Donnellan for poisoning Sir T. Boughton, Mr. John Hunter mentioned that he had met with two in-

* Recherches sur l'Apoplexie, p. 70.

stances of death from apoplexy in young women : my colleague Dr. Alison has related to me a similar case; Professor Bernt has described another of a young girl who died apoplectic from extravasation of blood over the whole brain and in the ventricles also ;[*] and Mr. Greenhow, a surgeon of London, has even noticed a case of apoplexy from effusion of blood over the surface of the brain in a child two years and a half old.[†] On this subject the treatise of Rochoux supplies excellent information : of his sixty-three cases sixty-one were above thirty years of age, two less than thirty, none younger than twenty.[‡] It is plain, therefore, that apoplexy in young people is rare. On the other hand, a great proportion of cases of poisoning with the narcotics when they have been taken intentionally (and such cases are most likely to lead to medico-legal questions), has occurred among the young, especially of the female sex.

3. The next criterion is, that apoplexy occurs chiefly among fat people. But it is here mentioned only that the medical jurist may be cautioned against the belief that it is in all circumstances a correct criterion. Upon this particular Rochoux has furnished some satisfactory data. Among his sixty-three patients thirty were of an ordinary habit, twenty-three were of a thin, meager habit, and ten only were large, plethoric and fat.[§] In receiving this statement, however, it is necessary to consider, that although the vulgar idea, that most apoplectic people are fat, does not apply to persons in the rank of Rochoux's patients, who were mostly hospital inmates, yet it may apply better to the upper ranks. For the same circumstances which predispose to apoplexy, namely, great strength, vigorous constitution and good digestive powers, likewise predispose to corpulency, so that whenever the condition of life permits the disposition to corpulency to be developed, the connexion of apoplexy with it will appear.

4. A fourth criterion is drawn from the relation which the appearance of the symptoms bears to the last article of food or drink that was taken. I believe that the effects of the common narcotics, in the cases where they prove fatal, begin not later than an hour, or at the utmost two hours, after they are taken ; and in a great majority of instances they begin in a much shorter time, namely, in fifteen or thirty minutes. Hence if it can be proved that the nervous symptoms, under which a person died, did not begin till several hours after he took food, drink or medicine, it appears almost, if not absolutely certain, that a narcotic poison cannot have been the cause of death. To some narcotic, or rather narcotico-acrid poisons this rule certainly will not apply, such as the poisonous fungi and spurred rye ; which seldom begin to act for several hours, sometimes for not less than a day and a half. Neither will the rule apply to poisoning with the deleterious gases, as their action has no connexion at all with eating or drinking. But these facts do not form a material objection to the rule laid down ; because the circumstances

[*] Beiträge zur Gerichtlichen Arzneikunde, iii. 40.
[†] London Medical and Physical Journal, xlvii. 181.
[‡] Recherches sur l'Apoplexie, 212.   [§] Ibidem, p. 214.

under which cases of the kind occur are generally so apparent, as at once to point out their real nature to a careful inquirer.

In regard to apoplexy as the disease which resembles most closely the effects of the narcotics, it was formerly stated that this disease is apt to occur soon or immediately after taking a meal (p. 95).* In the greater number of such cases, however, where the meal has been the exciting cause of the disease, the symptoms have begun *immediately* after, or even during a meal. This is very rarely the case with the symptoms of narcotic poisoning, and never happens in respect to those of the commonest of the narcotics, opium : An interval of 10, 15, 20 or 30 minutes always occurs. The deleterious gases and hydrocyanic acid, with its compounds, are the only familiar narcotic poisons which act more swiftly.

5. Another criterion relates to the progress of the symptoms. The symptoms of narcotic poisoning advance for the most part gradually : but those of apoplexy in general begin abruptly. Sometimes apoplexy commences at once with deep sopor. Narcotic poisoning never begins in that way, except in the instances of hydrocyanic acid and the narcotic gases ; the sopor is at first imperfect, and it increases gradually, though sometimes very rapidly. Apoplexy, however, does not always begin with deep sopor ; occasionally the sopor begins and increases like that of narcotism.

6. Although there is a great resemblance between the symptoms of apoplexy and those of narcotism, so far as regards their general features, there are particulars which are not indeed always present, but which when present will help to distinguish the one from the other. When the sopor of apoplexy is completely formed, it is rarely possible to rouse the patient to consciousness, and never, I believe, where the risk of confounding apoplexy with poisoning is greatest, — in the cases where death happens neither instantly, nor after the interval of a day, but in a few hours. On the other hand, in many cases of poisoning with the narcotics, and particularly with the commonest variety, opium, the person may be roused from the deepest lethargy, if he is spoken to in a loud voice, or forcibly shaken for some time, or if water is injected into his ear. Even in cases of poisoning with opium, however, the coma may have continued too long to admit of this temporary restoration to sense ; the susceptibility of being roused is not so often remarked in other varieties of narcotic poisoning ; and in some, such as poisoning with prussic acid, I am not aware that it has ever been remarked, at least in fatal cases.

There are some other symptoms which in special cases may help to distinguish narcotic poisoning from apoplexy. Thus in poisoning

* Instances of congestive apoplexy thus arising were then quoted. I may here add a very opposite instance of hemorrhagic apoplexy, occurring in similar circumstances. Dr Jennings, an American physician, mentions the case of a female fifty years of age, who, after a full meal, tumbled down in a fit of insensibility and immediately expired, and in whom after death there was found enormous distension of the stomach with food, an extensive effusion of blood into the central parts of the brain, and ossification of the cerebral arteries. (London Med. Gazette, xvi. 735.)

with opium convulsions are rare ; in apoplexy they are common enough. Bloating of the countenance is likewise much more common in apoplexy than in poisoning with opium. In apoplexy, too, the pupil is generally dilated, while in poisoning with opium the pupil is almost always contracted. But such distinctions do not apply either to the narcotics as a class, or to all cases of any one kind of narcotic poisoning.

7. In the last place, a useful criterion may be derived from the duration of the symptoms in fatal cases. I believe few people die of pure narcotic poisoning who outlive twelve hours ; and the greater number die much sooner, — in eight, or six hours. Apoplexy often lasts a whole day, or even longer. On the other hand, the narcotic poisons very rarely prove so rapidly fatal as apoplexy sometimes does. Apoplexy, according to the vulgar opinion, may prove fatal instantly or in a few minutes. The only late author of repute who maintains that opinion is M. Devergie. He mentions the case of an elderly man subject to somnolency, who, after complaining for a short time of headache, became suddenly pale, hung down his head, and expired immediately, and in whose body no other morbid appearance was found, except great congestion of the cerebral membranes.* The best modern pathologists, however, deny that apoplexy proves immediately fatal, and maintain with much apparent reason that when death is so sudden, the cause is commonly disease of the heart, and not apoplexy.† However this may be, it is at all events certain that apoplexy may occasion death in considerably less than an hour. Now the only narcotics in common use which can prove fatal so soon are the narcotic gases, and prussic acid. As to opium, the most common of the narcotic poisons, and by far the most important to the medical jurist, the shortest duration I have yet seen recorded is three hours. Apoplexy often proves fatal in a much shorter time.

From this enumeration of the criterions between apoplexy and the symptoms produced by narcotics, the toxicologist will conclude, that few cases can occur in which he will not be able to give a presumptive opinion of the real cause from the symptoms only, — that in many instances a diagnosis may be drawn with an approach to certainty, — and that on all occasions it will be possible to say without risk of error, whether there are materials for forming a diagnosis at all, — a point which is of great moment when the criterions are not universally applicable.

Of the Morbid Appearances. — The next subject of inquiry is the distinction between apoplexy and narcotic poisoning, as to the appearances after death. It has been already stated, that the narcotic poisons rarely produce very distinct morbid appearances, — that the greatest extent of unnatural appearance they cause in the brain is congestion of vessels, — and that the physical qualities of the blood appear to be altered, though not invariably.

* Annales d'Hygiène Publique. xx. 170.
† Rochoux, Recherches sur l'Apoplexie, 66.

Of Simple Apoplexy. — Apoplexy may, in the first place, occasion death without leaving any sign at all in the dead body. Cases of this sort were called nervous apoplexy by the older authors ; but for the purpose of avoiding a name that involves a theory as to their nature, they have been more appropriately termed by Dr. Abercrombie simple apoplexy. At one time they were believed to be common. The researches of modern pathologists, however, have shown that they are rare, and that the apparent absence of morbid appearances may be often with justice ascribed to an insufficient examination ; for it is not always easy to detect, without minute attention, two disorders little known till in recent times, and sometimes closely allied in their symptoms to apoplexy, — hypertrophy of the brain, and inflammation of its substance. On this account some have even gone so far as to deny altogether the existence of simple or nervous apoplexy ; and M. Rostan, who is of this opinion, has supported it by the fact, that in the course of his pathological researches he had examined no less than 4000 heads, and never met with an instance of it.* But although this statement, made by so eminent a pathologist, is sufficient to prove the rarity of the disease, it does not establish its non-existence in the face of positive observations, made by others after the phenomena and effects of cerebral inflammation were well known.

Among the modern authorities to whom reference may here be made for examples of simple apoplexy, Dr. Abercrombie, M. Louis, my colleague Dr. Alison, and M. Lobstein, may be particularized. Dr. Abercrombie has seen four cases,[†] M. Louis has recorded three,[‡] M. Lobstein one,[§] and Dr. Alison informs me, that he has seen one and got the particulars of another from the late Dr. Gregory. In several of these cases the individuals were at the time of the apoplectic seizure affected with other diseases, such as asthma, anasarca, or slight febrile symptoms ; but in four of them the coma commenced during a state of perfect health. I have myself seen two of the former class, one occurring during convalescence from a slight pleurisy, the other terminating a complicated case of pulmonary emphysema and catarrh, diseased kidneys and anasarca. Reference may be also made under this head to several cases of apoplexy described in Corvisart's Journal, as connected with the enormous accumulation of worms in the intestines. Such a connexion is said to be common on the coast of Brittany ; and one striking instance is related of a young man, who, after an attack of headache, vomiting, and loss of speech, died comatose in two days, and in whose body no unnatural appearance could be seen except a prodigious mass of worms in the small intestines.[||]

In none of all the cases of apoplexy now under consideration was

* Recherches sur le Ramollissement du Cerveau, p. 150.
† Pathological and Practical Researches on Diseases of the Brain, p. 210.
‡ Recherches Pathologiques, 460, 466, and 472.
§ Archives Gén. de Méd. xxiii. 260.
|| Journal de Médecine. xiii. 315.

there found within the head any appearance corresponding with the symptoms, except occasionally a slight turgescence of vessels.

This form of apoplexy, then, is a very important affection in a medico-legal point of view. The possibility of its occurrence is in fact the chief obstacle, which, in many cases involving the question of poisoning with narcotics, prevents the physician from coming to a positive decision on a review merely of symptoms and appearances after death. Instances will occur where it is impossible to draw a diagnosis between the natural and the violent form of death. And indeed it might even be a fair subject of inquiry, whether death from at least some narcotic poisons, such as opium, is any thing else than death from simple apoplexy.

It may be mentioned, — although too much importance ought not to be attached to the fact, as forming the ground of a diagnosis in certain rapid cases of narcotic poisoning, — that of the instances of simple apoplexy referred to above none proved fatal in less than five hours. This was Dr. Gregory's case. Dr. Alison's proved fatal in seven hours; M. Louis's cases in eight, nine, and ten hours; one of Dr. Abercrombie's in eight hours; the three others in about twenty-four hours; and M. Lobstein's in five days.

Another consideration is, that simple apoplexy is undoubtedly very rare, more particularly in persons who enjoy perfect health. Hence, although it is impossible to distinguish the effects of narcotics from this disease by the appearances in the body after death, yet, when the general evidence of poisoning is strong, and none of the medical circumstances are at variance with the supposition of narcotic poisoning, the evidence of poisoning, as judged of by the jury from the whole facts, medical and general, will be commonly sufficient, — so far as regards the possibility of death from simple apoplexy. For such a concurrence of circumstances as is here supposed can scarcely be outweighed by a mere possibility of death from so rare a natural disease.

It is worthy of remark, in reference to charges and suspicions of poisoning during a state of ill health, that simple apoplexy occurring in the course of a considerable period of indifferent health is far from uncommon. Such incidents, however, ought not to be confounded with narcotic poisoning, because the coma comes on gradually. From what I have myself frequently observed, cases of this nature are often connected with the granular disintegration of the kidneys, which has been brought under the notice of physicians by the able researches of Dr. Bright. I have related two instances of the kind,* and several others have been since published by Dr. James Arthur Wilson.† In none of these could there have been any risk of mistaking the phenomena for narcotic poisoning. But it may be well to advert to the subject here for the sake of turning the attention of the profession to the propriety of examining the state of the kidneys in all medico-legal cases of death in a state of coma.

* Edin. Med. and Surg. Journal, xxxii. 262.
† London Med. Gazette, xi. 777.

Of Congestive Apoplexy. — Apoplexy may, in the second place, leave in the dead body no other sign but congestion of vessels within the head. This form or variety of apoplexy is so generally admitted, that it is hardly necessary to mention special instances. But, for the sake of those who may prefer special facts to general propositions, the two following cases by M. Rostan are referred to. One of his patients, without any precursory symptom, was suddenly deprived of sense, soon became delirious and comatose, and expired in a day and a half. The other, also without any previous symptom, became rapidly comatose, and died in twenty-four hours. In both the whole membranes were minutely injected with blood ; and in one the whole brain had also a rose-red colour.* In regard to the diagnosis between such cases and poisoning with narcotics, it must be remembered, that congestion of the cerebral vessels is considered by many a common effect of such poisons, and that therefore the diagnosis cannot be rested on the appearances in the dead body. I have not perused a sufficient number of fatal cases of congestive apoplexy to enable me to attempt a diagnosis ; but, so far as I have gone, it appears to me, that this form of the disease, which is not often fatal without extravasation also being produced, does not cause death till after an interval of nearly a day at least. Should this prove a general fact, it would form the ground of a diagnosis between congestive apoplexy and many forms of narcotic poisoning, which, if death ensues, prove fatal much sooner.

Of Serous Apoplexy. — Apoplexy may, in the third place, produce serous effusion on the external surface, and in the ventricles of the brain. This form of the disease, which has been named serous apoplexy, although not very uncommon as an insulated affection, is for the most part united with inflammation of the cerebral substance. Serous effusion is more frequently the termination of an inflammatory disorder of the brain, than of that deranged state which constitutes the apoplectic attack. But nevertheless it does occur in connexion with pure apoplexy, as may be seen, for example, on referring to Dr. Abercrombie's work,† or to Bernt's Contributions to Medical Jurisprudence,‡ or to the Hospital Reports of Dr. Bright.§ In such cases the only appearances have been the effusion of an unusual quantity of serum on the surface of the brain, in its ventricles, and in the base of the skull. Cases of this sort agree very exactly as to the signs in the dead body with some cases of narcotic poisoning. When serous effusion is preceded by decided apoplectic symptoms, the disease, so far as I have been able to inquire, is always of several days' duration. But sometimes the symptoms are to the very last obscure and different from those of apoplexy, as in an instance related by Dr. Abercrombie.||

Of Apoplexy from extravasation. — The last variety of apoplexy

* Recherches sur le Ramollissement du Cerveau, p. 133 and 135.
† Pathological Researches, 214
‡ Beiträge zur gerichtl. Arzneik. ii. 61, iii. 42, iv. 42.
§ Reports of Medical Cases, ii. 240, 242, 244. || Pathological Researches, 216.

is that which leaves in the dead body extravasation of blood within the head. This, the most common of all its forms, is very rarely imitated by narcotic poisoning. A case, however, will be afterwards mentioned of extravasation produced apparently by poisoning with opium, another of extravasation caused by carbonic acid, another by poisonous fungus, and several by spirits. The existence, therefore; of extravasated blood is not absolutely certain proof, but supplies, in relation to most narcotics, a strong presumption of natural death.

Here it will be necessary to add a word or two of caution regarding what are called apoplectic cells or cavities, containing blood in the brain. If an apoplectic cell be found, it must not be at once considered as the cause of death. When blood is extravasated in the brain, the patient may gradually recover altogether, and the cell nevertheless continue full. Such persons often die of a subsequent attack of apoplexy, or of inflammation around the cell. We can say with certainty, that an apoplectic cell has been the occasion of death only when the blood is recent, or when it is surrounded by signs of recent inflammation.

So much, then, as to the criterions derived from morbid appearances within the skull, for distinguishing poisoning with narcotics from apoplexy.

It has been proposed to derive other criterions from the state of the blood. But on considering the effects of the individual poisons of the class, it will appear that the state of the blood is by no means characteristic.

It may be useful to conclude this view of the distinctions between poisoning and apoplexy with the particulars of an interesting case, in which the medical witnesses fell into an egregious error by disregarding the most palpable criterions. In 1841, an elderly gentleman at Chambéry in France, subject to apoplexy, one day after having made a hearty dinner and afterwards supped on bread, cheese, and white wine, was suddenly seized with staggering immediately after finishing his wine, and soon lost all consciousness. Emetics and stimulants restored his faculties so far as to enable him to say he felt better and had no pain; but the tongue and mouth were drawn to the left side, and there was great prostration. Four hours after his first seizure the countenance became livid; he again became unconscious and insensible; the twisting of the mouth increased; and the left arm presented spasmodic contraction. Blood-letting and other remedies were resorted to without avail; the pulse, previously strong and regular, became gradually feeble; and in six hours after his first illness he expired, without ever having had convulsions of any kind. On the body being examined seven days after death, great congestion was found in the vessels on the surface of the brain; on raising the brain, a dense dark clot of the size of a large egg escaped from the lower part of the ventricles; and an abundant extravasation of the same nature was found under the *tentorium cerebelli*.

It appears scarcely possible to find a more characteristic case than this of apoplexy from extravasation. The slight intermission in the symptoms was the only unusual circumstance. Yet because the inspectors remarked in various parts of the body a peculiar odour, which they could not at the time characterise, but which they afterwards thought was the odour of bitter almonds, — and misled by the sudden invasion of the symptoms instantly after a meal, — they gave their opinion that death had arisen from some narcotic poison ; a chemical examination was made of various textures of the body (not, however, of the contents of the stomach), which yielded obscure and very doubtful indications of hydrocyanic acid ; poisoning with hydrocyanic acid was accordingly declared to have been the cause of death ; and, in defiance of an able report by Professor Orfila, pointing out the error of the primary witnesses, the nephew and heir of the deceased was condemned.* It is almost unnecessary to point out the impossibility of death having arisen in this case from hydrocyanic acid. The length of time the deceased survived, the want of convulsions, the presence of deflexion of the mouth and tongue, the intermission of the symptoms, and the morbid appearances, all clearly indicate that death in the way supposed was impossible ; and the chemical evidence, which it would require too much space to analyze here, was proved by Orfila to be completely unsatisfactory.

Of the Distinction between Epilepsy and Narcotic Poisoning.

Of the Symptoms. — Epilepsy is distinguished from other diseases by the abolition of sense and by convulsions. It resembles closely the symptoms caused by prussic acid, and by some of the narcotic gases, such as carbonic acid gas and the asphyxiating gas of privies. It also bears the same resemblance to the effects of many narcotico-acrid poisons, such as belladonna, stramonium, hemlock, and others of the first group of that class, also camphor, cocculus indicus, and the poisonous fungi.

Epilepsy is in general a chronic disease, and for the most part ends slowly in insanity. But sometimes it proves fatal during a paroxysm. The circumstances by which an epileptic fit may be distinguished from narcotic poisoning are the following :

1. The epileptic fit *is sometimes preceded by certain warnings*, such as stupor, a sense of coldness, or creeping, or of a gentle breeze proceeding from a particular part of the body towards the head. Warnings, however, are by no means universal. M. Georget, indeed, has even stated that they do not occur in more than five cases in the hundred.† But this estimate probably underrates their frequency.

2. The symptoms of the epileptic fit *almost always begin violently and abruptly.* The individual is suddenly observed to cry out, often to vomit, and instantly falls down in convulsions. The effects of the narcotic poisons, if we except some cases of poisoning with hydrocyanic acid, the narcotic gases, and a few rare alkaloids, never begin otherwise than gradually, though their progress towards their extreme

* Annales d'Hygiène-Publique, 1841, xxvi. 399.
† Article Epilepsie in Dictionnaire de Médecine, viii. 209.

of violence is often rapid. This distinction is generally an excellent
one.   But it will not apply so well to some cases of epilepsy in which
the convulsions are trivial.   Esquirol says an epileptic fit may consist of nothing more than coma, with convulsive movements of the
eyes, or lips, or chest, or a single finger.*   Still even then the coma
generally begins abruptly, so that if the case is seen from the beginning, it can hardly be mistaken for narcotic poisoning.   Some forms
of epilepsy, in which the fit is constituted merely by giddiness, staring,
wandering of the mind, and imperfect loss of recollection,† might be
confounded with the milder forms of narcotic poisoning.   But collateral circumstances will scarcely ever be wanting to distinguish such
cases from one another.

The varieties of narcotic poisoning which, in the violence and ab-
ruptness of their commencement, bear the closest resemblance to an
epileptic attack, are some cases of poisoning with hydrocyanic acid
or with the deleterious gases.   Both of these varieties, however,
when they begin so abruptly, are distinguished from a fatal paroxysm
of epilepsy by the fourth characteristic to be mentioned presently ; and
besides, in abrupt cases of poisoning with hydrocyanic acid, the poison under certain conditions will be found in the body ; while in
sudden poisoning with the narcotic gases, the nature of the accident
is rendered obvious to a cautious inquirer by the collateral circumstances.

3. As in apoplexy, so in epilepsy the patient *in general cannot be
roused* by external stimuli.   This, as already observed, is often, although certainly not always, practicable in cases of poisoning with
narcotics.   Sometimes, too, in the epileptic fit a partial restoration
of consciousness may be effected by loud speaking, so that in reply
to questions the patient will roll his eyes or move his lips.   It is
therefore to be understood in applying the present criterion, that it is
only a safe guide when, as in many cases of poisoning with opium,
the individual can be roused to a state of tolerably perfect consciousness.

4. When a person dies in a fit of epilepsy, *the paroxysm generally
lasts long*, sometimes more than a day.   So far as I have been able
to ascertain (though on this point it must be confessed authors are
singularly silent), it never proves fatal in a shorter time than several
hours, unless there have been many previous fits ; and even then it
rarely proves fatal more rapidly.   I have met with a case which,
after many previous fits, proved fatal in little more than an hour.‡   In
an instance mentioned by Mr. Clifton of irregularly recurring epilepsy,
the patient after being exempt for four months was attacked twice
a day for four days, and during an interval of ease fell down in the
street and died.   General congestion and excessive softening of the
brain were found.§   I have met with a case very like this, where
death was owing to enormous extravasation of blood into the ventricles.

* Diction. de Med. xii. 512.   † Georget, *in loco cit.* 212.
‡ The body in this case was not examined.
§ Edin. Med. and Surg. Journal, x. 40.

So rapid a termination never occurs except after several paroxysms ; and probably never without well-marked appearances in the dead body. The variety of poisoning with which epilepsy is most apt to be confounded, poisoning with hydrocyanic acid, has hitherto always proved fatal within three-quarters of an hour, and can probably never prove fatal so late as a whole hour after the symptoms begin, unless the dose has been small and given repeatedly. Poisoning with the gas of privies, — another variety, which sometimes imitates precisely a fit of epilepsy, appears not to prove fatal in its convulsive form later than two hours after the exposure.

5. M. Esquirol, a writer of high authority, says that epilepsy *very rarely proves fatal in the first paroxysm.* I suspect it may be said that the first paroxysm never proves fatal. For the cases considered and described as such have been either inflammation of the brain or its membranes, or hypertrophy of the brain, or inflammation of the spinal cord, or effusion of serum or blood into the spinal canal, or worms in the intestines, — all of which may be known by the morbid appearances. I have also seen cases of continued fever with typhomania and convulsions, which might have been considered by a careless observer examples of epilepsy fatal in the first fit. On the present characteristic it would be wrong to speak with confidence, as the question regarding the possible fatality of epilepsy in the first fit must depend greatly on the degree of extension given to the term epilepsy. I can only say, that in the course of reading I have not hitherto met with an instance fatal in the first paroxysm, which might not have been referred by the morbid appearances to one or other of the diseases mentioned above.

Of the Morbid Appearances. — With regard to the morbid appearances found in the bodies of epileptics, much difference of opinion prevails among pathologists. The most frequent are tumours within the cranium, excrescences from the bone or dura mater, concretions in the brain itself, or abscesses there, and effusion into the ventricles or on the surface of the brain. Other appearances which have also been remarked are probably little connected with the disease ; and at all events have been often seen when epilepsy did not precede death.*

The morbid appearances connected with epilepsy are not always to be looked for within the head. The cause which produces the fit is often some irritation in distant organs. — The presence of worms in the intestines of children may occasion fatal epilepsy. It is believed also that they may cause fatal epilepsy even in adults ; and whether their presence has been the cause of death or not, it is certain that they have been found enormously accumulated in the stomach or intestines of adult epileptic subjects.† The most recent information on this subject is furnished by M. Gaultier de Claubry. In a girl seven years old, who died of convulsions in six days, he found eleven *lumbrici* in the general cavity of the belly, and the coats

* Esquirol, Dict. des Sciences Méd. xii. 528.
† Corvisart's Journ. de Méd. xiii. 315, and xl. 81 ; also Prost, la Médecine éclairée par l'ouverture des cadavres, ii. 382, 389, 394.

47

of the stomach perforated with holes, in some of which other worms were sticking.   In another child of the same age, who died in seven days of convulsions, he found thirty-six worms in the peritoneal sac, a great mass of them in the stomach, and twenty-seven making their way through holes in its coats.*   In a singular case related by M. Lepelletier of a boy twelve years old, who died of convulsions in four days, the only morbid appearance found was a perforation of the gullet six lines in diameter, through which two lumbrici had made their way into a cavity in the middle right lobe of the lungs, while another was sticking in the hole, six more occupied the lower part of the gullet, and three lay in the stomach.† — The irritation of teething may also excite epilepsy, and in cases where it has proved fatal may be recognized by the redness and swelling of the gum, by the tooth being on the point of piercing the alveolar process, and by the turgescence of vessels around.‡ — A well-known but rather rare cause is the presence of some hard substance in the course of a nerve. This variety, like those already mentioned, may prove fatal in the fit, as appears from the following interesting case.   A stout young woman became suddenly liable to epilepsy, and, after suffering repeated fits in the course of twenty months, died comatose in a paroxysm of thirty-three hours' duration.   The fits having always begun with acute pain in a particular part of the thigh, this part of the body was carefully examined, and a bony tumour as big as a nut was found on a branch of the sciatic nerve.§ — Other appearances might likewise be here enumerated, which have been supposed the cause of symptomatic epilepsy.‖   But few of these have been so thoroughly ascertained as to be allowed much influence on a medico-legal opinion.

It cannot, I apprehend, be denied, that in many cases of epilepsy no decided morbid appearance is to be found in the body; and that in many others the appearances are either so equivocal as not to be satisfactorily recognized in any circumstances, or so hidden in their situation that they may escape notice, unless the inspector's attention be drawn to the particular spot by a knowledge of the symptoms.

Hence in actual questions as to the occurrence of narcotic poisoning when the symptoms resemble epilepsy, it will be seldom possible to found on the absence of morbid appearances more than a presumptive opinion that death did not proceed from the natural cause.   It is right to remember, however, that in considering the absence of morbid appearances in reference to the diagnosis of narcotic poisoning and epilepsy, the attention should be confined to cases of epilepsy which prove fatal during the fit.   Now I suspect no such case ever occurs, at least in adults, without an adequate cause being discoverable in the dead body, either in the head, or in the course of some nerve, or in the accumulation of worms in the intestines.   This statement must not be considered as made with confidence; but it deserves investigation.

* Nouveau Journal de Médecine, ii. 269.
† Journal Hebdomadaire et Universel, iv. 366.
‡ Portal, Observations sur la nature et le traitement de l'Epilepsie, p. 65 and 67.
§ Memozie della Soc. Méd. di Genova, i. 89.   ‖ Portal, *passim.*

From all that has now been said on the subject of epilepsy as a disease which imitates many varieties of narcotic poisoning, the medical jurist will probably arrive at the conclusion, that, although a diagnosis cannot always be drawn with certainty, yet in numerous cases the consideration of the symptoms and appearances after death will enable him to say positively that poisoning is out of the question, and in many others that poisoning is highly probable.

Of the Distinction between Meningitis and Narcotic Poisoning.

Inflammation of the inner membranes of the brain, which constitutes the *acute hydrocephalus* or acute *meningitis* of authors, is not in general apt to cause much ambiguity ; for its progress is commonly gradual, well-marked and less rapid than most cases of narcotic poisoning : and the appearances in the dead body, such as effusion of serum, lymph or pus on the outer surface of the brain or in the ventricles, are for the most part obvious.

Dr. Abercrombie, however, has described a form of it occurring among children during the existence of other diseases, particularly of the chest, which might be the cause of perplexity ; for its course is sometimes finished within a day, its symptoms are delirium, convulsions and coma intermingled, and the only morbid appearance is congestion of vessels on the surface and in the substance of the brain.* The affection now alluded to imitates closely, both in its progress and in its signs after death, some varieties of poisoning with the vegetable narcotico-acrids, such as belladonna, stramonium, and hemlock. But the latter cases, when they prove fatal, seldom last nearly so long as a day, while the instances of meningitis under consideration rarely cause death within twenty-four hours. Dr. Abercrombie also notices a parallel disease occurring among adults ; but it is in them always marked by a considerably longer, though often more obscure course.†

Dr. Bright takes notice of a similar affection under the title of " Arachnitis with excessive irritability" occurring chiefly among very intemperate people, but independently of previous disease. In general the disorder has a well-marked course of at least several days' duration. But in two of the instances he has given the early stage was very obscure, the only symptoms having been headache and sickness of no great severity for four or five days ; after which delirium came suddenly on, and was followed by coma, and by death within thirty-six or forty hours. The sole appearances found within the head were some serous effusion and vascularity on the surface of the brain and in the ventricles.‡ To these illustrations may be added the heads of a remarkable case which occurred here in the person of an eminent lawyer, and for the particulars of which I am indebted to Dr. Maclagan. For three days there had been occasional headache, not great enough to prevent him pursuing his ordinary avoca-

* On Diseases of the Brain and Spine, Cases 18, 19, 20
† On Chronic Inflammation of the Brain, Ed. Med. and Surg. Journal, xiv.
‡ Reports of Medical Cases, ii. 14, 15.

tions, yet becoming so troublesome on the morning of the third day as to induce him to have leeches applied. But next morning he was seized rather suddenly with quickly increasing coma, and in forty hours more he expired. In this instance the whole surface of the arachnoid membrane, both over the hemisphere and in the ventricles, was found lined with soft, yellowish-green lymph.

In such cases it is apparent that an inspection after death will often unfold their real nature, where the history of the symptoms may leave it in doubt. But even without an inspection it is not likely that a careful physician could mistake them for narcotic poisoning; for independently of other considerations, the severe symptoms are ushered in by a precursory stage of ill health, commonly indicating an obscure affection of the head, and such as no one but a careless observer could fail to discover and appreciate.

It is not improbable, however, that acute meningitis may seem to prove suddenly fatal, in consequence of its course being in a great measure latent. The following case reported by Mr. Davies of Somers Town, seems of this nature. A woman, who had previously complained only of slight headache, was attacked after breakfast with violent vomiting for half an hour, when she fell down, and immediately expired. After death there was found great gorging of the vessels of the cerebral membranes, with opacity and thickening of the pia mater and arachnoid coats, and an effusion of nearly five ounces of bloody serum under the dura mater.* Such a case might give rise to great perplexity in a charge of poisoning, until the examination of the body unfolded its true nature.

I should scarcely have thought it necessary to mention *chronic meningitis* among the diseases apt to imitate the effects of narcotic poisons, because it is commonly marked by a long and distinct course. But the following case, for which I am indebted to Dr. Arnoldi of Montreal, will show that, like other diseases of the head, chronic meningitis may be latent in its early stage, and may, after developing itself, terminate in a day, and then in some measure imitate poisoning with narcotics. A middle-aged female, subject for a twelvemonth to a purulent discharge from the left ear, and occasional headache, which was supposed to be rheumatic, was seized one morning with acute pain in the head, followed in a few hours by convulsions and tendency to coma ; under which symptoms she died within twenty hours, although treated actively from the commencement. On dissection, the brain and pia mater were found healthy, except at the part corresponding with the petrous portion of the left temporal bone, where the brain was a little softened. The corresponding part of the temporal bone and the adjacent part of the occipital were completely denuded and covered with pus, which had established a passage for itself into the cavity of the ear.

Of the Distinction between Inflammation of the Brain and Narcotic Poisoning.

Inflammation of the brain itself, the *ramollissement* of French

* Lancet, 1838-39, ii. 236.

writers, occasionally excites symptoms not unlike those produced by some narcotic poisons; and in a few instances its course has appeared to be equally short. It requires particular notice, because the appearances left in the dead body are sometimes apt to escape observation.

This disease in its well-marked form has been noticed by various authors from Morgagni downwards. But the first regular accounts of it were given in 1818 by Dr. Abercrombie,[*] and in 1819 by M. Rostan[†] of Paris, and Professor Lallemand[‡] of Montpellier. Its symptoms are allied to those of apoplexy and epilepsy. But the comatose state is generally preceded by delirium or imperfect palsy, and often by a febrile state of the circulation. Contraction of the voluntary muscles, once supposed to be a distinguishing sign of this disease, is neither essential nor peculiar to it. In the dead body it is recognized by the presence either of an abscess in the brain, — or more commonly of a nucleus of disorganized cerebral tissue surrounded by unnatural redness or softness, — or sometimes of a clot of blood surrounded by similar softening. Occasionally, when the disease kills in its early stage, nothing is found but redness of a part of the brain, and slight softening of the tissue, recognizable only by scraping it with the edge of the scalpel.

In the form in which it is commonly seen, and as described by Rostan and Lallemand from a great number of cases, it can hardly be confounded with the effects of narcotic poisons ; for its course is much slower, being seldom less than several days when it proves fatal.[§] Yet in some instances it may prove fatal instantly. Lancisi notices the case of an Italian nobleman, who after an apoplectic fit became liable to frequent attacks of lethargy, — who at length died quite suddenly more than a year afterwards, — and in whose brain an organized clot was found, with extensive suppuration of the brain around it.[||] An unequivocal case of the same kind has been related by Mr. Dickson, a navy-surgeon. An elderly sailor, who for months before had done duty, eaten his rations, and drunk his grog as usual, suddenly dropped down while in the act of pulling his oar, and died at once ; and after death there was found in the middle lobes of the brain an extensive abscess, which had made its way to the surface.[¶] Such cases might, in certain circumstances, be mistaken for the effects of large doses of hydrocyanic acid ; but the morbid appearances are of course quite characteristic. M. Louis has related an instance like the last two, but where the disease was altogether latent. His patient after a long illness died of diseased heart, the ventricles of which communicated together. He never had a symptom of disorder of the head ; yet on dissection an extensive recent

---

[*] On Diseases of the Brain and Spine, Cases 16 and 17.
[†] Recherches sur le Ramollissement de Cerveau, 1819, 1823.
[‡] Recherches Anat. Pathol. sur l'Encephale. 1820.
[§] See also Dr. Abercrombie on Diseases of the Brain and Spinal Cord, p. 71.
[||] Opera varia, Venetiis, 1739. — De Mortibus Subitaneis, p. 12.
[¶] London Medical Repository, N. S. ii. 318.

47*

softening was found in the right *corpus striatum* and another in the right *thalamus*.*

None of the treatises I have seen on the subject make mention of a variety of this disease intermediate between suddenly fatal cases and those which last several days, — a form in which the patient's illness endures for a few hours only, and which, both in the special symptoms and in their course, imitates exactly the effects of some narcotics. Two such cases have come under my notice, both of them judicial, poisoning having been suspected. One of them proved fatal in an hour and a half, the individual having previously been in excellent health; and the only appearance of disease was softening of a considerable part of the surface of the brain where it lies over the left orbit. The other was more remarkable in its circumstances. In November, 1822, a man, who had previously enjoyed excellent health, was found one morning in a low lodging-house in the Lawn-market comatose, and convulsed; and he died seven hours afterwards. The neighbours spread a report, that the woman of the house had poisoned him, with the view of selling the body; and by an odd co-incidence the police, when they went to apprehend the woman, found an anatomist hid in a closet. The body was judicially examined by Sir W. Newbigging and myself; and we found an ulcer on the fore-part of the left hemisphere of the brain, and a small patch of softening on each middle lobe.

It is only in cases like the last two that the disease is likely to be mistaken for the effects of poison; and the morbid appearances will at once distinguish them. But it is requisite to remember that soften-ing of the brain when not far advanced is apt to escape notice, as it is not necessarily attended with a change in the colour of the dis-eased part. In the first of the two cases I have related, the cause of death was very nearly assumed to have been simple apoplexy, when at lenght the true disorder was unexpectedly noticed. I presume, indeed, that strictly speaking, both of the cases which came under my notice ought to be considered as simple apoplexy excited by pre-existing *ramollissement*.

Of the Distinction between Hypertrophy of the Brain and Narcotic Poisoning.

This disease is not here mentioned, because its symptoms and pro-gress resemble very closely those of poisoning with the narcotics; for it causes epileptic symptoms, which, besides that they are pre-ceded for some time by other head affections, very seldom prove fatal in less than three days. But some notice of it is necessary, because the disease is rare and of recent discovery, so that the appearances left by it in the dead body may escape observation. Besides, the physician is at present imperfectly acquainted with it, and therefore, when a more extensive collection of cases shall have been made, it may be found to prove at times fatal so rapidly as to admit of being

* Recherches Anatomico-Pathologiques, 313.

confounded with narcotic poisoning. Hypertrophy of the brain, it is true, is always a chronic or slow disease, but, like other diseases of the brain, its early stages may possibly be so completely latent that the patient may appear to die of a few hours' illness. This, however, must be left to the determination of future experience. The most rapid case yet published proved fatal twenty-four hours after the first appearance of symptoms.

The appearances left in the body are increased density and firmness of the whole brain or a part of it, — flattening of the convolutions on their outer surface, so that their grooves are almost obliterated and the investing membrane uncommonly dry, — unusual emptiness of the blood-vessels of the brain and its membranes, — and a protrusion of the brain upwards on removal of the skull-cap, as if the organ were too large for its containing cavity.*

Some pathologists doubt the existence of hypertrophy of the brain as a distinct disease, and conceive that the appearance of flattening of the convolutions is produced by serum effused between the dura mater and arachnoid membrane. But this explanation will not account for those cases in which it is expressly stated that little or no fluid was to be found in any part of the brain or in the base of the skull.

Of the Distinction between Diseases of the Spinal Cord and Narcotic Poisoning.

It is not necessary to say much on the acute diseases of the spinal cord, which are apt to be confounded with the effects of narcotic poisons. The diseases are extravasation of blood into the spinal canal, inflammation of the membranes, and inflammation [*ramollissement*] of the cord itself. These disorders are commonly marked by obvious and characteristic symptoms, as well as a much slower course than that of the affections induced by narcotic poisons. But occasionally they approach closely the characters of some of the slow cases of narcotic poisoning, — palsy being absent, the leading symptoms consisting of delirium, convulsions, and coma, and the fatal event occurring within the third day. Dr. Abercrombie and M. Ollivier have related examples of the kind arising from extravasation of blood,† serous effusion,‡ and softening of the cord.§ Such cases are exceedingly rare ; but the possibility of their occurrence should impose on the medical jurist the necessity of examining the spine with care in all judicial cases of alleged narcotic poisoning, especially when death has not been rapid.

Of the Distinction between syncopal Asphyxia, and Narcotic Poisons.

The only other natural disease requiring notice under the present

* Laennec, Revue Médicale, 1828, iv. Dance, Répertoire Gén. d'Anatomie Pathologique, vi. 197.

† On the Diseases of the Brain and Spinal Cord, Case 132.

‡ Ibidem, Case 131. Ollivier, Traité de la moelle épinière, Obs. 42.

§ Abercrombie, Case 138.

head is the *Asphyxia Idiopathica* of the late Mr. Chevallier. It may be the cause of embarrassment in questions regarding narcotic poisoning, when the course of the symptoms to their fatal termination is rapid, and was not witnessed by any person ; for it causes death with equal rapidity, and its signs in the dead body are very obscure. It has been observed chiefly among women in the latter months of pregnancy, or soon after delivery ; but it has also been known to attack the male sex. It generally commences during a state of perfect health, and is seldom preceded by any warning of danger. The person suddenly complains of slight sickness, giddiness, and excessive faintness, immediately seems to sleep or swoon away, and expires gently without a struggle. The only appearance of note found in the dead body is unusual flaccidity and emptiness of the heart.* But even these slight appearances are not constant ; for in a case related by Rochoux of a woman who, while in a state of perfect health, suddenly grew pale, slipped off her chair, and died on the spot, the auricles of the heart contained a great deal of blood.† This singular disorder appears to consist of nothing else than a mortal tendency to fainting ; and it may prove fatal either in the first fit of syncope, or after an hour and a half. — Under the same head are probably to be arranged the cases of sudden death described by M. Devergie under the title of Death by Syncope. He has given scarcely any account of the circumstances attending death ; but it may be inferred from his classification of the cases that fainting immediately preceded it. In all of them he found blood in both sides of the heart ; and the blood, contrary to what happens in other kinds of sudden death, had separated into clear serum, and fibrin free of colouring matter.‡ — Under the same head also may be noticed a denomination of cases, which, though alluded to before by various pathologists, were first distinctly characterized by M. Ollivier, where death is caused on a sudden, apparently by the disengagement of a large quantity of aëriform fluid from the blood in the heart and great vessels. Among the instances described by Ollivier, it appears that death repeatedly occurred quite suddenly while the individuals enjoyed sound health ; and the only appearances of any note found in the body were tympanitic distension of the heart, absence of blood there and in the great vessels, and the existence of a gaseous fluid in numerous globules throughout the blood-vessels of the brain. The circumstances of death and the appearances in the dead body are much the same with those observed from the admission of air into the veins during surgical operations. A case of this kind, owing to its suddenness, might be confounded with the effects of the more active narcotic poisons, such as hydrocyanic acid, especially as its characters in the dead body might escape notice.§

Death often takes place from sudden syncope in *organic diseases of the heart.* Such cases may be confounded with the most rapid variety of poisoning with hydrocyanic acid ; and if the duration of the symp-

---

* London Medico-Chirurgical Transactions, i. 157.
† Recherches sur l'Apoplexie, p. 159.
‡ Annales d'Hygiène-Publique, xx. 173.
§ Archives Gén. de Med. 1838, i. 40.

toms preceding death is unknown, they may give rise to a suspicion of poisoning generally. But they are at once distinguished by the morbid appearances. A trivial organic derangement may be the occasion of instant death.

The genera comprehended in the class of narcotics are opium, henbane, lettuce-opium, solanum, hydrocyanic acid, and the deleterious gases. Of these genera the last is by no means a pure one, for it includes many gases which act as irritants only; but it is more convenient to consider them together, than to distribute them into separate classes. Some other vegetable substances besides henbane, lettuce-opium, and solanum, possess nearly the same properties; but as they likewise cause irritation, they are arranged more appropriately in the next class, the narcotico-acrids.

Most narcotic vegetables owe their poisonous properties to a peculiar principle, probably of an alkaline nature, and slightly different in each. This discovery was made with regard to opium in 1812; and the discovery of the active principle in that drug has been followed by the detection of analogous principles in most narcotics, as well as in many narcotico-acrids.

These principles are generally crystalline, soluble in alcohol and the acids, little soluble in water, free from mineral admixture, and entirely destructible by heat. When purified with the greatest care, they still retain decided alkaline properties; but on account of their number and the low power of neutralization their alkaline nature was long denied; and they have been conventionally styled alkaloids.

In their natural state they exist in combination with various ternary acids, some of which are peculiar; and they are likewise intimately blended, or more probably united chemically, with other inert principles of the vegetable kingdom, particularly resinous and extractive matters, to which they adhere with great obstinacy.

They are all highly energetic, and generally concentrate in themselves the leading properties of the substance from which they are obtained.

The experiments, which have led to the conclusion, that the narcotic poisons act on the brain by entering the blood-vessels, have been repeated with their alkaloids, and have yielded similar results. But the alkaloids are in equal quantities much more energetic than the crude poisons. Their effects indeed are truly formidable, and some well-authenticated instances of their action appear hardly less marvellous than the most extravagant notions entertained in ancient times of the operation of poisons. One of them, the principle of nux vomica, which, however, does not belong to the present class, is so active that in all probability a man might be killed with the third part of a grain in less than fifteen minutes.

It is very difficult to detect some of the vegetable alkaloids; and it is fortunate, therefore, that they are rare, and not to be procured but by complex processes.

Chemical analysis does not by any means supply so good evidence of poisoning with the narcotics as it does of poisoning with the irritants. Their chemical properties are not very characteristic, and they are not well developed unless with a larger quantity of the poison than will usually be met with in medico-legal investigations. This remark, however, does not apply universally; and it is probable, that, as organic analysis goes on improving, better and more delicate processes will be discovered.

CHAPTER XXVII.

OF POISONING WITH OPIUM.

To the medical jurist opium is one of the most important of poisons; since there is hardly any other whose effects come more frequently under his cognizance. It is the poison most generally resorted to by the timid to accomplish self-destruction, for which purpose it is peculiarly well adapted on account of the gentleness of its operation. It has also been often the source of fatal accidents, which naturally arise from its extensive employment in medicine. It has likewise been long very improperly employed to create amusement. And in recent times it has been made use of to commit murder, and to induce stupor previous to the commission of robbery. Mr. Burnett, in his work on Criminal Law, has mentioned a trial for murder in 1800, in which the prisoners were accused of having committed the crime by poisoning with opium; and although a verdict of *not proven* was returned, there is little doubt that the deceased, an adult, was poisoned in the way supposed. A few years ago, a remarkable trial took place at Paris, where poisoning was alleged to have been effected by means of the alkaloid principle of opium; and the prisoner, a young physician of the name of Castaing, was condemned and executed.

In several parts of Britain during the last fifteen years many persons have been brought into great danger by opium having been administered as a narcotic to facilitate robbery; and some have actually been killed. In December, 1828, a conviction was obtained in the Judiciary Court of Edinburgh for this crime, in which instance the persons who had taken the opium recovered. A fatal case, which was strongly suspected to be of the same nature, was submitted to me by the sheriff of this county in 1828; but sufficient evidence could not be procured. In July, 1829, a man Stewart and his wife were condemned, and subsequently executed for the same crime, the person to whom they gave the opium having been killed by it. And about a year afterwards a similar instance occurred at Glasgow, for which a man Byers and his wife were condemned at the Autumn Circuit of 1831.

SECTION I. — *Of the Chemical History and Tests of Opium.*

Opium is the inspissated juice of the capsules of the *Papaver som-*

niferum. It has a reddish-brown colour, and a glimmering lustre on a fresh surface. It is soft and plastic when recent; but if pure, may be dried so as to become brittle. Its smell is strong and quite peculiar. It has a very bitter and most peculiar taste. In consequence of this taste one would suppose it no easy matter to administer opium secretly. The plan resorted to by thieves and robbers seems to be, to deaden the sense of taste by strong spirits, and then to ply the person with porter or ale drugged with laudanum, or the black drop, which possesses less odour.

The following account of the chemical history of opium will be confined in a great measure to the leading properties of the principles, in which its active qualities are concentrated, or which are likely by their chemical characters to supply proof of its presence.

The common solvents act readily on opium. Water dissolves its active principles even at low temperatures. So does alcohol. So particularly do the mineral and vegetable acids when much diluted. Ether removes from it little else than one of its active principles, narcotine. By the action of these agents are procured various preparations in common use. *Laudanum* is a spirituous infusion, and contains the active ingredients of a twelfth part of its weight of opium. *Scotch Paregoric Elixir*, a solution in ammoniated spirit, is only one-fifth of the strength of laudanum ; and *English Paregoric*, tincture of opium and camphor for its chief ingredients, is four times weaker still. *Wine of opium* contains the soluble part of a sixteenth of its weight. The *black drop* and *Battley's sedative liquor* are believed to be solutions of opium in vegetable acids, and to possess, the former four, the latter three times the strength of laudanum. But their strength has been greatly exaggerated ; neither of them, according to my own experience, being above half what is supposed. The juice and infusion of the garden poppy are also powerfully narcotic, so as even to have caused death both when given by the mouth and in the way of injection.* Many other pharmaceutic preparations contain opium.

If opium be infused in successive portions of cold water, the water dissolves all its poisonous principles, and also a peculiar acid possessing characteristic chemical properties. These principles are separated by means of the alkalis, the alkaline carbonates, or the alkaline earths. The most important of them are *morphia*, the chief alkaloid of opium, — *narcotine*, a feeble poison, not an alkaloid, — a peculiar acid, termed *meconic acid*, — and a *resinoid substance*. Other crystalline principles also exist in opium, though apparently in too small proportion either to affect its action or to be available in medico-legal analysis as the means of detecting the drug. These are codeïa, meconine, narceïne, paramorphia, and porphyroxine.

Of the various principles now indicated it is necessary to notice here only morphia, narcotine, codeïa, porphyroxine and meconic acid. They require mention either as being active poisons, or because a knowledge of their leading characters may be useful in conducting a medico-legal analysis in a case of poisoning with opium.

* Archives Gén. xiv. 406.

Meconic acid, as procured by evaporation, is usually in little scales of a pale brown or yellowish tint, being rendered so by adhering resin or extractive matter ; but when nearly colourless, it forms long, extremely delicate tabular crystals, which in mass have a fine silky appearance like spermaceti.   1. When heated in a tube, it is partly decomposed, and partly sublimed ; and the sublimate condenses in filamentous, radiated crystals.   2. When dissolved even in a very large quantity of water, the solution acquires an intense cherry-red colour with the perchloride of iron.   The sublimed crystals have the same property.   Only one other acid is so affected, namely, the sul-pho-cyanic, a very rare substance.   It has been repeatedly stated,[*] that the redness produced by meconic acid may be distinguished by the effect of an alkali, which is said to bleach the colour produced by sulpho-cyanic acid, but to deepen the cherry-red tint occasioned by the meconic.   This is not correct; an alkali added to the red so-lution of meconate of iron precipitates oxide of iron and renders the liquid colourless.   The best distinction yet proposed is the following which has been suggested by Dr. Percy.   Acidulate the red fluid with sulphuric acid, drop in a bit of pure zinc, and suspend at the mouth of the tube a bit of paper moistened with solution of acetate of lead : If the redness be caused by sulphocyanic acid, hydrosulphuric acid gas is evolved, and blackens the paper ; but no such effect ensues, if the redness be owing to meconic acid.[†] — According to Dr. Pe-reira, solutions of the acetates, an infusion of white mustard, decoc-tions of Iceland moss, and of the *Gigantina helminthocorton*, besides other more rare substances, are reddened, like solution of meconic acid, by the salts of peroxide of iron.[‡]   3. The solution of meconic acid gives a pale-green precipitate with the sulphate of copper, and, if the precipitate is not too abundant, it is dissolved by boiling, but re-appears on cooling.

Of the Tests for Morphia and its Salts. — Morphia, when pure, is in small, beautiful, white crystals.   Various forms have been ascribed to it ; but in the numerous crystallizations I have made, it has always assumed when pure the form of a slightly flattened hexangular prism. It has a bitter taste, but no smell.

A gentle heat melts it, and if the fluid mass is then allowed to cool, a crystalline radiated substance is formed.   A stronger heat reddens and then chars the fused mass, white fumes of a peculiar odour are disengaged, and at last the mass kindles and burns brightly. — Morphia is very little soluble in water.   It is more soluble, yet still sparingly so, in ether.   But its proper solvents are alcohol, or the diluted acids, mineral as well as vegetable.   All its solutions are intensely bitter, and that in alcohol has an alkaline reaction. — From its solutions in the acids crystallizable salts may be procured ; and morphia may be separated by the superior affinity of any of the inorga-nic alkalis ; but it is easily redissolved by an excess of potash. — Mor-phia when treated with nitric acid is dissolved with effervescence, and becomes instantly orange-red, which, if too much acid be used,

[*] London Medical Gazette, viii. 47.
[†] Lancet, July 31, 1841.   [‡] Elements of Materia Medica, 1842, p. 1738.

changes quickly to yellow. The coloration of morphia by nitric acid is a characteristic property; which, however, it possesses in common with some other alkaloids, such as brucia, and also strychnia when not quite pure. The change of colour is said by some chemists to depend on adhering resinoid matter, and not to be possessed by perfectly pure morphia; but this is a mistake. It is probable that some other vegetable substances besides the three alkaloids, morphia, brucia, and strychnia, may be turned orange-red by nitric acid. Dr. Pereira says that oil of pimento undergoes the same change.* — When suspended in water in the form of fine powder and then treated with a drop or two of perchloride of iron containing little or no free hydrochloric acid, it is dissolved and forms a deep-blue solution, the tint of which is more purely blue, the stronger the solution, and the purer the morphia. This is a property even more characteristic than the former, since no such effect is produced on any other known alkaloid. Like the effect of nitric acid, it is said not to be essential to morphia, but to depend on adhering resinoid matter; yet the blue colour is always strongly produced with powdered morphia of snowy-whiteness. — Another property by which morphia may be also distinguished is the decomposition of iodic acid. A solution of iodic acid is turned brown either by morphia or its salts, owing to the formation of iodine; and the test is so delicate that it affects a solution containing a 7000th of morphia.† So many other substances, however, possess the property of disengaging iodine from iodic acid, that little importance can be attached to this criterion.

Acetate of Morphia is in some countries the common medicinal form for administering morphia; but it has been almost entirely superseded in this city by the hydrochlorate, since Dr. W. Gregory pointed out a cheap mode of procuring that salt in a state of purity.‡ The acetate is in confused crystals, often of a brownish colour from impurities. The stronger acids disengage acetic acid. The alkalis throw down morphia from its solution in water. Nitric acid and perchloride of iron act on it as on morphia itself.

Hydrochlorate of Morphia. — The muriate or hydrochlorate must be carefully attended to by the medical jurist, because it is extensively used in medical practice instead of opium. As now prepared, it is snowy-white and apparently pulverulent, but is in reality a congeries of filiform crystals. It decrepitates slightly when heated, then melts, and at the same time chars, exhaling a strong odour somewhat like that of truffles. Nitric acid and perchloride of iron act on it as on morphia. Boiling water dissolves fully its own weight, and very easily three-fourths of its weight of hydrochlorate of morphia; and on cooling down to 60° F. it retains seven parts per cent., and deposits the rest in tufts of beautiful filiform crystals. The solution commonly employed in medicine contains one per cent. of the salt. Nitric acid turns the solution yellow, acting distinctly enough when

* London Medical Gazette, xviii. 930.
† Serullas Journ. de Chim. Méd. vi.
‡ Edin. Med. and Surg. Journal, xxxv. 331.

48

the water contains a hundredth, and perceptibly when it contains only a two-hundredth of its weight. Perchloride of iron strikes a deep blue with a solution containing a hundredth of its weight, very distinctly when the proportion is a two-hundredth, and even perceptibly when it is only a five-hundredth. A solution much more diluted than even the last has a strong bitter taste. When moderately concentrated, morphia is precipitated from it by the alkalis.

Of the preceding properties of morphia and its salts, those which constitute the most characteristic tests are the effects of perchloride of iron and of nitric acid on all of them, the effect of heat on morphia, and the effect of an alkali on its solutions in acids.

Of the Tests for Narcotine. — Narcotine is rather distinguished by negative than by positive chemical properties. When pure, it is in transparent colourless pearly crystals, which, as formed from alcohol, may be either very flat, oblique, six-sided prisms, or oblong four-sided tables obliquely bevelled on their sides. But when crystallized from sulphuric ether the crystals are prisms with a rhombic base. They fuse with heat, and concrete on cooling into a resinous-like mass. They are soluble in ether, and fixed oil, less so in alcohol, insoluble in water or the alkalis, very soluble in the diluted acids, but without effecting neutralization ; and if perfectly pure, they do not undergo the changes produced on morphia by perchloride of iron or nitric acid. Few specimens of narcotic, however, are so pure as not to render nitric acid yellow. Care must be taken not to confound narcotine with morphia. When crystallized together from alcohol and not quite pure, narcotine forms tufts of pearly thin tabular crystals, while morphia is in short, thick, sparkling prisms.

Of Codeïa — This substance is, like morphia, an alkaloid, capable of combining with acids. It differs from morphia and narcotine in being moderately soluble in water ; and from this solution it may be crystallized in large crystals affecting the octaedral form. It is unnecessary to detail its chemical properties.

Of the Tests for Porphyroxine. — This principle is a neutral crystalline body, insoluble in water, soluble in alcohol and ether, and also soluble in weak acids, which part with it unchanged on the addition of an alkali. When heated with hydrochloric acid, a fine purple or rose-red solution is produced ; whence its name. It is supposed that this property may be of use in medico-legal researches ; and the following mode of developing it has been proposed by Dr. Merck, its discoverer.* Decompose the suspected fluid with caustic potash ; agitate the mixture with sulphuric ether ; dip a bit of white filtering paper repeatedly in the etherial solution, drying it after each immersion ; then wet the paper with hydrochloric acid, and expose it to the vapour of boiling water; upon which the paper will become more or less acid.

Of the Process for detecting Opium in mixed fluids and solids.

Having stated these particulars of the chemical history of opium

* Buchner's Repertorium für die Pharmacie, 2te Reihe, xxxii. 104.

and its chief component ingredients, I shall now describe what has appeared to me the most delicate and satisfactory method of detecting it in a mixed state.

1. If there be any solid matter, it is to be cut into small fragments, water is to be added if necessary, then a little acetic acid sufficient to render the mixture acidulous, and when the whole mass has been well stirred, and has stood a few minutes, it is to be filtered, and evaporated at a temperature somewhat below ebullition to the consistence of a moderately thick syrup. To this extract strong alcohol is to be gradually added, care being taken to break down any coagulum which may be formed : and after ebullition and cooling, the alcoholic solution is to be filtered. The solution must then be evaporated to the consistence of a thin syrup, and the residue dissolved in distilled water and filtered anew.

2. Add now the solution of acetate of lead as long as it causes precipitation, filter and wash. The filtered fluid contains acetate of morphia, and the precipitate on the filter contains meconic acid united with the oxide of lead.

3. The fluid part is to be treated with hydrosulphuric acid gas, to throw down any lead which may remain in solution. It is then to be filtered while *cold*, and evaporated sufficiently in a vapour-bath. The solution in this state will sometimes be sufficiently pure for the application of the tests for morphia ; but in most cases it is necessary, and in all advisable, to purify it still farther. For this purpose the morphia is to be precipitated with carbonate of soda; and the precipitate having been collected, washed, and drained on a filter, the precipitate and portion of the filter to which it adheres are to be boiled in a little pure alcohol. The alcoholic solution, — filtered, if necessary, — will give by evaporation a crystalline residue of morphia, which becomes orange-red with nitric acid, and blue with perchloride of iron. The latter property I have sometimes been unable to develope when the former was presented characteristically.

4. It is useful, however, to separate the meconic acid also ; because, as its properties are more delicate, I have repeatedly been able to detect it satisfactorily, when I did not feel satisfied with the result of the search for morphia. Dr. Ure made the same remark in his evidence on the trial of Stewart and his wife. He detected the meconic acid, but could not separate the morphia. It may be detected in one of two ways, — by means of hydrosulphuric acid, or by sulphuric acid.

If the former method be chosen, suspend in a little water the precipitate caused by the acetate of lead (par. 2); transmit hydrosulphuric acid gas till the whole precipitate is blackened ; filter immediately without boiling; then boil, and if necessary filter a second time. A great part of the impurities thrown down by the acetate of lead will be separated with the sulphuret of lead ; and the meconic acid is dissolved. But it requires in general farther purification, which is best attained by again throwing it down with acetate of lead, and repeating the steps of the present paragraph. The fluid is now to be concentrated by evaporation at a temperature not exceed-ing 180° F., and subjected to the tests for meconic acid, more par-ticularly to the action of perchloride of iron, when the quantity is small. If there is evidently a considerable quantity of acid, a por-tion should be evaporated till it yields crystalline scales ; and these are to be heated in a tube to procure the arborescent crystalline sub-limate formerly described.   About a sixth of a grain of meconic acid, however, is required to try the latter test conveniently.

If the method of separating meconic acid by means of sulphuric acid be preferred, the precipitate formed by acetate of lead is to be treated with weak sulphuric acid, which forms insoluble sulphate of lead, and disengages the meconic acid.   The liquid obtained by filtration is then to be evaporated as above, to obtain crystals, which are to be examined by the tests for meconic acid.   Orfila thinks this method more delicate than the mode by hydrosulphuric acid gas. I am inclined from my own experiments to doubt his statement.

5. If there be a sufficiency of the original material, Merck's process for detecting porphyroxin may be tried [see p. 534].   But I doubt whether this process is sufficiently delicate for medico-legal purposes.

I wish I could add my testimony to the opinion, expressed on a remarkable occasion by Professor Chaussier, in favour of the delicacy of the tests for morphia and its compounds, that they might be de-tected "jusqu'à une molécule."*   In one sense this statement may be correct.   Morphia, separated from the complex mixture of prin-ciples with which it is combined in opium, may be detected in ex-tremely small quantities.   Accordingly, M. Lassaigne has supplied, for the discovery of acetate of morphia in mixed fluids, an excellent process, whence the chief part of the three first paragraphs of the preceding method for opium are borrowed ; and from the facts stated by him in his paper,† as well as from the experimental testimony of Professor Orfila,‡ it appears that Lassaigne's process will furnish strong indications, if not absolute proof of the presence of that salt, in the proportion of two grains to eight ounces of the most complex mixtures.   Hence the search for acetate of morphia in a suspected case is by no means hopeless.   But the detection of acetate of mor-phia is an object of small moment, compared with the detection of morphia in its natural state of combination in opium.   Now my own observations lead me to entertain serious doubts, whether the best method of operating hitherto known could be successfully applied to the detection of the equivalent opium in complex mixtures.   By the process I have recommended it is easy to procure, from an infusion of ten grains of opium in four ounces of water, satisfactory proof of the presence of morphia by the action of ammonia, perchloride of iron and nitric acid, and equally distinct proof of the presence of meconic acid by perchloride of iron, as well as sulphate of copper. But on proceeding to apply the process to organic mixtures, I have found that when the soluble part of ten grains of opium was mixed

* Procès de Castaing, p. 113.   † Ann. de Chim. et de Phys. xxv. 102.
‡ Toxicol. Gén. ii. 60.

with four ounces of porter or milk, I could develope no property of morphia but its bitterness, and no indication of meconic acid but the action of perchloride of iron. MM. Larocque and Thibierge, it is right to add, have in similar circumstances found the process somewhat more delicate.*

It is of great consequence, however, to remark, that in cases of poisoning with opium, the medical jurist will seldom have the good fortune to operate even upon so large a proportion of the poison as in my experiments; because the greater part of it disappears from the stomach before death. This will not happen always, as may be seen from various cases mentioned afterwards in the section on the morbid appearances caused by opium. But, according to my own observations, the poison will often disappear in a short time, so far as to render an analysis abortive. Thus in the case of a young woman who died five hours after taking not less than two ounces of laudanum, I could apply to the fluid, procured from the contents of the stomach, by paragraphs 1, 2, and 3 of my process, only the test of its taste, which had the bitterness of morphia. In the case of another young woman, whose stomach was emptied by the stomach-pump four hours after she took two ounces of laudanum, I could obtain from the evacuated fluid, when properly prepared, only the indications of the presence of morphia supplied by its bitterness and the imperfect action of nitric acid, — and the indication of the presence of meconic acid supplied by the imperfect action of perchloride of iron. In a third case, where the stomach was evacuated two hours after seven drachms of laudanum had been swallowed, even the first portions of fluid withdrawn had not any opiate odour, and did not yield any indication of the presence even of meconic acid. Now, on the one hand, the quantity taken in these instances is rarely exceeded in cases of poisoning with laudanum; and, on the other hand, the interval during which it remained in the stomach subject to vital operations is considerably less than the average in medico-legal, and above all in fatal cases. It may be laid down, therefore, as a general rule, that in poisoning with opium the medical jurist, by the best methods of analysis yet known, will often fail in procuring satisfactory evidence, and sometimes fail to obtain any evidence at all, of the existence of the poison in the contents of the stomach. In a case published by Dr. Bright from the experience of Mr. Walne of London, it is stated that the matter removed from the stomach only half an hour after an ounce and a half of laudanum had been taken, while the stomach was empty, did not smell of opium.† This case is quoted to put the reader on his guard. But at the same time it does appear extremely improbable that the whole opium had disappeared from the stomach in so short a time, and much more likely that it might have been found by analysis in the matter first withdrawn.

I have taken some pains to establish the proposition laid down above, because in a matter of such importance it is always essential,

---

* Orfila, Tox. Gén. 1813, ii. 254.
† Reports of Medical Cases, ii. 203.

that the medical inspector know the real extent of his resources; and it has appeared to me that, greatly as the hand of the chemist has been strengthened by late discoveries in vegetable analysis, his power has been overrated both by his scientific brethren, and by the medical profession generally. I am happy to find, since the first publication of these remarks, that they coincide with the experience and opinion of so eminent an authority as Professor Buchner; who has observed that a chemical analysis must often fail to detect opium where there could be no doubt of its having been administered in large quantity.*

It is of moment to add, that in two of the instances mentioned above the odour of laudanum was perceived in the subject of analysis, — faintly, however, and only for a few hours after it was removed from the stomach. Although the peculiar odour of opium is a delicate criterion of its presence, it does not follow that it should be preferred to an elaborate chemical analysis. For it is a test of extreme uncertainty. There is in the contents of the stomach such a complication of odours, that with a rather delicate sense of smell, I have sometimes been unable to satisfy myself of the presence of the opiate odour where others were sure it existed. At the same time the medical jurist should not neglect it as a subsidiary test. It is always strongest and most characteristic, first, when the stomach is just opened, or the contents just withdrawn, and again, when the fluid, in the course of preparation, as directed in paragraph 1 (p. 535), is just reaching the point of ebullition. The latter odour is somewhat different from the former, yet quite peculiar, and such as every chemist must have remarked on boiling an infusion of opium. It is further to be observed, that although the odour of opium is a very delicate test of its presence even in complex organic mixtures, chemical analysis may be successful, where this character fails. Dr. Morehead of the Bombay service, in applying my process to the fluid withdrawn by the stomach-pump, detected morphia both by nitric acid and perchloride of iron, although he could not detect any odour of opium in the fluid.†

So much for the delicacy of the process. As to its precision, — from what I have myself witnessed, as well as from the experience of Dr. Ure, it will often happen in actual practice, that the only indication of opium to be procured by the process consists in the deep

---

* Repertorium für die Pharmacie, xxxi. 174. — Professor Orfila, in the last edition of his Toxicologie Gén. [1843. ii. 253], has attacked in no very measured terms this opinion of Professor Buchner and myself. But, although he professes to give a literal translation of the passage above, he has translated it so incorrectly as wholly to misrepresent our opinion. The close of the paragraph, " chemical analysis must often fail to detect opium where there could be no doubt of its *having been administered* in large quantity," is rendered into French by the Parisian Professor in these words, — " l'analyse chimique, propre à constater l'existence de l'opium, est souvent inutile, même dans le cas *où il existe* une grande quantité de cette substance," — which is a very different proposition. Orfila clearly overrates the utility of the process for detecting opium, both in this criticism and in his whole observations on the subject, by losing sight of the tendency of absorption to remove the poison beyond reach.

† Bombay Med. Phys. Transactions, i. 322.

red colour struck by perchloride of iron with the meconic acid. Now, will this alone constitute sufficient proof of the presence of opium? On the whole, I am inclined to reply in the affirmative. Sulphocyanic acid, it is true, has the same effect, and this acid has been proved by Professors Gmelin and Tiedemann to exist in the human saliva,* — a fact which was called in question by Dr. Ure in his evidence on the trial of the Stuarts, but which at the time I had verified, and which Dr. Ure has since been compelled by experiments of his own to admit.† But it must be very seldom possible to procure a distinct blood-red coloration from the saliva, after it has been mixed with the complex contents of the stomach, and subjected to the process of analysis detailed above ;‡ and the check proposed by Dr. Percy (p. 532) will distinguish it.

SECTION II. — *Of the Action of Opium, and the Symptoms it excites in Man.*

The symptoms and mode of action of opium have been long made the subject of dispute, both among physicians and toxicologists ; and in some particulars our knowledge is still vague and insufficient.

Under the head of general poisoning, some experiments were related, from which it might be inferred that opium has the power of stupefying or suspending the irritability of the parts to which it is immediately applied. The most unequivocal of these facts, which occurred to Dr. Wilson Philip, was instant paralysis of the intestines of a dog, when an infusion of opium was applied to their mucous coat ;§ another hardly less decisive was palsy of the hind-legs of a frog, observed by Dr. Monro *Secundus*, when opium was injected between the skin and the muscles ;‖ and a third, which has been remarked by several experimentalists, is immediate cessation of the contractions of the frog's heart when opium is applied to its inner surface.¶

The poison has also powerful constitutional or remote effects, which are chiefly produced on the brain. Much discussion has arisen on the question, whether these constitutional effects are owing to the conveyance of the local torpor along the nerves to the brain, or to the poison being absorbed, and so acting on the brain through the blood. The question is not yet settled. It appears pretty certain, however, that the poison cannot act constitutionally without entering

* Die Verdauung nach Versuchen, &c.   † Journal of Science, N. S. vi. 56.

‡ Dr. Pereira states that he is obliged to differ from me upon this important subject for he "has several times obtained from the stomach of subjects in the dissecting-room a liquor which reddened the salts of iron" (Elements of Materia Medica, p. 1741). This fact, however, does not exactly touch the question. The reddening must be occasioned, not in the crude fluid, but with a substance obtained by the process of analysis for detecting meconic acid in complex organic mixtures, — otherwise the proposition in the text stands good.

§ Experiments on Opium. Appendix to Treatise on Febrile Diseases, vi. 697.

‖ Edin. Lit. and Phys. Essays, iii. 309.

¶ Monro, Ibidem, 331, and Philip, *ut supra*, p. 680.

the blood-vessels; although it is not so clear, that after it has entered them, it acts by being carried with the blood to the brain. The newest doctrine supposes that it enters the blood-vessels, and produces on their inner coat an impression which is conveyed along the nerves.

According to the experiments of Professor Orfila, it is more energetic when applied to the surface of a wound than when introduced into the stomach, and most energetic of all when injected into a vein.* The inference generally drawn from these and other analogous experiments† is, that the blood transmits the poison in substance to the brain. They certainly, however, do not prove more than that the poison must enter the blood before it acts.

The old doctrine, that the blood-vessels have no concern with its action, and that it acts only by conveyance along the nerves of a peculiar local torpor arising from its direct application to their sentient extremities, has been long abandoned by most physiologists as untenable. But some have adopted a late modification of this doctrine, by supposing that opium may act both by being carried with the blood to the brain, and by the transmission of local torpor along the nerves. They believe, in fact, that opium possesses a double mode of action, — through sympathy as well as through absorption. It would be fruitless to inquire into the grounds that exist for adopting or rejecting this doctrine, because sufficient facts are still wanting to decide the controversy. So far as they go, however, they appear adverse to the supposition of a conveyance of impressions along the nerves, without the previous entrance of the poison within the blood-vessels. The difficulties, in the way of the theory of the sympathetic action of opium, would be removed by the doctrine of Messrs. Morgan and Addison. According to their views, the experiments, which appear at first sight to prove that this substance operates by being carried with the blood to the part on which it acts, are easily explained by considering that the opium makes a peculiar impression on the inside of the vessels, which impression subsequently passes along the nerves to the brain.‡ But, as stated in the introductory chapter on the physiology of poisoning, this theory requires support.

The effects of opium, through whatever channel it may produce them, are exerted chiefly on the brain and nervous system. This appears from the experiments of a crowd of physiologists, as well as from the symptoms observed a thousand times in man. In animals the symptoms are different from those remarked in man. Some experimentalists have indeed witnessed in the higher orders of animals, as in the human subject, pure lethargy and coma. But the latest researches, among the rest those of M. Orfila, show that much more generally it causes in animals hurried pulse, giddiness, palsy of the

* Toxicol. Gén. ii. 77.

† Monro, Edin. Phys. and Lit. Essays, ii. 335, 324.— Charret, Revue Médicale, 1827, i. 515.

‡ On the Operation of Poisonous Agents on the Living Body, *passim.*

hind-legs, convulsions of various degrees of intensity, from simple tremors to violent tetanus, and a peculiar slumber, in the midst of which a slight excitement rouses the animal and renews the convulsions. These symptoms are produced in whatever way the poison enters the body, whether by the stomach, or by a wound, or by direct injection into a vein, or by the rectum. In man, convulsions are sometimes excited ; but much more commonly simple sopor and coma.

According to the inquiries of M. Charret, which were extended to every class of the lower animals, opium produces three leading effects. It acts on the brain, causing congestion, and consequently sopor ; on the general nervous centre as an irritant, exciting convulsions ; and on the muscles as a direct sedative. It is poisonous to all animals, — man, carnivorous quadrupeds, the *rodentia*, birds, reptiles, amphibious animals, fishes, insects, and the *mollusca*. But of its three leading effects some are not produced in certain classes or orders of animals. In the *mammalia*, with the exception of man, there is no cerebral congestion induced, and death takes place amidst convulsions. In birds there is some cerebral congestion towards the close ; but still the two other phenomena are the most prominent.*

It has been rendered probable, by what is stated above, that opium enters the blood. The question, therefore, naturally arises, whether its presence there can be proved by chemical analysis ? But considering the imperfection of the processes for detecting it when mixed with organic substances, no disappointment ought to be felt if this proof should fail in regard to so complex a fluid as the blood. The only person who has represented himself successful in the search is M. Barruel of Paris. He examined the urine and blood of a man under the influence of a poisonous dose of laudanum, amounting to an ounce and a half ; and procured indications of morphia in both. When three ounces of urine were boiled with magnesia, and the insoluble matter was collected, washed, dried, and boiled, in alcohol, the residue of the alcoholic solution formed a white stain, which became deep orange-red on the addition of nitric acid. The blood was subjected to a more complex operation. One pound and ten ounces of it were bruised in a mortar, diluted with two pounds of water, strongly acidulated with sulphuric acid, boiled, filtered, and washed. The filtered fluid was saturated with chalk, and the excess of carbonic acid driven off by heat. The fluid was then filtered again, and after being washed with water, was acted on by diluted acetic acid. The acetic solution left on evaporation a residue which was repeatedly acted on by alcohol ; and the residue of the alcoholic solutions was treated with pure alcohol and carbonate of lime. The new solution when filtered and evaporated left several small white stains, which became orange-red with nitric acid.† These results have been since contradicted by M. Dublanc. He in vain sought for morphia in the blood and urine of people who were taking

* Revue Médicale, 1827, i. 514 .   † Archives Gén. vii. 558.

acetate medicinally, or of animals that were killed by it.* Barruel's results are also at variance with some pointed experiments of M. Lassaigne, who could not detect any acetate of morphia even in blood drawn from a dog twelve hours after thirty-six grains were injected into the crural vein ;† nor any in the liver or venous blood of a dog poisoned with eight ounces of Sydenham's laudanum.‡

In investigating the effects of opium and its principles on man, the natural order of procedure is to consider in the first place those of opium itself in its various forms.

The effect of a small dose seems to be generally in the first instance stimulating : the action of the heart and arteries is increased, and a slight sense of fulness is caused in the head. This stimulus differs much in different individuals. In most persons it is quite insignificant. In its highest degree it is well exemplified by Dr. Leigh in his Experimental Inquiry, as they occurred to a friend of his who repeatedly made the experiment. If in the evening when he felt sleepy, he took thirty drops of laudanum, he was enlivened so that he could resume his studies ; and if, when the usual drowsiness approached, which it did in two hours, he took a hundred drops more, he soon became so much exhilarated, that he was compelled to laugh and sing and dance. The pulse meanwhile was full and strong, and the temporal arteries throbbed forcibly. In no long time the customary torpor ensued. The stimulant effect of opium given during a state of exhaustion is also well illustrated by Dr. Burnes in his account of Cutch. " On one occasion," says he, " I had made a very fatiguing night march with a Cutchee horseman. In the morning, after having travelled above thirty miles, I was obliged to assent to his proposal of haulting for a few minutes, which he employed in sharing a quantity of about two drachms of opium between himself and his jaded horse. The effect of the dose was soon evident on both, for the horse finished a journey of forty miles with great apparent facility, and the rider absolutely became more active and intelligent."§

By repeating small doses frequently, the stimulus may be kept up for a considerable time in some people. In this way are produced the remarkable effects said to be experienced by opium-eaters in the east. These effects seem to be in the first instance stimulant, the imagination being rendered brilliant, the passions exalted, and the muscular force increased ; and this state endures for a considerable time before the usual stage of collapse supervenes. A very poetical, but I believe also a faithful, picture of the phenomena now alluded to is given in the Confessions of an English Opium-eater, — a work well known to be founded on the personal experience of the writer. It is singular that our profession should have observed these phenomena so little, as to be accused by him of having wholly misrepresented the action of the most common drug in medical practice. In reply to this charge the physician may simply observe, that he seldom ad-

* Arch. Gén. i. 150.   † Ann. de Chim. et de Phys. 1824, xxv. 102.
‡ Journ. de Chim. Méd. 1841, 488.
§ Narrative of a Visit to the Court of Sinde, p. 231.

ministers opium in the way practised by the opium-eater; that when given in the usual therapeutic mode it rarely causes material excitement; that some professional people prefer giving it in frequent small doses, with the view of procuring its sedative effect, and undoubtedly do succeed in attaining their object; that in both of these medicinal ways of administering it, excitement is occasionally produced to a great degree and of a disagreeable kind; that the latter phenomena have been clearly traced to idiosyncrasy; and therefore that the effects on opium-eaters are probably owing either to the same cause, or to the modifying power of habit. This much at all events is certain,—that in persons unaccustomed to opium it seldom produces material excitement in a single small dose, and dose not always cause continuous excitement when taken after the manner of the opium-eater. The effect of a full medicinal dose of two or three grains of solid opium, or forty or sixty grains of the tincture, is to produce in general a transient excitement and fulness of the pulse, but in a short time afterwards torpor and sleep, commonly succeeded in six, eight, or ten hours by headache, nausea, and dry tongue.

The symptoms of poisoning with opium, administered at once in a dangerous dose, begin with giddiness and stupor, generally without any previous stimulus. The stupor rapidly increasing, the person soon becomes motionless and insensible to external impressions; he breathes slowly; generally lies still, with the eyes shut and the pupils contracted; and the whole expression of the countenance is that of deep and perfect repose. As the poisoning advances, the features become ghastly, the pulse feeble and imperceptible, the muscles excessively relaxed, and, unless assistance speedily arrive, death ensues. If recovery take place, the sopor is succeeded by prolonged sleep, which commonly ends in twenty-four or thirty-six hours, and is followed by nausea, vomiting, giddiness, and loathing of food.

The period which elapses between the taking of the poison and the commencement of the symptoms is various. A large quantity, taken in the form of tincture, on an empty stomach, may begin to act in a few minutes; but for obvious reasons it is not easy to learn the precise fact as to this particular. Dr. Meyer, late medical inspector at Berlin, has related a case of poisoning with six ounces of the saffron tincture of opium, where the person was found in a hopeless state of coma in half an hour,* and M. Ollivier has described another instance of a man who was found completely soporose at the same distance of time after taking an ounce and a half of laudanum.† In these cases, the symptoms must have begun in ten or fifteen minutes at farthest. In a case noticed by M. Desruelles the sopor was fairly formed in fifteen minutes after two drachms of solid opium were taken.‡ For the most part, however, opium, taken in the solid form, does not begin to act for half an hour or even almost a whole hour, — that period being required to allow its poisonous principles to be separated and absorbed by the bibulous vessels. It is singular that

* Rust's Magazin, iii. 24.   † Archives Gén. vii. 550.
‡ Journal Universel, xix. 340.

an interval of an hour was remarked in a case where the largest quantity was taken which has yet been recorded. The patient swallowed eight ounces of crude opium; but in an hour her physician found her able to tell connectedly all she had done; and she recovered.[*] In some rare cases the sopor is put off for a longer period: thus, in a case mentioned in Corvisart's Journal, there seems to have been no material stupor till considerably more than an hour after the person took two ounces and a half of the tincture with a drachm of the extract.[†]

The result of almost universal observation, however, is, that in pure poisoning with opium the commencement of the symptoms is not put off much beyond an hour. Such being the fact, it is extremely difficult to account for the following extraordinary case, which was communicated to me by Dr. Heude, of the East India Company's service. A man swallowed an ounce and a half of laudanum, and in an hour half as much more, and then lay down in bed. Some excitement followed, and also numbness of the arms and legs. But he continued so sensible and lively seven hours after the first dose was taken, that a medical gentleman, who saw him at that time and got from him a confession of what he had done, very naturally did not believe his story. It was not till at least the eighteenth hour that stupor set in; but two hours later, when Dr. Heude first saw him, he laboured under all the characteristic symptoms of poisoning with opium in an aggravated degree. The stomach-pump brought away a fluid quite free of the odour of opium. In seven hours more, under assiduous treatment, after having been in an almost hopeless state of insensibility, he had recovered so far as to be safely left in charge of a friend; and eventually he got quite well. No particular cause could be discovered for the long apparent suspension of the usual effects of opium.

Although the symptoms are very rarely postponed beyond an hour in pure poisoning with this substance, there is some reason for thinking that the interval may be much longer, if at the time of taking the opium the person be excited by intoxication from previously drinking spirits. Mr. Shearmen has related a striking case of an habitual drunkard, who took two ounces of laudanum while intoxicated to excitement with beer and spirits, and had no material stupor for five hours, during which period vomiting could not be induced. Five hours afterwards, he was found insensible, and he eventually died under symptoms of poisoning with opium.[‡]

The most remarkable symptom in the generality of cases of poisoning with opium is the peculiar sopor. This state differs from coma, in as much as the patient continues long capable of being roused. It may be difficult to rouse him; but unless death is at hand, this may be commonly accomplished by brisk agitation, tickling the nos-

* American Medical Recorder, xiii. 418, from Gemeinsame Deutsche Zeitschrift für Geburtshulfe, 1826, i. 1.
† Corvisart's Journal de Médecine, xvi. 22.
‡ Lond. Med. and Phys. Journal, xlix. 119.

trils, loud speaking, or the injection of water into the ear. The state of restored consciousness is always imperfect, and is speedily followed again by lethargy when the exciting power is withheld. — It has been already remarked, that the possibility of thus interrupt-ing the lethargy caused by opium is in general a good criterion for distinguishing the effects of this poison from apoplexy and epilepsy.

It was observed, in describing the mode of action of opium, that convulsions, although very frequently produced by it in animals, are rarely caused in man. It is not easy to account for this difference. Orfila has endeavoured to explain it, by supposing that convulsions are produced only by very large doses ; but there are many facts incompatible with that supposition.

While convulsions are certainly not common in the human subject, yet when they do occur they are sometimes violent. Tralles men-tions that he had himself several times seen convulsions excited in children by moderate doses.* The Journal Universel contains the case of a soldier who took two drachms of solid opium, and died in six hours and a half, after being affected with locked-jaw and dread-ful spasms.† A case is related in the Medical and Physical Journal of a young man, who, three hours after swallowing an ounce of laudanum, was found insensible, with the mouth distorted, the jaws fixed, and the hands clenched ; and who, soon after the insensibility was lessened by proper remedies, was seized with spasms of the back, neck, and extremities, so violent as to resemble opisthotonos.‡ Another good case of the kind is related by Mr. M'Kechnie, where the voluntary muscles were violently convulsed in frequent paroxysms, and affected in the intervals with subsultus, for three hours before the sopor came on.§ Two instances of convulsions alternating with sopor are shortly related by Dr. Bright.‖ The convulsions sometimes assume the form of permanent spasm, which may affect the whole muscles of the body, as in a case related in Corvisart's Journal¶ — Another rare symptom of poisoning with opium is delirium. It ap-pears to occur occasionally along with convulsions, as happened in Mr. M'Kechnie's case, and in one related by M. Ollivier.**

The state of the pulse varies considerably. In an interesting case described by Dr. Marcet it is mentioned that the pulse was 90, feeble and irregular ; and such appears to be its most common condition when the dose has been so large as seriously to endanger life.†† Fre-quently, however, it is much slower ; and then it is rather full than feeble, just as in apoplexy. In cases where convulsions occur, it is for the most part hurried, and does not become slow till the coma becomes pure. In Mr. M'Kechnie's case the pulse was at first 126 ; but when the convulsions ceased, and pure sopor supervened, it fell to 55. I

* De Usu Opii, iv. 149.   † Journal Universel, xix. 340.
‡ London Med. and Phys. Journal, xxxi. 468.
§ Edin. Med. and Surg. Journal, vii. 305.
‖ Reports of Medical Cases, ii. 205, 206.
¶ Journal de Médecine, xvi. 21.   ** Arch. Gén. vii. 552.
†† London Med. Chir. Trans. i. 77.

always becomes towards the close very feeble. and at length imperceptible.

The respiration is almost always slow. In Dr. Marcet's case, as in some others, it was stertorous; but this is not common. On the contrary, it is more frequently soft and gentle, as it has been in all the cases I have witnessed; and sometimes it can hardly be perceived at all, even in persons who eventually recover, as in an instance of recovery recorded by Dr. Kinnis.*

The pupils are always at least sluggish in their contractions, often quite insensible; — sometimes, it is said, dilated :† but much more commonly contracted, and occasionally to an extreme degree. In the case last noticed, they were no bigger than a pin's head. The pupils have been so invariably found contracted in all recent cases of poisoning with opium, that some doubt arises whether they are ever otherwise, and whether the earlier accounts, which represent them to have been dilated, may not be incorrect, and the result of hasty observation.

The expression of the countenance is for the most part remarkably placid, like that of a person in sound natural sleep. Occasionally there is an expression of anxiety mingled with the stupor. The face is commonly pale. Sometimes, however, it is flushed ;‡ and in rare cases the expression is furious.§

In moderately large doses opium generally suspends the excretion of urine and fæces; but it promotes perspiration. In dangerous cases the lethargy is sometimes accompanied with copious sweating. In a fatal case, which I examined judicially, the sheets were completely soaked to a considerable distance around the body.

A remarkable circumstance, which has been noticed by a late author, is the sudden death of leeches applied to the body. The patient was a child who had been poisoned by too strong an injection of poppy-heads.‖

In some instances the symptoms proper to poisoning with opium become complicated with those which belong rather to organic affections of the brain, in consequence of such affections being suddenly developed through means of the cerebral congestion occasioned by the poison. Thus, in a case related in Corvisart's Journal, there were convulsions and somnolency on the third day, and palsy of one arm for four days; and for nearly two months afterwards the patient complained of occasional attacks of weakness and numbness, sometimes of one extremity, sometimes of another.¶ Here the brain must have sustained some more permanent injury than usual. — A more remarkable illustration once occurred to Dr. Elliotson. A young man, seven hours after swallowing two ounces of laudanum, presented the usual effects of opium, such as contracted pupils, redness of the features, a frequent feeble pulse, coldness of the integuments, and

* Edin. Med. and Surg. Journ. xiv. 603.
† Journ. Universel, xix. 340.
‡ Edin. Med. and Surg. Journal, vii.   § Journ. Universel, xix. 340.
‖ Melier in Archives Gén. de Méd. xiv. 406.
¶ Corvisart's Journ. de Méd. xvi. 21.

stupor, from which he could be roused without particular difficulty. The stomach-pump brought away a fluid which had not any odour of opium ; powerful stimulants were given, such as ether, ammonia and brandy ; and he was kept constantly walking between two men. In an hour and a half, when sensibility had been materially restored, his head suddenly dropped down upon his breast, and he fell down dead. The sinuses and veins of the brain were turgid, and a moderately thick layer of blood was effused over the arachnoid membrane.*
— Under the same head must be arranged the following extraordinary case related by Pyl. That author admits it as one of simple poisoning, with a complete remission of the symptoms for several days. But the possibility of such a remission must be received with great hesitation. It is well known that most of the symptoms may be dispelled by vigorous treatment, and the patient nevertheless relapse immediately if left to himself, and even die. This is acknowledged on all hands. Pyl, however, admits the possibility of a much more complete and longer interval. His case is shortly as follows. A man who had taken a large quantity of opium, and became very dangerously ill, was made to vomit in twelve hours, and regained his senses completely. The bowels continued obstinately costive ; but he had for some days no other symptom referrible to the poison ; when at length the whole body became gradually palsied and stiff, and he died on the tenth day. No importance can be attached to a solitary case differing so widely from every other. The only way in which opium could cause death in such a manner, must be by calling forth some disposition to natural disease. Pyl's case was probably one of supervening *ramollissement,* or inflammation of the substance of the brain.†

Notwithstanding the purely narcotic or nervous symptoms, which opium produces in a vast proportion of instances, there is no doubt that it also excites in a few rare cases those of irritation. Thus, although it generally constipates the bowels, it has been known to induce diarrhœa or colic in particular constitutions. In the first volume of the Medical Communications, it is observed by Michaëlis that both diarrhœa and diuresis may be produced by it. The soldier, whose case was quoted as having been accompanied with convulsions, had acute pain in the stomach for some time after swallowing the poison ; and in the case just quoted from Corvisart's Journal, the accesssion of somnolency was attended with excruciating pain of two days' duration.

Another and more singular anomaly is the spontaneous occurrence of vomiting. Sometimes a little vomiting immediately succeeds the taking of the poison. This may not interrupt, however, the progress of the symptoms ;‡ but more commonly it is the means of saving the person's life, as in a striking case described by Petit of an English officer,§ who, in consequence of vomiting immediately after taking two ounces of laudanum, had only moderate somnolency. At

* Lance, 1836-37, i. 271.
† Aufsätze und Beobachtungen, i. 93.
‡ Ollivier's case in Arch. Gén. vii. 550.   § Corv. Journ. de Méd. xxxiv. 274.

other times vomiting occurs at a much later period. Pyl, in his Essays and Observations, gives a case in which, some hours after thirty grains were swallowed, vomiting took place spontaneously, and recurred frequently afterwards ; in the same paper is an account of another case by the individual himself, who attempted to commit suicide by taking a large dose of laudanum, but was disappointed in consequence of the poison being spontaneously vomited after the sopor had fairly set in ;* and a similar case is related by M. Mascarel, where, after seven ounces of Sydenham's laudanum had been taken, vomiting occurred spontaneously, and was followed only by inconsiderable stupor.† — Vomiting is a common enough symptom after the administration of emetics, or subsequent to the departure of the somnolency.‡

The ordinary duration of a fatal case of poisoning with opium is from seven to twelve hours.   Most people recover who outlive twelve hours.   At the same time fatal cases of longer duration are on record : Réaumur mentions one which proved fatal in fifteen hours,§ Orfila another fatal in seventeen hours,‖ Leroux another fatal in the same time,¶ Alibert another fatal in nearly twenty-four hours.**   An instance has even been related, which appeared to prove fatal not till towards the close of the third day ;†† but the whole course of the symptoms was in that case so unusual, that some other cause must have co-operated in occasioning death.   Sometimes, too, death takes place in a shorter time than seven hours ; six hours is not an uncommon duration ; I once met with a judicial case, which could not have lasted above five hours ; an infirmary patient of my colleague, Dr. Home, died in four hours ; in the 31st volume of the Medical and Physical Journal, there is one which proved fatal in three hours.‡‡ This is the shortest I have read of.

The dose of opium requisite to cause death has not been determined.   Indeed it must vary so much with circumstances, that it is almost vain to attempt to fix it.   Pyl relates a case, quickly fatal, where the quantity taken was 60 grains ;§§ Lassus an instance of

* Aufsätze und Beobachtungen, i. 94, 100.   † Archives Gén. de Méd. li. 495.

‡ These effects must not be confounded with those which poppy-juice has been known to cause when spoiled. A whole family of Jews were attacked with violent vomiting and purging, in consequence of partaking of a decoction of poppy-heads, which had been kept four days in a hot stove, and had consequently undergone decomposition. The usual narcotism was not produced at all. (Rust's Magazin, xxii. 484.)

§ Mém. de l'Acad. des Sciences, xxxviii. 1735.

‖ Toxicol Gén. from Bibliothèque Médicale, Aout, 1806.

¶ Corvisart's Journal de Médecine, iv. 3.

** Nouveaux Elémens de Thérapeutique, ii. 60.

†† London Med. and Phys. Journal, xxviii. 81. This patient took at 4 A.M. two ounces of wine of opium, became drowsy at 6, was capable of being roused at 9, vomited by emetics a liquid coloured with laudanum, and was kept awake for the rest of the day. But at 7 P.M. having previously had a cough and brown sputa from vinegar entering his windpipe, he became gradually more and more insensible, till at last he was quite comatose; and in this state he continued till his death on the evening of the third day. On dissection nothing was found in the brain or stomach attributable to opium.

‡‡ London Med. and Phys. Journal, xxxi. 468.

§§ Aufsätze und Beobachtungen, i. 85.

death from 36 grains ;* Wildberg has related a fatal case caused by little more than half an ounce of the Berlin tincture,† which contains the soluble matter of forty grains ; and Mr. Skae has mentioned a case fatal in about thirteen hours, where the dose seems to have been well ascertained not to have exceeded half an ounce of common laudanum, or about twenty grains of opium.‡ Dr. Paris, without quoting any particular fact, says four grains may prove fatal.§ I should have felt some difficulty in admitting this statement, as I have repeatedly known persons, unaccustomed to opium, take three or four grains without any other effect than sound sleep. But I have been favoured with the particulars of a case by Mr. W. Brown of this city, where a dose of four grains and a half, taken by an adult along with nine grains of camphor, was followed by the usual signs of narcotism, and death in nine hours. The man took the opium for a cough at seven in the morning ; at nine his wife found him in a deep sleep, from which she could not rouse him ; nothing was done for his relief till three in the afternoon, when Mr. Brown found him labouring under all the usual symptoms of poisoning with opium, contracted pupils among the rest; and death ensued in an hour, notwithstanding the active employment of remedies. On examining the body no morbid appearance was found of any note except fluidity of the blood, — a common appearance in those who have died of the effects of this drug.

It is more important than may at first sight be imagined to acquire an approximative knowledge of the smallest fatal dose. For, in consequence of the dread entertained of opium by many unprofessional persons, it is currently believed to be much more active than it is in reality; and instances of natural death have been consequently imputed to medicinal doses taken fortuitously a short time before. The facts stated above comprehend the only precise information I have been able to collect as to the smallest fatal doses in adults. I may add some farther observations, however, on the smallest fatal doses in children. Very young children are often peculiarly sensible to the poisonous action of opium, so that it is scarcely possible to use the most insignificant doses with safety. Sundeling states in general terms that extremely small doses are very dangerous to infants on account of the rapidity of absorption. This opinion is amply supported by the following cases. — An infant three days old got by mistake about the fourth part of a mixture containing ten drops of laudanum. No medical man was called for eleven hours. At that time there was great somnolency and feebleness, but the child could be roused. The breathing being very slow, artificial respiration was resorted to, but without advantage : the child died in twenty-four hours, the character of the symptoms remaining unchanged to the last. At the inspection of the body, which I witnessed, no morbid ap-

* Mémoires de l'Institut — Sc. Physiques, ii. 107.
† Practisches Handbuch für Physiker, iii. 329.
‡ Edin. Med. and Surg. Journal, liv. 151.
§ Paris and Fonblanque's Medical Jurisprudence, ii. 383.

49*

pearance was found. — Of the same kind was a case communicated to me by Dr. Simson of this city, where the administration of three drops of laudanum in a chalk mixture, for diarrhœa, to a stout child fourteen months old, was followed by coma, convulsions, and death in about six hours. Dr. Simson satisfied himself, as far as that was possible, that the apothecary who made up the mixture did not commit a mistake. — Dr. Kelso of Lisburn met with a similar case in an infant of nine months, who died in nine hours after taking four drops.* — My colleague, Dr. Alison, tells me he has met with a case where an infant a few weeks old died with all the symptoms of poisoning with opium after receiving four drops of laudanum, and that he has repeatedly seen unpleasant deep sleep induced by only two drops. — These remarks being kept in view, it will, I suspect, be difficult to go along with an opinion against poisoning expressed by a German medico-legal physician in the following circumstances. A child's maid, pursuant to a common but dangerous custom among nurses, gave a healthy infant, four weeks old, an anodyne draught to quiet its screams. The infant soon fell fast asleep, but died comatose in twelve hours. There was not any appearance of note in the dead body; and the child was therefore universally thought to have been killed by the draught. But the inspecting physician declared that to be impossible, as the draught contained only an eighth of a grain of opium and as much hyoscyamus.† In the first edition of this work an opinion was expressed to the same purport. But the facts stated above throw doubt on its accuracy, and rather show that the dose was sufficient in the circumstances to occasion death.

A very important circumstance to attend to in respect to the dose of opium required to prove fatal is the influence of constitutional circumstances in rendering this drug unusually energetic. In some persons this peculiar anomaly exists always, even during a state of health. Thus, I am acquainted with a gentleman on whom seven drops of laudanum act with great certainty as a hypnotic. In such a one doses, which are safely taken by many, might prove dangerous.

It is more usual, however, to meet with this anomaly in the course of some diseases. These have not yet been satisfactorily indicated. I have several times, however, met with unusually energetic action from medicinal doses in elderly persons affected with severe habitual catarrh; and in one instance death occurred after a dose of twenty-five drops in the advanced stage of acute catarrh supervening on its chronic form, the symptoms being those of poisoning with opium, succeeding apparently a state of comfortable sleep.— A case seemingly of the same nature, where the dose was fifteen drops of Battley's Sedative Liquor, occurred at Islington in 1841. An elderly lady, in delicate health, and affected severely with asthma, which for ten days prevented her from sleeping, got from a neighbouring druggist a draught of Battley's solution, syrup, and camphor-mixture. Next morning she was found insensible and livid in the face, with cold

* Lancet, 1837-38, i. 304.
† Pyl's Repert. für die gerichtl. Arzneiwissenschaft, iii. 145.

extremities and contracted pupils; and she died about twelve hours after taking the draught. There was no sign of natural disease in the dead body to account for death. The druggist was absurdly blamed for giving such a dose to a frail old lady ; for the dose was not more than would be generally given in such circumstances. This case was communicated to me by the druggist in question. — Another of the like kind has been communicated to me by Mr. Garstang of Clitheroe. An elderly female, long subject to severe cough, having enjoyed a comfortable night's rest after a dose of a preparation containing half a grain of opium, took in the morning the equivalent of two grains and a half, or three grains at the utmost, and fell asleep soon after. In no long time, her husband, alarmed because he could not rouse her, sent for Mr. Garstang, who found her husband labouring under all the symptoms of poisoning with opium ; and, notwithstanding active treatment, she died six hours after the second dose. Her husband took half a grain with her the evening before, but experienced no effect from it at all. Not the slightest ground could exist in this case for suspecting either foul play or pharmaceutic error. — As a farther illustration, the following incident deserves notice, which occurred last year in London, and was communicated to me by Dr G. Johnson, a former pupil. A little girl, five years and a half old, affected with violent cough, got a mixture containing opium, which was repeated six, thirteen, and twenty-six hours afterwards. She slept soundly after each dose, and awoke readily after the first three ; but after the fourth she had more stupor and much uneasiness ; in which state, but with at least one interval of sensibility, she died in nine hours more, or thirty-five hours after the first dose. According to the prescriber's intention, the child ought to have taken only two minims of laudanum in all ; but, according to a rough analysis by Mr. Alfred Taylor, each dose contained an eighth of a grain of opium. or a trifle more. In either view it is impossible that doses so small, and so distant, could produce these effects in ordinary circumstances.

Such cases are important in several respects, but especially because they naturally give rise to suspicions of an over-dose of opium having been incautiously given, and thus to misrepresentations injurious to the druggist or medical attendant. In the last case a Coroner's Jury brought in the preposterous verdict, that death was caused by " too much opium ordered without due instructions."

It is scarcely necessary to add, that the dose required to prove fatal is very much altered by habit. Those who have been accustomed to eat opium are obliged gradually to increase the dose, otherwise its usual effects are not produced. Some extraordinary, but I believe correct information on this subject, is contained in the confessions of an English opium-eater. The author took at one time 8000 drops daily, or about nine ounces of laudanum.

An important topic relative to the effects of opium on man is its operation on the body when used continuously in the manner practised by opium-eaters. This subject was brought forcibly under my notice in 1831, in consequence of a remarkable civil trial, in which I was concerned as a medical witness, — that of Sir W. F rbes and company against the Edinburgh Life Assurance Company. The late Earl of Mar effected insurances on his life to a large amount while addicted to the vice of opium-eating ; which was not made known at the time to the insurance company. He died two years afterwards of jaundice and dropsy. The company refused payment, on the ground that his lordship had concealed from them a habit which tends to shorten life ; and Sir W. Forbes and company, who held the policy of insurance as security for money lent to the earl, raised an action to recover payment.

In consequence of inquiries made on this occasion, I became for the first time aware of the frequency of the vice of opium-eating among both the lower orders and the upper ranks of society ; and at the same time satisfied myself, that the habit is often easily concealed from the most intimate friends, — that physicians even in extensive practice seldom become acquainted with such cases, — that the effects of the habit on the constitution are not always what either professional persons or the unprofessional would expect, — and generally that practitioners and toxicologists possess little or no precise information on the matter. In what is about to be offered on the subject, some facts will be stated which appear to me interesting, and may induce others to contribute their knowledge towards filling up so important a blank in medico-legal toxicology.

The general impression is, that the practice of opium-eating injures the health and shortens life. But the scientific physician in modern times has seen so many proofs of the inaccuracy of popular impressions relative to the operation of various agents on health and longevity,[*] that he will not allow himself to be hastily carried along in the present instance by vague popular belief. The general conviction of the tendency of opium-eating to shorten life has obviously been derived in part from the injurious effects which opium used medicinally has on the nervous system and functions of the alimentary canal, — and partly on the reports of travellers in Turkey and Persia, who have enjoyed opportunities of watching the life and habits of opium-eaters on a great scale. The statements of travellers, however, are so vague that they cannot be turned to use with any confidence in a scientific inquiry. Chardin, one of the earliest (1671) and best of modern travellers in Turkey, merely says the opium-eater becomes rheumatic at fifty, and " never reaches an extreme old age ;"[†] and his successors have seldom been more precise, — no one having given information as to the diseases which it tends to engender. By far the greater number of authorities, however, agree in representing the practice to be hurtful. Mr. Madden, a recent and professional authority, even alleges that it is very rare for an opium-eater at Constantinople to outlive his thirtieth year, if he began the practice early.

* See, for example, Parent-Duchatelet and D'Arcet on the health and longevity of Tobacco-manufacturers and Woodfloaters, in Annales d'Hyg. Publ. et de Méd. Lég. L 169, and iii. 245.

† Voyages en Perse, iii. 93.

On the other hand, a few late observers deny altogether the accuracy of these statements. To this number belongs Dr. Burnes of the Bombay army; whose opinion is worthy of notice, because he had ample opportunities of observation during his residence in Cutch and at the Court of Sinde for several years prior to 1831. From what he there witnessed, Dr. Burnes is inclined to think "it will be found in general that the natives do not suffer much from the use of opium," — that " this powerful narcotic does not seem to destroy the powers of the body, nor to enervate the mind to the degree that might be imagined."* Dr. Macpherson of the Madras army, who had occasion to observe the effects of the parallel practice of opium-smoking in China, coincides in opinion with Dr. Burnes. He says, " were we to be led away by the popular opinion that the habitual use of opium injures the health and shortens life, we should expect to find the Chinese a shrivelled, emaciated, idiotic race. On the contrary, although the habit of smoking opium is universal among rich and poor, we find them to be a powerful, muscular, and athletic people, and the lower orders more intelligent and far superior in mental acquirements to those of corresponding rank in our own country."†

The familiar effects of the medicinal use of opium in disordering the nervous system and the digestive functions constitute a better reason, than the loose statements of eastern travellers, for the popular impression of the danger of its habitual and long-continued use. Yet this consideration ought not to be allowed too much weight ; because the functions of the nervous system and of digestion may be deranged by other causes, for example by hysteria, without necessarily and materially shortening life. It is desirable therefore to appeal if possible to precise facts.

The following is a summary of twenty-five cases, the particulars of which I have obtained from various quarters. The general result rather tends to throw doubt over the popular opinion. — 1. A lady about thirty, in good health, has taken it largely for twenty years, having been gradually habituated to it from childhood by the villany of her maid, who gave it frequently to keep her quiet. 2. A female who died of consumption at the age of forty-two, had taken about a drachm of solid opium for ten years, but had given up the practice for three years before her death, and led in other respects a licentious life from an early age. 3. A well-known literary author, about sixty years of age, has taken laudanum for thirty-five years, with occasional short intermissions, and sometimes an enormous quantity, but enjoys tolerable bodily health. 4. A lady, after being in the practice of drinking laudanum for at least twenty years, died at the age of fifty, — of what disease I have been unable to learn. 5. A lady about fifty-five, who enjoys good health, has taken opium many years, and at present uses three ounces of laudanum daily. 6. A lady about sixty gave it up after using it constantly for twenty years, during which she enjoyed good health ; and subsequently she resumed it.

* Narrative of a Visit to the Court of Sinde, p. 230.
† Two Years in China, 1843, p. 243.

7. Lord Mar after using laudanum for thirty years, at times to the amount of two or three ounces daily, died at the age of fifty-seven of jaundice and dropsy; but he was a martyr to rheumatism, and besides lived rather freely.   8. A woman, who had been in the practice of taking about two ounces of laudanum daily for very many years, died at the age of sixty or upwards.   9. An eminent literary character, who died about the age of sixty-three, was in the practice of drinking laudanum to excess from the age of fifteen ; and his daily allowance was sometimes a quart of a mixture consisting of three parts of laudanum and one of alcohol.   10. A lady, who died lately at the age of seventy-six, took laudanum in the quantity of half an ounce daily for nearly forty years.   11. An old woman died not long ago at Leith at the age of eighty, who had taken about half an ounce of laudanum daily for nearly forty years, and enjoyed tolerable health all the time.   12. Visrajee, a celebrated Cutchee chief, mentioned by Dr. Burnes, had taken opium largely all his life, and was alive when Dr. Burnes drew up his Narrative, at the age of eighty, " paralyzed by years, but his mind unimpaired."[*]

For the particulars of the remaining cases I am indebted to Dr. Tait, surgeon of police in this city.   13. M. C., a ruddy, healthy-looking woman, sixty years of age, has taken laudanum for twenty-five years to the extent of half an ounce daily in a single dose.   14. M. H., a flabby, dissipated-looking woman of thirty-six, has taken for ten years thirty grains of opium daily in three doses.   15. M. T., a widow, forty-eight years of age, who takes twice daily a dose of one fluidrachm of laudanum, and has done so for fourteen years, cannot observe any permanent injury except diminution of appetite.   16. Mrs. G., aged twenty-four, has taken a single dose of sixty drops regularly at bed-time for five years, and has not suffered in health in any respect, except that she is costive.   17. F. S., a thin, sallow woman of forty-six years of age, has taken a fluidrachm of laudanum three times a day for ten years, cannot take food without it, but is so well as to be able to get up regularly at six in the morning.   18. H. S., a shrivelled old-looking woman, who for thirty-eight years had taken daily towards a drachm of opium in one dose, and who latterly was strong, lively, and of good appetite, died recently at the age of sixty-nine.   19. Mrs. S., who has taken about a scruple of opium for twenty-one years, is a tall, active, old-looking woman of fifty-seven, enjoys good health when she uses the opium, but suffers from an affection like delirium tremens, when she cannot get her usual quantity.   20. M. A., aged thirty-one, has taken half a drachm of opium daily in two doses for ten years, was a thin, drunken, starved-looking prostitute some years ago, but, having reformed her ways, is now " a fine-looking, bouncing woman," younger in appearance than formerly, and not liable to any suffering either before or after her doses, except that she cannot take food without them.   21. Miss M., who has taken ten grains of opium three times a day for five years, is a healthy, florid young woman of twenty-seven, liable to costive-

* Narrative, &c. p. 231.

ness, and, when without her opium, to languor and want of appetite, but otherwise free of complaint. 22. Mrs. ——, a plump, hale-looking old lady of seventy, has taken opium for six and twenty years, and for some years to the extent of a drachm daily in two doses. She thinks her health improved by it, and has suffered no inconvenience except merely costiveness, and always aversion to food till she gets her dose. 23. J. B., aged 23, has taken laudanum since she was fourteen, and some time past to the amount of an ounce or ten drachms in three or four doses daily. She has only menstruated twice since first using the laudanum, has bilious vomiting once a month, and looks older than her years, but is otherwise quite healthy, and has two children. 24. Mrs. M'C., a ruddy young-looking woman of forty-two, has taken opium during two years for cough and pain in the stomach, latterly to the extent of ten grains twice a day. She has never menstruated since, but has enjoyed better health, and in particular has a good appetite after her dose, and has got entirely quit of a former tendency to constipation. 25. An army officer's widow, fifty-five years old, healthy and young-looking, although subject to costiveness and rather defective appetite, has taken laudanum for eleven years, and latterly opium to the extent of fifteen grains morning and evening.

These facts tend on the whole rather to show, that the practice of eating opium is not so injurious, and an opium eater's life not so un-insurable, as is commonly thought; and that an insured person, who did not make known this habit, could scarcely be considered guilty of concealment to the effect of voiding his insurance. But I am far from thinking, — as several represent who have quoted this work, — that what has now been stated can with justice be held to establish such important inferences; for there is an obvious reason, why in an inquiry of this kind those instances chiefly should come under notice where the constitution has escaped injury, cases fatal in early life being more apt to be lost sight of, or more likely to be concealed.

Meanwhile, insurance companies and insurance physicians ought to be aware, that not a few persons in the upper ranks of life are con-firmed opium-eaters without even their intimate friends knowing it. And the reason is, that at the time the opium-eater is visible to his friends, namely, during the period of excitement, there is frequently nothing in his behaviour or appearance to attract particular attention. From the information I have received, it appears that the British opium-eater is by no means subject to the extraordinary excitement of mind and body described by travellers as the effect of opium-eating in Turkey and Persia; but that the common effect merely is to remove torpor and sluggishness, and make him in the eyes of his friends an active and conversible man. The prevailing notions of the nature of the excitement from eating opium are therefore very much exag-gerated. Another singular circumstance I have ascertained is, that constipation is by no means a general effect of the continued use of opium. In some of the cases mentioned above no laxatives have been required; and in others a gentle laxative once a week is sufficient.

In the civil suit regarding Lord Mar's insurances, the insurance company was at first found not entitled to refuse payment,— not, however, on the ground that the habit of opium-eating is harmless to longevity,— but chiefly on a technical ground, implying that they did not make inquiry into his habits with the care usually observed by insurance companies, and were therefore to be understood as accepting the life at a venture. A new trial was granted by the court on the ground of the judge's charge having been not according to evidence; but on this occasion the parties compromised the case.*

The previous remarks on the symptoms of poisoning with opium in man have been confined to its effects when swallowed. But it was mentioned under the head of its mode of action, that this poison has been known to act with energy upon animals through every channel by which it can be introduced into the system. It is natural to expect that the same will be the case with man also.

The only other modes in which poisoning with opium is reported to have been produced in man, besides administration by the mouth, have been by injections into the anus, by application to the skin deprived of its cuticle, perhaps even also to the unbroken skin, and by its introduction into the external opening of the ear.

In the Journal de Chimie Médicale, an instance is shortly noticed of a lady who was poisoned by the administration of too strong an anodyne injection prepared by herself from fresh poppy-heads. She recovered.†

It is generally believed in France that opium acts more energetically through the medium of the rectum, than through the stomach. Orfila in particular has endeavoured to establish this proposition by experiments on animals, and quotations from cases recorded by some authors of its action upon man.‡ But neither the experiments nor the quotations appear to me satisfactory; and the rule they go to support is completely at variance with the practice pursued in the medicinal administration of the drug in Britain. It is the custom to give at least twice as much in an enema as in a draught. I have given by injection, without producing more than the usual somnolency, one drachm and even two drachms by measure of laudanum, a dose which, were Orfila's statement correct, would prove fatal.

As to the action of opium through the skin when deprived of its cuticle, I am not acquainted with any fatal case of the kind, but have no doubt that such may happen. One of my friends very nearly lost his life in the way alluded to. He had applied an opium-poultice to the scrotum to allay the violent irritation caused by a blister, and fell into a state of profound sopor, which was luckily interrupted by a visitor, so that the cause was discovered before it was too late. An instance of the same kind has also been published by M. Pelletan. A child two months old very nearly perished, in consequence of a cerate containing fifteen drops of laudanum having been kept for twenty-four hours on a slight excoriation produced by a fold of the skin. When the cause of illness was discovered, the child had been

* Edin. Medical and Surgical Journal, xxxvii. 123.
† Journal de Chimie Méd. iii. 24.   ‡ Toxicologie Gén. ii. 81, 82.

for some hours almost completely insensible, with a slow, obscure pulse, and occasional convulsions.*

But perhaps opium may in some circumstances act even through the unbroken skin. It has certainly been often applied in this way to relieve local pain without avail. Yet on the other hand its effect is at times unequivocal; and the following incidents seem to show, that it may even prove fatal, both when the skin is healthy, and in certain diseased states of the integuments. A young dramatic writer in Paris was directed by his father, a physician, to apply over the stomach a poultice moistened with a few drops of laudanum. The patient, in order to relieve his pain more quickly, poured the whole contents of the bottle over the poultice, and soon fell into a deep sleep. Prompt assistance was obtained, but proved of no avail, and death is said to have ensued with great rapidity.† A soldier affected with erysipelas of the leg, had a linseed poultice applied, which his surgeon ordered to be sprinkled with 15 drops of laudanum. Next morning the patient was found in a state of deep sopor, accompanied with convulsive twitches of the muscles of the face and limbs; and in no long time he expired. His soporose state turned the surgeon's attention to the poultice, which he found coloured yellow and smelling strongly of opium; and on removing it he discovered that it was completely soaked with laudanum, which the attendant had carelessly poured on it to the extent of an ounce. The patient died notwithstanding all the remedies which his state called for; and the viscera were found quite healthy; but in many places the blood is said to have had a strong odour of opium.‡

In an instance reported by M. Tournon of Bordeaux, death is supposed to have arisen from the introduction of opium into the external opening of the ear, as a remedy for ear-ache. It is possible that fatal poisoning may thus be induced by laudanum too freely and frequently renewed: but it seems very unlikely that death was owing to opium in the instance in question, since it was used in the solid form, and in the quantity of four grains; so that the dose was small, and absorption must have been very slow. The account merely states that the patient fell asleep, but his sleep was that of death.§

Of the Action of Morphia, Narcotine, Codeïa, and Meconic Acid.

The action and symptoms caused by two active principles of opium, morphia, and narcotine, have been examined by many experimentalists.

The action of *morphia* is nearly the same as that of opium, but more energetic. In its solid state it has little effect, being nearly insoluble. But when dissolved in olive oil, or in alcohol, or in weak acids, it excites in animals the same symptoms as opium. Experimentalists are not yet agreed as to its power. The trial of Castaing

---

* Journal de Chim. Méd. vii. 250.   † Ibidem, 1842. 583.
‡ Journal de Chimie Médicale, Avril, 1827, and Edin. Med. Journ. xxix. 450.
§ Ibidem, vii. 114.

gave rise to a physiological inquiry by three French physicians, De-
guise, Dupuy, and Leuret, who assigned to it feeble properties; but
more reliance is usually placed in the experiments of Orfila, who
found that one part of morphia is equal in energy to two parts of the
watery extract, and to four parts of crude opium.   The observations
I have made on the medicinal effects of morphia and its muriate, lead
me to believe that half a grain is fully equal in power to three grains
of the best Turkey-opium.   Probably those who have observed but
slight effects from it have accidentally used narcotine instead of it;
for at one time they were often confounded together.

On man morphia acts like opium ; it produces somnolency.   It
was at one time thought that in medicinal doses it does not produce
either the disagreeable subsequent or idiosyncratic effects of opium ;
Magendie made some observations to this purport ;* and Dr. Quadri
of Naples was led to the same conclusion.†   Others, however, have
doubted the accuracy of these authors, and opposite results appear to
have been procured by some.   My own experience with the muriate
of morphia inclines me to concur in opinion with Magendie and
Quadri.

The effects of morphia on man in fatal doses have hitherto been
observed in a few cases only.   An instance, which was the occasion
of a criminal trial at Aberdeen in 1842, has been communicated to me
by Dr. Traill, who was consulted in the case on the part of the crown.
A schoolmaster gave ten grains of the muriate to a girl immediately
after she came out of an epileptic fit.   In fifteen minutes she seemed
to fall asleep ; she continued in this state for some hours before it
was discovered that she was in a state of stupor, from which she could
not be roused ; and she expired twelve hours after the poison was
administered.   A similar case occasioned by ten grains, and also
fatal, occurred at Cheltenham in 1839.

Orfila relates the particulars of the case of a young Parisian graduate, who swallowed twenty-two grains for the purpose of self-destruction.   In ten minntes he felt heat in the stomach and hindhead,
with excessive itchiness ; in three hours and a half he had also a
sense of pricking in the eyes, with dimness of vision ; and in an
hour more he for the first time felt approaching stupor. Half an hour
afterwards, when the people of the house entered his room he could
not see them, though he was sensible enough to be able to reply to
their inquiries, that he lay in bed because he had not slept the night
before.   Soon after this he fell into a state of profound stupor and
lost all consciousness.   In thirteen hours he was visited by Orfila,
who found him cold, quite comatose, and affected with locked-
jaw ; the pupils were feebly dilated, the pulse 120, the breathing
hurried and stertorous, the belly tense and tympanitic ; and there
were occasional convulsions, with intense itching of the skin.   By
means of copious venesection, sinapisms, ammoniated friction, stimu-

* Bulletins de la Société Philomatique, 1818, p. 54. — Journal de Chimie Médicale,
Avril, 1827.
† Annali Universali di Med. xxxi. 169, xxxiv. 100.

lant clysters, ice on the head, and acidulous drinks, he was gradually roused, so that in six hours he recognised his physician. In the subsequent night and following day he had difficult and scanty micturition, with pain in the kidneys and bladder, and difficulty in swallowing; but these symptoms went off during the second night; and on the third morning he was quite well.* The itching of the skin remarked in this case is considered by M. Bally an invariable symptom of the operation of morphia even in medicinal doses.† It is not, however, always produced.

Another case, which occurred at Lunéville, is very remarkable in its circumstances. A young man addicted to opium-eating, but who had left off the practice for a twelvemonth, took first ten grains, and in ten minutes forty grains more of acetate of morphia. In five minutes he had excessive general feebleness and a sense of impending dissolution, which forced him to confess what he had done. In fifteen minutes more M. Castara, who describes the particulars, found him motionless, almost comatose, and breathing laboriously. The limbs were flaccid, the pupils contracted, the face and lips livid, the skin warm and moist, the pulse full and hard, and deglutition impossible. Tartar-emetic was ordered, but could not be administered. He was then bled at the arm to eighteen ounces; upon which he started as from sleep, rubbed his eyes, said every thing turned round him, and that he could not see the people present. When left to himself he quickly fell into a calm slumber; but if kept awake, he told collectedly all that happened before he became comatose. He complained chiefly of intense itching and a general sense of bruising. In an hour, by keeping him constantly roused, consciousness was almost restored, and this without vomiting having been produced, though two grains of tartar-emetic had been swallowed and three administered by the rectum. In four hours after he swallowed the poison he vomited freely and had diarrhœa. He then steadily recovered, the sleepiness continued all next day, and the itching of the skin even longer.‡

M. Julia-Fontenelle met with a case of poisoning with this alkaloid, in consequence of its having been administered with a clyster in the form of sulphate. The subject was a child five years old, the dose five grains, the symptoms those of apoplexy, and death supervened within twenty-four hours.§

Another case worthy of particular mention is that of the French gentleman who was supposed to have been poisoned by Dr. Castaing. It is not a pure one, for besides the symptoms of a consumptive complaint under which he had laboured for some time, there were circumstances in his last illness which indicated the administration of other deleterious substances. About thirty-six hours before his death, however, they were exactly such as might be expected from a large dose of morphia. About five minutes after the admi-

---

* Journal de Chim. Méd. v. 410. † Mém. de la Soc. Roy. de Médecine, i. 142.
‡ Journal de Chim. Méd. vii. 135. § Revue Médicale, 1829, iii. 424.

nistration of a draught by the prisoner, the gentleman was attacked with convulsions, and not long afterwards his physician found him quite insensible, unable to swallow, bathed in a cold sweat, with a small pulse, a burning skin, the jaws locked, the neck rigid, the belly tense, and the limbs affected with spasmodic convulsions. In this state he seems to have continued till his death. The only appearances found in the dead body, which bore any relation to the poison suspected, were congestion of blood and serous effusion in the vessels of the cerebral membranes. If morphia was the cause of death, it is highly probable that, besides what was administered thirty-six hours before he died, several doses were given subsequently; otherwise, from what is known of the action of opium, the narcotism could scarcely have lasted uninterruptedly for so long a period.[*]

For the following extraordinary case I am indebted to one of my pupils, Mr. Clark of Montrose: A woman took one morning by mistake ten grains of pure muriate of morphia, which had been prepared not long before by Mr. Clark in my laboratory, and was freed of codeïa. The mistake having been discovered almost immediately, means were taken to prevent any ill effects from the accident, and within half an hour after the poison was swallowed, the stomach was completely cleared by the stomach-pump. At this time she was quite sensible. But stupor quickly came on after the poison was evacuated, and deep imperturbable coma gradually formed, so that nothing could rouse her in the slightest degree except cold affusion of the head and chest, which caused faint signs of returning consciousness. Before night she expired, though all the usual remedies were resorted to. An inspection of the body was not obtained, which is much to be regretted, since without it the case is quite obscure. I do not know a single instance of fatal coma from opium where the proper remedies were resorted to before the stupor commenced; and death in such circumstances is so inconceivable, that we must ascribe the result in this case to apoplexy, either incidentally concurring, or brought on by the operation of the poison.

Morphia, like opium, may occasion serous effects when too freely applied to a blistered surface. In a case related by M. Dupont, four-tenths of a grain of acetate of morphia, applied to a blister on the side, caused in twenty minutes dimness of vision, vomiting, and delirium; and though it was then removed, the patient had afterwards continued vomiting, dilated pupils, and great feebleness of the pulse. Recovery took place, but the patient was not quite free of incoherence next day.[†] The dose here was so small, and the symptoms were so unlike the usual effects of morphia, that doubts arise whether the case was really one of poisoning.

The effects of *narcotine* have been examined experimentally by Magendie and Orfila; but their results do not coincide. According to Orfila it is not easy to poison dogs with it, as it excites vomiting and is discharged. But when the gullet is tied, the animal dies in

* Procés Complet d'Edme-Samuel Castaing, p. 31.
† Edinburgh Med. and Surg. Journal, lvi 296.

two, three or four days, without any remarkable symptom but languor and hard breathing.* In these experiments it was dissolved in olive oil; it does not act at all in the solid state. Magendie found that it produces in dogs a state like reverie, accompanied with convulsions. They lie still except when convulsed, and they are apparently asleep or dreaming; but they are really alive to external objects, and even in a state of acute irritability. In short, he considers the symptoms to constitute an aggravated form of the subsequent and idiosyncratic effects caused by opium on man. Vinegar, he says, destroys altogether the poisonous properties of narcotine. According to Orfila it only weakens them. Muriatic acid would seem to annihilate them entirely; for Orfila found no effect in dogs from forty grains dissolved in water with the aid of muriatic acid; and Bally gave sixty grains in like manner to a patient without injury.† Forty grains dissolved by sulphuric acid, proved fatal to a dog in twenty-four hours.‡

Narcotine, like other narcotic poisons, is more powerful when introduced at once into the blood, but produces nearly the same effects as when it is swallowed. Orfila found that a single grain was as powerful through the former, as eight grains through the latter channel.§ Dieffenbach observed that half a grain dissolved in water by means of a drop or two of hydrochloric acid killed cats in five minutes when injected into a vein, and always produced congestion within the head, and extravasation on the surface of the cerebellum. A remarkable circumstance observed in the course of his experiments was, that leeches, applied to a rabbit under the influence of narcotine, died immediately in convulsions; and that a portion of the blood of the same rabbit when injected into the vein of another produced drowsiness, languor, and pandiculation for nearly a day.‖

The effects of narcotine on man have not been much inquired into. From the only researches on the subject I have yet seen, those of Dr. Wibmer of Munich, it appears to be but a feeble poison. He found by experiment on himself, that two grains dissolved in olive oil produced merely slight transient headache; that eight grains dissolved by means of muriatic acid had no effect at all; and that the same quantity of solid narcotine occasioned temporary headache, and in twenty-eight hours a singular state of excitement, with trembling of the hands, restlessness, and inability to fix the thoughts on any object. These effects went off in a few hours.¶

The effects of codeïa have been examined by Dr. Kunkel. He found that twelve grains, dissolved in water and introduced into the stomach, killed a rabbit in three minutes; that six grains in solution when injected into the cellular tissue occasioned death in little more than two hours; that the same quantity administered by the mouth sometimes had little effect; that when given in powder its action

* Toxicol. Gén. ii. 70
† Traité de Médecine Légale, iii. 353.   ‡ Ibidem, iii. 356.
§ Toxicol. Générale, ii. 70.
‖ Meckel's Archiv für Anat. und Physiol. xiv. 19.
¶ Buchner's Repertorium für die Pharmacie, xxxvi. 204.

was very feeble; and that the symptoms were excitement of the pulse, convulsions, and tetanus, without any tendency to sopor or somnolency.* Hence codeïa is conceived to be a stimulant of the nervous system, and consequently the cause of the excitant effects sometimes produced by opium. It may be doubted, however, whether its proportion in opium is sufficient for explaining these effects.

Meconic acid is inert. Sertuerner, indeed, thought the meconate of soda acted as a powerful poison in some experiments made on himself and on dogs; but more careful researches have since proved that he was misled by some error. Sömmering found that ten grains of meconic acid or meconate of soda had no effect whatever on dogs.† Subsequently, in consequence of two people having died suddenly at Turin after taking each a grain of the acid, some careful experiments were made by Drs. Feneglio and Blengini, who gave eight grains to dogs, crows, and frogs, and four grains to various men, without remarking any injurious effects whatever.‡

The *distilled water* of opium was formerly considered an active poison; but Orfila found it nearly or altogether inert. Two pounds introduced into the stomach of a dog, and two ounces and a half injected into a vein, had no effect whatever.§

SECTION III. — *Of the Morbid Appearances caused by Opium.*

In discussing this subject the appearances in the best marked cases will be first noticed; and then some account will be given of the variations to which they are liable.

In Knape's Annals there is a good example of the most aggravated state of the appearances left by opium. It is the case of an infant who was killed in the course of a night by a decoction of poppy-heads. There was much lividity over the whole back part of the body. All the sinuses and vessels of the brain were gorged with fluid blood; and a good deal of serosity was found in the ventricles and base of the skull. The pharynx was red. The lungs were distended, and so gorged with fluid blood, that it ran out in a stream when they were cut. The cavities of the heart contained the same fluid blood. There was some redness in the villous coat of the stomach and intestines; and poppy-seeds were found in the stomach. Although the body had been kept only two days in the month of February, the belly emitted a putrid odour when it was laid open.||

In commenting upon these appearances, it may be first remarked, that turgescence of the vessels in the brain, and watery effusion into the ventricles, and on the surface of the brain, are generally met with. Dr. Bright mentions an instance where unusual turgescence

* Journal de Chim. Méd. ix. 223.   † Buchner's Toxicologie, p. 203.
‡ Henke's Zeitschrift für die Staatsarzneikunde, xiv. 456.
§ Toxicologie Générale, ii. 86.
|| Krit, Annalen der Staatsarzn. I. iii. 501.

was found, and on the surface of the brain a spot of slight ecchymosis as big as a crown piece.* I have seen turgescence of vessels and serous effusion in one instance to a considerable extent: each ventricle contained three drachms of fluid, the arachnoid membrane on the surface of the brain was much infiltered, and the vessels both in the substance and on the surface of the brain were considerably gorged with blood. But congestion and effusion are by no means universal: in a case I examined judicially in November, 1822, which proved fatal in about seven hours, there was neither unusual congestion nor effusion. In the remarks on the diseased appearances caused by the narcotics generally, it was observed that extravasation of blood is a very rare effect of opium. A good example of the kind, however, is related by Mr. Jewel of London. It was the case of a young married female, who died eight hours after taking two ounces of laudanum. Several clots were found in the substance of the brain, one of which, in the anterior right lobe, was an inch long.† A similar case, which occurred to Dr. Elliotson, has been mentioned already at p. 546. There is little doubt that poisoning with opium may cause extravasation, by developing a disposition to apoplexy; but considering the very great rarity of this appearance in persons killed by opium, it may reasonably be questioned whether extravasation can be produced without some predisposition co-operating.

The lungs are sometimes found gorged with blood, as in many cases of apoplexy. They were so in the soldier mentioned in the Journal Universel, who died in convulsions. They were in the same state in a patient of Dr. Home, a man who died in the Infirmary here in 1825, four hours after taking two ounces of laudanum in six ounces of whisky; and likewise in the case quoted from Pyl, in which sixty grains of solid opium were taken. But this appearance is not more constant than congestion in the brain. Orfila never found it in dogs, and in three cases I have examined the lungs were perfectly natural. Perhaps they are more usually turgid when death is preceded by convulsions. They were particularly so in the case of the soldier above mentioned, and likewise in another case of the same nature recorded in Rust's Magazin.‡

The stomach, as in Knape's case, is occasionally red, and in the woman mentioned by Lassus, who died after swallowing thirty-six grains, it is said to have been inflamed. But even redness is rare, and decided inflammation probably never occurs. In four cases I have examined, the villous coat was quite healthy; and it was equally so in another related in Knape and Hecker's Register.§

Lividity of the skin is almost always present more or less, and sometimes it is excessive. In one of the cases I examined it was universal over the depending surface of the body.

It has been said that the blood is always fluid. This certainly

* Reports of Medical Cases, ii. 203.   † Lond. Med. and Phys. Journal, Feb. 1816.
‡ Magazin für die Gesammte Heilkunde. xvii. 121.
§ Kritische Jahrbucher, ii. 100. When inflammation is found, it is not improbably owing to irritants given to produce vomiting, but failing to act. This was apparently the cause in a case described by Mr. Stanley, Trans. London Coll. of Phys. vi. 414.

appears to be very generally the case. For example, the blood was fluid in the case of the soldier who died in convulsions, in Dr. Home's patient, in four adults I have examined, in Dr. Traill's case of death from morphia, and likewise in Pyl's case. But at the same time this condition of the blood is not invariable : In the case related in Knape and Hecker's Register, it was coagulated in the left cavities of the heart ; in another related by Petit in Corvisart's Journal, there were clots in both ventricles ;[*] and in the case of the first infant mentioned in page 549, clots were also found in both ventricles. In Alibert's case a large fibrinous concretion was found in the heart, clearly showing that the blood had coagulated after death as usual.

It appears that the body is often apt to pass rapidly into putrefaction. In one of the cases I examined, although the body had been kept only thirty hours in a cool place in the month of December, the cuticle was easily peeled off, the joints were flaccid, and an acid smell was exhaled. In Réaumur's case, that of a young man who died in fifteen hours, in consequence of his companions in a drunken frolic having mixed a drachm of opium in his wine, the body soon became covered with large blue stains, and gave out an insupportable odour. A French physician has related in the Journal de Médecine a still more pointed case of a lady who died seven hours after taking a large quantity of laudanum by mistake, and whose body was so far gone in putrefaction fourteen hours after death, that the dissection could not be delayed any longer. The hair and cuticle separated on the slightest friction, and the stomach, intestines, and large vessels were distended with air.[†]

It is doubtful whether this is a constant appearance or not. In one case I examined, the body was free from putrefaction forty-eight hours after death.

Although opium is generally believed to suspend all the secretions and excretions but the sweat, instances have been met with where a great collection of urine was found in the bladder after death. In a paper on the signs of death by opium, in Augustin's Repertorium, it is stated that Welper of Berlin always found the bladder full of urine, and the kidneys gorged with blood, both in man and animals.[‡] I am not prepared to say how far this is a common condition, as the state of the urinary organs is seldom noticed in published cases.

In the examination of the dead body unequivocal evidence will sometimes be procured by the discovery of a portion of the poison in the stomach. But it must not always be concluded that opium has not been swallowed, because the sense of smell, chemical analysis, and experiments on animals fail to detect it. For, as previously remarked, the opium may not remain in the stomach after death, though a large quantity was swallowed, and not vomited. This may arise from two causes. It may be all absorbed, as will often happen when it has been taken in the liquid form : or it may be partly absorbed and partly

---

[*] Journ. de Méd. xxxiv. 267.

[†] The reference to this case has been lost.   [‡] Augustin's Repertorium, i. 2, 12.

decomposed by the process of digestion. But in one or other of these ways it may certainly disappear, and that in a very few hours only. Several instances to this effect have been already mentioned (pp. 57, 537). These remarks are important, because the fact is generally believed to be the reverse. Dr. Paris, in his work on Medical Jurisprudence, has tended to propagate the misconception, by asserting that in all fatal cases opium may be detected in the stomach;* and in the last edition of his Toxicology, Orfila has over-rated the facility and frequency with which an analysis may be conducted successfully. [See p. 538.]

At the same time there is no doubt that the poison may sometimes be found in the stomach. In Knape 'and Hecker's Register there is the case of a girl who died about eight hours after taking half an ounce of laudanum ; and the reporters found that an extract prepared from the contents of the stomach caused deep sleep in frogs, chickens, and dogs, and threw some of them into a comatose state, which proved fatal.† Wildberg has related a very interesting case of a young lady of Berlin, who had been seduced, and finding herself pregnant, swallowed about half an ounce of laudanum in the evening, and died during the night. In this instance the contents of the stomach had a narcotic odour, and their extract when given to a young dog caused excessive sleep, reeling, palsy of the legs, convulsions, and death.‡

M. Petit has related another case fatal in about ten hours, where the contents of the stomach had the smell of opium ; and their alcoholic extract had a bitter taste, and killed guinea-pigs, with symptoms of narcotism.§ In a case related by Mayer in Rust's Magazin, which also proved fatal after an interval of ten hours, the poison, which in this instance was the saffron-tincture, was distinctly detected in the stomach by a strong odour of opium and saffron.‖ In a case where the patient lived between thirteen and fourteen hours, that of the individual for whose murder Stewart and his wife were executed at Edinburgh, Dr. Ure succeeded in detecting meconic acid in the contents of the stomach, which had been removed by the pump about three hours after the opium was swallowed.¶ In another case published by Mr. Skae of this city, where death was caused by half an ounce in thirteen hours, without any attempt having been made to evacuate the stomach, the contents of that organ, treated according to the process at p. 534, yielded evident indications of morphia, and obscure evidence of meconic acid.** Lastly, it may be added that in Dr. Traill's case of poisoning with ten grains of muriate of morphia, when the contents of the stomach were decomposed by magnesia, a solution was obtained from the precipitate by rectified spirit, which, when concentrated, had the strong bitter taste of morphia, and became yellow with nitric acid ; and yet the individual survived no less than twelve hours.

* Medical Jurisprudence, ii. 394.　　　　† Kritische Jahrbücher, ii. 100.
‡ Praktisches Handbuch für Physiker, iii. 331.
§ Corvisart's Journal de Médecine, xxxiv. 263.
‖ Magazin für die gesammte Heilkunde, iii. 24.
¶ Oral evidence at the Trial, also London Journal of Science, N. S. vi. 56.
** Edinburgh Med. and Surg. Journal, liv. 151.‍j

An important fact, ascertained by MM. Orfila and Lesueur, is that neither opium nor the salts of morphia undergo decomposition by being long in contact with decaying animal matter. Even after many months they may be discovered ; at least the putrefaction of the matter with which they are mingled does not add any impediment in the way of their discovery. It is only necessary to observe that the alkaloid may be rendered insoluble by the evolution of ammonia, which separates it from its state of combination.*

SECTION IV. — *Of the Treatment of Poisoning with Opium.*

The treatment of poisoning with opium, owing partly to the numerous cases that have been published, and partly to the experiments of Orfila on the supposed antidotes, — is now well understood.

The primary object is to remove the poison from the stomach. This is proper even in the rare cases in which vomiting occurs spontaneously. It is by no means easy to remove all the opium by vomiting, especially if it was taken in the solid state ; for it becomes so intimately mixed with the lining mucus of the villous coat, that it is never thoroughly removed till the mucus is also removed, which is always effected with difficulty.

The removal of the poison is to be accomplished in one of three ways, by emetics administered in the usual manner, by the stomach-pump, or by the injection of emetics into the veins.

By far the best emetic is the *sulphate of zinc* in the dose of half a drachm or two scruples, which may be repeated after a short interval, if the first dose fails to act. In order to insure its action it is of great use to keep the patient roused as much as possible, — a point which is often forgotten. — The *sulphate of copper* has been used by some as an emetic ; but it is not so certain as the sulphate of zinc. Besides, as it is a much more virulent poison, it may prove injurious, if retained long in the stomach. In Dr. Marcet's case the patient, after recovering from the lethargic symptoms, suffered much from pain in the throat and stomach, occasioned probably by the sulphate of copper which he took remaining some time undischarged. *Tartar emetic*, from the uncertainty of its action when given in considerable doses, is even worse adapted for such cases. This is illustrated by a case in the seventh volume of the Medical and Surgical Journal, the same which has already been referred to as exemplifying the occasional occurrence of convulsions and delirium in poisoning with opium. A scruple of tartar emetic was administered to cause vomiting, but to no purpose. When it had remained fifteen minutes, sulphate of zinc was also given, and with immediate effect. But the patient, after recovering from the sopor, was attacked with pains in the stomach and bowels, and with tenesmus, which lasted several days.

Emetics should be preferred for evacuating the stomach, provided the case be not urgent. Even then, however, they sometimes fail altogether. The best practice in that case is to endeavour to remove

* Revue Médicale, 1828, ii. 473, 475.

the poison with the stomach-pump ; and this in urgent cases should be the first remedy employed. The treatment by the stomach-pump has now become so generally known, that it is unnecessary to describe it particularly. It was recommended in this country by the late Dr. Monro in his lectures ; but does not appear to have been tried by him. In 1803 it was first published by Renault in his treatise on the counter-poisons of arsenic ; and he had tried it on animals.* But the first person who used it in an actual case of poisoning with opium was Dr. Physick of Philadelphia. He saved the life of a child with it in 1812 ; and not long afterwards his countryman, Dr. Dorsey, cured two other individuals.† More lately it was again proposed in London by Mr. Jukes, who does not appear to have been acquainted with these prior trials and experiments. Although he cannot be considered in the light of a discoverer, the profession is much indebted to him for having recalled their attention to this treatment, and for having by his success and activity fairly established its reputation. An account will be seen of his apparatus and of several cases in the Medical and Physical Journal for September and November, 1822. In using the stomach-pump care must be taken not to injure the stomach by too forcible suction. — When it is not at hand, Mr. Bryce of this city recommended the substitution of a long tube with a bladder attached. After the stomach has been filled with warm water from the bladder, the tube is to be turned down so as to act upon the contents of the stomach as a syphon. Dr. Alison cured a patient in this way.‡

Another method of removing opium from the stomach, which has been practised successfully where the patient could not be made to submit to the common treatment, is the injection of tartar-emetic into the rectum. A case is related by Dr. Roe of New York where this treatment proved successful. Fifteen grains in half a gallon of water excited free vomiting, and ten grains more renewed it. Care was taken to insure the discharge of the whole tartar-emetic by a subsequent purgative injection.§

The last method for removing opium from the stomach is a desperate one, which can only be recommended when emetics by the mouth have utterly failed, and when a stomach-pump or Mr. Bryce's substitute, cannot be procured. It is the injection of an emetic into the veins. Tartar-emetic answers best for this purpose, and its effect is almost certain. A grain is the dose. While injecting it, care must be taken by the operator not to introduce air into the vein.

The next object in conducting the treatment of poisoning with opium is to keep the patient constantly roused. This alone is sufficient when the dose is not large, and the poison has been discharged by vomiting ; and in every case it forms, next to the evacuation of the stomach, the most important of the treatment.

The best method of keeping the patient roused is to drag him up

* Sur les Contrepoisons de l'Arsénic, 93.
† Beck's Medical Jurisprudence, 435.
‡ Edin. Med. and Surg. Journal, xxiii. 416.
§ American Journal of the Med. Sciences, vii. 555.

and down between two men, who must be cautioned against yielding
to his importunate entreaties and occasional struggles to get free and
rest himself. For the sopor returns so rapidly, that I have known a
patient answer two or three short questions quite correctly on being
allowed to stand still, and suddenly drop the head in a state of insensibility while standing. The duration of the exercise should vary
according to circumstances from three, to six, or twelve hours.
When he is allowed at length to take out his sleep, the attendants
must ascertain that it is safe to do so by rousing him from time to
time ; and if this should become difficult, he must be turned out of
bed again and exercised as before.

It appears from some cases published not long ago by Mr. Wray[*]
and Dr. Copland,[†] and more lately also by Dr. Bright,[‡] that the most
insensible may be roused to a state of almost complete consciousness
for a short time, by dashing cold water over the head and breast.
This treatment can never supersede the use of emetics : and as its effect
is but temporary, it ought not to supersede the plan of forced exercise.
But it appears to be an excellent way to insure the operation of
emetics. If the emetic is about to fail in its effect, cold water
dashed over the head restores the patient for a few moments to sensibility, during the continuance of which the emetic operates.
Dashing cold water over the head may perhaps be dangerous in the
advanced stage, when the body is cold and the breathing imperceptible ; but the most desperate remedies may be then tried, as the
patient is generally in almost a hopeless state. In one of the cases
mentioned by Dr. Bright from the experience of Mr. Walne, complete recovery was accomplished, mainly by cold affusion of the
head, where there appeared reason to believe that more than an
ounce and a half of laudanum had disappeared from the stomach
before evacuating remedies were used. — This treatment seems to
have been first proposed in 1767 by a German physician, Dr. Gräter.[§]
A suggestion, which is probably an improvement, has been recently
made by Dr. Boisragon of Cheltenham, to alternate the use of cold
with that of warm water, applied to children in the shape of warm
bath, and to adults in the form of warm-sponging and the foot-bath.
The alternating impression of heat and cold may act better as a stimulant than either agent singly ; and the occasional employment of
heat prevents the risk of collapse from too continuous exposure to
cold. Dr. Boisragon saved in this way two cases in very unpromising circumstances.[‖]

In some cases internal stimulants have been given with advantage,
such as assafœtida, ammonia, camphor, musk, &c. It is always useful
to stimulate the nostrils from time to time, by tickling them or holding
ammonia under the nose ; but the application should be neither

* London Med. Repository. xviii. 26.
† London Med. and Phys. Journal, xlviii. 225.
‡ Reports of Medical Cases, ii. 203.
§ Diss. Inaug. de Venenis in genere. Argentorati, 1767, quoted by Marx, die Lehre
von den Giften, I. ii. 237.
‖ London Med. Gazette, 1839-40, i 878.

frequent nor long continued, as the ammonia may cause deleterious effects when too freely inhaled. Pulling the hair and injecting water into the ears are also powerful modes of rousing the patient.

Venesection has been recommended and successfully used by some physicians. If the stomach be emptied, and the patient kept roused, as may almost always be done when means are resorted to in time, venesection will be unnecessary. Sometimes, however, when the pulse is full and strong, it may be prudent to withdraw blood; and it certainly appears that in most cases where this remedy has been employed the sensibility began to return almost immediately after. This is very well shown in a case of poisoning with opium related by Mr. Ross* in the Edinburgh Medical Journal, in another described in the same journal by Mr. Richardson,† and also in two cases of poisoning with acetate of morphia mentioned in a former page. Sometimes, on the contrary, it has seemed injurious, probably because it was not had recourse to till the patient was moribund. It is a sound general rule that blood-letting ought not to be resorted to until the poison is thoroughly removed from the stomach; for it favours absorption. And yet facts are not wanting to show that this rule, now generally admitted since the researches of Magendie on absorption, is not infallible. Dr. Young of the United States has given the particulars of a case where imperturbable coma was formed, together with puffing stertorous respiration, in consequence of an ounce of laudanum having been swallowed,— and where recovery took place, without the poison having been removed at all, simply under the employment of three blood-lettings to the amount of twenty-eight ounces altogether, of cold to the head, and of sinapisms to the legs.‡

Galvanism has been sometimes resorted to, but seldom with decided advantage. I saw it tried, with dubious utility, a few years ago in an urgent case which was treated in the Edinburgh Infirmary. Six ounces of laudanum had been swallowed, but most of it was removed in three-quarters of an hour by the stomach-pump. A stage of deep sopor followed, after which sensibility was restored, and maintained for four hours by forced exercise. A state of pure and extreme coma then ensued, during which galvanism was for some time of great service, in rousing the patient. Gradually, however, it ceased to have any effect of the kind. Recovery took place eventually under the use of external and internal stimuli. Mr. Erichsen of the University-College Hospital, London, has related a case, in which electro-magnetism was of undoubted service. The usual symptoms had been occasioned by an ounce of laudanum. The poison had been withdrawn by the stomach-pump, when unavailing attempts were made to restore sensibility by means of various stimulants. At length several electro-magnetic shocks were passed from the forehead to the upper part of the spine, with the effect of speedily eliciting signs of consciousness; in twenty minutes the pa-

* Edin. Med. and Surg. Journal, xix. 247. † Ibidem, xvii. 226.
‡ London Medical Gazette, xiv. 655.

51

tient could answer questions and walk a little ; and eventually complete recovery took place.*

In desperate circumstances artificial respiration may be used with propriety. After the breathing has been almost or entirely suspended the heart continues to beat for some time ; and so long as its contractions continue, there is some hope that life may be preserved. But it is essential for the continuance of the heart's action, that the breathing be speedily restored to a state of much greater perfection than that which attends the close of poisoning with opium. It is not improbable that the only ultimate cause of death from opium is suspension of the respiration, and that if it could be maintained artificially so as to resemble exactly natural breathing, the poison in the blood would be at length decomposed and consciousness gradually restored. The following is an interesting example by Mr. Whately, in which artificial respiration proved successful. A middle-aged man swallowed half an ounce of crude opium and soon became lethargic. He was roused from this state by appropriate remedies, and his surgeon left him. But the poison not having been sufficiently discharged, he fell again into a state of stupor ; and when the surgeon returned, he found the face pale, cold and deadly, the lips black, the eyelids motionless, so as to remain in any position in which they were placed, the pulse very small and irregular, and the respiration quite extinct. The chest was immediately inflated by artificial means, and when this had been persevered in for seven minutes, expiration became accompanied with a croak, which gradually increased in strength till natural breathing was established. Emetics were then given, and the patient eventually recovered.† — Dr. Ware of Boston (U. S.) has more lately described another case, where artificial respiration was employed with marked advantage, and would probably have saved the patient's life in very unfavourable circumstances, but for the disease on account of which the opium was given.‡ — Another has been lately described by Mr. C. J. Smith of Madras. The patient was not seen for four hours, and received no benefit from the ordinary remedies during the next hour and a half. Artificial respiration was then resorted to and maintained for nearly five hours with an hour of interval ; and this measure certainly seems to have brought the case to a favourable termination under most unpromising circumstances.§ — Dr. Watson of Glasgow has mentioned to me the particulars of an instructive case in the person of an infant three weeks old, in whom, after the breathing had stopped and the heart had nearly ceased to beat, the occasional inflation of the chest with the breath at intervals of two or three minutes restored for a time the action both of the heart and lungs, and eventually accomplished recovery. On physiological principles it appears probable, that this simple mode of procedure may prove more frequently successful than might at first be thought.

* Lond. Med. Gaz., 1840-41, i. 390.   † London Med. Obs. and Inq. vi. 331.
‡ North American Med. and Surg. Journal, July 1826.
§ London Med. and Chir. Transactions, xx. 86.

It would be a fruitless task to examine into the merits of the numerous antidotes which have from time to time been proposed for poisoning with opium. Professor Orfila has examined many of them with great care, such as vinegar, tartaric acid, lemonade, infusion of coffee, decoction of galls, solution of chlorine, camphor, diluents; and he has found them all useless before the poison is expelled from the stomach, with the single exception of decoction of galls. As he remarked that this fluid throws down the active principles of an infusion of opuim, and subsequently found that such a mixture acts more feebly on the animal system than the opiate infusion itself, he thinks the decoction of galls may with propriety be used as an imperfect antidote, till the poison can be evacuated from the stomach.* His experiments, however, do not assign to it very material activity as a remedy; and certainly the whole efforts of the physician ought in the first instance to be directed to the removal of the opium, and to keeping the patient roused. When the opium has been completely removed, the vegetable acids and infusion of coffee have been found useful in reviving the patient, and subsequently in subduing sickness, vomiting, and headache; but till the poison is completely removed the administration of acids is worse than useless, provided the opium was given in the solid state, because its solution in the juices of the stomach is accelerated. It has been maintained that iodine, chlorine, and bromine are all antidotes for poisoning with the vegetable alkaloids.† Some notice will be taken of this statement in the chapter on Nux Vomica. It has also been lately alleged in the United States that opium has no effect when given with acetate of lead; and an hospital case is reported as having occurred at New York, where the poison was swallowed in this way to the extent of thirty grains, without any injurious effect.‡ There must have been some mistake here, however. When given with acetate of lead in medicinal doses, opium exerts its usual sedative and anodyne action; and indeed there is no chemical or physiological reason why it should not do so.

CHAPTER XXVIII.

OF POISONING WITH HYOSCYAMUS, LACTUCA, AND SOLANUM.

Of Poisoning with Hyoscyamus. — Of the narcotic poisons none bears so close a resemblance to opium in its properties as the *hyoscyamus* or henbane. Several species are poisonous; but the only one that has been examined with care is the *H. niger*, from which the extract of the apothecary is prepared.

The hyoscyamus has been analyzed by various chemists, and found to contain a peculiar alkaloid, in which the properties of the plant

* Toxicol. Gén. ii. 110.   † Le Globe, vii. 525. Août, 1829.
‡ London Medical Gazette, 1840-41, i. 318.

are concentrated. It is named hyoscyamia. This substance in its pure state, as first obtained by MM. Geiger and Hesse, is a solid body, in fine silky crystals, without odour, of a strong acrid taste like tobacco, partially volatilizable with boiling water, entirely volatilizable alone at a somewhat higher heat, very soluble in alcohol and ether, but sparingly so in water.[*]

Farther, hyoscyamus, like many other narcotic vegetables, stramonium, digitalis, opium, tobacco, and hemlock, has been found by Mr. Morries Stirling to yield by destructive distillation an empyreumatic oil of great activity. Its poisonous properties, however, are not essential to the oil, but reside in a volatile principle which may be detached by weak acetic acid. The relation of this principle to hyoscyamia has not been ascertained ; but it is an active poison, small doses producing in rabbits, convulsions, coma, and speedy death.[†]

Runge proposes as evidence of poisoning with hyoscyamus, in common, however, with stramonium and belladonna, to concentrate a solution of the contents of the stomach, and apply it to a cat's eye to dilate the pupil. Dilatation, he says, was even produced by an extract obtained from the urine of a rabbit which had been fed some time on hyoscyamus.[‡]

According to the experiments of Professor Orfila, the juice or extract procured from the leaves, stems, and especially the root, produces in animals a state of sopor much purer than that caused by opium. It is most active when injected into the jugular vein, less so when applied to the cellular tissue, and still less when introduced into the stomach. Except occasional paralysis of the heart, indicated by florid blood in its left cavities, no morbid appearance is to be found in the dead body. Six drachms of the pharmaceutic extract of the leaves killed a dog in two hours and a quarter when swallowed ; and three drachms killed another in four hours through a wound in the back. Its action appears to be exerted through the medium of the blood-vessels, and is purely narcotic.[§]

It is probable that the activity of this plant is much affected by season; and the energy of its preparations varies greatly with the manner of obtaining them. The information, however, which is at present possessed on these two points is vague, because the influence of the two circumstances has seldom been viewed carefully apart.

The leaves, from which the pharmaceutic preparations of hyoscyamus are obtained, are commonly held to be most active during the inflorescence of the plant in the second summer of its existence. On general principles this appears probable ; but there are no satisfactory experiments on the subject, even the late researches of Mr. Houlton having left much still to be determined.[‖]

[*] Annalen der Pharmacie, 1833, vii. 270.
    Edinburgh Medical and Surg. Journal, xxxix. 381.
[‡] Orfila, Médecine-Légale, iii. 374.
[§] Orfila, Toxicologie Gén. ii. 137.
[‖] Pharmaceutic Journal, 1843-44, 578.

Orfila has made some important remarks as to the effect of season and vegetation on the energy of the root as a poison. The root he maintains is the most active part of the plant; but in the spring it is nearly inert. Thus the juice of three pounds of the root collected near the end of April, when the plant has hardly begun to shoot, killed a dog in somewhat less than two days; while a decoction of an ounce and a half collected on the last day of June, when the plant was in full vegetation, proved fatal in two hours and a half.

The extract of the leaves, procured from different shops, was found by Orfila to vary greatly in point of strength, some samples being absolutely inert.* The causes of these differences have been ascertained experimentally by Brandes to be, that the herb loses its active principle in part by decomposition in the process of simple desiccation, and also when long kept; and that the greater part is also similarly decomposed in preparing an extract, unless the process be finished quickly, and at a low heat.

The seeds of hyoscyamus are poisonous, as well as the leaves and root. Indeed the whole plant is so. The seeds contain much more hyoscyamia than the leaves.

The effects of hyosciamus on man differ somewhat from those on animals, and vary greatly with the dose.

In medicinal doses it commonly induces pleasant sleep. This indeed has been denied by M. Fouquier, who infers from his experiments that it never causes sleep, but always headache, delirium, nausea, vomiting, and feverishness.† I have certainly seen it sometimes have these effects; but much more generally it has acted as a pleasant hypnotic and anodyne.

Its effect in large doses have been well described by M. Choquet as they occurred in two soldiers who ate by mistake the young shoots dressed with olive-oil. They presently became giddy and stupid, lost their speech, and had a dull, haggard look. The pupils were excessively dilated, and the eyes so insensible that the eyelids did not wink when the cornea was touched. The pulse was small and intermitting, the breathing difficult, the jaw locked, and the mouth distorted by *risus sardonicus.* Sensibility was extinct, the limbs were cold and palsied, the arms convulsed, and there was that singular union of delirium and coma which is usually termed typhomania. One of the men soon vomited freely under the influence of emetics, and in a short time got quite well. The other vomited little. As the palsy and somnolency abated, the delirium became extravagant, and the patient quite unmanageable till the evening of the subsequent day, when the operation of brisk purgatives restored him to his senses. In two days both were fit for duty.‡

In a treatise on vegetable poisons, Mr. Wilmer has related the history of six persons in a family, who were poisoned by eating at dinner the roots of the hyoscyamus by mistake instead of parsneps. Several were delirious and danced about the room like maniacs, one

---

* Orfila, Toxicol. Gén. ii. 137.
† Archives Gén. de Méd. i. 297.　　　‡ Corvisart's Journal de Méd. xxvi. 353.

appeared as if he had got drunk, and a woman became profoundly and irrecoverably comatose. Emetics could not be introduced into the stomach, stimulant clysters had no effect, external stimuli of every kind failed to rouse her, and she expired next morning at six.[*] The roots in this instance were gathered in the winter time, — a fact, which does not quite coincide with the conclusions of Orfila, that the plant must be in full vegetation before the energy of the root is considerable.

From these and other cases, the abstracts of which are to be seen in Orfila's Toxicology, or in Wibmer's Treatise on the Operation of Medicines and Poisons, it follows that hyoscyamus in a poisonous dose causes loss of speech, dilatation of the pupil, coma, and delirium, commonly of the unmanageable, sometimes of the furious kind. In general a stage of delirium precedes coma ; and sometimes as the coma passes off, delirium returns for a time. It has been known to act powerfully in the form of clyster.[†] It has also been known to act with considerable energy even through the sound skin, as appears from a case which occurred to Wibmer. He was called to a lady affected with great stupor, dilated pupils, flushed face, loss of speech, full hard pulse, and swelling of the abdomen ; and he found that these symptoms were owing to several ounces of henbane leaves having been applied to the belly in a poultice, on account of strangury and tympanitis. She was still capable of being roused by speaking loudly close to her ear; and under proper treatment she recovered.[‡]

Henbane seldom causes any distinct symptoms of irritant poisoning. In several, however, of the cases related by the older modern authors some pain in the belly, a little vomiting, and more rarely diarrhœa, appear to have occurred.[§] Plenck quotes, from a Swedish authority, an instance of its having produced burning in the stomach, intense thirst, watching, delirium, depraved vision, and next day a crowded eruption of dark spots and vesicles, which disappeared on the supervention of a profuse diarrhœa.[||] The same author alludes to cases where it proved fatal ; but this event is rare in the present day, obviously because the precursory stage of delirium gives an opportunity of removing the poison, before the stage of coma is formed. A fatal case, which occurred to Mr. Wibmer, has been mentioned above ; and another has been related in Pyl's Magazin. Two boys a few minutes after eating the seeds were attacked with convulsions and heat in the throat ; and one of them, who could not be made to vomit, died in the course of the ensuing night.[¶]

The accidents it has occasioned have commonly arisen from the individuals confounding the root with that of the wild chicory or with the parsnep, the latter of which it somewhat resembles.

Of the other species of the hyoscyamus, the *H. albus* has been known to cause symptoms precisely the same with those above

[*] On the Poisonous Vegetables of Great Britain, p. 3.
[†] Foderé, Médecine-Légale, iv. 25.
[‡] Die Wirkung der Arzneimittel und Gifte, iii. 154.
[§] Acta Curiosorum Naturæ. Also Wibmer, Die Wirkung, &c. 146-154.
[||] Toxicologia, p. 87.   [¶] Neues Magazin, ii. 3, p. 100.

described. Professor Foderé has given a good example of its effects on man, as they occurred in the crew of a French corvette in the Archipelago. The plant was boiled and distributed among the whole ship's company, as several of the sailors said they knew it to be eatable and salubrious. But in no long time they were all seized with giddiness, vomiting, convulsions, colic, purging, and delirium of the active kind. They were all soon relieved by emetics and purgatives.[*]

Dr. Archibald Hamilton has described a case of the same nature, which was caused by the seeds of this plant. A young medical student, who took about twenty-five grains of the seeds, was seized in half an hour with lassitude and somnolency, and successively with dryness of the throat, impeding deglutition, convulsive movements of the arms, incoherency, total insensibility of the skin, and loss of recollection. These symptoms continued about twelve hours, and then slowly receded.[†]

Three other species, the *H. aureus, physaloides* and *scopolia* are represented by Orfila to be equally deleterious.

The alkaloid hyoscyamus possesses in an intense degree the active properties of the plant. It has not been hitherto examined in this respect with much care. But extremely minute quantities produce excessive enlargement of the pupil, when put within the eyelids in the form of neutral salt.

Treatment. The treatment of poisoning with hyoscyamus consists in removing the poison, diminishing cerebral congestion, and restoring sensibility. It is therefore substantially the same as in poisoning with opium, except that general or local evacuation of blood is more frequently required, in consequence of the greater tendency of hyoscyamus to induce determination of blood towards the head and congestion there. It has been lately alleged by an Italian author that a large dose of lemon juice is an immediate antidote for the effects of too large a medicinal dose, even when the poison was administered in the form of injection.[‡] This does not seem probable.

Of Poisoning with Lactuca.

Allied in its effects, but greatly inferior in power to opium and hyoscyamus, is the *Lactuca virosa*, together with the *Lettuce-opium*, or inspissated juice of *L. sativa*, and *L. virosa*.

Orfila found that three drachms of the extract of *L. virosa* introduced into the stomach of a dog killed it in two days, without causing any remarkable symptom ; that two drachms applied to a wound in the back induced giddiness, slight sopor, and death in three days; and that thirty-six grains injected in a state of solution into the jugular vein caused dulness, weakness, slight convulsions, and death in

* Foderé, Médecine-Légale, iv. 23. For another instance of the effects of the seeds, not however fatal, see Acta Helvetica, v. 333.
† Edin. Phys. and Lit. Essays, ii. 268.
‡ Medoro in Edinburgh Med. and Surg. Journal, lv. 265.

eighteen minutes.* This poison, therefore, like other narcotics, acts through absorption. But it is far from being energetic. The extract is very uncertain in strength, — as may indeed be inferred from the variable nature of the processes by which it is prepared.

Lactucarium, the inspissated juice, especially that obtained from *L. virosa*, is obviously a more active preparation than the extract. Doses of no great magnitude kill small animals. But there is a want of good observations on its effects and energy as a poison.

Of Poisoning with Solanum.

Different species of *solanum*, a genus of the same natural order with the hyoscyamus, have been considered by Orfila to possess the same properties, though in a much feebler degree. The *S. dulca-mara* or bittersweet has been erroneously believed by some to pos-sess distinct narcotic properties.† M. Dunal found that a dog might take 180 of the berries or four ounces of the extract without any inconvenience, and quotes an experiment on the human subject where thirty-two drachms of extract were taken in two doses also without injury.‡ If it has any power at all, therefore, it must possess too little to be entitled to the name of a poison. Chevallier says he knew an instance of a druggist's apprentice being attacked with deep somnolency for ten hours after carrying a large bundle of it on his head ;§ but some other cause may be justly suspected to have here been in operation. The *S. nigrum* or common nightshade has been made the subject of experiment by Orfila, who found its extract to possess nearly the power and energy of lettuce-opium.‖ The follow-ing seems a genuine case of poisoning with the berries of this species. Three children near Nantes in France were seized with severe headache, giddiness, colic, nausea, and vomiting. One of them then had excessive dilatation of the pupils, sweating and urgent thirst ; loss of voice, stertorous breathing, and tetanic spasms ensued ; and in twelve hours he died. Another had swelling of the face, alternate contraction and dilatation of the pupils, repeated vomiting, and eventually coma ; but he recovered. The third was similarly, but more slightly affected, and also recovered. The children who reco-vered pointed out the berries they had eaten ; which were found to be those of *S. nigrum*.¶ The *S. fuscatum* is rather more active, fifteen berries having caused hurried breathing and vomiting.** The *S. mammosum* is also probably an active species, the capsule of the berries having been known to excite vomiting, giddiness, and confu-sion of mind.†† In the *S. nigrum* and *dulcamara*, M. Desfosses dis-covered in 1821 a peculiar alkaloid, which induces somnolency in animals, but is not a very active poison.‡‡

    * Toxicol. Gén. ii. 184.   † Dr. Schlegel, in Hufeland's Journal, liv. ii. 29.
    ‡ Histoire des Solanum.   1813.
    § Annales d'Hyg. Publique et de Méd. Légale, viii. 334.
    ‖ Toxicol. Gén. ii. 190.
    ¶ Journal de Chimie Médicale, 1840, 142.   ** Dunal, &c.
    †† M. Des-Alleurs in Journ de Chim. Méd. ii. 30.
    ‡‡ Bulletins de la Soc. Méd. d'Emul. — Mars, 1821.

It has been supposed by some that the tubers of *Solanum tuberosum*, the common potato, may acquire in certain circumstances poisonous qualities of no mean energy. Dr. Kabler of Prague has described the cases of four individuals in a family who were seized with alarming narcotic symptoms after eating potatoes which had begun to germinate and shrivel. The father of the family, who had eaten least of them all, appeared as if tipsy, and soon became insensible. The mother and two children became comatose and convulsed. All had vomited before becoming insensible. They recovered under the use of ether, frictions, and coffee; and in two hours were out of danger.†

An alkaloid has been indicated by several chemists in various species of solanum. The most recent account, that of Otto, represents it to be a pearly, white, pulverulent substance, alkaline in reaction, and capable of uniting with acids. One grain of sulphate of solania killed a rabbit in six hours, and three grains a stronger rabbit in nine hours, — the symptoms being those of narcotic poisoning,†

Violent effects have often been assigned to the genus Solanum, in consequence of its similarity to a powerful poison, the *Atropa belladonna;* which indeed is described by the older authors under the name of *Solanum furiosum.* It will be noticed among the Narcotico-acrid Poisons.

CHAPTER XXIX.

OF POISONING WITH HYDROCYANIC ACID.

The poisons, whose energy depends on the presence of the prussic or hydrocyanic acid, are of great interest to the physiologist as well as the medical jurist. Some of them are natural productions, derived from the leaves, bark, fruit-kernels, and roots of certain plants; others are formed artificially by complex chemical processes. The species to be here noticed are the *hydrocyanic acid* itself, and the essential oils and distilled waters of the *bitter almond, cherry-laurel, peach-blossom, cluster-cherry, mountain-ash,* and *bitter cassava.* These poisons have for some time attracted great attention on account of their extraordinary power. And indeed in rapidity of action, or the minuteness of the quantity in which they operate, no poison surpasses and very few equal them. They are exceedingly interesting to the medical jurist, because, as they are now generally known, their effects often become the subject of medico-legal investigation: they have been repeatedly taken by accident; they have often been resorted to for committing suicide; and they have likewise been employed as the instruments of murder. A remarkable instance occurred in England towards the close of last century, where murder was committed with the cherry-laurel water;

* Journal de Chimie Médicale, 1837, 130.   † Journal de Pharmacie, xx. 96.

and two cases have been tried in England where death arose from hydrocyanic acid, and the prisoners were charged with administering it, but were found not guilty. These cases will be noticed presently.

Of the Hydrocyanic Acid.

Section I. — Of its Chemical History and Tests.

This singular substance was discovered some time ago by Scheele; but Gay-Lussac was the first who obtained it in a state of purity. It is familiarly known to chemists under two forms, — as a pure acid, and diluted with water.

The pure acid is liquid, limpid, and colourless. It has an acrid, pungent taste, and a very peculiar odour, which, when diffused through the air, has a very distant resemblance to that of bitter almonds, but is accompanied with a peculiar impression of acridity on the nostrils and back of the throat. It is an error, however, to suppose, as is very generally done, that the odour is the same with that of the almond. It boils at 80°; freezes at 5°; and is very inflammable. I have kept it unchanged for a fortnight in ice-cold water; but at ordinary temperatures it decomposes spontaneously, and becomes brown, sometimes in an hour, and commonly within twelve hours. On this account it is extremely improbable that a case will ever happen, in which the medical jurist will have to examine it in its concentrated form.

When united with water it forms the acid discovered by Scheele, and now kept in the druggist's shop. In this state it has the same appearance, taste, and smell as the pure acid; but it is less volatile, does not burn, and may be preserved long without change, if excluded from the light. In consequence of its volatility, however, it becomes weak, unless kept with great care; many samples of it also undergo decomposition, and deposit brown flakes, if not excluded from the light; and hence the acid of the shops is very variable in point of strength. The acid prepared by decomposing the solution of the ferrocyanate of potass by sulphuric acid may be kept for years, even exposed to diffuse light, without being decomposed at all. A French physician made some experiments not long ago on the uncertainty of the strength of the medicinal acid; and he found that he could swallow a whole ounce of one sample, and a drachm of a stronger sample, without sustaining any injury; but on trying some which had been recently prepared by Vauquelin, he was immediately taken ill, as will be related presently, and narrowly escaped with his life.* — The acid of commerce differs much in strength, according to the process by which it has been prepared, and independently of decomposition by keeping. The medicinal acid long used in this country is intended to be an imitation of that of Vauquelin, which contains 3·3 per cent.;† but the London College of Physicians, in adopting it in their last Pharmacopœia, improperly altered the strength to 2 per

* Revue Médicale, xvii. 265.
† Schubarth in Journal der Praktischen Heilkunde, li. i. 125.

cent. That of Giese, which keeps well, is of the same strength as the first; that of Schrader contains only one per cent.; that of Göbel 2·5 per cent.; that of Ittner 10 per cent.;* that of Robiquet 50 per cent.† Of the alcoholic solutions the best known are that of Schrader, which contains about 1·5 per cent. of pure acid, — that of the Bavarian Pharmacopœia, which contains 4 per cent., — that of Duflos, 9 per cent., — that of Pfaff 10 per cent., — and that of Keller, 25 per cent.* These statements are necessary for understanding the cases of poisoning published in foreign works.

The tests for hydrocyanic acid has been examined by M. Lassaigne of Paris, by Dr. Turner of London, and by Professor Orfila. They are its odour, the salts of copper, the salts of iron, and nitrate of silver.

The *peculiar odour* of the acid is a very characteristic and delicate test of its presence. According to Orfila, the smell is perceptible when no chemical reagent is delicate enough to detect it.‡ But I doubt the accuracy of this statement, and may farther observe, that I have known some persons nearly insensible of any smell, even in a specimen which was tolerably strong. Hence, when the odour is resorted to as a test, it ought to be tried by several persons.

Sulphate of copper forms with hydrocyanic acid, when rendered alkaline with a little potass, a greenish precipitate, which becomes nearly white, on the addition of a little hydrochloric acid. The purpose of the hydrochloric acid is to re-dissolve some oxide of copper thrown down by the potass. The precipitate is then the cyanide of copper. This test, according to Lassaigne, will act on the poison when dissolved in 20,000 parts of water. But as the precipitate is not coloured, the test is an insignificant one compared with the next.

If the acid be rendered alkaline by potass, the *salts of the mixed peroxide and protoxide of iron* produce a grayish-green precipitate, which, on the addition of a little sulphuric acid, becomes of a deep prussian blue colour. Common green vitriol answers very well for this purpose. The salts of the peroxide of iron will also often answer, because, unless carefully prepared, they are never altogether free of protoxide. But the salts of the pure peroxide of iron have no such effect. They cause with the potass a brownish precipitate, which is redissolved on the addition of sulphuric acid, leaving the solution limpid. Mr. Ilott of Bromley has pointed out to me, that the iron test does not act on a weak solution of hydrocyanic acid, if there be an excess of ammonia present, either such from the first, or disengaged by potash from muriate of ammonia; that the blue precipitate is produced by driving off the ammonia with heat; but not by neutralizing it with an acid.

The *nitrate of silver* is a delicate and characteristic reagent for hydrocyanic acid. A white precipitate, the cyanide of silver, is produced in a very diluted solution; and this precipitate is distin-

* Fechner's Repertorium der Organischen Chemie, ii. 70, 75.
† Codex Medicamentarius, 389.
‡ Archives Gén. de Médecine, xx. 386.

guished from the other white salts of silver, by being insoluble in
nitric acid at ordinary temperatures, but soluble in that acid at its
boiling temperature.   In this action it is necessary to observe that
something more is accomplished than simple solution ; the cyanide
is decomposed, nitrate of silver is formed, and hydrocyanic acid is
disengaged by the ebullition.   A more characteristic property is,
that the precipitate when dried and heated emits cyanogen gas ;
which is easily known by the beautiful rose-red colour of its flame.*

Sometimes it is necessary to determine the strength of diluted
hydrocyanic acid ; because, on account of its tendency to decomposition, doubts may be entertained whether a mixture which contains
it is strong enough to be dangerously poisonous.   According to
Orfila, the best method of ascertaining the strength either of a pure
solution or of a mixture in syrup, is to throw down the acid with the
nitrate of silver and dry the precipitate ; a hundred parts of which
correspond to 20·33 of pure hydrocyanic acid.

Process for Mixed Fluids. — Some important observations have
been made by MM. Leuret and Lassaigne on the effect of mixing
animal matters with hydrocyanic acid.   The most material of their
results are, that if the body of an animal poisoned with the acid is
left unburied for three days, the poison can no longer be detected ;
and that if it is buried within twenty-four hours the poison may be
found after a longer interval, but never after eight days.   The reason
is either that the acid volatilizes, or that it is decomposed.   The
possibility thus indicated of detecting the poison in the body some
days after death has been since confirmed by actual examination in
a medico-legal case.   In a case of poisoning with hydrocyanic acid,
followed by dismemberment of the body for the purpose of concealment, distinct proof of the presence of the poison seven days after
death was obtained by the second of the succeeding processes, although the trunk of the body had never been buried, but had been
for some time lying in a drain.†

For detecting the poison in mixed fluids Orfila has lately advised
the following process.   The fluid may be treated with animal charcoal without heat.   The colour being thus generally destroyed, the
test will sometimes act as usual.   Or, without this preparation, a slip
of bibulous paper moistened with pure potass, may be immersed in
the suspected fluid for a few minutes, and then touched with a solution of sulphate of iron : upon which the usual blue colour will be
produced on the paper.   If neither of these methods should answer,
the fluid is to be distilled.‡

Distillation of the fluid is on the whole the best mode of procedure.
It was proposed some time before by Lassaigne and Leuret for detecting the poison in the stomach after death.   The steps of their
process, which appears to me the best yet proposed, are as follows.
The contents after filtration are to be neutralized with sulphuric acid

* Archives Gén. de Méd. xx. 386.
† Chevallier, Annales d'Hygiène Publique, &c. ix. 337.
‡ Archives Gen. de Méd. xx. 387.

if they are alkaline, in order to fix the ammonia which may have been disengaged by putrefaction ; the product is then to be distilled from a vapour-bath till an eighth part has passed over into the receiver ; and the distilled fluid is to be tested with the sulphate of iron in the usual way.* Orfila maintains that from hydrocyanized syrup only two-thirds of the acid can be distilled over ; and cautions the analyst against estimating quantity by such means.† M. Ossian Henry has proposed to condense the acid in distillation by a much more complex process, which consists in obtaining it in the first instance in the form of cyanide of silver.‡ But with a good refrigeratory there is no difficulty in condensing every particle of acid with no other aid than cold water.

By this process Lassaigne could detect the poison in a cat or dog killed by twelve drops and examined twenty-four or forty-eight hours after death.§ But Dr. Schubarth has objected to it, — and the same objection will apply to every process in which heat is used, — that hydrocyanic acid may be formed during distillation by the decomposition of animal matter.‖ His objection, however, appears only to rest on conjecture or presumption at farthest ; and I doubt whether, supposing the distillation to go on slowly in the vapour-bath, the heat is sufficient to bring about the requisite decomposition. The force of the objection must be decided by future researches.

It is worthy of remark that hydrocyanic acid is apt to be formed in the course of the changes produced by various agents in organic matters. These are probably more numerous than the toxicologist is at present exactly aware of. An instance of its formation in the course of the decay of unsound cheese has been ascertained lately by Dr. Witling ;¶ and another example will be mentioned under the head of spurred rye.

Cyanide of Potassium. — The only compound of hydrocyanic acid which requires notice is the cyanide of potassium. This is, when pure, a white salt, bitter, not decomposable by a red heat unless in contact with air, very soluble in water, and sparingly so in rectified spirit. Its watery solution restores the blue of reddened litmus, and does not precipitate lime-water : the mixed sulphates of the two oxides of iron form with it Prussian blue : nitrate of silver causes a white precipitate insoluble in cold nitric acid, but disappearing when the acid is boiled : sulphate of copper causes an apple-green precipitate, which becomes white on the addition of hydrochloric acid : chloride of platinum or perchloric acid will indicate the potash. In a complex organic mixture it is difficult to detect the potash ; but hydrocyanic acid may be obtained from it by distilling the suspected fluid with tartaric acid.**

* Journ de Chim. Méd. ii. 561.
† Médecine-Légale, iii. 385.
‡ Journal de Pharmacie, 1837, p. 27.
§ Ann. de Chim. et de Phys. xxvii. 200.
‖ Hufeland's Journal der Praktischen Heilkunde, lii. i. 92.
¶ Journal de Chim. Méd. vi. 723.   ** Ibidem, 1843, 94.

SECTION II. — *Of the Action of Hydrocyanic Acid and the Symptoms it excites in Man.*

The effects of hydrocyanic acid on the animal system have been examined by several physiologists. The best experiments with the concentrated acid are those of M. Magendie; who says that, if a single drop be put into the throat of a dog, the animal makes two or three deep hurried respirations, and instantly drops down dead; that it causes death almost as instantaneously when dropped under the eyelid; and that when it is injected into the jugular vein, the animal drops down dead at the very instant, as if struck with a cannon-ball or with lightning.*

On repeating these experiments in order to determine less figuratively the shortest period which elapses before the poison begins to operate, as well as the shortest time in which it proves fatal, — two points it will presently be found important to know, — I remarked that a single drop, weighing scarcely a third of a grain, dropped into the mouth of a rabbit, killed it in eighty-three seconds, and began to act in sixty-three seconds, — that three drops weighing four-fifths of a grain, in like manner killed a strong cat in thirty seconds, and began to act in ten, — that another was affected by the same dose in five and died in forty seconds, — that four drops weighing a grain and a fifth did not affect a rabbit for twenty seconds, but killed it in ten seconds more, — and that twenty-five grains, corresponding with an ounce and a half of medicinal acid, began to act on a rabbit as soon as it was poured into its mouth, and killed it outright in ten seconds at farthest. Three drops injected into the eye acted on a cat in twenty seconds, and killed it in twenty more; and the same quantity dropped on a fresh wound in the loins acted in forty-five and proved fatal in 105 seconds. Dr. A. T. Thomson says he has seen the concentrated acid kill a strong dog in two seconds.† Mr. Blake on the other hand alleges that all the accounts which represent the action of the poison to begin in less than ten seconds are exaggerated, because he could never find it to act more quickly, even when thirty minims of concentrated acid were injected at once into the femoral vein.‡ But it is impossible that any negative results can outweigh positive observations, especially when made, as mine were, expressly with the view of ascertaining the shortest interval. In the slower cases enumerated above there were regular fits of violent tetanus; but in the very rapid cases the animals perished just as the fit was ushered in with retraction of the head. In rabbits opisthotonos, in cats emprosthotonos, was the chief tetanic symptom. — The practical application of these experiments will appear presently.

Of all the forms in which the pure acid can be administered, that of vapour appears the most instantaneous in operation. M. Robert found, that when a bird, a rabbit, a cat, and two dogs were made to

* Ann. de Chim. et de Phys. vi. 347.
† Lancet, 1836-37, ii. 324.
‡ Edinburgh Med. and Surg. Journal, li. 339.

breathe air saturated with its vapour, the first died in one second, the second also in a single second, the cat in two, one dog in five, and the other dog in ten seconds.*

The effects of the diluted acid are the same when the dose is large, but somewhat different when inferior doses are given. These effects have been observed by many physiologists; but the most accurate and extensive experiments are those of Emmert published in 1805,† those of Coullon in 1819,‡ and those of Krimer in 1827.§ They found that when an animal is poisoned with a dose not quite sufficient to cause death, it is seized in one or two minutes with giddiness, weakness and salivation, then with tetanic convulsions, and at last with gradually increasing insensibility ; that after lying in this state for some time, the insensibility goes off rapidly and is succeeded by a few attacks of convulsions and transient giddiness; and that the whole duration of such cases of poisoning sometimes does not exceed half an hour, but may extend to a whole day or more. — When the dose is somewhat larger the animal perishes either in tetanic convulsions or comatose ; and death for the most part takes place between the second and fifteenth minute. I have seen the diluted acid, however, prove fatal with a rapidity scarcely surpassed by the pure poison. Thus in an experiment with Vauquelin's acid, made on a strong cat at the same time with the second and third of the experiments with the pure acid detailed above, I found that thirty-two grains, which contain one of real acid, began to act in fifteen seconds, and proved fatal in twenty-five more. According to Schubarth's experiments death may be sometimes delayed for thirty-two minutes;‖ but if the animal survives that interval, it recovers. He farther states, that during the course of the symptoms the breath exhales an odour of hydrocyanic acid.¶ Coullon once saw a dog die after nineteen hours of suffering; but cases of this duration are exceedingly rare.** When the dose is very large Mr. Macaulay, as will afterwards be mentioned (p. 590), has found death take place in a few seconds, exactly as when the pure acid is given.

The body presents few morbid appearances of note. The brain is generally natural. Yet occasionally its vessels are turgid; and Schubarth once found even an extravasation of blood between its external membranes in the horse.†† The heart and great vessels are distended with black blood, which is commonly fluid, but occasionally coagulated as usual. The lungs, according to Schubarth, are sometimes pale, but much more generally injected and gorged with blood.‡‡ The pure acid, according to Magendie, exhausts the irritability of the heart and voluntary muscles so completely, that they are insensible

---

* Annales de Chimie, xcii. 59.
† Diss. Inaug. de Venenatis Acidi Borussici in Animalia effectibus. Tubingæ, 1805.
‡ Recherches et Considérations sur l'Acide Hydrocyanique. Paris, 1819.
§ Journal Complementaire, xxviii. 33.
‖ Bemerkungen über die Wirkungen der Blausaure. Hufeland's Journal der Praktischen Heilkunde, lii. . 88.
¶ Bemerkungen, &c. 85.　　　　　** Recherches, &c. p. 136.
†† Bemerkungen, &c. 81.　　　　　‡‡ Ibid. 82.

even to the stimulus of galvanism.* The diluted acid has not always this effect. In the experiments of Coullon the heart and intestines contracted, and the voluntary muscles continued contractile, after death as usual.† So too Mr. Blake remarked both by inspection of the body after death, and by means of the hæmadynamometer during life, that, when the poison is introduced directly into a vein, so as to prove fatal in forty-five seconds, the contractions of the heart, though irregular, are not materially impaired in energy.‡ On the other hand Schubarth states that the heart is never contractile, although the intestines and voluntary muscles retain their contractility.§ The reason of these discrepant statements is that, as I have had occasion to observe, a considerable difference really prevails in experiments conducted under circumstances apparently the same. In eight experiments on cats and rabbits with the pure acid the heart contracted spontaneously, as well as under stimuli, for some time after death, except in the instance of the rabbit killed with twenty-five grains, and one of the cats killed by three drops applied to the tongue. In the last two the pulsations of the heart ceased with the short fit of tetanus which preceded death; and in the rabbit, whose chest was laid open instantly after death, the heart was gorged and its irritability utterly extinct. The later researches of Dr. Lonsdale likewise show great varieties in the condition of the heart; and he has been led to conclude that the diluted acid does not perceptibly influence the heart, while the pure acid enfeebles it, if introduced into the stomach, but arrests it, if injected into the wind-pipe.‖

The experiments of Emmert, Coullon, and Krimer show that the diluted acid acts most energetically through the serous membranes, and next upon the stomach; that it also acts with energy on the cellular tissue; that it has no effect when applied to the trunks or cut extremities of nerves, or to a fissure made in the brain or spinal marrow; that its action is prevented when the vessels of any part are tied before the part is touched with the poison; that its action is not prevented by previously dividing the nerves; and that it may sometimes be discovered in the blood after death by chemical analysis,¶ and frequently by the smell when analysis cannot succeed in separating it.** These results favour the supposition that hydrocyanic acid acts through the medium of the blood-vessels. But the extreme rapidity of its operation in large doses is usually considered incompatible with an action through the blood, or any other channel except direct conveyance along the nerves. The tremendous rapidity of action indicated by the experiments of Magendie, or of Mr. Macaulay (p. 543), of M. Robert, as well as in some of those performed by myself,—certainly appears rather inconsistent with the notion, that the acid must enter the blood-vessels before producing its effects.

This acid acts on the brain and also on the spine independently

* Ann. de Chim. et de Phys. vi.   † Recherches, &c. 146.

‡ Edin. Med. and Surg. Journal, li. 339.   § Bemerkungen, &c. 83.

‖ Edin. Med. and Surg. Journal, li. 39.

¶ Krimer detected the acid in the blood of the heart of an animal killed in 36 seconds by a few drops put on the tongue. Journ. Complementaire, xxviii. 37.

** Lassaigne, Journ. de Chim. Méd. ii.

of its action on the brain.   Its action on both is clearly indicated by the combination of coma with tetanus.   The independent action on the spine is well shown by the following experiment of Wedemeyer. In a dog the spinal cord was divided at the top of the loins, so that no movement took place when the hind-legs were pricked : hydrocyanic acid being then introduced into a wound in the left hind-leg, symptoms of poisoning commenced in one minute, and the hind-legs were affected with convulsions as well as the fore-legs.*

Hydrocyanic acid affects all animals indiscriminately.   From the highest to the lowest in the scale of creation all are killed by it; and all perish nearly in the same manner.   Such is the result of a very extensive series of experiments by Coullon.

It is scarcely necessary to observe that hydrocyanic acid acts energetically as a poison, through whatever channel it is introduced into the body.   Whether it be swallowed, or injected into the rectum, or dropped into the eye, or applied to a fresh wound, or inhaled in the form of vapour, its action is exerted with tremendous energy. Perhaps it may even act through the sound skin.   It has not, hitherto, indeed, been found to affect animals in this way, evidently because their skin is too thick and impermeable.   But M. Robiquet informed me that once, while he was making some experiments on the tension of its vapour, his fingers, after being some time exposed to it, became affected with numbness, which lasted several days ; I have repeatedly remarked the same effect when handling tubes which contained the concentrated acid ; and Emmert found that the essential oil of bitter almond, applied to the uninjured skin of the back of a rabbit, produced the usual symptoms and death : and that the peculiar odour of the poison was quite distinct after death in the deep-seated muscles of the back.†

This substance is poisonous in all its chemical combinations. Coullon remarked that two drops of the hydrocyanate of ammonia killed a sparrow in two minutes ;‡ Robiquet and Magendie found that a hundredth part of a grain of the cyanide of potassium killed a linnet in thirty seconds, and five grains a large pointer in fifteen minutes ;§ Orfila has related an instance of death in the human subject within an hour after the administration of six grains of cyanide of potassium in an injection ;‖ and in a recent experimental investigation the same author found that this salt produces all the effects of hydrocyanic acid.¶ Schubarth killed a dog in twenty minutes with twenty drops of the diluted acid neutralized by ammonia,** and another in three hours with twenty-five drops neutralized by potass. These facts are a sufficient answer to a statement made by Mr. Murray of London, to the effect, that a considerable dose of the acid

* Versuche ueber das Nervensystem, 271, quoted by Marx, die Lehre von den giften, I. ii. 154.
† Ueber das Amerikanische Pfeilgift.   Meckel's Archiv. für Anat. und Physiol. iv. 203.
‡ Recherches, &c. 221.   § Journal de Physiol. iii. 230.
‖ Annales d'Hyg. Publique et de Méd. Légale, xi. 240.
¶ Journal de Chim. Médicale, 1843, 94.   ** Horn's Archiv. 1824, i. 75.

may be given without injury to a rabbit,* if previously rendered alkaline by ammonia. But, nevertheless, as will be seen under the head of the treatment, ammonia, as Mr. Murray stated, is a good antidote when administered after the poison as a stimulant.

The *ferrocyanates*, or prussiates, do not possess deleterious properties. These salts were at one time considered compounds of hydrocyanic .acid with a double oxidized base, oxide of iron being one. Thus the prussiate of potass was considered a compound of hydrocyanic acid with potass and oxide of iron. But since the investigations of Mr. Porrett, it has been admitted that there is only one base, potash; and that it is in union with a hydracid, called ferrocyanic acid, the radicle of which is a ternary body composed of carbon, azote, and iron. The physiological effects of this substance, which have been examined by many experimentalists, are favourable to Porrett's opinion; for although some have found it poisonous, all agree in assigning it very feeble properties, and some have not been able to discover in it any deleterious quality at all. Coullon observes that Gazan killed a dog with two drachms, and Callies another with three drachms of the salt met with in commerce.† Schubarth found that half an ounce had not any material effect on dogs, even when vomiting did not occur for half an hour;‡ and Callies, who found the salt of commerce somewhat poisonous, also remarked, that when it was carefully prepared, several ounces might be given without harm.§ D'Arcet once swallowed half a pound of a solution without any injury.‖ Similar results were obtained previously with smaller doses by Wollaston, Marcet,¶ and Emmert,** as well as afterwards by Dr. Macneven,†† and Schubarth,‡‡ who found that a drachm or even two drachms might be taken with impunity by man and the lower animals.

The *sulpho-cyanic acid*, another substance analogous in chemical nature to the ferrocyanic, was once supposed like it to be a poison of great activity, but this is doubtful. Professor Mayer of Bonn ascertained that a drachm and a half of a moderately strong solution of the acid sometimes killed a rabbit in ninety seconds when injected into the windpipe, and that the same quantity of a solution of sulphocyanate of potassa might occasion death in the course of four hours; but that some rabbits took half an ounce of the former and three drachms of the latter without material harm, both when administered through the windpipe, when injected into the rectum, and when introduced into the stomach by a gullet-tube. In the fatal cases death took place under symptoms of oppressed breathing, rarely attended with convulsions; and extensive traces of irritation were found in the alimentary canal.§§ Dr. Westrumb of Hammeln,

---

* Edin. Journal of Science, ii. 215.   † Recherches, &c. 221.
‡ Horn's Archiv für Medizinische Erfahrung, 1827, i. 73.   § Coullon, 221.
‖ Revue Médicale, xvii. 271.   ¶ Nicholson's Journal, xxxi. 191.
** Ueber die giftige Wirkungen der unächten Angustura. — Hufeland's Journal, xl. iii. 68.
†† Archives Gén. de Méd. iii. 269.   ‡‡ Hufeland's Journal, lii. i. 93.
§§ Wibmer. Die Wirkung der Arzneimittel und Gifte, iii. 138, from Harless, Jahrbuch der Medizin, ix. 1.

however, seems to have found it more active in the form of sulpho-cyanate of potassa. Two scruples in an ounce of water produced in a dog spasmodic breathing, convulsions, efforts to vomit, and death in seven minutes; and forty grains killed another in less than two hours. In the latter animal he detected the poison by the sulphate of iron in the blood, lungs, liver, spleen and kidneys.* Some experiments by Soemering would even make it out to be a poison of very great energy ; for half a drachm of concentrated sulpho-cyanic acid given to a dog occasioned immediate death ; and the same quantity of sulpho-cyanate of potassa killed another in one minute.†

Cyanic and cyanous acids are not poisonous, according to the experiments of Hünefield ;‡ but *cyanogen* is a powerful poison, as will be mentioned under the head of the Narcotic Gases.

The symptoms of hydrocyanic acid observed in man are very similar to those witnessed in animals.

Coullon has given a good account of the effects of small doses as ascertained by experiment on himself. When he took from 20 to 86 drops of a diluted acid, he was attacked for a few minutes with nausea, salivation, hurried pulse, weight and pain in the head, succeeded by a feeling of anxiety, which lasted about six hours.§ Such symptoms are apt to be induced by too large medicinal doses. Another remarkable symptom which has been sometimes observed during its medicinal use is salivation with ulceration of the mouth. Dr. Macleod thrice had occasion to remark this in patients who had been using the drug for about a fortnight, and twice in one individual ; and Dr. Granville says he had also twice witnessed the same effect.‖

As to the effects of fatal doses, it is probable that in man, as in animals, two varieties exist. When the dose is very large, death will in general take place suddenly, without convulsions. But for obvious reasons the symptoms in such cases have not been hitherto witnessed.

The most complete account of the symptoms from fatal doses when convulsions occur, is given in a case reported by Hufeland of a man, who, when apprehended for theft, swallowed an ounce of alcoholized acid, containing about forty grains of the pure acid. He was observed immediately to stagger a few steps, and then to sink down without a groan, apparently lifeless. A physician, who instantly saw him, found the pulse gone and the breathing for some time imperceptible. After a short interval he made so forcible an expiration that the ribs seemed drawn almost to the spine. The legs and arms then became cold, the eyes prominent, glistening, and quite insensible ; and after one or two more convulsive expirations he died, five minutes after swallowing the poison.

In Horn's Journal is recorded another case which also proved fatal

* Meckel's Archiv für Anat. und Physiol. vii. 543, 545.
† Wibmer. Die Wirkung der Arzneimittel, &c. iii. 136.
‡ Horn's Archiv für Medizinische Erfahrung. 1830, ii. 858.
§ Recherches, &c. 127.   ‖ London Med. and Phys. Journal, xlvi. 359 and 363.
¶ Journal der Praktischen, Heilkunde, xl. i. 85.

in five minutes, with precisely the same symptoms.*   A short notice
of what appears to have been a similar case is given in the Annales
de Chimie.   The person was a chemist's servant, who swallowed a
large quantity of the alcoholic solution by mistake for a liqueur, the
poison having been accidentally left on the table by her master, who
had been showing it as a curiosity to some friends.   No account is
given of the symptoms, farther than that she died apoplectic in two
minutes.†   To these cases may be also added a short notice of the
French physician's case mentioned at the commencement of this chapter.   It will convey a good idea of the operation of the poison when
not quite sufficient to kill.   Very soon after swallowing a tea-spoonful of the diluted acid he felt confusion in the head, and soon fell
down insensible, with difficult breathing, a small pulse, a bloated
countenance, dilated insensible pupils, and locked jaw.   Afterwards
he had several fits of tetanus, one of them extremely violent.   In two
hours and a half he began to recover his intellects and rapidly
became sensible ; but for some days he suffered much from ulceration of the mouth and violent pulmonary catarrh, which had evidently
been excited by the ammonia given for the purpose of rousing him.
This gentleman had eructations with the odour of the acid three or
four hours after he took it ; and during the earlier symptoms the same
odour was exhaled by his breath.‡   The hydrocyanic odour of the
breath is of course an important distinguishing character, which
would appear, from the observations of Dr. Lonsdale on animals,§ to
occur more frequently than might be supposed from the silence observed on the subject by the reporters of cases.

Hydrocyanic acid is not considered a cumulative poison, — that is,
the continued use of frequent small doses is not believed to possess
the power recognised in iodine, mercury, and foxglove, of gradually
and silently accumulating in the body, and then suddenly breaking
out with dangerous or fatal violence.   The frequent experience of
practitioners in this and other countries seems to prove that hydrocyanic acid possesses no such property.   It is right at the same time
to mention, that a case published by Dr. Baumgärtner of Freyburg
has been thought by some‖ to establish the reverse.   A man had
taken for two months, on account of chronic catarrh, ten drops of
Ittner's acid daily in doses of one grain, without experiencing the
slightest toxicological effect.   At length he was found one morning
in bed apparently labouring under the poisonous operation of the
acid.   He had headache, blindness, dilated insensible pupil, feeble
irregular pulse, occasional suspension of the breathing, and rapidly
increasing insensibility.   The cold affusion and ammonia were immediately resorted to, and at first with advantage.   But in no long time
spasms commenced in the toes, and gradually affected the rest of the
body, till at length violent fits of general tetanus were formed, lasting
for six or ten minutes, and alternating in the intervals with coma.   Vene-

* Archiv für Mediz. Erfahrung, 1813, 510.
† Ann. de Chimie, xcii. 63.   ‡ Revue Médicale, 1825, i. 265.
§ Edinburgh Med. and Surg. Journal, li. 51.
‖ Such as Sobernheim in his Handbuch der Toxicologie, 1838, 455.

section was next resorted to; after which the spasms were confined to the jaw and eyes. Delirium succeeded, but was removed by a repetition of the bloodletting. At four in the afternoon he was tolerably sensible; during the night delirium returned; at ten next morning he recovered his sight; and on the subsequent morning he had no complaint but headache and pain in the eyes.* This case differs so much from every other in the collateral circumstances, as well as in duration, that, although the symptoms themselves correspond with those of poisoning with hydrocyanic acid, we may justly suspect either some other cause, or the accidental administration of too large a dose. It ought, however, to turn the attention of practitioners to the possibility of this poison acting by the accumulation of the effects of small doses frequently repeated for a great length of time.

The period within which hydrocyanic acid usually proves fatal is fixed with considerable accuracy, not only by the cases observed in the human subject, but likewise by the experiments of many physiologists, and more especially those of Schubarth (p. 583). It is probable that very large doses occasion death in a few seconds; and at all events a few minutes will suffice to extinguish life when the dose is considerable; but if the individual survive forty minutes, he will generally recover. In the course of a dreadful accident which happened a few years ago in one of the Parisian hospitals, when seven epileptic patients were killed at one time by too large doses of the medicinal acid, it was found that several did not die for forty-five minutes.‡ But the researches of Schubarth would certainly justify the expectation that recovery will take place under active treatment when the patient survives so long. — These facts may be highly important in the practice of medical jurisprudence.

The period within which it begins to operate ought also to be accurately ascertained for the same reason. Indeed in a very interesting trial, which took place a few years ago in this country, the fate of the prisoner depended in a great measure on the question, within how short a time the effects of this poison must show themselves ?‡ The nature of the case was as follows: An apothecary's maid-servant at Leicester who was pregnant by her master's apprentice, was found one morning dead in bed; and she had obviously been poisoned with hydrocyanic acid. Circumstances led to the suspicion that the apprentice was accessary to the administration of the poison. On the other hand, it was distinctly proved that the deceased had made arrangements for a miscarriage by artificial means on the night of her death; and it was therefore represented, on the part of the prisoner, that she had taken the poison of her own accord. But the body was found stretched out in bed in a composed posture, with the arms crossed over the trunk, and the bed-clothes pulled smoothly up to the chin; and at her right side lay a small narrow-necked phial,

* Medinisch-chirurgische Zeitung, 1829, i. 377.
† Annales d'Hyg. Publ. et de Med. Lég ii. 497.
‡ Trial of Freeman for the murder of Judith Buswell at Leicester, April 2, 1829.

from which about five drachms of the medicinal prussic acid had been taken, and which was corked and wrapped in paper. There naturally arose a question, whether the deceased, after drinking the poison out of such a vessel, could, before becoming insensible, have time to cork up the phial, wrap it up, and adjust the bed-clothes ?* To settle this point, experiments were made at the request of the judge, by Mr. Macaulay, Mr. Paget, and several other medical men of Leicester ; and on the trial they, with the exception of Mr. Paget, gave it as their opinion, founded on the experiments, that the supposed acts of volition, although within the bounds of possibility, were in the highest degree improbable.   The chief experiments were three in number, from which it appeared that one dog was killed with four drachms in eight seconds, another with four drachms in seven seconds, and another with four drachms and a half in three seconds ; but in other experiments the interval was greater. — For these particulars I am indebted to Mr. Macaulay.

In the first edition of this work I expressed my concurrence with the majority of the witnesses. But some facts, which came subsequently under my notice, led me to think that this concurrence was given rather too unreservedly. I still adhere so far to my original views as to think it improbable that, if the deceased, after swallowing the poison, had time to cork the phial, wrap it in paper, pull up the bed-clothes, and place the bottle at her side, the progress of the symptoms could have been so rapid and the convulsions so slight, as to occasion no disorder in the appearance of the body and the bed-clothes, — and I still likewise think, that after swallowing so large a dose it was improbable she could have performed all the successive acts of volition mentioned above — with ordinary deliberation. But I am informed on good authority, that some gentlemen interested in the case found by actual trial, that all the acts alluded to might be accomplished, if gone about with promptitude, within the short period, which, in some of their experiments, the witnesses found to elapse, before the action of the poison commenced. And such being the fact, we ought not perhaps to attach too great importance to the other argument I have employed, — the probability of disorder in the body and bed-clothes from the convulsions ; for if the poisoning commenced very soon, the convulsions might have been slight. The results of my own experiments related in p. 582, although on the whole confirmatory of those of Mr. Macaulay and his colleagues, are never-

* Profsesor Amos of the London University, in criticizing in his Lectures what I have said of this case in the first edition of the present work, has accused me of mis- stating the evidence, and grounds the charge on a Report by a professional Reporter, where no notice is taken of the phial having been wrapped up in paper, or of the bed- clothes having been pulled up to the chin, or of the arms being crossed over the trunk [Lond. Med. Gazette, viii. 577]. I have nevertheless thought it right to retain my original statement of the evidence, as it was derived from what I still consider the best authority, — the medical witness, who mentions the special fact on which he founded the most important, indeed the only important professional opinion in the case, and to which therefore his attention must have been more pointedly turned than that of any Law-Reporter. The Report alluded to by Professor Amos was afterwards published in the Medical Gazette, viii. 759.

theless sufficient to prove that large doses occasionally do not begin to operate with such rapidity as was observed in their experiments ; for in one instance four drops of concentrated acid, equivalent to two scruples of medicinal acid, did not begin to act on a rabbit for twenty seconds; and certainly, for so small an animal, two scruples are as large a dose as five drachms for a grown-up girl.

The two following cases will throw some farther light on the time within which this poison begins to act on man when taken in large quantity. The first case shows, that even when an enormous dose is taken, a few simple voluntary acts may be executed before the symptoms begin. In this instance which is related by Dr. Gierl of Lindau, the dose was no less than four ounces of the acid of the Bavarian Pharmacopœia, which contains four per cent. of pure acid, and is equivalent to five ounces at least of that commonly used in Britain and France. The subject, an apothecary's assistant, was found dead in bed, with an empty two-ounce phial on each side of the bed, — the mattrass, which is used in Germany instead of blankets, pulled up as high as the breast, — the right arm extended straight down beneath the mattrass, — and the left arm bent on the elbow.* The second case proves that, although one or two acts of volition may be accomplished, the interval is so very brief that these acts can only be of the simplest kind. An apothecary's apprentice-lad was sent from the shop to the cellar for some carbonate of potass ; but he had not been a few minutes away, when his companions heard him cry in a voice of great alarm, " Hartshorn ! Hartshorn !" On instantly rushing down stairs, they found him reclining on the lower steps and grasping the rail ; and he had scarcely time to mutter " Prussic acid !" when he expired, — not more than five minutes after leaving the shop. On the floor of the cellar an ounce-phial was found, which had been filled with the Bavarian hydrocyanic acid, but contained only a drachm. It appeared that he had taken the acid ignorantly for an experiment ; and from the state of the articles in the cellar, it was evident that, alarmed at its instantaneous operation, he had tried to get at the ammonia, which he knew was the antidote, but had found the tremendous activity of the poison would not allow him even to undo the coverings of the bottle.†

When the quantity of the poison is small, a much longer interval may elapse before the commencement of its action. Thus, when the dose is barely short of what is required to occasion death, the effects may be postponed even for fifteen minutes, as in a case which occurred to Mr. Garson of Stromness.‡ This, so far as I am at present aware, is the extreme limit of interval hitherto observed.

In the trial related above the prisoner Freeman was found *Not Guilty*.

It is important to fix, if possible, the smallest fatal dose of hydrocyanic acid. This will vary with particular circumstances, such as the strength of the individual, and the fulness or emptiness of the stomach

* Medizinisch-chirurgische Zeitung, 1829, i. 396.
† Buchner's Repertorium für Pharmacie, xxi. 313.
‡ Edinburgh Medical and Surg. Journal, lix. 72.

at the time. The cases of the Parisian epileptics, who were killed each by a draught containing two-thirds of a grain of pure acid,* will supply pointed information. For, on the one hand, considering the long time they survived, it is not probable that a dose materially less would have a fatal effect on man. And on the other hand repeated instances of recovery have been observed, where the dose was as great or even greater. Thus Dr. Geoghegan had a patient who recovered from a state of extreme danger after taking two-thirds of a grain ;† and Mr. Banks of Lowth met with a case of recovery in similar circumstances, where the dose was very nearly a whole grain.‡

It is almost unnecessary to add, that in man, as in animals, this poison will act violently, through whatever channel it may be introduced into the body. It has not been positively ascertained to act with force through the unbroken skin. The chemist Scharinger indeed was supposed to have been killed in consequence of accidentally spilling the acid on his naked arm ;§ but this was in all probability a mistake. Should the skin be freely exposed to the air it seems reasonable to expect that the poison will evaporate before it could act with energy ; but if confined by pledgets or otherwise, a different result might ensue. Through every other surface, however, besides the unbroken skin, hydrocyanic acid acts with very great power ; and it is in particular important to remember that its power is very great when inhaled, so that dangerous accidents have ensued even from its vapour incautiously snuffed up the nostrils. I have known a strong man suddenly struck down in this way ; a French physician, M. Damiron, has related the case of an apothecary who remained insensible for half an hour subsequently to the same accident ;‖ and cases of the kind are more apt to occur than might at first view be thought, because, contrary to what is generally believed and stated in chemical as well as medico-legal works, its smell is for a few seconds barely perceptible, and never of the kind which these accounts would lead one to anticipate. Accidental death may readily arise from its action on a wound or an abraded surface. Sobernheim mentions that Mr. Scharring, a druggist at Vienna, was poisoned in consequence of a phial of the acid breaking in his hand and wounding it ; and he expired in an hour.¶

The only case with which I am acquainted of poisoning with the artificial compounds of hydrocyanic acid is that formerly alluded to as having been occasioned by the cyanide of potassium. Six grains dissolved in a clyster amounting to six ounces, occasioned general convulsions, palpitations, slow laboured breathing, coldness of the limbs, dilated pupil, fixing of the eyeballs, and death in one hour, — phenomena much the same with those produced by the acid itself.** — Another case has been published, in which a French physician, igno-

* Orfila, Annales d'Hyg. Publ. et de Méd. Lég. i. 507.
† Dublin Medical Journal, viii. 308.
‡ Edinburgh Med. and Surg. Journal, xlviii. 44.
§ Coullon, Recherches, &c. p. 200.
‖ Journ. de Chim. Médicale, vii. 426.
¶ Handbuch der Toxikologie, 1838, 443.
** Annales d'Hyg. Publique, &c. xi. 240.

rant of the correct dose, prescribed a potion with three grains of cyanide of potassium twice a day. Immediately after the first dose the patient was seized with the usual symptoms of poisoning with hydrocyanic acid ; and expired in three-quarters of an hour.* In noticing the first of these cases, Orfila draws the attention of practitioners particularly to the fact, that not long before a similar dose of a sample of cyanide, which had been moist for some time, was twice administered with impunity. The reason is that the cyanide of potassium undergoes decomposition when acted on by water, or when long kept.

SECTION III. — *Of the Morbid Appearances produced by Hydrocyanic Acid.*

Under this head the appearances in a special case will first be mentioned, and then the varieties to which they are liable.

In *Hufeland's* case [p. 587] the inspection was made the day after death. The eyes were still glistening, like those of a person alive ; but the countenance was pale and composed like one asleep. The spine and neck were stiff, the belly drawn in, the back alone livid. The body generally, the blood even within the head, and especially the serous cavities, exhaled a hydrocyanic odour, so strong as to irritate the nostrils. The blood was every where very fluid, so that two pounds flowed from the incision in the scalp and twelve ounces from that of the dura mater ; and it had a glimmering bluish appearance, as if Prussian blue had been mixed with it. The vessels of the brain were gorged, the substance of the brain natural, and the left ventricle distended with half an ounce of serum. The villous coat of the stomach was red, easily removed with the nail, and gangrenous.† The intestines were reddish, and the liver gorged. The lungs were also turgid, and to such a degree in the depending parts as to resemble the liver. The arteries and left cavities of the heart were empty, the veins and right cavities distended.

In commenting on this description it is first to be remarked, that the blood, as in the preceding case, is generally altered in nature. Ittner, who made some good experiments on the subject, found it in animals black, viscid, and oily in consistence.‡ Emmert found it fluid and of a cochineal colour. In a case related by Mertzdorff of an apothecary's apprentice, who was found dead in bed after swallowing three drachms and a half of diluted acid,§ in the case recorded in Horn's Archiv, and in that related by Dr. Gierl, it was fluid. It was also perfectly fluid every where in the bodies of the seven epileptic patients poisoned at Paris. Yet this state is not invariable. Coullon, though his results tally in general with those of Ittner and Emmert, has given some experiments in which the blood coagulated after flowing from the body ;‖ and in the case of an apothecary related in Rust's Journal it was found coagulated in the heart.¶

* Journal de Chimie Médicale, 1843, 95, 98.
† See Note at p. 365.   ‡ Beiträge zur Geschichte der Blausäire, 1809.
§ Journal Complémentaire, xvii. 366.   ‖ Recherches, &c.
¶ Magazin für die ges. Heilkunde, xiv. 104.

53

In the next place, Magendie and other physiologists have observed that, as in Hufeland's case, the blood and cavities of the body in animals exhale a hydrocyanic odour, even though the quantity taken was small. The blood did so likewise in the heart of the apothecary just mentioned as well as throughout the whole body in the case described in Horn's Journal. The odour, however, is not always present. For example, there was none in the case of another German apothecary, who poisoned himself with an ounce, as recorded in a later volume of Rust's Journal ;* neither was there any odour in the blood in Mertzdorff's case, although it was strong in the stomach; nor in the blood nor any other part of the body in the Parisian epileptics. It also appears from an experiment by Schubarth,† and from a case by Leuret where life was prolonged above fifteen minutes,‡ — that the odour may be distinct in the blood, brain, or chest, when hardly any is to be perceived in the stomach. Schubarth has inquired with some care into the circumstances under which the hydrocyanic odour may, or may not, be expected. He states, as the result of his researches, that if the dose is sufficient to cause death within ten minutes, the peculiar odour will always be remarked in the blood of the heart, lungs, and great vessels, provided the body have not been exposed to rain or to a current of air, and the examination be made within a moderate interval, — for example, twenty-one hours for so small an animal as a dog ; but that, if the dose is so small that life is prolonged for fifteen, twenty-seven, or thirty-two minutes, then even immediately after death it may be impossible to remark any of the peculiar odour, evidently because, as already mentioned, the acid is rapidly discharged by the lungs ; and that even when the dose is large enough to cause death in four minutes, the smell may not be perceived if the carcase has been left in a spacious apartment for two days, or exposed to a shower for a few hours only. These facts explain satisfactorily why no odour could be perceived in the bodies of the Parisian epileptics : for they lived from half an hour to forty-five minutes. The poison may exist in the stomach, though not appreciable by the sense of smell. In Chevallier's case mentioned above, the contents of the stomach had not any odour of hydrocyanic acid ; which, however, was evident to the sense of smell, and plainly indicated by various tests, in the fluid obtained by distilling the contents.

The presence of this odour in the blood may be accounted strong evidence of poisoning with hydrocyanic acid, if it is unequivocal to the sense of several individuals. An exhalation of the same kind is occasionally formed by natural processes in the excrement. Itard once remarked in a case of inflammation of the intestines, and again in a case of inflamed liver, a strong smell of bitter almonds in the fæces, although no medicine containing hydrocyanic acid had been given.§ Mr. Taylor mentions that he once observed a sort of hydrocyanic odour in the brain of a person who died of natural disease.‖

* Magazin für die ges. Heilkunde, xxiii. 375.
† Bemerkungen, &c. Hufeland's Journal, lii. i. 76.
‡ Annales d'Hyg. Publ. et de Méd. Lég. iv. 422.
§ Rust's Magazin, xx. 577.   ‖ Manual of Medical Jurisprudence, 251.

These facts will render the inspector cautious, but can scarcely throw a doubt over evidence derived from an unequivocal hydrocyanic odour in the blood.

Few successful attempts have yet been made to detect the acid in the blood by chemical analysis. The odour may be present, although chemical analysis fails in eliciting any indication. This follows from the observations of Dr. Lonsdale,[*] as well as of various authors quoted by him in his paper. The cyanide of potassium has been detected by Mayer not merely in the blood, but likewise in the serous secretions and sundry soft solids.[†]

In most instances, — for example, in the Parisian epileptics, the state of the brain, as to turgescence of vessels, has corresponded with the description given by Hufeland. Venous turgescence and emptiness of the arterial system are commonly remarked throughout the whole body. Thus in the epileptic patients, the heart and great arteries were empty ; the great veins gorged ; the spleen gorged, soft, and pultaceous ; the veins of the liver gorged ; and the kidneys of a deep violet colour, much softened, and their veins gorged with black blood.

It is impossible that hydrocyanic acid could cause gangrene of the stomach, which is said to have been witnessed in Hufeland's case. But there are often signs of irritation in that organ. The villous coat has been found red in animals ; it was shrivelled, and its vessels were turgid with black blood in the instance of the apothecary mentioned in the fourteenth volume of Rust's Journal ; in Mertzdorff's case it was red and checkered with bloody streaks ; and in the case related by Dr. Gierl, where four ounces were swallowed, it was dark-red, as it were tanned or steeped in spirits, and easily separated from the subjacent contents. The contents of the stomach have in every instance had a strong hydrocyanic odour, except in the cases of the Parisian epileptics, and in those related by Leuret and by Chevallier. According to the experiments of Lassaigne and Schubarth, formerly noticed, it is not to be looked for when the body has been kept a few days, more especially if the individual lived some time. Dr. Lonsdale generally found it eight or nine days after death in animals, which had been either buried during that time, or kept in an apartment at the temperature of 50^{C} F.[‡] In a case which occurred not long ago in London the poison was found in the stomach five days after death. A coroner's inquest had terminated in a verdict of natural death. But suspicions having arisen, that the man had poisoned himself in anticipation of a charge of forgery, another inquiry was made ; when the odour of hydrocyanic acid was evolved from the contents of the stomach, and the distilled water obtained from them yielded decisive chemical evidence of its being present.[§] It is important to observe, in reference to the evidence of

[*] Edinburgh Med. and Surg. Journal, li. 52.
[†] Archiv für Anatomie und Physiologie, iii. 485, vi. 37.
[‡] Edinburgh Medical and Surgical Journal, li. 53.
[§] Lancet, 1838-39, i. 880, and ii. 14

hydrocyanic acid in the stomach, that here, as in the instance of the blood, the odour may be strong, and yet the poison may not be discoverable by analysis. This fact rests on the united testimony of Coullon, Vauquelin, Leuret, Turner, and Dr. Lonsdale ; the last of whom mentions that he could not detect it chemically after the fourth day in the bodies of some animals, in which it was perceptible by its odour even four or five days later.[*] It is possible, however, that these failures to detect the poison by analysis may have sometimes arisen from imperfections in the method of analysis employed ; for it was detected by the process formerly mentioned in the stomach of the apothecary last alluded to, in Chevallier's case, though not perceptible to the smell, and frequently by Lassaigne in animals.

Mertzdorff remarked both in his case of poisoning with hydrocyanic acid, and likewise in a parellel instance of poisoning with the essential oil of bitter almonds,[†] a singular appearance in the bile, the colour of which was altered to deep blue.

Coullon and Emmert say they have observed, that the bodies of animals resist putrefaction. The latter in particular mentions, that he had left them several days in a warm room without perceiving any sign of decay. This certainly would not à priori be expected, considering the state of the blood. And it is not universal ; for in one instance, the case of Mertzdorff, putrefaction commenced within thirty hours after death. In the Parisian epileptics, the bodies passed through the usual stage of rigidity.

It appears that even long after death the eye, as in Hufeland's case, has a peculiar glistening and staring expression, so as to render it difficult to believe that the individual is really dead ; and this appearance has been considered by Dr. Paris so remarkable, as even alone to supply " decisive evidence of poisoning by hydrocyanic acid."[‡] But the accuracy of this opinion may be questioned. The appearance is indeed very general in cases of poisoning with preparations containing hydrocyanic acid. Besides occurring in the case of Hufeland, and in that which gave occasion to Dr. Paris's statement, it was witnessed by Mertzdorff, and in the instance described in Horn's Journal. But it is not a constant appearance ; for it was not observed in the seven Parisian epileptics. Neither is it peculiar ; for death from carbonic acid has the same effect ; I have remarked it six hours after death in a woman who died of cholera ; and it has been observed in cases of death during the epileptic paroxysm.

SECTION IV. — *Of the Treatment of Poisoning with Hydrocyanic Acid.*

Much attention has been lately paid to the treatment of this variety of poisoning ; and the object of those who have studied it has naturally been the discovery of an antidote.

An antidote to hydrocyanic acid must either be a substance which

[*] *Ut supra,* p. 52.　　　　　[†] Journal Complémentaire, xvii. 366.
[‡] London Med. and Phys. Journal, lvii. 151.

renders it immediately insoluble, or one which exerts upon the body
an action contrary to that excited by the poison, that is, a powerful
stimulant action on the nervous system.   Hence all such remedies as
oil, milk, soap, coffee, treacle, turpentine, at one time thought serviceable, are quite inert.*

Antidotes have hitherto been chiefly sought for among the powerful,
diffusible stimulants.   And it is plain, that even although a chemical
antidote were known, a stimulant antidote is indispensable also, because the mischief done, before the poison can be rendered inert, is
generally sufficient to cause death, unless counteracted by treatment.

Of the diffusible stimulants, *ammonia* is considered by many the
most energetic antidote.   The first who made careful experiments
with it was Mr. John Murray of London ; and he was so convinced
of its efficacy, that he expressed himself ready to swallow a dose of
the acid large enough to prove fatal, provided a skilful person were
beside him to administer the antidote.†   The favourable results obtained by Murray were afterwards confirmed by M. Dupuy.‡   Afterwards, however, the efficacy of ammonia was called in question.
Orfila stated in the third edition of his Toxicology that he had several
times satisfied himself of the complete inutility of this as well as
many other antidotes.§   And Dr. Herbst of Göttingen made some
careful experiments, from which he concludes that ammonia, though
useful when the dose of poison is not large enough to kill, and even
capable of making an animal that has taken a fatal dose jump up and
run about for a little, yet will never save its life.‖   But farther experiments by Orfila have led him to modify his former statement, and
to admit, that, although liquid ammonia is of no use when introduced into the stomach, yet if the vapour from it is inhaled, life may
sometimes be preserved, provided the dose of the poison be not large
enough to act with great rapidity.   He remarked, that when from
eight to fourteen drops of the medicinal acid were given to dogs of
various sizes, they died in the course of fifteen minutes if left without
assistance, but were sometimes saved by being made to inhale ammoniacal water, and recovered completely in little more than an
hour.¶   As this is very nearly the conclusion to which Mr. Murray
was led by his experiments performed in 1822, it is rather extraordinary, that his name, as the undoubted discoverer of the remedy,
has never been mentioned by the Parisian Professor.   Buchner, it is
right to add, had found this remedy useful in the same year in which
Mr. Murray's experiments were made.**   A gentleman who took an
over-dose of two drachms of hydrocyanic acid while using it medicinally, and who seems to have been in great danger, owed his recovery to the assiduous use of carbonate of ammonia held to the
nostrils, and spirit of ammonia internally.   Relief was obtained im-

* Coullon. Recherches sur l'Acide Hydrocyanique, 225, *et passim.*
† Edin. Philosoph. Journal, vii. 124, and Edin. Journal of Science, ii. 214.
‡ Archives Gén. de Méd. xi. 30.   § Toxicologie Gén. ii. 167.
‖ Archiv für Anatomie und Physiologie, 1828, p. 208.
¶ Annales d'Hyg. Publ. et de Méd. Lég. i. 511.
** Repertorium für die Pharmacie, xii. 144.

53*

mediately.* Orfila suggests an important caution, — not to use a strong ammoniacal liquor, otherwise the mouth, air-passages, and even the alimentary canal may be attacked with inflammation, — as indeed happened to the French physician whose case was formerly mentioned. The strong *aqua ammoniæ* should be diluted with several parts of water.

Another remedy of the same kind with ammonia as to action is *chlorine*. This substance was first proposed as a remedy in 1822 by Riauz, a chemist of Ulm, who found that, when a pigeon, poisoned with hydrocyanic acid, was on the point of expiring, it immediately began to revive, on being made to breathe chlorine, and in fifteen minutes was able to fly away.† Buchner repeated Riauz's experiments and arrived at the same results. More lately M. Simeon, apothecary to the hospital of St. Louis at Paris, apparently without being acquainted with the observations of the German chemists, was likewise led to suppose, that this gas might prove a useful antidote ;‡ and MM. Cottereau and Vallette have formed the same conclusion.§ Orfila in his paper already quoted expresses his conviction, that this remedy is the most powerful antidote of all hitherto proposed. His experiments have convinced him, that animals, which have taken a dose of poison sufficient to kill them in fifteen or eighteen minutes, will be saved by inspiring water impregnated with a fourth part of its volume of chlorine, even although the application of the remedy be delayed till the poison has operated for four or five minutes. In some of his experiments he waited till the convulsive stage of the poisoning was passed, and the stage of flaccidity and insensibility had supervened ; yet the animals were obviously out of danger ten minutes after the chlorine was first applied, and recovered entirely in three-quarters of an hour.‖

The last remedy of this nature which deserves notice is the *cold affusion*. This was first recommended by Dr. Herbst of Göttingen, who, on account of the success he witnessed from it in animals, considers it the best remedy yet proposed. When the dose of the poison was insufficient to prove fatal in ordinary circumstances, two affusions he found commonly sufficient to dispel every unpleasant symptom. When the dose was larger, it was necessary to repeat the effusion more frequently. Its efficacy was always most certain when resorted to before the convulsive stage of the poisoning was over ; yet even in the stage of insensibility and paralysis it was sometimes employed with success. In the latter instance the first sign of amendment was renewal of the spasms of the muscles. Many experiments are related by the author in support of these statements. But the most decisive is the following. Two poodles of the same size being selected, hydrocyanic acid was given to one of them in repeated small doses till it died. The whole quantity administered being

* Dr. Geoghegan, in Lancet, 1835-36, i. 174.
† Repertorium für die Pharmacie, xii. 141.   ‡ Ibidem, xii. 144.
§ London Med. and Surg. Journal. iii. 58.
‖ Annales d'Hyg. Publ. et de Méd. Leg. 525.

seven grains of Ittner's acid, this dose was given at once to the other dog. Immediately it fell down in convulsions, violent opisthotonos ensued, and in half a minute the convulsive stage was followed by flaccidity, imperceptible respiration, and failing pulse. The cold affusion was immediately resorted to, but at first without any amendment. After the second affusion, however, the opisthotonos returned, and was accompanied by cries ; and on the remedy being repeated every fifteen minutes, the breathing gradually became easier and easier, the spasms abated, and in a few hours the animal was quite well.* Professor Orfila repeated Dr. Herbst's experiments, with analogous results; but he considers the cold affusion inferior to chlorine.†— It is probably advantageous to apply the cold water rather in the form of cold douche to the head and spine than to the body at large. Dr. Robinson of Sunderland found that rabbits, which had taken doses adequate to occasion death, might be saved by pouring on the hindhead and along the spine cold water impregnated with common salt and nitre.‡ A case, which seems to have been cured in this way, has been published by Mr. Banks of Lowth. A young woman took by mistake a solution containing very nearly a grain of real acid, and immediately became insensible and convulsed. Ordinary stimulants were of no use. But in fifteen minutes, when the convulsions had ceased, and she lay in a state of complete coma and general paralysis, the cold douche on the head first renewed the convulsions, then strengthened the pulse and restored some appearance of consciousness, and finally roused her, so that in a few hours she was quite well.§

It is probable, that *bleeding from the jugular vein* deserves more attention as a remedy than it has yet received. The right side of the heart is almost invariably found much gorged with blood in animals examined at the moment of death ; and the contractions of the heart, in such circumstances imperfect or arrested altogether, have often been observed by experimentalists to be instantly restored on promptly removing the state of turgescence. Accordingly Dr. Cormack found that a dog, at the point of death after receiving a fatal dose of the acid, was speedily roused and eventually saved by bleeding from the jugular vein.‖ And in a careful inquiry by Dr. Lonsdale, it was ascertained that the turgescence of the heart might be effectually diminished in this way, and that recovery might frequently be accomplished when the poison was otherwise amply sufficient to have occasioned speedy death.¶ In a case treated by Magendie, that of a young lady poisoned by too large a medicinal dose, the chief remedies were ammonia and blood-letting from the jugular vein ; and she recovered.**

* Archiv für Anatomie und Physiologie, 1828, p. 208.
† Annales d'Hyg. Publ. et de Méd. Lég. i. 518.
‡ Buchner's Repertorium für die Pharmacie, lxxv. 403.
§ Edinburgh Med. and Surg. Journal, xlviii 44.
‖ Prize Thesis— On the Presence of Air in the Organs of Circulation." Edinburgh, 1837.
¶ Edinburgh Medical and Surgical Journal. li. 57.
** Formulaire pour les Nouveaux Médicamens.

Few observations have hitherto been made on the chemical antidotes for hydrocyanic acid, or those substances which render it innoxious by converting it into an insoluble compound. It is plain that several probable antidotes of this kind exist. But toxicologists have been apparently deterred from trying them by the fearful rapidity with which the poison acts, and the consequent improbability that in practice any such antidote can be administered in time. It has lately been shown, however, by Messrs. T. and H. Smith of this city, that the effects of a fatal dose may be warded off by the timely administration of the re-agents necessary for converting the acid into Prussian blue. They found that if a solution of carbonate of potash followed by a solution of the mixed sulphates of iron be given to animals very soon after the administration of a dose of thirty drops of the Edinburgh medicinal acid, containing three per cent. of real acid, recovery in general takes place, and sometimes little inconvenience seems to be sustained. The solutions they used were one of 144 grains of carbonate of potash in two ounces of water, and another composed of a drachm and a half of sulphate of protoxide of iron, together with two drachms of the same salt converted into sulphate of sesquioxide by means of sulphuric and nitric acids in the usual way. About 52 minims of each of these solutions will remove the whole acid contained in 100 grains of the Edinburgh medicinal acid ; but for certainty, three or four times as much should be used, — which may be done with perfect safety.*

On the whole, then, it appears that the proper treatment of a case of poisoning with hydrocyanic acid consists in the cold affusion applied to the head and spine, the inhalation of diluted ammonia or chlorine, venesection at the jugular vein, and the administration of carbonate of potash and the mixed sulphates of iron, if aid has been obtained in good time.

It is right to remember, however, that on account of the dreadful rapidity of this variety of poisoning, it will rarely be in the physician's power to resort to any treatment soon enough for success ; — and farther, that his chance of success must generally be feeble even though the case be taken in time, because when hydrocyanic acid is swallowed by man, the dose is commonly so large as not to be counteracted by any remedies.

On the Vegetable Substances which contain Hydrocyanic Acid.

Hydrocyanic acid exists in several plants ; which are consequently poisonous. I have considered it advisable to describe their effects separately from those of the pure acid.

The plants which have been thoroughly examined and found to yield it belong chiefly to the division *Drupaceæ*, of Decandolle's Natural Family the *Rosaceæ*. These are the bitter almond, cherry-laurel, bird-cherry, and peach. The leaves and seeds of the nectarine and apricot, and the seeds of the plum and cherry, have the

* Lancet, 1844, October 5.

same taste with these four, and therefore will certainly be found to contain the acid also. The same inference may be drawn from the taste of some pomaceous seeds; and accordingly I have obtained a hydrocyanated oil from the seeds of the New York pippin, and those of the white-beam-tree, the *Pyrus aria.* The poison procured from these sources exists in two forms, — as a distilled water, and as an essential oil. Further, the acid has been discovered to constitute the active poison of the juice of the *Janipha manihot,* or bitter cassava [see p. 457].

The distilled waters yield hydrocyanic acid, as is shown by the blue precipitate they give with potass and the mixed sulphates of iron. They have a powerful, peculiar, grateful odour, which is usually likened to that of pure hydrocyanic acid. But the smell really bears very little resemblance to that of hydrocyanic acid, and is not owing to its presence : the odour remains equally strong after the acid is thrown down by the test now mentioned. The active part of the distilled water may be separated in the form of a volatile oil. This is colourless at first, afterwards yellowish or reddish, acrid, bitter, heavier than water, and very volatile. The essential oil of the bitter almond has been carefully examined by various chemists. Vogel, by subjecting it twice to distillation from caustic potass, procured hydrocyanate of potass in the residue ; and a volatile oil was distilled over, which no longer contained hydrocyanic acid, but nevertheless had the odour of the original oil.* This purified oil he considered equally poisonous with that which contains hydrocyanic acid, a single drop of it having killed a sparrow ; and his opinion was confirmed by the experiments of Professor Orfila. But according to some careful experiments by Stange,† which have been amply confirmed by Dr. Göppert of Breslau,‡ and also by MM. Robiquet and Boutron-Charlard,§ — if the purified oil retains active poisonous properties, this must be owing to the acid not having been entirely removed. Göpmert in particular remarked that twenty-five drops of the purified bitter-almond oil, cherry-laurel oil, or bird-cherry oil had very little effect on rabbits, not more indeed than the same quantity of the common essential oils. The purified oil, according to all these chemists, possesses the odour of the original oil, as Vogel first stated.

Of the Bitter Almond.

The bitter almond was once extensively used in medicine, and is still much employed by confectioners for flavouring puddings, sweatmeats, and liqueurs. It is the kernel of the fruit of the *Amygdalus communis.* This species has too varieties, the *dulcis* and the *amara;* which differ from one another in the fruit only. The fruit of the former yields the sweet, and of the latter the bitter almond. The bitter almond is the smaller of the two. The two plants, according

* Journal de Pharmacie, vii. 465.
† Buchner's Repertorium für die Pharmacie, xvi. 100.
‡ Rust's Magazin für die gesammte Heilkunde, xxxii. 494.
§ Annales de Chim. et de Phys xliv. 352.

to Murray, are convertible into each other, — the sweet variety becoming bitter by neglect, — the bitter becoming sweet by cultivation,
or certain modes of management not well known, — and the seed of
either variety producing plants of both.* These statements as to the
mutual convertibility of the two varieties require confirmation.

The bitter almond depends for its activity on the essential oil,
which is common to all the vegetable poisons belonging to the
present tribe. According to the researches of Robiquet and Boutron-
Charlard, followed up by Liebig, the oil does not, like common essential oils, exist ready formed in the almond, but is only produced
when the almond-pulp comes in contact with water. It cannot be
separated by any process whatever from the almond without the co-
operation of water, — neither, for example, by pressing out the fixed
oil, nor by the action of ether, nor by the action of absolute alcohol.
After the almond is exhausted by ether, the remaining pulp gives the
essential oil as soon as it is moistened ; but if it is also exhausted by
alcohol, the essential oil is entirely lost. The reason is that alcohol
dissolves out a peculiar crystalline principle, named amygdalin,
which, with the co-operation of water, forms the essential oil by
reacting on a variety of the albuminous principle in the almond,
called emulsion or synoptase.

In some respects, therefore, the essential oil of almonds is quite
peculiar in its nature, and quite different from the common essential
or volatile oils. — The presence of hydrocyanic acid in it is easily
proved by dissolving it with agitation in water, and treating the solution with caustic potass, followed by the mixed sulphates of iron
and sulphuric acid. — The quantity of essential oil which may be
procured from the bitter almond amounts, according to Krüger of
Rostock, to four drachms from five pounds or a ninety-sixth part.†
The quantity of hydrocyanic acid in the oil varies considerably :
Schrader got from an old sample 8·5 per cent., from a new sample
10·75 ;‡ but Göppert got from another specimen so much as 14·33
per cent.§

Effects on Animals. — The bitter almond is a powerful poison,
which acts in the same way as hydrocyanic acid, but likewise excites
at times vomiting and other signs of irritation. The first good experiments on it are those related in Wepfer's treatise on the Cicuta ;
but its properties seem to have been known even to Dioscorides.
The symptoms it induces in animals are trembling, weakness, palsy,
convulsions, often of the tetanic kind, and finally coma. But frequently it occasions vomiting before these symptoms begin, and the
animal in that way may escape.‖ According to Orfila, twenty
almonds will kill a dog in six hours by the stomach if the gullet be
tied ; and six will kill it in four days when applied to a wound.¶

* Murray, Apparatus Medicaminum, iii. 257.
† Buchner's Repertorium für die Pharmacie, xii. 135.
‡ Fechner's Repertorium der Organischen Chemie, ii. 65.
§ Rust's Magazin für die gesammte Heilkunde, xxxii. 500.
‖ Wepferi, Cicutæ aquaticæ Historia et Noxæ, 244 ; and Coullon, Recherches sur
l'Acide Hydrocyanique, 55.   ¶ Toxicol. Gén. ii. 179.

The essential oil is not much inferior in activity to the pure hy-drocyanic acid. A single drop of it applied by Sir B. Brodie on the tongue of a cat caused violent convulsions and death in five minutes.* But more generally a larger dose, or about seven drops, has been found necessary to kill a middle-sized dog. Five drops, according to Göppert, will kill a rabbit in six minutes. When entirely freed of hydrocyanic acid, it becomes, as already mentioned, not more poi-sonous than common volatile oils.

Symptoms in Man. — The effects of the almond and of the oil upon man are equally striking with those of hydrocyanic acid.

In small doses the bitter almond produces disorder of the digestive organs, nausea, vomiting, and sometimes diarrhœa. These symptoms are occasionally brought on by the small quantities used for flavouring sweetmeats, if the confectioner has not been careful in compounding them. Virey says that accidents occasionally happen to children at Paris from their eating freely of macaroons, which are sometimes too strongly flavoured with the bitter almond.† In this country accidents from the same cause may be with justice apprehended, as confec-tioners now generally use, not the bitter almond, but its essential oil, which is distilled for the purpose in London, and sold in the drug-gists shops under the name of peach-nut oil. Göppert suggests that this oil ought to be freed of its hydrocyanic acid by repeated distil-lation with caustic potassa, because the flavour is not in the least in-jured by the process, while its activity as a poison is greatly lessened.

In peculiar constitutions the minutest quantity, even a single almond, will cause a state resembling intoxication, succeeded by an eruption like nettle-rash. The late Dr. Gregory was subject to be affected in this way. Other vegetable bitters had the same effect on him, but none so remarkably as bitter almonds. They caused first sickness, generally tremors, then vomiting, next a hot fit with an eruption of urticaria, particularly on the upper part of the body. At the same time the face, and head swelled very much, and there was generally a feeling like intoxication. The symptoms lasted only for a few hours. The rash did not alternately appear and disappear as in common nettle-rash.‡ A lady of my acquaintance is liable to be attacked with urticaria even from eating the sweet almond.

The quantity of bitter almonds which may be eaten with impunity is unknown ; but Wibmer mentions an experimentalist who took half an ounce without any other effect besides headache and sickness.§ Two cases of death in the human subject from eating them have been quoted by Coullon from the Journal de Médecine of Montpel-lier. One is a doubtful case, but the other is unequivocal. A bath-woman gave her child the " expressed juice" of a handful of bitter almonds to cure worms. The child, who was four years old, was immediately attacked with colic, swelling of the belly, giddiness, locked jaw, frothing at the mouth, general convulsions, and insen-

* Philosophical Transactions, 1811, p. 184.
† Journal de Pharmacie, ii. 204. ‡ Dr. Alison's Manuscript Lectures.
§ Die Wirkung der Arzneimittel und Gifte, i. 166.

sibility, and died in two hours.* Murray, however, asserts in his Apparatus Medicaminum that the expressed juice is sweet and not poisonous.† But this apparent contradiction is easily explained by referring to the chemical relations of the almond, — the oil expressed without water being free from essential oil, while the milky fluid expressed from the pulp beat up with water is strongly impregnated with it. — Another case was published not long ago by Mr. Kennedy of London ; but the symptoms were imperfectly ascertained. The person, a stout labourer, appeared to have eaten a great quantity of bitter almonds, which were subsequently found in the stomach. He was seen to drop down while standing near a wall ; soon after which the surgeon who was sent for found him quite insensible, with the pulse imperceptible, and the breath exhaling the odour of bitter almonds ; and death took place in no long time.‡

Coullon has noticed many other instances where alarming symptoms were produced by this poison, but were dissipated by the supervention of spontaneous vomiting.

The effects of small doses of the oil have been tried by Sir B. Brodie on himself ; and a fatal case of poisoning with it has been recorded by Mertzdorff. In the course of his experiments Sir B. Brodie once happened to touch his tongue with the end of a glass rod which happened to be dipped in the oil ; and he says he had scarcely done so before he felt an uneasy, indescribable feeling in the pit of the stomach, great feebleness of his limbs, and loss of power to direct the muscles, so that he could hardly keep himself from falling. These sensations were quite momentary.§

Mertzdorff's case is interesting, not only as being accurately related, but likewise on account of the exact resemblance of the symptoms to those observed in the celebrated case of Sir Theodosius Boughton, which will presently be mentioned. A hypochondriacal gentleman, 48 years old, swallowed two drachms of the essential oil. A few minutes afterwards, his servant, whom he sent for, found him lying in bed, with his features spasmodically contracted, his eyes fixed, staring, and turned upwards, and his chest heaving convulsively and hurriedly. A physician, who entered the room twenty minutes after the draught had been taken, found him quite insensible, the pupils immoveable, the breathing stertorous and slow, the pulse feeble and only 30 in a minute, and the breath strongly impregnated with the odour of bitter almonds, death ensued ten minutes afterwards.‖ A fatal case occurred lately in London, where the individual, intending to compound a nostrum for worms with beech-nut oil, got by mistake from the druggist peach-nut oil, which is nothing else than the oil of bitter almond. — A singular case of recovery from a very large dose of this poison has been lately published by M. Chevasse. A shopkeeper, who swallowed half an ounce by mistake for

* Recherches, &c. 60.   † Apparatus Medicaminum, iii. 257.
‡ London Med. and Phys. Journal, lvii. 150.
§ Philosophical Transactions, 1811, p. 183.
‖ Journal Complémentaire, &c. xvii. 366.

spirit of nitric ether, had an attack of spontaneous vomiting, which was forthwith encouraged by sulphate of zinc. He nevertheless became pale and convulsed ; the pulse disappeared ; and delirious muttering ensued, with *risus sardonicus*, sparkling of the eyes, and panting respiration. Recovery, however, took place under the use of brandy and ammonia.*

The morbid appearances are the same as in poisoning with the pure acid. In Mertzdorff's case the whole blood and body emitted a smell of almonds ; putrefaction had begun, though the inspection was made twenty-nine hours after death; the blood throughout was fluid, and flowed from the nostrils and mouth ; the veins were every where turgid ; the cerebral vessels gorged ; the stomach and intestines very red. — In the case from the Medical and Physical Journal of poisoning with the almond itself, the vessels of the brain were much gorged, and the eyes glistening and staring as if the person had been alive.

Of the Cherry-Laurel.

The cherry-laurel, or *Cerasus lauro-cerasus*, was at one time much used for flavouring liqueurs and sweetmeats. But it is now less employed than formerly, as fatal accidents have happened from its having been used in too large quantity. The custom, however, has not been altogether abandoned; for there is an account in an English newspaper in 1823 of two persons killed by ratifia'd brandy, which had been flavoured with this plant ; and Dr. Paris has mentioned an instance of several children at an English boarding-school having been dangerously affected by a custard flavoured with the leaves.†
Almost every part of the plant is poisonous, especially the leaves and kernels ; but the pulp of the cherry is not. The flower has a totally different odour from the leaves. The healthy vigorous shoots in the early part of summer, and the inner bark, both then and in autumn, smell strongly of the bitter almond when broken across. The kernels of the seeds have a strong taste of bitter almonds. — The plant yields a distilled water and an essential oil, which Robiquet found to have all the chemical properties of the oil of bitter almond.‡ — A very peculiar source of danger in using the leaves of this plant, for imparting a ratafia flavour to sweetmeats and liqueurs, is that the proportion of oil varies excessively according to the age of the leaf. It abounds most in the young undeveloped leaves, and diminishes gradually afterwards. Hence, the leaves being evergreen and outliving more than two summers, the young leaves in May or June contain, as I have found, nearly ten times as much oil as the old ones at the same moment.

Cherry-laurel oil, according to Schrader, contains 7·66 per cent. of hydrocyanic acid;§ but according to Göppert, a specimen supposed

* Journal de Chimie Médicale, 1840, 92.
† Medical Jurisprudence, ii. 402.   ‡ Journal de Pharmacie, viii. 304
§ Buchner's Repertorium, xii. 130.

to be genuine gave only 2·75 per cent.* It is probably therefore a weaker poison than the oil of bitter almond. The latest experiments made with this oil are those of some Florentine physicians, performed at the laboratory of the Marquess Rodolphi, and described by Professor Taddei.† Sixteen drops put on the tongue of rabbits killed them in nine, fifteen, or twenty minutes; and ten or twelve drops injected in oil into the anus killed them in four minutes. The symptoms were slow breathing, palsy of the hind-legs, then general convulsions; and death was preceded by complete coma. A very extraordinary appearance was found in the dead body, — blood extravasated abundantly in the trachea and lungs.

The cherry-laurel water, prepared by distillation from the leaves of this plant, was long the most important of the poisons which contain the hydrocyanic acid, as it was the most common before the introduction of the acid itself into medical practice. Water dissolves by agitation 3·25 grains of oil per ounce; which may be considered the proportion in a saturated distilled water. The water contains, according to Schubarth, only 0·25 per cent. of hydrocyanic acid;‡ according to Schrader§ only half as much; and by long keeping even that small proportion will gradually disappear, as I have ascertained by experiment. Hence its strength must vary greatly, — a fact which will explain the very different effects of the same dose in different instances.

From experiments on animals by a great number of observers, it appears that, whether it is introduced into the stomach, or into the anus, or into the cellular tissue, or directly into a vein, it occasions giddiness, palsy, insensibility, convulsions, coma, and speedy death; — that the tetanic state brought on by the pure acid, is not always so distinctly caused by cherry-laurel water; — and that tetanus is most frequently induced by medium doses.

The attention of physicians was first called to this poison by an account, published by Dr. Madden in the Philosophical Transactions for 1737, of several accidents which occurred at Dublin in consequence of strong ratifia'd brandy having been prepared with it. Foderé has also given an account of two cases, caused by servants having stolen and drunk a bottle of it, which they mistook for a cordial.‖ Being afraid of detection, they swallowed it quickly, and in a few minutes expired in convulsions. Murray has noticed several others in his Apparatus Medicaminum.¶ In most of these cases the individuals suddenly lost their speech, fell down insensible, and died in a few minutes. Convulsions do not appear to have been frequent. Coullon has also related an instance where a child seems to have been killed by the leaves applied to a large sore on the neck.**

* Rust's Magazin für die gesammte Heilk. xxxii. 497.

† Bericht über einige Versuche über die Wirkung des Oleum Essentiale Laurocerasi. — Hufeland's Journal der Praktischen Heilkunde, liv. iii. 27.

‡ Bemerkungen, &c. Journal der Praktischen Heilkunde, li. i. 125.

§ Fechner's Repertorium der Org. Chemie, ii. 65.

‖ Médecine Légale, iv. 27.

¶ Apparatus Medicaminum, iii. 216.   ** Recherches, &c. p. 95.

The dose required to occasion these effects, and more especially to prove fatal, has not been determined with care. It must vary with the age of the sample used. It will vary also according as the water has been filtered or not; for what is not filtered often presents undissolved oil suspended in it or floating on its surface. One ounce has proved fatal;[*] and half an ounce has caused only temporary giddiness, loss of power over the limbs, stupor, and sense of pressure in the stomach.[†]

The appearances found in the dead body have varied. In general the blood has been fluid. The smell of bitter almond has commonly been distinct in the stomach.

The cherry-laurel water has attracted much attention in this country, in consequence of being the poison used by Captain Donnellan for the murder of Sir Theodosius Boughton. The trial of Donnellan, the most important trial for poisoning which ever took place in Britain, has given rise to some discrepance of opinion both among barristers and medical men, as to the sufficiency of the evidence by which the prisoner was condemned.[‡] For my part, taking into account the general, as well as medical circumstances of the case, I do not entertain a doubt of his guilt.

Leaving the general evidence out of view, however, as foreign to the objects of the medical jurist's regard, it must be admitted that the medical evidence, taken by itself, was defective. It may be summed up shortly in the following terms: — Sir Theodosius was a young man of the age of twenty, and in perfect health, except that he had a slight venereal complaint of old standing, for which he occasionally took a laxative draught. On the morning of his death, his mother, Lady Boughton, remarked, while giving him his draught, that it had a strong smell of bitter almonds. Two minutes after he took it, she observed a rattling or gurgling in his stomach; in ten minutes more he seemed inclined to doze; and five minutes afterwards she found him quite insensible, with the eyes fixed upwards, the teeth locked, froth running out of his mouth, and a great heaving at his stomach and gurgling in his throat. He died within half an hour after swallowing the draught. The body was examined ten days after death, and the inspectors found great congestion of the veins every where, gorging of the lungs, and redness of the stomach. But the examination was unskilfully conducted. For the head was not opened; the fæces were allowed to rush from the intestines into the stomach; and, as a great quantity of fluid blood was found in each cavity of the chest, the subclavian veins must have been divided during the separation of the clavicles. Very little reliance, therefore, can be placed in the evidence from the inspection of the body.[§]

* Philosophical Transactions, 1739, No. 452.
† Wibmer, die Wirkung der Arzneimittel und Gifte, ii. 90.
‡ Considerations on the criminal proceedings of this country, on the danger of convictions on circumstantial evidence, and on the case of Mr. Donnellan. By a Barrister of the Inner Temple, 1781. — Phillips's Treatise on the Law of Evidence, Appendix, p. 30. — Male's Juridical Medicine, p. 86. — These authorities all consider the guilt of the prisoner doubtful.
§ Trial, &c. taken in short hand by Gurney.

On comparing these particulars with what has been said above regarding the effects of hydrocyanic acid and this whole genus of poisons, it will be seen that every circumstance coincides precisely with the supposition of poisoning with the cherry-laurel water. The symptoms were exactly the same as in Mertzdoff's case of poisoning with the essential oil of almonds (p. 604). When to this are added, the smell of the draught, which Lady Boughton could hardly mistake, the rarity of apoplexy in so young and healthy a person as Sir Theodosius, and the improbability of either that or any other disease of the head proving fatal so quickly, — the conclusion at which, in my opinion, every sound medical jurist must arrive is, that poisoning in the way supposed was very probable. But I cannot go along with those who think that it was certain ; nor is it possible to see on what grounds such an opinion can be founded, when the general or moral circumstances are excluded.

The medical evidence in Donnellan's case has been much canvassed, and especially that of Mr. John Hunter. It would be foreign to the plan hitherto pursued in this work to analyze and review what was said by him and his brethren. But I must frankly observe, that Mr. Hunter's evidence does him very little credit, and that his high professional eminence is the reverse of a reason for palliating his errors, or treating them with the lenity which they have experienced from his numerous critics.

Of the Peach, Cluster-Cherry, Mountain-Ash, &c.

Little need be said of the other plants formerly mentioned among those which yield hydrocyanic acid, and act on the system in consequence of containing that substance.

The *Amygdalus persica* or peach is the most active of them. Most parts of the plant exhale the odour of the bitter-almond, but particularly the flowers and kernels. According to the chemical researches of M. Gauthier, the fresh young shoots of the peach collected in July contain, weight for weight, even more essential oil than the bitter almond, or cherry-laurel leaves ; for 250 grains yielded nearly five grains of it or two per cent. ; and he found the oil may be easily procured by distilling the shoots without addition till the product begins to pass over clear.* The kernels of the peach, when distilled with water, yield nearly one grain of hydrocyanic acid per ounce.†

Coullon has collected two instances of poisoning with the peach-blossom. One is the case of an elderly gentleman, who swallowed a sallad of the flower to purge himself. Soon afterwards he was seized with giddiness, violent purging, convulsions, and stupor ; and he died in three days. Here the poison must have proved fatal by inducing true apoplexy in a predisposed habit ; at least poisoning with hydrocyanic acid never lasts nearly so long. The other, a child eighteen months old, after taking a decoction of the flowers to destroy worms, perished with frightful convulsions, efforts to vomit, and

* Buchner's Repertorium für die Pharmacie, xxviii. 416.
† Geiseler in Repertorium für die Pharmacie, lxix. 291.

bloody diarrhœa.* The peach-blossom would therefore appear to be rather a narcotico-acrid, than a narcotic. — Peach-leaves are represented to have produced even purely irritant effects. A man, who took a decoction of a handful boiled in a quart of water down to a third, — when of course no hydrocyanic acid could remain, — was attacked with tightness in the chest, a sense of suffocation, violent colic, pain in the stomach and frequent desire to vomit, followed by a hard pulse, restlessness, and flushing of the face. But he recovered slowly under the use of fomentations and opiates.†

The bark of the *Prunus padus*, or cluster-cherry, a native of this country, owes its poisonous qualities to the same substance as the preceding plants. Heumann found that the distilled water obtained from two ounces of bark in March contains two grains of acid, two ounces of developed leaves half a grain, and two ounces of the seed a trifle less.‡ Its distilled water has the odour of bitter almonds, contains the same essential oil with that of the bitter almond, and yields more hydrocyanic acid than the cherry-laurel water.§ The oil, according to Schrader, contains 9·25‖ per cent. of hydrocyanic acid, according to Göppert only 5·5 per cent.¶ Bremer, who has examined this plant with great care, found that both the distilled water and the essential oil kill mice when put into the mouth, eye, nose, ear, anus, or a wound ; and that half an ounce of the water killed a dog in twelve minutes.** The fruit is also poisonous. It has a nauseous taste, but communicates a pleasant flavour to spirituous liquors. The kernels yield by expression a transparent, fixed oil, concrete at 41° F., which contains a small quantity of the essential oil ; and the cake which is left yields so much of the latter, that, as we are informed by M. Chancel of Briançon, a handful has proved fatal to cows in a short time.†† In these kernels, as in the bitter almond, the essential oil does not exist ready formed, but is developed only in consequence of the contact of water ; and hence, if the fixed oil by expression contains a little of it, as Chancel says, this must arise from the kernels having been moist when squeezed.

The *Sorbus aucuparia*, mountain-ash, or Rowan-tree as it is called in Scotland, has been lately added to the list of plants which abound in the same poisonous principle. M. Grassmann of St Petersburgh has found that many parts of this tree, such as the flowers and the bark of the trunk and branches, contain more or less of the peculiar essential oil; and that the root in particular contains so much in the month of May as to smell strongly of it when broken across, and to yield a distilled water which holds fully as much hydrocyanic acid as that procured from an equal weight of cherry-laurel leaves.‡‡

* Recherches, &c. p. 74.   † Journal de Chimie Médicale, 1837, 99.
‡ Repertorium für die Pharmacie, lxxv. 220.
§ Bremer, Bermerkungen und Erfahrungen über die Wirksamkeit des Trauben-Kirsch-baums. — Archiv für Medizinische Erfahrung, 1812, i. 41.
‖ Buchner's, Repertorium, xii. 130.   ¶ Rust's Magazin, xxxii. 500.
** Bemerkungen, &c. Horn's Archiv, 1812, i. 71.
†† Journal de Pharmacie, iii. 275.
‡‡ Buchner's Repertorium für die Pharmacie, xxvii. 238.

Several other plants of the same natural order possess similar though weaker properties, such as the *Prunus avium*, or black-cherry, or mazzard, the *Prunus insititia*, or bullace, the *Prunus spinosa*, or sloe, the *Amygdalus nana*, or dwarf-almond, and even the leaves and kernels of the common cherry, the *Cerasus communis*. Twelve ounces of cherry kernels distilled with water, yield, according to Geiseler, seven grains of hydrocyanic acid.* I have no doubt, from my experiments, that the seeds of *Pyrus malus*, the apple, *Pyrus aria*, the white-beam, and also, if the taste may be taken for a criterion, the whole seeds of the *Pomaceæ*, yield by distillation with water a large quantity of hydrocyanic acid.

CHAPTER XXX.

OF POISONING WITH CARBAZOTIC ACID.

A substance long known to chemists by the name of indigo-bitter, which is procured by the action of nitric acid on indigo, silk, and other azotized substances, and which has been found to consist chiefly of a peculiar acid, termed by Liebig, from its composition, the carbazotic acid, appears to be a pure narcotic poison of considerable activity.† It is in the form of shining crystals, of an excessively bitter taste, and of a yellow colour so singularly intense that it imparts a perceptible tint to a million parts of water. The pure crystals are composed of carbon, azote, and oxygen.

The only account I have seen of the physiological properties of this substance is a full analysis by Buchner in his Toxicology, of some interesting experiments by Professor Rapp of Tübingen.‡ He found that sixteen grains in solution, when introduced into the stomach, killed a fox, ten grains a dog, and five grains a rabbit, in an hour and a half; that the injection of a watery solution into the windpipe occasioned death in a few minutes; that the introduction of it into the cavity of the pleura or peritonæum occasioned death in several hours; that a watery solution of ten grains injected into the jugular vein of a fox killed it instantaneously, and in like manner five grains affected a dog in three minutes and killed it in twenty-four hours; and that thirty grains applied to a wound killed a rabbit. The symptoms remarked from its introduction into the stomach of the fox were in half an hour tremors, grinding of the teeth, constant contortion of the eyes and convulsions, in an hour complete insensibility, and death in half an hour more. In the dog there was also remarked an attack of vomiting and feebleness of the pulse.

In the dead body no particular alteration of structure was remarked. The heart, examined immediately after death from the introduction of the poison into the stomach, was found much gorged and motionless;

---

* Buchner's Repertorium für die Pharmacie, lxix. 293.
† Annales de Chim. et de Phys. xxxv. 72.   ‡ Toxikologie, 373.

but the irritability of the voluntary muscles remained. The stomach was not inflamed, but dyed yellow. A very interesting appearance was dyeing of various textures and fluids throughout the body. In the fox killed by swallowing sixteen grains the conjunctiva of the eyes, the aqueous humour, the capsule of the lens, the membranes of the arteries, in a less degree those of the veins, the lungs, and in many places the cellular tissue, had acquired a lemon-yellow colour. The dog killed in the same manner presented similar appearances, also those killed by injection of the poison into the pleura or peritonæum ; and in the latter animals the urine was tinged yellow. In a rabbit killed by the application of the poison to a wound the same discoloration was also every where remarked, together with yellowness of the fibrin of the blood. But no yellowness could be seen any where in the dog, which died in twenty-four hours after receiving five grains into the jugular vein. In no instance was there any yellow tint perceptible in the brain or spinal cord.

These facts form an interesting addition to the physiology of poisons. They supply unequivocal proof that this substance is absorbed in the course of its operation, and furnish strong presumption that other poisons, which act on organs remote from the place where they are applied, and which have been sought for without success in the blood, as well as in other fluids and solids throughout the body, have not been detected, merely because the physiologist does not possess such simple and extremely delicate means of searching for them.

The researches of Professor Rapp have been arranged under the title of carbazotic acid, because this acid forms the most prominent substance in the matter with which his experiments appear to have been made. But it is right to state, that the article actually used was, if I understand correctly the abstract given by Buchner, not the pure crystals, but the yellow fluid, from which the crystals are procured, and which contains also a resinous matter and artificial tannin. — The bitter principle of Welther produced by the action of nitric acid on silk, and that formed by Braconnot by the action of the same acid on aloes, appear to be impure carbazotic acid.

CHAPTER XXXI.

OF THE POISONOUS GASES.

THE subject of the poisonous gases is one of great importance in relation to medical police, as well as medical jurisprudence. They are objects of interest to the medical jurist, because their effects may be mistaken for those of criminal violence, and because they have even been resorted to for committing suicide. They are interesting as a topic of medical police, since some trades expose the workmen to their influence.

It has hitherto been chiefly on the continent that use has been made of the deleterious gases for the purpose of self-destruction.

Osiander mentions, that Lebrun, a famous player on the horn, suffocated himself at Paris in 1809 with the fumes of sulphur ; and that an apothecary at Pyrmont killed himself by going into the *Grotto del Cane* there, which, like that near Naples, is filled with carbonic acid gas.* Many instances have lately occurred in France of suicide caused by the emanations from burning charcoal in a close chamber.

But these poisons come under the notice of the medical jurist chiefly because their effects may be mistaken for those of other kinds of violent death. Several mistakes of this nature are on record. Zacchias mentions the case of a man, who was found dead in prison under circumstances which led to the suspicion, that he had been privately strangled by the governor. But Zacchias proved this to be impossible, and ascribed death to the fumes from a choffer of burning charcoal left in the room.† A more striking instance of the kind occurred a few years ago at London. A woman, who inhabited a room with other five people, alarmed the neighbours one morning with the intelligence that all her fellow-lodgers were dead. On entering the room they found two men and two women actually dead, and another man quite insensible and apparently dying. This man, however, recovered ; and as it was said that he was too intimate with the woman who gave the alarm, a report was spread that she had poisoned the rest, to get rid of the man's wife, one of the sufferers. She was accordingly put in prison, various articles in the house were carefully analysed for poison, and an account of the supposed barbarous murder was hawked about the streets. At last the man who recovered remembered having put a choffer of coals between the two beds, which held the whole six people ; and the chamber having no vent, they had thus been all suffocated.‡ — The following is a similar accident not less remarkable in its circumstances. Four people in *Gerolzhofen* in Bavaria, were found one morning in bed, some dead, others comatose ; and only one recovered. A neighbour who had supped with them, but slept at home, did not suffer. The stomach and intestines were found very red and black ; and the coats of the stomach brittle. The contents of the stomach, the remains of their supper, and the wine were analysed without any suspicious substance being found. A little smoke having been noticed in the room by those who first entered it, the stove and fuel were examined, but without furnishing any insight into the cause of the accident. At last the cellar was examined, and then it was found that one of the sufferers had heated a copper vessel there so incautiously, that the fire communicated with the unplastered planks of the floor above. The planks had burnt with a low smothered flame, and the vapours passed through the crevices in the floor.§

What Irrespirable Gases are Poisonous?

Some gases act negatively on the animal system by preventing the

---

* Ueber den Selbstmord, p. 176.
† Quæstionum Medico-legalium, T. iii. 63. Consilium 44.
‡ London Courier, Jan. 16, 1823.   § Buchner's Toxikologie, 331.

access of respirable air to the lungs ; others are positively poisonous. The first point, therefore, is to ascertain which are negatively, and which positively hurtful.

M. Nysten, who has made the most connected train of experiments on this subject, conceived that a gas will not act through any other channel besides the lungs, if it exerts merely a negative action : — and that, on the contrary, it certainly possesses a direct and positive power, if it has nearly the same effects, in whatever way it is introduced into the body.* He therefore thought the best way to ascertain the action of the gases would be, to inject them into the blood, — conceiving that, after allowance is made for the mere mechanical effects of an aëriform body, the phenomena would point out the true operation of each.

His first object then was to learn what phenomena are caused by the mechanical action of atmospheric air. He found that four cubic inches and a half, injected into the jugular vein of a dog, killed it immediately amidst tetanic convulsions, by distending the heart with frothy blood ; — that a larger quantity introduced gradually caused more lingering death, with symptoms of oppressed breathing, which arose from gorging of the lungs with frothy blood ; — and that a small quantity, injected into the carotid artery towards the brain, occasioned speedy death by apoplexy, which arose from the brain being deprived by means of the air of a due supply of its proper stimulus, the blood. Numerous experimental inquiries have been since made on this subject, the latest of which, those of Dr. Cormack, coincide with the first results of Nysten, that air injected into the veins causes death by arrestment of the action of the heart.†

Proceeding with these data, Nysten found that *oxygen* and *azote* had the same effect when apart, as when united in the form of atmospheric air ; that *carburetted hydrogen, hydrogen, carbonic oxide*, and *phosphuretted hydrogen* likewise seemed to act in the same way ; and that the *nitrous oxide*, or intoxicating gas, although it does not cause so much mechanical injury as the others, on account of its superior solubility in the blood, has the same effect when injected in sufficient quantity, and produces little or none of the symptoms of intoxication excited by it in man.‡ As to *carbonic acid gas*, he found that, on account of its great solubility in the blood, it is difficult to produce mechanical injury with it ; that sixty-four cubic inches are absorbed, and do not excite any particular symptoms ; but that when injected into the carotid artery, it occasions death by apoplexy, although it is rapidly absorbed by the blood.§

The other gases he tried were hydrosulphuric acid, nitric oxide, ammonia and chlorine ; and all of these proved to be positively and highly deleterious.

Two or three cubic inches of *hydrosulphuric acid gas* caused tetanus

* Nysten, Recherches Chimico-Physiologiques, p. 11.
† On the Presence of Air in the Organs of Circulation. Prize Thesis at Edinburgh, 1837.
‡ Nysten, Recherches Chimico-Physiologiques, *passim.*   § Ibidem, p. 81.

and immediate death, when injected into the veins, although the gas was at once absorbed by the blood. The same quantity acted with almost equal rapidity when injected into the cavity of the chest. Similar results were obtained when it was injected into the cellular tissue, or even when it was left for some time in contact with the sound skin.[*] The last important fact has been since confirmed by Lebküchner in his Thesis on the permeability of the tissues ;[†] and it had previously been observed also by the late Professor Chaussier, whose experiments will be mentioned presently (p. 617). In none of Nysten's experiments with this gas was the blood changed in appearance.

Nitric oxide gas, according to Nysten, is the most energetic of all the poisonous gases. A very small quantity causes death by tetanus, when introduced into a vein, the cavity of the chest, or the cellular tissue ; and it always changes the state of the blood, giving it a chocolate-brown colour, and preventing its coagulation. In one of Nysten's experiments a cubic inch and three-quarters injected into the chest killed a little dog in 45 minutes.[‡] Dr. John Davy appears to have found this gas not so active.[§]

Nysten found the two other gases, *ammonia* and *chlorine*, to be acrid in their action. When injected into the veins they kill by over-stimulating the heart; and when injected into the cavity of the chest, they excite inflammation in the lining membrane.[||] Hébréart farther remarked in his experiments relative to the action of irritants on the windpipe, that chlorine when inspired, produces violent inflammation in the windpipe and its great branches, ending in the secretion of a pseudo-membrane like that of croup ;[¶] and that a very small quantity of ammonia has the same effect.

From this abstract of Nysten's researches, it appears to follow, that ammonia and chlorine are irritants ; hydrosulphuric acid and nitric oxide, narcotics; oxygen, azote, hydrogen, carburetted hydrogen, phosphuretted hydrogen, carbonic oxide, and nitrous oxide, negative poisons ; and carbonic acid, doubtful in its nature. Some of these conclusions do not correspond with the effects observed in man ; which will presently be found to lead to the inference, that not only carbonic acid, but likewise carbonic oxide, nitrous oxide, and carburetted hydrogen are narcotics. The reason Nysten did not find these gases injurious was probably, that, before they could pass from the vein into which they were injected, to the brain on which they act, they were in a great measure exhaled from the lungs. The experiments of physiologists since Nysten's time likewise tend to show that oxygen gas is a positive poison when pure, and that even hydrogen possesses active properties. The inquiries of Mr. Broughton led him to consider hydrogen a positive poison, because animals die in it in half a minute, and the heart immediately after death is found

---

[*] Rech. Chemico-Physiologiques, p. 114.

[†] Diss. Inaug. utrum, per viventium adhuc animalium membranas materiæ ponderabiles permeare queant. Tubingæ, p. 10.

[‡] Nysten, Recherches, &c. p. 137.   [§] Philosophical Transactions, cxiii. 508.

[||] Nysten, Recherches, &c. p. 140.   [¶] Corvisart's Journal de Méd. xxiv. 249.

to have lost its contractility. Previous experimentalists had also remarked hypnotic effects from the inhalation of it diluted with oxygen.[*] As to oxygen, the same physiologist ascertained that when pure, it is a narcotic poison, though a feeble one, as at least five hours of continuous respiration in the pure gas are required to prove fatal.[†]

Of the Effects of the Poisonous Gases on Man.

According to the effects of the poisonous gases on man, they may be arranged in two groups, the first including the *irritants*, the second the *narcotics*. It might have been therefore a more philosophical mode of arrangement, if the former had been considered under the irritant class of poisons ; but it is more convenient to examine the whole deleterious gases together.

The *irritant gases* are nitric oxide gas and nitrous acid vapour, hydrochloric acid gas, chlorine, ammonia, sulphurous acid, and some others of little consequence.

Of Nitric oxide gas and Nitrous acid vapour. — Before nitric oxide gas can be breathed in ordinary circumstances, it is transformed by the oxygen of the air into nitrous acid vapour, of a ruddy colour and irritating odour. Hébréart found that in animals killed by inhaling it the windpipe was much inflamed.[‡] Sir H. Davy tried to inhale it, and with this view took the precaution of previously breathing the nitrous oxide or intoxicating gas, in order to expel the atmospheric air as much as possible from his lungs. But he found that the small quantity of nitrous acid fumes formed with the remaining air was sufficient to cause a sense of burning in the throat, and at once stimulated the glottis to contract, so that none of the nitric oxide gas could pass into the larynx. The subsequent entrance of the external air into the mouth, which Sir Humphrey unluckily had not provided for, was of course attended by the immediate formation of more acid fumes, by which his tongue, cheeks, and gums, were irritated and inflamed ; and there is no doubt, as Sir Humphrey himself remarks, that if he had succeeded in inhaling the nitric oxide gas, the same chemical change would have happened in the lungs and excited pneumonia.[§]

The following cases will prove that nitrous acid vapour, disengaged from the fuming nitrous acid, is a very violent and dangerous poison when inhaled. A chemical manufacturer, in endeavouring to remove from his store-room a hamper in which some bottles of nitrous acid had burst, breathed the fumes for some time, and was seized in four hours with symptoms of inflammation in the throat and stomach. At night the urine was suppressed ; the skin then became blue ; at last he was seized with hiccup, acute pain in the diaphragm, con-

[*] Allen and Peys, also Wetterstedt. See Dr. Apjohn's article on Toxicology in Cycl. of Pract. Med. iv. 238.
[†] London Quarterly Journal of Science, vi. N. S.
[‡] Corvisart's Journal de Méd. xxiv. 246.
[||] Researches, Chemical and Philosophical, concerning nitrous oxide gas, p. 475.

vulsions, and delirium ; and he died twenty-seven hours after the accident.* Another case has been described in the Bulletins of the Medical Society of Emulation. It proved fatal in two days, and the symptoms were those of violent pneumonia. In this instance there was pneumonia of one side, and pleurisy of the other ; the uvula and throat were gangrenous, and the windpipe and air-tubes dark-red ; the veins throughout the whole body were much congested, the skin very livid in many places, and the blood fluid in the heart, but coagulated in the vessels.† Dr. Reitz, a writer in Henke's Journal, met with two cases of death from the same cause in hatters. They had incautiously exposed themselves too much to the fumes, which are disengaged during the preparation of nitrate of mercury for the operation of felting, and which are well known to be nitric oxide gas converted into nitrous acid vapour by contact with the air. Two men died of inflammation of the lungs excited in that manner ; and a third, a boy of fourteen, after sleeping all night in an apartment where the mixture was effervescing, was attacked in the morning with yellowness of the skin, giddiness, and colic, which ended fatally in six days.‡

Of Poisoning with Chlorine. — The experiments of Nysten and Hébréart with chlorine, and its well-known irritating effects when inhaled in the minutest quantities, show that it will produce inflammation of the lungs and air-passages. The following is the only instance of poisoning with it in man which has come under my notice. A young man, after breathing diluted chlorine as an experiment, was instantly seized with violent irritation in the epiglottis, windpipe, and bronchial branches, cough, tightness, and sense of pressure in the chest, inability to swallow, great difficulty in breathing or articulating, discharge of mucus from the mouth and nostrils, severe sneezing, swelling of the face, and protrusion of the eyes. Ammonia was of no use ; but singular relief was obtained from the inhalation of a little sulphuretted hydrogen, so that in an hour and a half he was tolerably well.§

Although this gas is very irritating to an unaccustomed person, yet by the force of habit one may breathe with impunity an atmosphere much loaded with it. I have been told by a chemical manufacturer at Belfast, that his men can work in an atmosphere of chlorine, where he himself could not remain above a few minutes. The chief consequences of habitual exposure are acidity and other stomach complaints, which the men generally correct by taking chalk. He has likewise observed that they never become corpulent, and that corpulent men who become workmen are soon reduced to an ordinary size. It is not probable, however, that the trade is an unhealthy one ; for several of this gentleman's workmen have lived to an advanced age ; one man, who died not long ago at the age of eighty,

* Desgranges in Corvisart's Journal de Méd. viii. 487.
† Bulletins de la Soc. Méd. d'Emulation, Oct. 1823.
‡ Zeitschrift für die Staatsarzneikunde, xvii. 383.
§ Wibmer. Die Wirkung der Arzneimittel und Gifte, ii. 109, from Archiv des Apothekers-Vereins, xviii. 101.

had been forty years in the manufactory; and I have seen in Mr. Tenant's manufactory at Glasgow a healthy-looking man who had been also about forty years a workman there. It is an interesting fact, that during the epidemic fever which raged over Ireland from 1816 to 1819, the people at the manufactory at Belfast were exempt from it.

Of Poisoning with Ammonia. — For an account of the effects of *ammonia*, which, when in the state of gas, acts violently as an irritant on the mouth, windpipe, and lungs, the reader is referred to the chapter on ammonia and its salts in page 193. It appears to form one of the gases disengaged from the soil of necessaries, as will be noticed presently, and excites inflammation in the eyes of workmen who are incautiously exposed to it.[*]

Of Poisoning with Hydrochloric Acid Gas. — I have not met with any account of the effects of *hydrochloric acid gas* on man. But no doubt can be entertained that it will likewise act as a violent and pure irritant.

It is exceedingly hurtful to vegetable life. In the course of some experiments performed in 1827 by Dr. Turner and myself on the effects of various gases on plants, we found that a tenth of a cubic inch diluted with 20,000 times its volume of air, so as to be quite imperceptible to the nostrils, shrivelled and killed all the leaves of various plants, which were exposed to it for twenty-four hours.[†] These experiments were repeated in 1832 by Messrs. Rogerson, apparently in ignorance of them. Their results are on the whole the same; and the slighter effect obtained by them from minute proportions of the gas was evidently owing to the small size of their glass-jars not allowing them to use a sufficient quantity of it.[‡] They farther found that proportions of hydrochloric acid gas, amounting to a twentieth of the air, kill small animals in half an hour with symptoms of obstructed respiration. Their experiments with less proportions are not precise, yet warrant the inference that even a thousandth part of the gas will probably prove fatal in no long time.[§]

Of Poisoning with Hydrosulphuric Acid Gas. — The *narcotic gases* are of much greater importance than the irritants, on account of the singularity of their effects, and the greater frequency of accidents with them. This group includes hydrosulphuric acid, carburetted-hydrogen, carbonic acid, carbonic oxide, nitrous oxide, cyanogen, and oxygen.

Hydrosulphuric acid gas is probably the most deleterious of all the gases. According to Thenard and Dupuytren, air containing only an 800th of it will kill small birds in a few seconds; and a 290th is sufficient to kill a dog; which, however, will sustain so much as a 400th.[‖] Chaussier previously found, that a horse was killed by breathing atmospheric air which contained a 250th of hydrosulphuric

[*] Hallé, Recherches sur la nature du Méphitisme des fosses d'aisance, p. 137.
[†] Edin. Med. and Surg. Journal, xxviii. 361.
[‡] London Medical Gazette, x. 314.   [§] Ibidem, 352.
[‖] Dictionnaire des Sciences Médicales, ii. 391.

acid gas ; and that it acts with energy on animals, whether it be inhaled, or injected into the stomach, anus, or cellular tissue, or even
simply applied to the skin.   Nine quarts of the gas injected into the
anus of a horse killed it in one minute ; and a rabbit, whose skin
alone was exposed to it, died in ten minutes.*   Ulterior inquiries by
MM. Parent-Duchâtelet and Gaultier de Claubry, — scarcely so precise however as those of their predecessors, — appear to lead to the
conclusion, that its energy is in some circumstances not so great.
While superintending the clearing out of some of the choked drains
of Paris, they found that the workmen suffered no harm, though they
habitually breathed an atmosphere containing from 25 to 80 ten-
thousandths of hydrosulphuric acid gas, and on some occasions even
so much as one per cent. ; nay, on one occasion Gaultier remained
several minutes without injury, collecting air for chemical analysis
in an atmosphere, which proved to be loaded with three per cent. of
the gas.†   None of these researches point out the precise manner of
death.   Dr. Percy of Nottingham informs me he found in 1839,
that dogs, which breathed air, containing this gas, quickly died in
convulsions like those caused by hydrocyanic acid ; that in some
instances the heart's action was observed to have ceased, when
the body was opened immediately after death ; but that in general
it either continued to beat for some time, or could be made to do so
when its state of congestion was relieved by withdrawing a little
blood.

Dr. Turner and I found that hydrosulphuric acid gas is very injurious to vegetables, and that it acts differently from muriatic acid
gas, as it appeared to exhaust the vitality of plants and to cause in
them a state analogous to narcotic poisoning in animals.   Four cubic
inches and a half, diluted with eighty volumes of air, caused drooping of the leaves of a mignonette plant in twenty-four hours; and
the plant, though then removed into the open air, continued to droop
till it bent over altogether and died.‡

The best description of the effects of this gas on man has been
given by M. Hallé,§ in his account of the nature and effects of the
exhalations from the pits of the Parisian necessaries ; which exhalations appear, from the experiments of Thenard and Dupuytren, to
be mixtures chiefly of ammonia and sulphuretted-hydrogen.   The
symptoms, in cases where the vapours are breathed in a state of concentration, are sudden weakness and all the signs of ordinary asphyxia.
The individual becomes suddenly weak and insensible ; falls down ;
and either expires immediately, or, if he is fortunate enough to be
quickly extricated, he may revive in no long time, the belly remaining tense and full for an hour or upwards, and recovery being
preceded by vomiting and hawking of bloody froth.‖   When the

* Sedillot's Journal de Médecine, xv. 28, 34.
† Annales d'Hygiène Publique, 1829, ii. 83, 143.
‡ Edin. Med. and Surg. Journal, xxviii. 361.
§ Recherches sur la nature du Mephitisme des fosses d'aisance, 1785.
‖ Recherches, &c. p. 55.

noxious emanations are less concentrated, several affections have been noticed, which may be reduced to two varieties, the one consisting of pure coma, the other of coma and tetanic convulsions. In the comatose form, the workman seems to fall gently asleep while at work, is roused with difficulty, and has no recollection afterwards of what passed before the accident. The convulsive form is sometimes preceded by noisy and restless delirium, sometimes by sudden faintness, heaving or pain in the stomach, and pains in the arms, and almost always by difficult breathing, from weakness in the muscles of the chest. Insensibility, and a state resembling asphyxia rapidly succeed, during which the pupil is fixed and dilated, the mouth filled with white or bloody froth, the skin cold, and the pulse feeble and irregular. At last convulsive efforts to breathe ensue ; these are followed by general tetanic spasms of the trunk and extremities ; and if the case is to prove fatal, which it may not do for two hours, a state of calm and total insensibility precedes death for a short interval.* When the exposure has been too slight to cause serious mischief, the individual is affected with sickness, colic, imperfectly defined pains in the chest, and lethargy.†

The appearances in the bodies of persons killed by these emanations are fluidity and blackness of the blood, a dark tint of all the internal vascular organs, annihilation of the contractility of the muscles, more or less redness of the bronchial tubes, and secretion of brown mucus there as well as in the nostrils, gorging of the lungs, an odour throughout the whole viscera like that of decayed fish, and a tendency to early putrefaction.‡ Chaussier in his experiments also remarked in animals, that when a plate of silver or bit of white lead was thrust under the skin it was blackened.§ Dr. Percy could not detect the gas in the brain of animals killed by inhaling it.

These extraordinary accidents may be occasioned not only by exposure to the vapours from the *fosses*, but likewise by the incautious inhalation of the vapours proceeding from the bodies of persons who have been asphyxiated there. Sickness, colic, and pains in the chest, are often caused in the latter mode ; and Hallé has even given an instance of the most violent form of the convulsive affection having originated in the same manner.‖

In order that the reader may comprehend the exact cause of these accidents, — as it is not easy for an Englishman to comprehend how suffocation may arise from the fumes of a privy, — it may be necessary to explain, that in Paris the pipe of the privy terminates under ground in a pit, which is usually contained in a small covered vault, or is at the bottom of a small square tower open at the roof of the house ; and that the pit is often several feet long, wide and deep. Here the filth is sometimes allowed to accumulate for a great length of time, till the pit is full ; and it is in the process of clearing it out that the workmen are liable to suffer. Hallé has given an interest-

* Recherches, &c. pp. 57, 99, 144 ; and Nouv. Journ. de Méd. i. 237.
† Nouv. Journal, &c. ‡ Ibidem
§ Sedillot's Journ. de M'd. xv. 25. ‖ Recherches, &c. p. 57.

ing narrative of an attempt made to empty one of these pits in presence of the Duc. de Rochefoucault, the Abbé Tessier, himself, and other members of the Academy of Sciences, who were appointed by the French government to examine into the merits of a pretended discovery for destroying the noxious vapours. The pit chosen was ten feet and a half long, six wide, and at least seven deep; and repeated attempts had been previously made without success to empty it. For some time the process went on prosperously; when at last one of the workmen dropped his bucket into the pit. A ladder being procured, he immediately proceeded to descend, and would not wait to be tied with ropes. " But hardly," says Hallé, " had he descended a few steps of the ladder, when he tumbled down without a cry, and was overwhelmed in the ordure below, without making the slightest effort to save himself. It was at first thought he had slipped his foot, and another workman promptly offered to descend for him. This man was secured with ropes in case of accident. But scarcely had he descended far enough to have his whole person in the pit except his head, when he uttered a suppressed cry, made a violent effort with his chest, slipped from the ladder, and ceased to move or breathe. His head hung down on his breast, the pulse was gone; and his complete state of asphyxia was the affair of a moment. Another workman, descending with the same precautions, fainted away in like manner, but was so promptly withdrawn that the asphyxia was not complete, and he soon revived. At last a stout young man, secured in the same way as the rest, also went down a few steps. Finding himself seized like his companions, he re-ascended to recover himself for a moment; and still not discouraged, he resolved to go down again, and descended backwards, keeping his face uppermost, so that he was able to search for his companion with a hook and withdraw the body." It was impossible to go on with the operation of clearing out; and the pit was shut up again. The first workman never showed any sign of life; the second recovered after discharging much bloody froth; all the persons in the vault were more or less affected; and a gentleman who, in trying to resuscitate the dead workman, incautiously breathed the exhalations from his mouth, was immediately and violently seized with the convulsive form of the affection.[*]

The same kind of accident has been observed at Paris in the vaults of cemeteries, owing to the same cause, — the disengagement of hydrosulphuric acid and hydrosulphate of ammonia during putrefaction. A remarkable instance is related by Guerard.[†] Analogous accidents have happened in this country in clearing out drains.

In none of the French investigations on this singular subject has any allusion been made to the question, whether the health sustains any injury from long-continued exposure to the gas in very minute proportion. It is probably injurious however. At one time, while in the practice of not using any precautions against inhaling the gas

[*] Hallé, Recherches, &c. p. 50.
[†] Annales d'Hygiène Publique, 1840, xxiii. 131.

in chemical researches, I used to remark that daily exposure to it in minute quantity caused in a few weeks an extraordinary lassitude, languor of the pulse, and defective appetite. Strohmeyer in the like circumstances was liable to severe headache. Mr. Taylor says that the workmen in the Thames Tunnel suffered severely for some time from a similar exposure. Many of them became affected with giddiness, sickness, general debility and emaciation, then with a low fever attended with delirium, and in the course of a few months several died. No cause could be discovered for their illness except the frequent escape of sulphuretted-hydrogen from the roof. The affection only disappeared, when the communication from bank to bank was completed, so that the tunnel could be thoroughly ventilated.*

The presence of hydrosulphuric acid in all such emanations is best proved by exposing to them a bit of filtering paper moistened with a solution of lead. The smell alone must not be relied on, as putrescent animal matter exhales an odour like that of hydrosulphuric acid, though none be present. Workmen ought to be aware that hydrosulphuric acid may be quickly fatal where lights burn with undiminished brilliancy; and that in places where it is apt to accumulate, the degree of purity of the air may vary so much in the course of working, as to be wholesome only a few minutes before, as well as a few minutes after a fatal accident.†

In the present place, some notice may be taken of an extraordinary accident, which happened in 1831 near London. Great doubts may be entertained whether hydrosulphuric acid was the cause of it; and while these exist, it is not possible to arrange it under a proper head. It is too important, however, in relation to Medical Jurisprudence, to be omitted in this work; and I take the opportunity of mentioning it here, as the accident was ascribed to hydrosulphuric acid by those who witnessed it.

In August, 1831, twenty-two boys living at a boarding-school at Clapham were seized in the course of three or four hours with alarming symptoms of violent irritation in the stomach and bowels, subsultus of the muscles of the arms, and excessive prostration of strength. Another had been similarly attacked three days before. This child died in twenty-five, and one of the others in 'twenty-three hours. On examination after death, the Peyerian glands of the intestines were found in the former case enlarged, and as it were tuberculated; in the other there were also ulcers of the mucous coat of the small intestines, and softening of that coat in the colon. A suspicion of accidental poisoning having naturally arisen, the various utensils and articles of food used by the family were examined but without success. And the only circumstance which appeared to explain the accident was, that two days before the first child took ill, a foul cess-pool had been opened, and the materials diffused over a garden adjoining to the children's play-ground. This was consi-

* Manual of Medical Jurisprudence, 1844, p. 559.
† Hallé, Recherches, &c. pp. 46, 58.

55*

dered a sufficient cause of the disease by Dr. Spurgin and Messrs.
Angus and Saunders of Clapham, as well as by Drs. Latham and
Chambers, and Mr. Pearson of London, who personally examined
the whole particulars.*   Their explanation may be the only rational
account that can be given of the matter.   But as no detail of their
chemical inquiries was ever published, their opinion cannot be received with confidence by the medical jurist and the physician;
since it is not supported, so far as I am aware by any previous account of the effects of hydrosulphuric acid gas.

Of Poisoning with Carburetted Hydrogen. — Of the several species of carburetted hydrogen gas it is probable that all are more or
less narcotic ; but they are much inferior in energy to sulphuretted
hydrogen.

Sir H. Davy found that when he breathed a mixture of two parts
of air and three of carburetted hydrogen, procured from the decomposition of water by red-hot charcoal, he was attacked with giddiness, headache, and transient weakness of the limbs.   When he
breathed it pure, the first inspiration caused a sense of numbness in
the muscles of the chest; the second caused an overpowering sense
of oppression in the breast, and insensibility to external objects;
during the third he seemed sinking into annihilation, and the mouth-
piece dropped out of his hand.   On becoming again sensible, which
happened in less than a minute, he continued for some time to suffer
from a feeling of impending suffocation, extreme exhaustion, and
great feebleness of the pulse.   Throughout the rest of the day he
was affected with weakness, giddiness and rending headache.†
These experiments show that the gas is deleterious.   Yet Nysten
found it inert when injected into the veins, and what is more to the
point, colliers breathe the air of coal mines without apparent injury
when strongly impregnated with it.

The mixed gases of coal-gas or oil-gas appear likewise to be inert
when considerably diluted ; for gas-men breathe with impunity an
atmosphere considerably loaded with them ; and in the course of
some researches on the illuminating power and best mode of burning
these gases, Dr. Turner and myself daily, for two months, breathed
air strongly impregnated with them, but never remarked any unpleasant effect whatever.

It would seem, however, from several accidents in France and
England, that when the impregnation is carried a certain length,
poisonous effects may ensue ; and that the symptoms then induced
are purely narcotic.   The first case, which occurred at Paris in 1830,
has been related by M. Devergie.   In consequence of a leak in the
service-pipe which supplied a warehouse, five individuals who slept
in the house were attacked during the night with stupor ; and if one
of them had not been awakened by the smell and alarmed the rest,
it is probable that all would have perished.   As it was, one man
was found completely comatose and occasionally convulsed, with

* London Medical Gazette, pp. 375, 410, 448.
† Researches on Nitrous Oxide Gas, p. 467.

froth issuing from the mouth, occasional vomiting, stertorous respiration, and dilated pupils. Some temporary amendment was procured by blood-letting, but the breathing continued laborious, and he expired about nine hours after the party went to bed, and six hours after the alarm was given. On dissection the vessels of the brain were found much gorged, the blood in the heart and great vessels firmly coagulated, one of the lungs congested, and its bronchial tube blocked up by a kidney bean. The immediate cause of death in this case is therefore doubtful.* A similar set of cases happened at Leeds in 1838. An old woman and her grand-daughter were found dead in bed one morning at nine o'clock, ten hours and a half after they had been seen alive and well. The air of the apartment was loaded with coal-gas from a leak in a street-pipe ten feet from the bedroom. One body was cold and stiff when found, -and the other became rigid very soon. The attitude and expression were calm, the integuments pale, the cerebral membranes natural, the brain itself turgid, and its ventricles distended, in the case of the girl, with an ounce and a half of serosity, the lungs congested, the alimentary mucous membrane red, and the blood every where fluid, and unusually florid, even in the right side of the heart.† Another accident of the same kind, which proved fatal to five individuals, occurred at Strasbourg in 1841. Four were found dead, another survived twenty-four hours after the accident was discovered, and a sixth recovered. It appears from the statement of this person, that the first symptoms were headache and giddiness, then nausea and vomiting, afterwards confusion of ideas, and at length insensibility. General prostration, partial palsy, coma, and convulsions were the leading symptoms after the accident was observed. In the four people found dead the most remarkable appearances were cerebral congestion, redness of the bronchial membrane, accumulation of bloody, frothy mucus in the air tubes, scarlet redness of the lungs, coagulation and darkness of the blood. In the person who was found alive, but did not recover, there was no cerebral congestion, gorging of the air tubes, or redness of the lungs. Professor Tourdes, who reports these cases, ascertained that air containing a fiftieth of coal-gas kills rabbits in twelve or fourteen minutes, and that even a thirtieth proves fatal, though slowly. The gas which caused the accident, and which was prepared from a mixture of water and slate coal, consisted of 22·5 per cent. light carburetted hydrogen, 6·0 bicarburetted hydrogen, 21·9 carbonic oxide, 31 hydrogen, 14 azote, and 4·6 carbonic acid ; and by experiment the author found that the most energetic of these gases as a poison is the carbonic oxide, and that the action of the two carburetted-hydrogens is quite feeble.‡ It is somewhat remarkable that no such accident has ever happened in Edinburgh, where nevertheless coal-gas is more used for purposes of illumination in private houses than in any other city. The fine quality of the gas, — for it contains a mere trace of carbonic acid, and

* Annales d'Hyg. Publ. et de Méd. Lég. iii. 457.
† Mr. Pridgin's Teale in Guy's Hospital Reports, 1839, iv. 106.
‡ Annales d'Hygiène Publique, 1842, xxvii. 232.

probably less than four per cent. of carbonic oxide, — may be the reason why accidents are not occasioned by it. It is a singular fact, however, that the powerful odour of the gas, when it accidentally escapes in the night-time, generally awakes very soon those who are exposed to inhale it.

Of Poisoning with Carbonic Acid Gas. — Carbonic acid gas is the most important of the deleterious gases; for it is the daily source of fatal accidents. It is extricated in great quantity from burning fuel; it is given out abundantly in the calcining of lime; it is disengaged in a state of considerable purity in brew-houses by the fermentation of beer; it is often met with in mines and caverns, particularly in coal-pits and draw-wells; it may collect in apartments where fuel is burnt without a proper outlet for the vitiated air, or where persons are crowded too much for the capacity of the room. Hence many have been killed by descending incautiously into draw-wells, by falling into beer-vats, and by sleeping before the traps of lime-kilns, or in apartments without vents and heated by choffers. Instances have even occurred of the same accident from sleeping in green-houses during the night, when plants exhale much carbonic acid; and some dreadful cases have occurred of suffocation from confinement in small crowded rooms.

Physiologists, as already remarked, are not quite agreed as to the action of carbonic acid gas, — whether it is a positive poison, or simply an asphyxiating gas. But in my opinion reasons enough exist for believing that it is positively and energetically poisonous. This is perhaps shown by its effects being much more rapidly produced, and much more slowly and imperfectly removed, than asphyxia from immersion in hydrogen or azote.[*]   Thus immersion for twenty-five seconds in an atmosphere of carbonic acid gas has been found sufficient to kill an animal outright; and fifteen seconds will kill a small bird.[†] But it is more unequivocally established by the three following facts:

In the first place, if, instead of the nitrogen contained in atmospheric air, carbonic acid gas be mixed with oxygen in the same proportion, animals cannot breathe this atmosphere for two minutes without being seized with symptoms of poisoning.[‡] Even a much less proportion has the same effect. Five per cent. in the air will affect small birds in two minutes, and kill them in half an hour.[§] Persons have become apoplectic in an atmosphere of carbonic acid gas, which to those who entered it appeared at first quite respirable.[||]

Secondly, Professor Rolando of Turin having found that the land tortoise sustained little injury when the great air-tube of one lung was tied, — he contrived to make it breathe carbonic acid gas with one lung, while atmospheric air was inhaled by the other; and he remarked that death took place in a few hours.[¶]

[*] M. Collard de Martigny in Arch. Gén. de Méd. xiv. 209.
[†] Journal der Praktischen Heilkunde, 1831, iv. 119.   [‡] Collard de Martigny, 204.
[§] Dr. Bird in Guy's Hospital Reports, 1839, iv. 81.
[||] Nouv. Biblioth. Méd. 1827, iii. 91.   [¶] Archives Gén. de Med. v. 132.

Thirdly, the symptoms caused by inhaling the gas may be also produced by applying it to the inner membrane of the stomach or to the skin. On the one hand aërated water has been known to cause giddiness or even intoxication when drunk too freely at first;[*] and the sparkling wines probably owe their rapid intoxicating power to the carbonic acid they contain. And, on the other hand, M. Collard de Martigny has found that, if the human body be enclosed in an atmosphere of the gas, due precautions being taken to preserve the free access of common air to the lungs, the usual symptoms of poisoning with carbonic acid are produced, such as weight in the head, obscurity of sight, pain in the temples, ringing in the ears, giddiness, and an undefinable feeling of terror; and that if the same experiment be made on animals and continued long enough, death will be the consequence.[†]

When a man attempts to inhale pure carbonic acid gas, for example by putting the face over the edge of a beer-vat, or the nose into a jar containing chalk and weak muriatic acid, the nostrils and throat are irritated so strongly, that the glottis closes and inspiration becomes impossible. Sir H. Davy in making this experiment, farther remarked, that the gas causes an acid taste in the mouth and throat, and a sense of burning in the uvula.[‡] I have remarked the same effects from very pure gas disengaged by tartaric acid from carbonate of soda. Hence, when a person is immersed in the gas nearly or perfectly pure, as in a beer-vat, or old well, he dies at once of suffocation.

The effects are very different when the gas is considerably diluted; for the symptoms then resemble apoplexy. As they differ somewhat according to the source from which the gas is derived, and the admixtures consequently breathed along with it, it will be necessary to notice separately the effects of the pure gas diluted with air, — of the emanations from burning charcoal, tallow, and coal, — and finally of air vitiated by the breath.

1. M. Chomel of Paris has related a case of poisoning with the gas diluted with air, in the person of a labourer, who was suddenly immersed in it at the bottom of a well, and remained there three-quarters of an hour. He was first affected with violent and irregular convulsions of the whole body and perfect insensibility, afterwards with fits of spasm like tetanus; and during the second day, when these symptoms had gone off, he continued to be affected with dumbness.[§] — It is worthy of particular remark that, contrary to general belief, these effects may be produced in situations where the air is not sufficiently impure to extinguish lights. Thus M. Collard de Martigny relates the case of a servant, who, on entering a cellar where grape-juice was fermenting, became suddenly giddy, and, under a vague impression of terror, fled from the place, dropping her candle on the floor and shutting the door behind her. She fell down

---

[*] Foderé, Méd. Légale, iv. 37.   [†] Archives, &c. p. 211.
[‡] Recherches on Nitrous Oxide, p. 472.
[§] Nouv. Journal de Méd. ii. 196.

insensible outside the door, and those who went to her assistance found on opening the door that the light continued to burn.[*] — Mr. Taylor indeed has since ascertained that a candle will burn in air, which contains ten, or even twelve per cent. of carbonic acid,[†] — a proportion more than sufficient to cause poisoning in no long time. It is also important to observe, that, contrary to what would be expected from the statements of Sir H. Davy and other experimentalists on the effects of the pure gas, it will often happen that no odour or taste is perceived. M. Bonami, in an account of an accident which happened at Nantes to two workmen who descended an old well, says that the first while descending uttered a piercing cry and fell down; and that as soon as his comrade, who tried to rescue him, was lowered ten or twelve feet, he felt as if he was about to be suffocated for want of breath, but perceived no strong or disagreeable smell.[‡]   It should be remembered therefore by workmen, that there may be danger in descending pits where none is indicated by the sense of smell, or by the extinguishing of a light.

2. The fumes of burning charcoal have been long known to be deleterious. The early symptoms caused by them have been little noticed; for, as this variety of poisoning generally occurs during sleep, the patient is seldom seen till the symptoms are fully formed.   In an attempt at self-destruction described in a French journal, the first effects were slight oppression, then violent palpitation, next confusion of ideas, and at last insensibility.[§]   Tightness in the temples, and an undefinable sense of alarm have also been remarked;[||] and others have, on the contrary, experienced a pleasing sensation that seduced them to remain on the fatal spot.[¶]   The best account of the incipient symptoms has been given by Mr. Coathupe of Wraxhall, in an account of an experiment he made with Joyce's stove, — a preposterous invention, the fuel of which was supposed by the inventor to burn without contaminating the air, although it was neither more nor less than prepared charcoal.'   Having closed every aperture in a room of the capacity of eighty cubic yards, Mr. Coathupe kindled the stove and watched the results.   In four hours he had slight giddiness, in five hours and a half intense giddiness, the desire to vomit without the power, excessive prostration and incapability of muscular effort, a frequent full throbbing pulse, a sense of distention of the cerebral arteries, agonizing headache, chiefly in the hind-head, but no sense of suffocation.   At this time he experienced great difficulty in opening the window and removing the stove; and in seven hours, when his wife entered the room, he was unable to tell what was the matter, although quite conscious of all that was passing.   He then slowly recovered.[**]   A similar account has also been given by Mr. Chapman of Tooting of the effects of this notorious stove.   A young

* Archives Gén. de Médecine, xiv. 205.
† Manual of Medical Jurisprudence, 1844, 555.
‡ Histoire de la Soc. Roy. de Med. i. 353.
§ Nouv. Biblioth. Méd. 1827, iii. 91.
|| Collard de Martigny, Arch. Gén. de Méd. xiv. 205.
¶ Orfila, Toxicol. Gen. ii. 475.   Note.   ** Lancet, 1838-39, i. 260.

gentleman, after being only one hour in a chamber heated by it, felt first slight giddiness and headache, and afterwards violent pain in the head and tightness round the forehead and temples; the pupils became excessively dilated and nearly insensible; there was constant ringing in the ears, a feeble frequent pulse, paleness of the features and lividity of the lips and hands, coldness of the extremities, laborious irregular breathing, and extreme prostration. A temporary relief, obtained by stimulants, was succeeded by violence; which, however, was subdued by blood-letting; and he recovered.* A set of cases, 70 in number, similar to the last two, but milder, occurred in January, 1836, in the church of Downham in Norfolk, which was heated by two of these stoves.†

The following abstract of a case by Dr. Babington will convey an accurate idea of the advanced symptoms. The waiter of a tavern and a little boy, on going to bed, left a choffer of charcoal burning beside it; and next morning were found insensible. The boy died immediately after they were discovered. The waiter had stertorous breathing, livid lips, flushing of the face, and a full, strong pulse ; for which affections he was bled to ten ounces. When Dr. Babington first saw him, however, the pulse had become feeble, the breathing imperfect, and the limbs cold ; the muscles were powerless but twitched with slight convulsions, the sensibility gone, the face pale, the eyelids closed, the eyes prominent and rolling, the tongue swollen and the jaw locked upon it, and there was a great flow of saliva from the mouth. The employment of galvanism at this time caused an evident amendment in every symptom. But it was soon abandoned ; because each time it was applied, the excitement was rapidly followed by corresponding depression. Cold water was then dashed upon him, ammonia rubbed on his chest, and oxygen thrown into the lungs ; through which means a warm perspiration was brought out, and his state rapidly improved. He was nearly lost, however, during the subsequent night by hemorrhage from the divided vein ; but next day he was so well that he could even speak a little. For two days afterwards the left side of the face was paralyzed, and his mental faculties were somewhat disordered.‡ — In such cases as this the stupor is generally very deep. There is a case in a French Journal of a girl, who, after remaining some time in a small close chamber heated by a charcoal choffer, fell down insensible, remained in that state for three hours, and found, on recovering from her lethargy, that the choffer had fallen, and burnt the skin and subjacent fat of the thighs to a cinder.§

Occasionally the stage of stupor is followed, as in some other varieties of narcotic poisoning, by a stage of delirium, at times of the furious kind, or by a state resembling somnambulism.‖ It does not follow that recovery is certain because coma has thus given place to

* Lond. Med. Gazette, 1838-39, i. 427.

† Dr. G. Bird in Guy's Hospital Reports, 1839, iv. 84.

‡ London Med. Chir. Transactions, i. 83.   § Nouv. Journ. de Méd.

‖ Nouv. Biblioth. Med. 1827, iii. 91.

delirium, — an alteration, which in most varieties of narcotic poisoning is considered a sure sign of recovery. Collard de Martigny has
related a case which eventually proved fatal, notwithstanding this sign
of improvement.*

The narcotism induced by breathing charcoal fumes often lasts a
considerable length of time, — much longer indeed than the effects of
other narcotic poisons. This will appear sufficiently from the case
described by Dr. Babington. One of the people, mentioned at the
commencement of this chapter as having been suffocated at Gerolzhofen,
lingered five days in a state of coma before he expired.

Commonly in cases of recovery, there is found to have been no consciousness of any thing going on around, or recollection of what passed
subsequently to the first impressions of poisoning. The reverse, however,
occurred in Mr. Coathupe's experiment ; and a similar instance has
been published, where the individual, though apparently insensible,
knew when the room was first entered by strangers, and heard them
call him by name and bid him put out his tongue, and stretch forth
his arm, — without, however, his having the power to answer, or in
any way to express the consciousness of understanding them.†

Poisoning with charcoal vapour has become a subject of great
importance in French medical jurisprudence, partly on account of the
frequency with which it is resorted to for the purpose of committing
suicide, and partly because repeated attempts have been made to conceal murder by arranging matters so as to present the appearances of
suicide. M. Devergie says, that in the years 1834 and 1835 no fewer
than 360 cases of poisoning with charcoal-vapour occurred in Paris,
of which nearly four-fifths proved fatal ; and he has given the particulars of two attempts to conceal murder under the appearance of death
from this cause.‡

The subject has therefore been carefully examined by various authors, but by none so successfully as by M. Devergie ; of whose important researches the following is a brief analysis.

In stating the various sources whence charcoal-vapour may become
incidentally the cause of death, he dwells particularly on the risk of
its admission from adjoining vents, even in other houses from that
where the accidents happen, — because there may be currents in the
apartment which occasion back-draught. Three remarkable cases of
this kind, very obscure in their origin, have been related by M.
d'Arcet.§

The very discrepant effects of the poison on different individuals,
simultaneously and to appearance alike exposed to it, have usually
been explained by reference to the great density of the gas, which
consequently accumulates near the floor. Some, however, have doubted the fact that the gas is unequally diffused. Mr. Taylor in particular says he ascertained by analysis, that air collected above and below
a choffer of burning charcoal was equally contaminated, that what

* Archives Gén. de Méd. xiv. 210.
† Fallot, in Journal Complémentaire. Mai, 1829.
‡ Annales d'Hygiène Publique, 1840, xxiii. 176.   § Ibidem, xvi. 30.

was collected a foot above its level contained 4·65 per cent., and that another portion taken the same distance below it contained 4·5 of carbonic acid.* M. Devergie has discovered the source of these discrepant opinions. He has found,† that, notwithstanding the high density of carbonic acid gas, the currents caused by the heat, disengaged when charcoal is burnt in a room, without an issue for the products of combustion, produce an equable mixture of gases at all elevations in the apartment, provided the air be examined while still warm, and not long after the charcoal has burnt out ; but that, at a later period, such as twelve hours, the carbonic acid partly separates and sinks, so that, while the air at the top contains only a 78th, that near the floor contains four times as much, or a 19th of carbonic acid gas.

Disputes have also arisen as to the precise nature of the emanations from burning charcoal,— some believing that carbonic acid is alone discharged in such quantity as to prove injurious, and is singly sufficient to account for the effects which have been observed, — while others maintain that carbonic oxide, carburetted-hydrogen, or some peculiar pyrogenous vapour, may be also formed, and prove the real cause of the active properties of the vapour. According to the researches of Orfila, charcoal in a state of vivid ignition emits carbonic acid only, a hundred parts of the consumed air having been ascertained by him to be composed of 42 azote, 46 common air, and 12 carbonic acid. But when the combustion is low, a hundred parts consist of 52 azote, 20 common air, 14 carbonic acid, and 14 carburetted-hydrogen ; so that not only is the air more thoroughly consumed ; but likewise an additional poisonous gas is brought into action.‡ The difference thus indicated has been supposed to account for what is often observed in countries where charcoal choffers are much in use for warming close apartments, — namely, that the practice is attended with most danger when the combustion is low, and that it is unsafe to close the doors of an apartment till the fuel is in a state of vivid ignition. M. Guérard again maintains, that when the supply of air is incomplete and combustion low, carbonic oxide gas is formed in considerable quantity ; and that this gas, confessedly a much more powerful narcotic than carbonic acid, is probably the cause of many cases of poisoning with charcoal fumes.§ M. Devergie doubts the exactness of Orfila's experiments on this head, but gives no new analysis. He observes that charcoal-vapour gives the air of a room a peculiar odour and bluish misty appearance, the latter of which slowly diminishes, and in twelve hours disappears ; and that possibly there may be both a little carbonic oxide and carburetted-hydrogen in the air. But nevertheless he is of opinion that the carbonic acid alone is adequate to occasion all the effects observed in man or animals.‖ Professor Hünefeld is of a different opinion, and has supplied the most satisfactory explanation of the important fact, that charcoal fumes are most noxious when the fuel has been just kindled and burns low ; for he

---

* Manual of Medical Jurisprudence, 1844, p. 557.   † Annales, ut supra, 186.
‡ Toxicologie Gén. 1826, ii. 474.   § Annales d'Hygiène Publique, xxix. 53.
‖ Annales, ut supra, p. 191.

ascertained that at first it gives out a pyrogenous acid, which occasions headache and tendency to sickness, and which is not a product of combustion at the moment, but exists ready formed ; and that when charcoal is at a full red heat, this noxious substance is no longer given off.* Mr. Coathupe also thinks the cause of poisoning by charcoal fumes is an unknown pyrogenous body, and not carbonic acid gas.† — This department of inquiry is obviously susceptible of more precise information. But meanwhile, whatever may be the probability that, besides carbonic acid, some other gases, or some peculiar pyrogenous body, may occasionally exist in charcoal fumes, and increase their poisonous property, little doubt can exist that the carbonic acid is singly sufficient to account for all the leading phenomena.

M. Devergie has been led to the opinion that air, in which a fourth part of its oxygen has been converted into carbonic acid, and which therefore contains five per cent of that gas, is amply enough impregnated to occasion death.‡ This corresponds with the observations of M. Ollivier, who found that three per cent. was as much as could be breathed with impunity even for a moderate length of time.§ Less, however, will suffice to prove injurious or even fatal, if the air be breathed long. Mr Coathupe inferred from a rough estimate, that in the dangerous experiment he made upon himself, the carbonic acid, if uniformly diffused in the apartment, which was probably the case, amounted to only two per cent. ; but his data were inadequate.‖

Proceeding from the fact that five per cent. of carbonic acid is sufficient to cause death, Devergie points out what quantity of charcoal is required to form that proportion, — a question of no small moment in respect to charges of murder, concealed under the semblance of suicide by suffocation with charcoal fumes. And he shows, that a French bushel, or decalitre, weighing 3000 grammes, is sufficient for a close apartment of 1275 cubic mètres, that is 6·6 pounds avoirdupois for a space of 1666 English cubic yards, provided the gas be uniformly diffused.¶ The quantity of charcoal burnt in a given case may be arrived at pretty nearly from the weight of ashes left, which is estimated in round numbers at a twenty-fifth by himself,** and at a twentieth by Ollivier.††

It is important to remark that complete closure of an apartment is by no means essential for the action of carbonic acid, whether disengaged within it or introduced from without. For poisoning has occurred, even where a window was partially open.‡‡

3. It is probable that in some circumstances a very small quantity of the mixed gases proceeding from the slow combustion of tallow and other oily substances will produce dangerous symptoms. Dr. Blackadder remarked in the course of his experiments on flame, that the vapour into which oil is resolved, previous to its forming flame

* Annalen der Pharmacie, 1836, xx. 156.
† Lancet, *ut supra.*   ‡ Annales, &c. *ut supra*, p. 197.
§ Annales, &c. xx. 134.   ‖ Lancet, *ut supra.*
¶ Annales, *ut supra*, 197.   ** Ibidem, p. 199.
†† Ibidem, xx. 132.   ‡‡ Devergie, *ut supra,* 200.

round the wick, excites in minute quantities intense headache.[*] The emanations from the burning snuff of a candle, which are probably of the same nature, seem to be very poisonous. An instance indeed has been recorded in which they proved fatal. A party of iron-smiths, who were carousing on a festival day at Leipzig, amused themselves with plaguing a boy, who was asleep in a corner of the room, by holding under his nose the smoke of a candle just extinguished. At first he was roused a little each time. But when the amusement had been continued for half an hour he began to breathe laboriously, was then attacked with incessant epileptic convulsions, and died on the third day.[†] — The effects of such emanations are probably owing to empyreumatic volatile oil, which will be presently seen to be an active poison.

4. The vapours from burning coal are the most noxious of all kinds of emanations from fuel, and cause peculiar symptoms. But they are less apt to lead to accidents than the vapour of charcoal, as they are much more irritating to the lungs. This effect depends on the sulphurous acid gas which is mingled with the carbonic acid.

Sulphurous acid gas is exceedingly deleterious to vegetable life, being hardly inferior in that respect to hydrochloric acid. Dr. Turner and I found that a fifth of a cubic inch diluted with ten thousand times its volume of air destroyed all the leaves of various plants in forty-eight hours.[‡] I am not acquainted with any experiments on animals or observations on man regarding the effects of the pure gas. But it will without a doubt prove a powerful irritant.

Some of the peculiarities in the cases now to be mentioned were possibly owing to the admixture of sulphuric acid gas with the carbonic, both being inhaled in a diluted state. The cases are described by Mr. Braid, at the time surgeon at Leadhills. In March, 1817, several of the miners there were violently affected, and some killed, in consequence, it was supposed, of the smoke of one of the steam-engines having escaped into the way-gates, and contaminated the air in the workings. Four men who attempted to force their way through this air into the workings below were unable to advance beyond, and seem to have died immediately. The rest attempted to descend two hours after, but were suddenly stopped by the contaminated air. As soon as they reached it, although their lights burnt tolerably well, they felt difficulty in breathing, and were then seized with violent pain and beating in the head, giddiness and ringing in the ears, followed by vomiting, palpitation and anxiety, weakness of the limbs and pains above the knees, and finally with loss of recollection. Some of them made their escape, but others remained till the air was so far purified that their companions could descend to their aid. When Mr. Braid first saw them, some were running about frantic and furious, striking all who came in their way, — some ran off terrified whenever any one approached them, —

* On the Constitution of Flame — Edin. New Philos. Journal, i..224, 226.
† Ammann. — Medicina Critica, Cas. 59, p. 365.
‡ Edin. Med. and Surg. Journal, xxviii. 359.

some were singing, — some praying, — others lying listless and insensible. Many of them retched and vomited. In some the pulse
was quick, in others slow, in many irregular, and in all feeble. All
who could describe their complaints had violent headache, some of
them tenesmus, and a few diarrhœa. In a few days all recovered
except the first four and three others who had descended to the
deeper parts of the mine.* — Another accident of the same nature,
and followed by the same phenomena, happened more lately at
Leadhills.† Similar accidents have been also witnessed by Mr.
Bald, civil engineer, among the coal-miners who work in the neighbourhood of a burning mine belonging to the Devon Company. It
is worthy of remark, that the men sometimes worked for a considerable length of time before they were taken ill. Such being the case,
it will be readily conceived that the burning of the lights was not a
test of the wholesomeness of the air. Here, as at Leadhills and in
other instances already mentioned, the lights continued to burn where
the men were poisoned.‡

5. Somewhat analogous to the symptoms now described are the
effects of the gradual contamination of air in a confined apartment.
Every one must have read of the horrible death of the Englishmen
who were locked up all night in a close dungeon in Fort William at
Calcutta. One hundred and forty-six individuals were imprisoned
in a room twenty feet square, with only one small window ; and
before next morning all but 23 died under the most dreadful of tortures, — that of slowly increasing suffocation. They seem to have
been affected nearly in the same way as the workmen at Leadhills.§
A similar accident happened in London in 1742. The keeper of
the round-house of St. Martin's, crammed 28 people into an apartment
six feet square and not quite six feet high ; and four were suffocated.‖

The morbid appearances left on the body after poisoning with
carbonic acid gas have been chiefly observed in persons killed by
charcoal vapour. According to Portal the vessels of the brain are
congested, and the ventricles contain serum ; the lungs are distended,
as if emphysematous ; the heart and great veins are gorged with
black fluid blood ; the eyes are generally glistening and prominent,
the face red, and the tongue protruded and black.¶ — Gorging of the
cerebral vessels seems to be very common. Yet sometimes it is inconsiderable, as in two cases related by Dr. Bright, where, except
in the sinuses and in the greater veins of the ventricles and substance
of the brain, no particular gorging or vascularity seems to have been
met with, — the external membranes in particular having been very
little injected.** This, however, is certainly a rare occurrence. Serous effusion in the ventricles and under the arachnoid membrane is
very general, yet not invariable. — Dr. Schenck, medical inspector

* Edinburgh Med. and Surg. Journal, xiii. 353.   † Ibidem, xxxii. 315.
‡ Edin. New Phil. Journal, v. 110.
§ Holwell, Narrative of the deplorable Deaths of the English gentlemen and others
who were suffocated in the Black Hole at Fort William.
‖ Smith's Principles of Forensic Medicine, 221.
¶ Instruction sur le traitement des Asphyxiés, 25.
** Reports of Medical Cases, ii. 226, 227.

of Siegen, in reporting two cases of death caused by the vapours of burning wood, notices paleness of the countenance as a singular accompaniment of cerebral congestion ; and calls the attention of medical jurists to the extreme calmness of the features as a general character of this variety of poisoning.[*] Although the same appearance has also been noticed by others,[†] the countenance nevertheless is often livid. But whether livid or pale, it is always composed. — It appears from an account in Pyl's Essays of several cases of suffocation from the fumes of burning wood, that besides the appearances mentioned by Portal, there is usually great livor of the back, frothiness as well as fluidity of the blood, and more or less gorging of the lungs with blood.[‡] — A common appearance where the poisonous emanation has been charcoal vapour, is a lining of dark, or sometimes actually black dust on the mucous membranes of the air passages, thickest near the external opening of the nostrils, and disappearing towards the glottis. There are obvious reasons why this appearance cannot always be expected to occur; but when present, it may be in doubtful circumstances a very important article of evidence.[§] In Wildberg's collection of cases there is a report on two people who were suffocated in bed, in consequence of the servant having neglected to open the flue-trap when she kindled the stove in the bed-chamber ; and in each of them Wildberg found all the appearances now quoted from Portal and Pyl. The tongue was black and swelled.[‖] — Mertzdorff has related a case of death from the same cause, in which, together with the preceding appearances, an effusion of blood was found between the arachnoid and pia mater over the whole surface of both hemispheres.[¶] In one of Dr. Bright's cases there was a small ecchymosis in the cortical substance on the outer side of the anterior lobe, and not extending into the medullary matter. Fallot mentions an instance of suffocation from charcoal vapour, where a little coagulated blood was found between the layers of the arachnoid membrane of the cerebellum in the region of the left occipital hollow.[**] Three instances of extravasation are enumerated in a list of German cases analysed by Dr. Bird.[††] Such appearances might be expected more frequently, considering the manifest tendency of this kind of poisoning to cause congestion in the head. — The blood is generally described as being liquid and very dark. But M. Ollivier has lately called attention to the fact, that the blood both before and after death is not unusually more florid in the veins than natural.[‡‡] In a case mentioned by M. Rayer globules of an oily-looking matter were found swimming on the surface of the blood and urine.[§§] This is a solitary

* Horn's Archiv für Medizinische Erfahrung, 1823, i. 93.
† London Medical Gazette, 1838-39, i. 943.
‡ Aufsätze und Beobachtungen, i. 1. and vii. 95.
§ See various cases quoted in detail in Wibmer, die Wirkung der Arzneimittel, &c. ii. 49, 51, 55
‖ Practisches Handbuch für Physiker, iii. 278.
¶ Beiträge zur gerichtl. medizin.— Horn's Archiv für Medizinische Erfahrung, 1823, i. 296.
** Journal Complémentaire, Mai, 1829.   †† Guy's-Hospital Reports, *ut supra,*
‡‡ Annales d'Hygiène-Publique, xx. 114.   §§ Revue Médicale, 1827, iii. 528.

observation. — The body usually remains flaccid, and the customary stage of rigidity is imperfect. In some instances, however, as in those related by Dr. Schenck, the stage of rigidity is passed through in the usual manner. It is not uncommon to find vomited matter lying beside the body, a circumstance which may naturally mislead the unpractised. This is represented by Professor Wagner of Berlin to have occurred uniformly in his experience ;[*] and it is also mentioned in many of the cases reported by others ;[†] but it is not invariable. — A red appearance in the stomach and intestines has been noticed in many cases,[‡] and often ascribed to inflammation ; but it is probably nothing more than the result of the venous congestion, which pervades most of the membranous surfaces of the body.

The least variable appearances according to Dr. Bird are general lividity, protrusion of the tongue, a calm expression and attitude, cerebral congestion, and serous effusion. This author's paper in the Medical Gazette, 1838-39, i., or in Guy's Hospital Reports, iv., enters very fully into the appearances after death, and may be consulted with advantage for further details.

The treatment of poisoning with carbonic acid consists chiefly in the occasional employment of the cold affusion, and in moderate blood-letting either from the arm or from the head. In a case which happened at Paris, where a lady tried to make way with herself by breathing charcoal fumes, and was found in a state of almost hopeless insensibility, various remedies were tried unsuccessfully, till cupping from the nape of the neck was resorted to ; and she then rapidly recovered.[§] Another instance where blood-letting was also singularly successful deserves particular mention ; because for three hours the patient remained without pulsation in any artery, and without the slightest perceptible respiration. At first neither by cupping nor by venesection could any blood be obtained ; and it was only after the long interval just mentioned, and constant artificial inflation of the lungs, that the blood at length trickled slowly from the arm. The pulse and breathing were after this soon re-established ; but it was not till eight hours later that sensibility returned.[||]

Of Poisoning with Carbonic Oxide Gas. — Carbonic oxide gas, according to Nysten, has not any effect on man when injected into the pleura ; but when thrown slowly into the veins, it gives the arterial blood a brownish tint, and induces for a short time a state resembling intoxication.[¶] The quantity injected into the veins was probably too small to produce the full effect, or it was discharged in passing through the lungs ; for this gas certainly appears to be very deleterious when breathed by man, or the lower animals. M. Leblanc found by experiment that a sparrow was killed almost imme-

* Horn's Archiv. für Medizinische Erfahrung, 1834, 746.
† Bird, *ut supra*, iv. 93.
‡ Wibmer, die Wirkung der Arzneimittel, &c. ii. 47, *et seq.*
§ Nouvelle Bibliothèque Méd. 1829, i. 374.
|| Réné-Bourgeois, Archives Gén. de Méd. xx. 508.
¶ Nystem, Recherches Chimico-Physiologiques, pp. 88, 92, 96.

diately in air containing only a twentieth of it, and that so little even
as a hundredth part proved fatal in two minutes.*

A set of interesting but hazardous experiments were made with it
in 1814 by the assistants of Mr. Higgins of Dublin. One gentleman,
after inhaling it two or three times, was seized with giddiness, tremors, and an approach to insensibility, succeeded by languor, weakness, and headache of some hours' duration. The other had almost
paid dearly for his curiosity. Having previously exhausted his lungs,
he inhaled the pure gas three or four times, upon which he was suddenly deprived of sense and motion, fell down supine, and continued
for half an hour insensible, apparently lifeless, and with the pulse
nearly extinct. Various means were tried for rousing him, without
success; till at last oxygen gas was blown into the lungs. Anima-
tion then returned rapidly: but he was affected for the rest of the
day with convulsive agitation of the body, stupor, violent headache,
and quick irregular pulse; and after his senses were quite restored,
he suffered from giddiness, blindness, nausea, alternate heats and
chills, and then feverish, broken, but irresistible sleep.[†] A French
aëronaut, who used for his balloon a mixture of carbonic oxide and
hydrogen, obtained by decomposing water with red-hot charcoal,
lately suffered from similar symptoms in a milder degree, in consequence of the gas being disengaged upon him from the safety-valve
of his balloon.[‡]

Of Poisoning with Nitrous Oxide Gas. — The nitrous oxide or intoxicating gas is the last of the narcotic gases to be noticed. Nysten
found, that, when slowly injected in large quantity into the veins of
animals, it only caused slight staggering.[§] Frequent observation,
however, has shown that it is by no means so inert when breathed
by man. Sir H. Davy, who first had the courage to inhale it, observed that it excited giddiness, a delightful sense of thrilling in the
chest and limbs, acuteness of hearing, brilliancy of all surrounding
objects, and an unconquerable propensity to brisk muscular exertion.
These feelings were of short duration, but were generally succeeded
by alertness of body and mind, never by the exhaustion, depression,
and nausea, which follow the stage of excitement brought on by
spirits or opium.[||] Although many have since experienced the same
enticing effects, yet they are by no means uniform. For others have
been suddenly seized with great weakness, tendency to faint, loss of
voice, and sometimes convulsions; and two of Thenard's assistants,
on making the experiment, fainted away, and remained some seconds
motionless and insensible.[¶] It is a remarkable circumstance in the
operation of this gas, that, unlike other stimulants, it does not lose
its virtues under the influence of habit. Neither does the habitual
use of it lead to any ill consequence. Sir H. Davy, in the course of

* Annales d'Hygiène-Publique, xvix. 54.
† Mr. Witter in London Philosophical Journal, 1814, xliii. 367.
‡ Guérard in Annales d'Hygiène-Publique, xxix. 52.
§ Nysten, Recherches, &c.
‖ Davy's Chemical and Philosophical Researches, *passim.*
¶ Thenard, Traité de Chimie, iii. 675.

his researches, which were continued above two months, breathed it occasionally three or four times a day for a week together, at other periods four or five times a week only ; yet at the end his health was good, his mind clear, his digestion perfect, and his strength only a little impaired.*

Nitrous oxide gas is one of the few gases that are not injurious to vegetables. Dr. Turner and I found that seventy-two cubic inches, diluted with six times their volume of air, had no effect on a mignionette plant in forty-eight hours.†

Of Poisoning with Cyanogen Gas. — *Cyanogen gas* has been proved by the experiments of M. Coullon to be an active poison to all animals, — the guinea-pig, sparrow, leech, frog, wood-louse, fly, crab ; and the symptoms induced were coma, and more rarely convulsions.‡ These results are confirmed by the later experiments of Hünefeld, who found that it produces in the rabbit anxious breathing, slight convulsions, staring of the eyes, dilated pupils, coma, and death in five or six minutes.§   Buchner likewise found that small birds, held for a few seconds over the mouth of a jar containing cyanogen, died very speedily ; and on one occasion remarked, while preparing the gas, that the fore-finger, which was exposed to the bubbles as they escaped, became suddenly benumbed, and that this effect was attended with a singular feeling of pressure and contraction in the joints of the thumb and elbow.‖   It would undoubtedly be most dangerous to breathe this gas, except much diluted, and in very small quantity.

Of all narcotic gases it is the most noxious to vegetables.   Dr. Turner and I found that a third of a cubic inch, diluted with 1700 times its volume of air, caused the leaves of a mignionette plant to droop in twenty-four hours.   As usual with the effects of narcotic gases on vegetables, the drooping went on after the plant was removed into the open air ; and in a short time it was completely killed.¶

Of Poisoning with Oxygen Gas. — Of all the narcotic gases, none is more singular in its effects than oxygen.   When breathed in a state of purity by animals, they live much longer than in the same volume of atmospheric air.   But if the experiment be kept up for a sufficient length of time, symptoms of narcotic poisoning begin to manifest themselves.   For an hour no inconvenience seems to be felt ; but the breathing and pulse then become accelerated ; a state of debility next ensues ; at length insensibility gradually comes on, with glazing of the eyes, slow respiration and gasping ; coma is in the end completely formed ; and death ensues in the course of six, ten, or twelve hours.   If the animals are removed into the air before the insensibility is considerable, they quickly recover.   When the body is examined immediately after death, the heart is seen beating strongly,

---

* Researches, &c., p. 462.   † Edin. Med. and Surg. Journal, xxviii. 363.
‡ Journal Universel des Sc. Méd. ii. 240.
§ Archiv für Medizinische Erfahrung, 1830, ii. 859.
‖ Toxikologie, 382.   ¶ Edin. Med. and Surg. Journal, xxviii. 363.

but the diaphragm motionless ; the whole blood in the veins as well as the arteries is of a bright scarlet colour ; some of the membranous surfaces, such as the pulmonary pleura, have the same tint, and the blood coagulates with remarkable rapidity.   The gas in which an animal has died rekindles a blown out taper.   These experiments, which physiology owes to the researches of Mr. Broughton,* furnish a solitary example of death from stoppage of the respiration, although the heart continues to pulsate, and the lungs to transmit florid blood. Death is probably owing to hyper-arterialization of the blood.

CHAPTER XXXII.

CLASS THIRD.

OF NARCOTICO-ACRID POISONS GENERALLY.

THE third class of poisons, the narcotico-acrids, includes those which possess a double action, the one local and irritating like that of the irritants, the other remote, and consisting of an impression on the nervous system.

Sometimes they cause narcotism ; which is generally of a comatose nature, often attended with delirium ; but in one very singular group there is neither insensibility nor delirium, but merely violent tetanic spasms.

At other times they excite inflammation where they are applied. This effect, however, is by no means constant.   For Orfila justly observes, that under the name of narcotico-acrids several poisons are usually described which seldom excite inflammation.   Those which inflame the tissues where they are applied rarely occasion death in this manner.   Some of them may produce very violent local symptoms ; but they generally prove fatal through their operation on the nervous system.

For the most part, their narcotic and irritant effects appear incompatible.   That is, when they act narcotically, the body is insensible to the local irritation ; and when they irritate, the dose is not large enough to act narcotically.   In large doses, therefore, they act chiefly as narcotics, in small doses as irritants.   Sometimes, however, the narcotic symptoms are preceded or followed by symptoms of irritation ; and more rarely both exist simultaneously.

Most, if not all, of them, to whatever part of the body they are applied, act remotely by entering the blood-vessels ; but it has not been settled whether they operate by being carried with the blood to the part on which they act, or by producing on the inner membrane of the vessels a peculiar impression, which is conveyed along the nerves.   Some of them produce direct and obvious effects where they are applied.   Thus monkshood induces a peculiar numbness

* London Quarterly Journal of Science, January, 1830.

and tingling of the part with which it is placed in contact. The organs on which they act remotely are the brain and spine, and sometimes the heart also.

The appearances in the dead body are, for the most part, inconsiderable; more or less inflammation in the stomach or intestines, and congestion in the brain; but even these are not constant.

As a distinct class, they differ little from some poisons of the previous classes. Several of the metallic irritants, and a few vegetable acrids are, properly speaking, narcotico-acrids: they excite either narcotism or irritation, according to circumstances. But still, the poisons about to be considered form a good natural order when contrasted with these irritants. For the irritants which possess a double action are nevertheless characterized by the symptoms of inflammation being at least their most prominent effects; while the most prominent feature in the effects of the poisons now to be considered is injury of the nervous system. It is more difficult to draw the line of separation between the present class and the pure narcotics; for many narcotico-acrids rarely cause any symptom but those of narcotism.

The narcotico-acrids are all derived from the vegetable kingdom. Many of them owe their power to an alkaloid, consisting of oxygen, hydrogen, carbon, and azote.

The characters which distinguish the symptoms and morbid appearances of the narcotico-acrids from those of natural disease, do not require special mention; for almost all the remarks made in the introduction to the class of narcotics are applicable to the present class also. A few of the characters, however, which have been laid down, do not apply so well to the narcotico-acrids as to the narcotics. In particular, it appears that what was said on the short duration of the effects of the narcotics does not apply so well to the present class of poisons; some of which, in a single dose, continue to cause symptoms even of narcotism for two or three days. But the rule, that they seldom prove fatal if the case lasts above twelve hours, is still applicable, — at all events they rarely prove fatal after that interval by their narcotic action. The poisonous fungi, however, have proved fatal as narcotics so late as thirty-six hours, or even three days, after they were taken; and perhaps digitalis has proved fatal narcotically at the remote period of three weeks. But such cases are extremely rare.

Some narcotico-acids, such as the different species of *strychnos*, are quite peculiar in their effects; so that their symptoms may be distinguished at once from natural disease.

Orfila divides the narcotico-acrids into six groups, and this arrangement will be followed in the present work; but they are not all very well distinguished from one another.

CHAPTER XXXIII.

OF POISONING WITH NIGHTSHADE, THORN-APPLE, AND TOBACCO.

The first group of the narcotico-acrids comprehends these whose principal symptom in the early stage of their effects is delirium.   All the plants of the group belong to the natural order *Solanaceæ*, and Linnæus's class Pentandria Monogynia. Those which have been particularly examined are deadly nightshade, thorn-apple, and tobacco.

Of Poisoning with Deadly Nightshade.

The deadly nightshade, or *Atropa belladonna*, is allied in physiological and botanical characters to the *hyoscyamus* and *solanum* formerly mentioned ; and by the older writers, indeed, was confounded with the latter.   It is a native of Britain, growing in shady places, particularly on the edge of woods.   The berries, which ripen in September, have a jet-black colour.   Their beauty has frequently tempted both children and adults to eat them, although they have a mawkish taste; and many have suffered severely.   It is not the berry alone which is poisonous ; the whole plant is so ; and the root is probably the most active part.*   From one to four grains of the dried powder of the root will occasion dryness in the throat, giddiness, staggering, flushed face, dilated pupils, and sometimes even delirium.†   The juice of the leaves is very energetic, two grains of its extract being, when well prepared, a large enough dose to cause disagreeable symptoms in man.   It is a very uncertain preparation, unless when procured by evaporation *in vacuo ;* for some samples from the Parisian shops have been found by Orfila to be quite inert.

It contains a peculiar alkaloid, named *atropia.*   In the belladonna Brandes obtained a volatile, oily-like, alkaloidal fluid, of a penetrating narcotic smell, and bitterish, acrid taste, which he supposed to be the active principle of the plant.‡   The ulterior researches of Geiger and Hesse, however, as well as the simultaneous analysis of Mein, have proved that this fluid is not the pure alkaloid of belladonna, and that the real atropia is a solid substance, forming colourless, silky crystals, soluble in ether and alcohol, sparingly so in water, slightly bitter, liable to decomposition under contact with air and moisture, volatilizable, but with some decomposition, a little above 212°, and capable of forming definite crystallizable salts with acids.§ The aqueous solutions of its salts exhale during evaporation a narcotic vapour, which dilates the pupil, and causes sickness, giddiness, and headache.‖

The ordinary extract of belladonna in the dose of half an ounce will

---

* Buchner's Toxikologie, 188.
† Wibmer, Die Wirkung der Arzneimittel, &c. i. 360, 362.
‡ Annalen der Pharmacie, i. 68.
§ Ibidem, 1833, or Journal de Pharmacie, xx. 87.
‖ Buchner's Repertorium für die Pharmacie, ix. 71 and 77.

kill a dog in thirty hours when introduced into the stomach.   Half
that quantity applied to a wound will kill it in twenty-four hours.
And forty grains injected into the jugular vein prove even more
quickly fatal.   Convulsions are rarely produced, but only a state like
intoxication.*

The oleaginous atropia of Brandes in a dose of two or three drops
kill small birds instantaneously like concentrated hydrocyanic acid; in
less doses it occasions staggering, gasping, and in a few minutes death
amidst convulsions; and the dead body presents throughout the internal
organs great venous turgescence and even extravasation of blood, but
more especially excessive congestion within the head.†   The pure
crystalline atropia of Mein, when dissolved in water and greatly diluted, causes extreme and protracted dilatation of the pupils.

Symptoms in Man. — On man the effects of belladonna are much
more remarkable.   In small doses, whatever be the kind or surface
to which it is applied, — such as the skin round the eye, or the surface of a wound, or the inner membrane of the stomach, — it causes
dilatation of the pupil.   This effect may be excited without any con-
siitutional derangement.   When the extract is rubbed on the skin
round the eye, or a solution of it dropped upon the eyeball, vision
is not impaired ; but when it is taken internally so as to affect the
pupils, the sight is commonly much obscured.   The effects of large
or poisonous doses have been frequently witnessed in consequence of
children and adults being tempted to eat the berries by their fine
colour and bright lustre.   From the cases that have been published
the leading symptoms appear in the first instance to be dryness in
the throat, then delirium with dilated pupils, and afterwards coma.
Convulsions are rare, and, when present, slight.

The dryness of the throat is not a constant symptom.   It is often,
however, very distinct.   It occurred, for example, in 150 soldiers
who were poisoned near Dresden, as related by M. Gaultier de Claubry,‡ and in six soldiers whose cases have been described by Mr.
Brumwell.§   The former had not only dryness of the throat, but
likewise difficulty in swallowing.

The delirium is generally extravagant, and also most commonly
of the pleasing kind, sometimes accompanied with immoderate un-
controllable laughter, sometimes with constant talking, but occasionally with complete loss of voice, as in the cases of the 150 soldiers.
At other times the state of mind resembles somnambulism, as in the
instance of a tailor who was poisoned with a belladonna injection,
and who for fifteen hours, though speechless and insensible to external objects, went through all the customary operations of his trade
with great vivacity, and moved his lips as if in conversation.‖   Sometimes frantic delirium is almost the only symptom of consequence
throughout the whole duration of the poisoning.   Thus a gentleman

* Orfila, Toxicol. Gén. ii. 261.   † Annalen der Pharmacie, i. 71.
‡ Sedillot's Journ. Gén. de Méd. Dec. 1813, 364.
§ Lond. Med. Obs. and Inquiries, vi. 223.
‖ Journ. Universel, xxii. 239.

at Perigueux in France, who took by mistake a mixture containing a drachm and a half of extract, was attacked in half an hour with delirium, which soon became furious, and continued till next day, when it gradually left him.* In others the delirium is attended with a singular and total loss of consciousness, but without coma, as in the following case which occurred not long ago at St. Omer. A young man having taken by mistake an infusion of two drachms of dried leaves, was seized in an hour with great dryness of the mouth and throat, afterwards slight delirium, loss of consciousness, and dilatation of the pupil, next with retention of urine, convulsive twitches of the face and extremities, and incessant tendency to walk up and down. In three hours, after the action of an emetic and a clyster, he lay down, but still in a state of total unconsciousness and muttering delirium. Blood-letting being at last resorted to as a remedy, he speedily recovered his senses, and eventually got well, after suffering for some time from headache, fatigue, and much debility.†

The pupil is not only dilated in all cases, but likewise for the most part insensible ;‡ and, as in the soldiers at Dresden, the eyeball is sometimes red and prominent. The vision also, as in these soldiers, is generally obscure ; sometimes it is lost for a time ;§ and so completely that even the brightest light cannot be distinguished.||

The sopor or lethargy, which follows the delirium, occasionally does not supervene for a considerable interval. In a case related by Munnik it did not begin till twelve hours after the poison was taken.¶ Sometimes, as in the same case, the delirium returns when the stupor goes off. A patient of my colleague Dr. Simpson, after using a belladonna suppository consisting of two grains of extract, was attacked with dryness of the throat and delirium, followed soon by drowsiness and stupor ; and in five or six hours more, as the stupor wore off, the delirium returned, prompting to constant movements as if she was busy with her toilette and various other ordinary occupations. Sometimes the relation of the delirium to the coma is reversed, as in a case related by Mr. Clayton, where sopor came on first, and delirium ensued in six hours. The dose in this instance was forty grains of the extract.** Frequently the stupor is not distinct at any stage. — Even the delirium is not always formed rapidly. A man whose case is described by Sir John Hill did not become giddy for two hours after eating the berries, and the delirium did not appear till five hours later.†† In Mr. Brumwell's cases, the delirium was not particularly noticed till the morning after the berries were taken.

Convulsions, it has been already stated, are rare. In the case from the 24th volume of Sedillot's Journal, the muscles of the face were somewhat convulsed : there is also at times more or less locked-

* Journal de Chimie Médicale, 1837, p. 591.
† Ibid. 1839, 122.   ‡ Sedillot's Journ. de Méd. xxiv. 228.
§ Edin. Med. and Surg. Journal, ix. 380. || Journ. de Chim. Méd. ii. 586.
¶ Sedillot's Journal de Médecine, xxiv. 228.
** London Medical Gazette, 1838-39, i. 681.   †† British Herbal, 329.

jaw,[*] or subsultus tendinum ;[†] and occasionally much abrupt agitation of the extremities.[‡] But well-marked convulsions do not appear to be ever present.

The effects now detailed are by no means so quickly dissipated as those of opium. Almost every person who has taken a considerable dose has been ill for a day at least. The case from Sedillot's Journal lasted three days, delirium having continued twelve hours, the succeeding stupor for nearly two days, and the departure of the stupor being attended with a return of delirium for some hours longer. One of Mr. Brumwell's patients, too, was delirious for three days ; and Plenck has noticed several instances where the delirium was equally tedious.[§] Sage has related a case in which the individual was comatose for thirty hours.[‖] Blindness is also a very obstinate symptom, which sometimes remains after the affection of the mind has disappeared. This happened in Plenck's cases. In two children whose cases have been described in a late French journal, the eyes were insensible to the brightest light for three days.[¶] In general, the dilated state of the pupils continues long after the other symptoms have departed. It further appears from an official narrative in Rust's Journal, that dilated pupil is not the only symptom which may thus continue, but that various nervous affections, such as giddiness, disordered vision, and tremors, may prevail even for three or four weeks.[**]

Hitherto little or no mention has been made of symptoms of irritation from this poison. They are in fact uncommon, and seldom violent. In the cases related by Gaultier de Claubry and by Mr. Brumwell, dryness and soreness of the throat and difficult deglutition were remarked, and appear not unusual. These symptoms were especially noticed by Buchner, who by way of curiosity took half a drachm of seeds digested in beer. The sense of dryness and constriction of the throat were such as to prevent him swallowing even the saliva.[††] Sage's patient passed blood by stool ; and after the symptoms of narcotic poisoning ceased, he had aphthous inflammation in the throat, and swallowing was so difficult as for some time to excite convulsive struggles. Aphthæ in the throat and swelling of the belly also succeeded the delirium in Munnik's case. Mr. Wibmer alludes to the case of a man who, besides difficult deglutition at the beginning, had violent strangury towards the close.[‡‡] An instance of violent strangury with suppression of urine and bloody micturition is also related by M. Jolly. In the early stage, the patient had redness of the throat and burning along the whole alimentary canal, combined with the customary delirium and loss of consciousness. The symptoms were caused by forty-six grains of the extract given by mistake instead of jalap.[§§] Nausea and efforts to vomit are not infrequent at the commencement.

If the accident be taken in time, poisoning with belladonna is

* Journ. Universel, xxii. 239. — Edin. Med. and Surg. Journal, xxix. 452.
† Plenck's Toxicologia, 109.   ‡ Roux's Journal de Med. xxiv. 310.
§ Toxicologia, 109,   ‖ Moyens de remedier aux Pois Végét.
¶ Journ. de Chim. Méd. iii. 586.
** Magazin für die gesammte Heilkunde, xxi. 550.   †† Toxikologie, p. 220.
‡‡ On Vegetable Poisons, 17.   §§ Nouvelle Biblioth Méd. 1828, iii.

rarely fatal ; for, as the state first induced is delirium, not sopor, suspicion is soon excited, and emetics may be made to act before a sufficient quantity of the poison has been absorbed to prove fatal. Hence few fatal instances have occurred in recent times. Mr. Wilmer, however, has mentioned two fatal cases occurring in children, and terminating within twenty-four hours.[*] M. Boucher, a writer in the old French Journal of Medicine, has referred to several cases of the same nature ;[†] Gmelin has described the particulars of a good example ;[‡] and many others have been succinctly quoted by Wibmer, chiefly from the older authors.[§]

Cases of poisoning with this plant have occurred in man through other channels besides the stomach. Allusion has already been made to the instance of a tailor who was poisoned by an injection. A small quantity will sometimes suffice when administered in that way. A woman, whose case is mentioned in Rust's Journal, was attacked with wild delirium, flushed face and glistening eyes, in consequence of receiving, during labour, a clyster, that contained six grains of the common extract;[||] and Dr. Simpson's patient, who was severely affected, had only two grains.

Perhaps the berry is in some circumstances not very active. A French physician, M. Gigault of Pontcroix, says he has frequently had occasion to treat cases of poisoning with it, as accidents of the kind are extremely common in his neighbourhood ; that he never knew it prove fatal ; and that in one instance a young man took a pound of the berries before going to bed, and was not subjected to treatment till next morning, when he was found in a state of delirium, but speedily recovered after the free operation of emetics.[¶]

Morbid Appearances. — I have hitherto seen but one good account of the appearances after death from poisoning with belladonna. It is described by Gmelin. The subject was a shepherd who died comatose twelve hours after eating the berries. When the body was examined twelve hours after death, putrefaction had begun, so that the belly was swelled, the scrotum and penis distended with fetid serum, the skin covered with dark vesicles, and the brain soft. The blood-vessels of the head were gorged, and the blood every where fluid, and flowing profusely from the mouth, nose, and eyes.[**] In the only other fatal case I have read, where the body was inspected, there appears to have been no unusual appearance at all.[††]

As the husks and seeds of the berries are very indigestible, some of them will almost certainly be found in the stomach, as happened in the instance last quoted. It should likewise be remembered that the best possible evidence of the cause of the symptoms may be derived during life from the presence of the seeds, husks, or even entire berries, in the discharges. If vomiting has not been brought on at

---

[*] On Vegetable Poisons, p. 18.   [†] Roux's Journal de Méd. xxiv. 321.
[‡] Geschichte der Pflanzengifte, p. 538.
[§] Die Wirkung der Arzneimittel und Gifte, i. 347-364.
[||] Mag. für die gesammte Heilk. xxv. 578.
[¶] Journal de Chim. Méd. iv. 390.   [**] Geschichte der Pflanzengifte, p. 538.
[††] Histoire de l'Acad. de Paris, 1703, p. 69.

an early period, we may expect to find these remains both in the vomited matter and in the alvine evacuations. Mr. Wilmer mentions an instance. in which the black husks appeared in the stools brought away by laxatives at least thirty hours after the poison was swallowed.* One of Mr. Brumwell's patients vomited the seeds towards the close of the third day.† Several patients of M. Boucher vomited fragments of the fruit on the second day, and passed more by stool and injections on the third, although they had been treated with activity from the commencement.‡

While most of the cases of poisoning with belladonna have originated in accident, at the same time they have not been all of this description. Gmelin has quoted an instance of intentional and fatal poisoning by the juice of the berries being mixed with wine; and another singular case of poisoning with the decoction of the buds, given by an old woman for the purpose of committing theft during the stupor of the individual.§

Other species of atropa are probably similar to belladonna in properties. Wibmer quotes a single instance of frantic delirium occurring among several shepherds, as well as their cattle, from eating the herb of the *A. mandragora.*‖ This is well known to have been used anciently as a medicinal narcotic.

Of Poisoning with Thorn-Apple.

The thorn-apple, or *Datura stramonium,* is another plant of the same natural order, which it is proper to notice, because people have often been poisoned with it, and it has become a common ornament of our gardens. The cases of poisoning which have occurred in recent times in this country have been all accidental. But not long ago the thorn-apple appears to have been extensively used in Germany to cause loss of consciousness and lethargy, preparatory to the commission of various crimes.¶ It was also proved to have been used lately in France for this purpose. Some thieves made a man insensible with wine in which stramonium seeds had been steeped, and robbed him of five hundred francs while in this state. For twenty-four hours the victim knew nothing of what became of him; he was met wandering in a wood, affected with delirium, unconsciousness, staring of the eyes, and oppression of the breathing; and for some time he was taken for a madman.** In the Eastern Archi-

---

* On Vegetable Poisons, p. 21   † Med. Obs. and Inq. vi. 224.
‡ Roux's Journ. de Méd. xxiv. 317.
§ Geschichte des Pflanzengifte, 527.
‖ Die Wirkung der Arzneimittel, &c. i. 378.
¶ Gmelin, Geschichte der Pflanzengifte, 416. As examples of such crimes he mentions the following. Diebe und Huren um ihr Verbrechen desto ungehinderter zu begehen, wenn sie die Leute damit eingeschläfert haben ; Hurenwirthinnen, um in ihren gemietheten Mägdchen alles Gefühl der natürlichen Schaam zu ersticken ; alte Hurer um junge Mägdchen zu verführen; Missethäter um ihre Wächter sinnlos zu machen ; Ehebrecherinnen, um ihre Männer zu ruhigen Zuschauern ihrer Schandthaten zu machen. For most of these purposes gin and whisky are the instruments of villany in Britain ; and of late, as already mentioned, opium has been resorted to.
** Journal de Chimie Médicale, 1836, 319.

pelago, according to Mr. Crawford, this is a common mode of committing theft and robbery.*

It is chiefly the fruit and seeds that have hitherto been examined; but the whole plant is probably poisonous. Brandes discovered in it a volatile, oleaginous, alkaline substance, which he supposed to be its active principle.† But, though his observations were confirmed by Bley,‡ it now appears that the real principle is a colourless, crystalline alkaloidal substance, of an acrid taste like tobacco, which was discovered more lately by Geiger and Hesse; this is named daturine, or daturia.§

The physiological effects of the extract have been determined by Orfila. He found that half an ounce killed a dog within twenty-four hours after being swallowed, that a quarter of an ounce applied to a wound killed another in six hours, and that thirty grains killed another when injected into the jugular vein. The symptoms were purely nervous, and not very prominent. Hence this poison, like the former, acts through the blood-vessels, and probably on the brain.‖ Bley's daturia proves quickly fatal to small animals in the dose of a few drops. The crystalline daturia of Geiger and Hesse kills a sparrow in the dose of an eighth of a grain, and occasions great and persistent dilatation of the pupil when applied to the eye.

Symptoms in Man. — The symptoms produced by a poisonous dose in man are variable. The leading features are great delirium, dilatation of the pupils, and stupor; but sometimes spasms occur, and occasionally palsy.

Dr. Fowler has related the case of a little girl who took a drachm and a half of the seeds. In less than two hours she was attacked with maniacal delirium, accompanied with spectral illusions; and she remained in this state most of the following night, but had some intervals of lethargic sleep. Next morning, after the operation of a laxative, she fell fast asleep, and after some hours she awoke quite well.¶ In a case somewhat like this, related in Henke's Journal, the child had general redness of the skin, swelling of the belly, locked jaw, tremors of the extremities, and an attitude and expression as if about to tumble into a pit. Recovery took place after the action of an emetic.**

In two instances, one related by Vicat in his treatise on the poisonous plants of Switzerland,†† the other by Dr. Swaine‡‡ in the Edin. Phys. and Lit. Essays, the leading symptoms were furious delirium and palsy of the whole extremities. In the instances of three children related by Alibert there were delirium, restlessness, constant incoherent talking, dancing and singing, with fever and flushed face.§§ In another recorded by Dr. Young, there were some convulsions, and

* History of the Eastern Archipelago, i. 466.
† Schweigger's Journal, xxvi. 98.   ‡ Annalen der Pharmacie, iii. 135.
§ Journal de Pharmacie, xx. 94.   ‖ Orfila, Tox. ii. 271.
¶ Edin. Medical Commentaries, v. 163.
** Braun in Henke's Zeitschrift für die Staatsarzneikunde, xxix 177.
†† Orfila, Toxicol. Gén. ii. 247.   ‡‡ Edin. Phys. and Lit. Essays, ii. 272.
§§ Corvisart's Journ. de Méd. xxiii. 157.

57*

livid suffusion of the countenance.*   In an instance communicated
to me by my colleague Dr. Traill, where eighteen or twenty grains
of extract of stramonium were taken by mistake for sarsaparilla, the
symptoms were dryness of the throat immediately afterwards, then
giddiness, dilated pupils, flushed face, glancing of the eyes, and incoherence, so that he seemed to his friends to be intoxicated: and
subsequently there was incessant unconnected talking, like that of
demency.   Emetics were given without effect, and little amendment
was obtained from blood-letting, leeches on the temples, cold to the
head, or purgatives.   But after a glass of strong lemonade vomiting
took place, the symptoms began to recede, in ten hours he recognized those around him, and next day he was pretty well.   Kaauw
Boerhaave has related with great minuteness the case of a girl who
very nearly lost her life in consequence of a man having given her
the powder in coffee with the view of seducing her.   The symptoms
were redness of the features, delirium, nymphomania, loss of speech;
then fixing of the eyes, tremors, convulsions, and coma; afterwards
tetanic spasm and slow respiration with the coma.   She was with
much difficulty roused for a time by the operation of emetics, and
eventually got well after her lethargy had lasted nearly a day.†   In
another related in Rust's Magazin, and caused by a decoction of the
fruit, which was mistaken for thistle-heads, the leading symptoms
were spasmodic closing of the eyelids and jaws, spasms also of the
back, complete coma, and excessive dilatation and insensibility of the
pupil.‡   This case, which seems to have been a very dangerous one,
was rapidly cured by free blood-letting.   Blood-letting, indeed, seems
peculiarly called for in poisoning with thorn-apple, on account of the
strong signs of determination of blood to the head. — Gmelin has
quoted several fatal cases, one of which endured for six hours only;§
and Dr. Young says, that a child has been killed by a single apple.‖
The most complete account yet published of the phenomena of poisoning with stramonium when fatal is given by Mr. Duffin of London.
A child of his own, two years old, swallowed about 100 seeds without chewing them.   Soon after she became fretful and like a person
intoxicated; in the course of an hour efforts to vomit ensued, together with flushed face, dilated pupils, incoherent talking, and afterwards wild spectral illusions and furious delirium.   In two hours and
a half she lost her voice and the power of swallowing, evidently
owing to spasms of the throat.   Then croupy breathing and complete
coma set in, with violent spasmodic agitation of the limbs, occasional
tetanic convulsions, warm perspiration, and yet an imperceptible
pulse.   Subsequently the pulse became extremely rapid, the belly
tympanitic, and the bladder paralyzed, but with frequent involuntary
stools, probably owing to the administration of cathartics; and death
took place in twenty-four hours.   At an early period twenty seeds

* Edin. Med. and Surg. Journal, xv. 154.
† Gmelin, Gesch. der Pflanzengifte, 421.
‡ Magazin für die gesammte Heilkunde, xvii. 564.
§ Gmelin, 420.   ‖ Edin. Med. and Surg. Journal, xv. 154.

were discharged by an emetic: the stools contained eighty; and none were found in the alimentary canal after death. There was never any marked sign of congestion of blood in the head, except flushed face at the beginning.* Dr. Droste of Osnaburg has related a fatal case occasioned by a decoction of 125 seeds given to remove colic. In fifteen minutes the patient became delirious, but soon fell apparently fast asleep, and died in seven hours without again awaking.†

Dangerous effects may result from the application of the thorn-apple to the skin when deprived of the cuticle. An instance has been lately published of alarming narcotism from the application of the leaves to an extensive burn.‡

Morbid Appearances. — As to the *morbid appearances*, Droste found in his case redness of the cardiac end of the stomach, which contained two table-spoonfuls of a pulpy matter mixed with black and white grains, the remains of the teguments of the seeds ; and there was also lividity of the back, lividity of the lungs, emptiness of the cavities of the heart, and gorging of the vessels of the brain. Haller says he once found general congestion of the brain and sinuses,§ — an appearance which may naturally be expected, considering the signs of strong determination of blood towards the head, which often prevail during life. In Mr. Duffin's case, however, the brain was healthy, not congested ; the stomach and intestines presented no morbid appearance ; and the only unusual appearances observed were a slight blush over the pharynx, larynx, and upper third of the gullet, thickening and swelling of the rima glottidis, and a semi-coagulated state of the blood.

Of Poisoning with Tobacco.

A plant of the same natural order with the two former, tobacco, the *Nicotiana tabacum* of botanists, is familiarly known to be in certain circumstances a virulent poison. Every part of the plant possesses active properties. It has been used as a poison in this country for criminal purposes.

Vauquelin analyzed it some time ago, and procured an acrid volatile principle which he called nicotine.‖ This substance, which was afterwards obtained in a purer state as a crystalline body by Hermbstädt, has been more recently ascertained by MM. Posselt and Reimarus to be nothing else than essential oil of tobacco, which is sold at ordinary temperatures ; and they succeeded in procuring another principle which they consider the true nicotina. This is fluid at 29° F., volatile, extremely acrid, alkaline, and capable of forming crystallizable salts with some of the acids.§ Tobacco then appears to contain an acrid alkaline principle, and an essential oil to which the alkaloid

* London Medical Gazette, xv. 320.
† Henke's Zeitschrift für die Staatsarzneikunde, xxxiii. 129.
‡ Journal de Chim. Méd. ʀi. 722.   § Hist. Stirp. Helvet. Indig. i. 259.
‖ Vauquelin — Annales de Chimie, lxxi. 139.
¶ Bulletin des Scien. Méd. xii. 177, from Geiger's Magazin für Pharmacie, Nov. und Dec. 1828.

adheres with great obstinacy.   The relation of the empyreumatic oil
of tobacco to these principles has not been accurately ascertained,
though it probably contains one or other of them.   It is well known
to be an active poison, which produces convulsions, coma and death.
Mr. Morries-Stirling found that its active part is removed from the oil
by washing with weak acetic acid, as he also observed in the instance
of similar oils obtained from various narcotic vegetables.[*]

Process for detecting Tobacco in Organic mixtures. — In a medico-
legal case which happened at Aberdeen in 1834, and of which some
notice is taken at page 651, Dr. Ogston of that city successfully employed the following process for detecting tobacco in the contents of
the stomach.   The contents, consisting of a pulpy fluid, were acidulated with acetic acid, digested, and filtered ; the liquid was treated
with di-acetate of lead, filtered again, freed of lead by hydrosulphuric
acid, filtered a third time, treated with caustic potash, and then allowed to settle.   The supernatant liquid, which had the taste of to-
bacco-juice, was separated and distilled to half its volume.   The distilled liquor had a strong tobacco odour and taste, and some acridity,
and gave a precipitate with infusion of galls.   The residuum in the
retort presented oily particles on its surface, and when heated in an
open basin filled the apartment with a vapour which had a strong
odour of tobacco smoke, and caused in several persons present a sense
of acridity of the throat, watering of the eyes, and tendency to sneeze.
Various additional experiments confirmatory of these results were also
performed ; and a simultaneous examination of tobacco-powder gave
precisely the same indications.   I am indebted to Dr. Ogston for
these particulars and a detailed narrative of his investigation ; which
appears to supply a convenient and conclusive process for the detection of tobacco. — Perhaps the ordinary process for obtaining nicotina
may also be employed with advantage.   This consists in distilling the
suspected substance with caustic potash, neutralizing the distilled
liquor with sulphuric acid, concentrating the product to a thin syrup,
exhausting this with etherized alcohol, evaporating off the solvent, and
distilling the extract with strong solution of potash.   Nicotina passes
over, and may be recognized by its sensible and chemical qualities.

The effects of tobacco are somewhat different from those of belladonna and thorn-apple ; but it is here arranged with them, as it
belongs to the same natural family.   Orfila remarked that $5\frac{1}{2}$ drachms
of common rappee, introduced into the stomach of a dog and secured
by a ligature, caused nausea, giddiness, stupor, twitches in the muscles of the neck, and death in nine hours ; and that two drachms and
a quarter applied to a wound proved fatal in a single hour.   Mr. Blake
thinks tobacco has no direct action on the heart, even when admitted
directly into the blood by the jugular vein ; — that it acts primarily on
the capillary circulation of the lungs, by obstructing which it prevents
the blood from reaching the left cavities of the heart, and thus acts
on that organ indirectly.   For he observed, that laboured respiration
always preceded any sign of depressed action of the heart, that forci-

* Edinburgh Med. and Surg. Journal, xxxix. 382.

ble action of the heart often returned after its first cessation, and that its contractility continued after death.* An infusion of ten grains caused laborious breathing in ten seconds, and in twenty seconds temporary arrestment of the heart's action, which then returned, and was attended for a time with increased arterial pressure. Soon afterwards the animal recovered, without any convulsions or loss of sensibility. Two scruples had the 'same effect. But when three drachms were used, convulsions succeeded similar phenomena, and death ensued in two minutes, the heart continuing to act for some time after respiration had ceased, until at length it was stopped by the usual consequences of asphyxia.† On the other hand, Sir B. Brodie found that the effects are very different, according to the form in which the poison is used. Thus four ounces of a strong infusion, when injected into the anus of a dog, killed it in ten minutes by paralyzing the heart; for after death the blood in the aortal cavities was arterial. But the empyreumatic essential oil does not act in that manner : it excites convulsions and coma, without affecting the heart. It may prove fatal in two minutes.‡ Like other violent poisons, tobacco has no effect when applied directly to the brain or nerves.§ Two drops of the alkaloid, nicotina, injected into the jugular vein of a dog, begin to act in ten seconds, and will prove fatal in a minute and a half.||

Symptoms in Man. — The effects observed in man are allied to those produced in dogs by the infusion. In a slight degree they are frequently witnessed in young men, while making their first efforts to acquire the absurd practice of smoking. The first symptoms are acceleration and strengthening of the pulse, with very transient excitement, then sudden giddiness, fainting and great sickness, accompanied with a weak, quivering pulse. These effects are for the the most part transient and trifling, but not always. Some degree of somnolency is not uncommon. Dr. Marshall Hall has given an interesting account of a young man who smoked two pipes for his first debauch, and in consequence was seized with nausea, vomiting, and syncope, then stupor, stertorous breathing, general spasms and insensible pupils. Next day the tendency to faint continued, and in the evening the stupor, stertor and spasms returned ; but from that time he recovered steadily.¶ Gmelin has quoted two cases of death from excessive smoking, — caused in one by seventeen, in the other by eighteen pipes, smoked at a sitting.** It is likewise mentioned by Lanzoni that an individual fell into a state of somnolency and died lethargic on the twelfth day in consequence of taking too much snuff;†† Dr. Cheyne says, " he is convinced apoplexy is one of the evils in the train of that disgusting practice ;"‡‡ and I have met with an instance where the excessive use of snuff, occasioned twice, at distant intervals, an attack

* Edinburgh Med. and Surg. Journal, li. 340. † Ibidem.
‡ Philosophical Transactions, ci. 186, 181.
§ Macartney. — Orfila, Toxicol. Gén. ii. 282.
|| Blake, in Edin. Med. and Surg. Journal, liii. 44.
¶ Edin. Med. and Surg. Journal, xii. 11. ** Pflazengifte, 550.
†† Ephem. Cur. Nat. Dec. ii. — Ann. x. p. 222.
‡‡ On Apoplexy and Lethargy, p. 150.

resembling imperfect apoplexy, united with delirium. Such cases, however, must be admitted to be rare ; and the practice of taking snuff is in general unattended with injury.

Serious consequences have resulted from the application of tobacco to the abraded skin. In the Ephemerides an account is given of three children who were seized with giddiness, vomiting, and fainting from the application of tobacco-leaves to the head for the cure of ring-worm.[*] Dr. Merriman has also alluded to an instance of death in a child from the incautious employment of a strong decoction of tobacco as a lotion for ring-worm of the scalp.[†] And in Leroux's Journal there is an account of a man, who, after using a tobacco decoction for the cure of an eruptive disease, was seized with symptoms of poisoning, and died in three hours.[‡]

In recent times poisoning with tobacco has been often produced by the employment of too large doses in the way of injection. Richard has mentioned a case, not fatal, which arose from an infusion of five leaves in a choppin of water, used as an injection by a lady for cos-tiveness. She was immediately seized with colic, giddiness, buzzing in the ears, headache, nausea, and then syncope of seven hours' duration. During this period the breathing was difficult, the pulse very slow, the pupils dilated, the skin cold and moist, the urine sup-pressed, the efforts to vomit constant, and the belly depressed, con-tracted, and affected with constant borborygmus. She recovered under the use of emollient injections and fomentations.[§] Dr. Grahl of Hamburg has related minutely a fatal case, which arose from an ounce of rather more, boiled for fifteen minutes in water, and admi-nistered by advice of a female quack. The individual, who laboured merely under dyspepsia and obstinate costiveness, was seized in two minutes with vomiting, violent convulsions, and stertorous breath-ing, and died in three-quarters of an hour.[‖] Another accident of the same kind is noticed in the Journal de Chimie Médicale, where the person became as it were intoxicated, and died immediately. In-stead of an infusion of two drachms she had used a decoction of two ounces.[¶] — M. Tavignot describes the following remarkable case oc-casioned by a similar dose. An infusion prepared by mistake with two ounces and one drachm, instead of a drachm and a half, was used as an injection for a stout man affected with ascarides. In seven minutes he was seized with stupor, headache, paleness of the skin, pain in the belly, indistinct articulation, and slight convulsive tremors, at first confined to the arms, but afterwards general. Extreme prostra-tion and slow laborious breathing soon ensued, and then coma, which ended fatally in eighteen minutes.[**] — Even two drachms, however, or a drachm and a half, are by no means a safe dose. An

* Ephem. Cur. Nat. Dec. ii. — Ann. iv. p. 467.
† London Medical Gazette, 1839-40, i. 561.
‡ Journal de Chimie Médicale, 1839, 329.   § Ibidem, 165.
‖ Hufeland's Journal der Praktischen Heilkunde, lxxi. iv. 100.
¶ Journal de Chimie Médicale, iii. 23.
** Gazette Med. de Paris, 28 Novembre, 1840, or Edinburgh Med. and Surg. Journal, lv. 558.

anonymous writer in the Medical and Surgical Journal says a patient of his died in convulsions an hour or two after receiving a clyster composed of two drachms infused in eight ounces.* Nay, in the Acta Helvetica there is an account by an anonymous writer of the case of a woman, who, after an injection made with one drachm only, was seized with pain in the belly, anxiety and faintings, proving fatal in a few hours.† And a case, fatal in thirty-five minutes, which was occasioned by the same dose, occurred not long ago in Guy's Hospital, London.‡

Tobacco is an equally deadly poison when swallowed in large quantity. M. Caillard has related the particulars of the case of a lunatic, who, having swallowed half an ounce of snuff during a lucid interval, was seized with vomiting, and afterwards with oppression, incoherence, cold sweats, a slow full pulse, and dilated pupils; but he slowly recovered.§ The French poet Santeuil was killed in this way by a practical joker at the Prince of Condé's table. When the bottle had circulated rather freely, a boxful of Spanish snuff was emptied into a large glass of wine, and thus administered to the unlucky victim, who was in consequence " attacked with vomiting and fever, and expired in two days amidst the tortures of the damned."‖ The following important case has been communicated to me by Dr. Ogston of Aberdeen, who was employed in the judicial investigations connected with it. An elderly man, a pensioner, was seen to enter a brothel, while in perfect health; and in an hour he was carried out insensible and put down in a passage, where he was found by the police unable to speak or move. While carrying him to the watch-house hard by, the officers observed him attempt to vomit; but he was scarcely laid down before the fire, when he expired. It was ascertained, that he had drunk both rum and whisky in the brothel, and that something had been given him " to stupefy him or set him asleep." On dissection the blood was found every where very fluid, and four ounces of serosity were collected from the lateral ventricles and base of the skull. But there was no other unusual appearance, except that the stomach contained about four ounces of a thick brownish pulp, in which were seen several pellets of a powder resembling snuff. In these contents Dr. Ogston could not detect any opium; but he detected tobacco by the process mentioned above. No doubt could exist that the man died of poisoning with tobacco; but as no evidence could be obtained to inculpate any one in particular of many individuals who were in the brothel with him, the case was not made the subject of trial.

Evidence is not wanting, therefore, to prove that this plant is a very active poison; yet every one knows that under the influence of habit it is used in immense quantities over the whole world as an article of luxury, without any bad effect having ever been clearly traced to it. Its poisonous qualities were known in Europe as soon

* Edin. Med. and Surg. Journal, ix. 159.   † Acta Helvetica, 1762, v. 330.
‡ Journal de Chim. Médicale, 1839, 328.   § Ibidem, 327.
‖ Julia-Fontenelle, Ibidem, 1836, 652.   From Mémoires du Duc de St. Simon.

as it was brought from America ; and the belief that such properties could not fail to be attended, as in the case of spirits and opium, with evil consequences from its habitual use, led to much opposition on the part of various governments to its introduction.   Soon after it was brought to England by Sir W. Raleigh, King James wrote a philippic against it, entitled " The Counter-blaste to Tobacco." Some countries even prohibited it by severe edicts.   Amurath the 4th in particular made the smoking of tobacco capital ; several of the Popes excommunicated those who smoked in the church of St. Peter's ; in Russia it was punished with amputation of the nose ; and in the Canton of Bern it ranked in the tables next to adultery, and even so lately as the middle of last century a particular court was held there for trying delinquents.*   Like every other persecuted novelty, however, smoking and snuff-taking passed from place to place with rapidity; and now there appear to be only two luxuries which yield to it in prevalence, spirituous liquors and tea.

The only accounts I have seen of the morbid appearances after poisoning with tobacco are contained in the cases of Dr. Grahl and Dr. Ogston.   In the former there was great lividity of the back, paleness of the lips, flexibility of the joints (two days after death), diffuse redness of the omentum without gorging of vessels, similar redness with gorging of vessels both on the outer and inner coats of the intestines, in some parts of the mucous coat patches of extravasation, unusual emptiness of the vessels of the abdomen ; while the stomach was natural, the lungs pale, the heart empty in all its cavities, and the brain natural.   The appearances in Dr. Ogston's case have been already stated.

Writers on the diseases of artisans have made many vague statements on the supposed baneful effects of the manufacture of snuff on the workmen.†   It is said they are liable to bronchitis, dysentery, ophthalmia, carbuncles and furuncles.   At a meeting of the Royal Medical Society of Paris, however, before which a memoir to this purport was read, the facts were contradicted by reference to the state of the workmen at the Royal Snuff Manufactory of Gros-Caillou, where 1000 people are constantly employed without detriment to their health.‡   This subject was afterwards investigated with care by MM. Parent-Duchatelet and D'Arcet, who inquired minutely into the state of the workmen employed at all the great tobacco-manufactories of France, comprising a population of above 4000 persons ; and the results at which they arrived are, — that the workmen very easily become habituated to the atmosphere of the manufactory, — that they are not particularly subject either to special diseases, or to disease generally, — and that they live on an average quite as long as other tradesmen.§   These facts are derived from accurate statis-

* Paris and Fonblanque's Medical Jurisprudence, ii. 415.
† Rammazini, de Morb. Opificum, 535. — Fourcroy, Essai sur les Mal. des Artizans, 89. — Patissier, Traité des Mal. des Art. 202.
‡ Revue Médicale, 1827, iii. 168.
§ Annales d'Hygiène Publique et de Med. Lég. i. 169. 1829.

tical returns, showing the number of days each person was annually off work from sickness, the ages at which superannuated allowances were granted, the period of death, and the prevalent diseases.

CHAPTER XXXIV.

OF POISONS OF THE UMBELLIFEROUS ORDER OR PLANTS.

THE Natural Order *Umbelliferæ* contains a variety of plants, to which narcotico-acrid properties have been at different times ascribed. But these properties have been satisfactorily traced in the instance of four species only, the *Conium maculatum, Œnanthe crocata, Cicuta virosa,* and *Æthusa cynapium.* It is supposed that others may be poisonous. But the facts on the subject are equivocal ; for the several species of the family are very apt to be confounded with one another, and there is reason to think that other species have repeatedly been mistaken for one of the four already mentioned.

The symptoms caused by the umbelliferous narcotics comprehend chiefly coma, convulsions, paralysis, and delirium. But the knowledge possessed on this head is rather vague, and the phenomena are not unfrequently complex and difficult to observe with accuracy ; so that their nature has been sometimes misunderstood. The irritant properties of the poisons of this tribe of narcotico-acrids are seldom well defined.

Of Poisoning with Hemlock.

The first to be mentioned is the common hemlock, or *Conium maculatum,* one of the most abundantly diffused of umbelliferous vegetables. It is distinguished from all those which it resembles by its tall, smooth, spotted stem, — its smooth leaves, — the rugged edge of the five ribs of its fruit, — its singular mousy odour, — and the very peculiar odour of conia, emitted when the pulp or juice of the leaves is mixed with caustic potash. The only other umbelliferous native which has a spotted stem, the *Myrrhis temulenta,* is easily distinguished from hemlock by the whole plant being very hairy.

Cases of poisoning with hemlock are not infrequent on the continent, the root having been mistaken for fennel, asparagus, parsley, but particularly parsnep.* It is generally believed to have furnished the poison which was used in ancient times, and especially among the Greeks, for despatching criminals; but we have not any precise information on the subject.

A peculiar alkaloid was indicated in hemlock not long ago by Brandes, half a grain of which killed a rabbit with symptoms like those of tetanus.† Other chemists were unable to obtain his results.

---

* Gmelin's Pflanzengifte, S. 598.
† Philosophical Magazine, N. S. iv. 231.

But the subject was afterwards taken up with success by Geiger, who obtained from the plant a volatile, oleaginous alkaloid, which possesses great energy as a poison.* Mr. Morries-Stirling procured from hemlock by destructive distillation an empyreumatic oil similar in properties to those of hyoscyamus, stramonium and tobacco, but producing in animals a state of pure coma.†

The effects of hemlock on the animal system have been variously described by different observers. Sometimes they have appeared to be purely soporific like those of opium ; at other times they have resembled the effects of belladonna and thorn-apple ; and in the lower animals they are quite different, as I have witnessed them, from what they have been described to be in man, — the phenomena being simply those of asphyxia from paralysis of the muscles, without material convulsions and without insensibility. Its irritant action is not well established.

Orfila observed that an ounce of the extract of the leaves killed a dog in forty-five minutes when swallowed, ninety grains killed another through a wound in an hour and a half, and twenty-eight grains another through a vein in two minutes. It therefore acts by entering the blood-vessels. The extract is a very uncertain preparation ; the reason of which is, that the alkaloid conia is very easily decomposed in its natural state of mixture by heat or age, being converted into an inert resinoid matter, — that the dried leaves of hemlock contain scarcely any of it, — and that even an extract of the fresh leaves contains little, unless prepared with a gentle heat, yet speedily.‡ The symptoms remarked by Orfila were convulsions and insensibility; and in the dead body the blood of the left cavities of the heart was sometimes found arterial.— The result of my observations is quite at variance with this statement. In various experiments with a strong extract prepared from the green seeds with absolute alcohol, the only effect I could remark were palsy, first of the voluntary muscles, next of the chest, lastly of the diaphragm,— asphyxia in short from paralysis, without insensibility, and with slight occasional twitches only of the limbs, and the heart was always found contracting vigorously for a long time after death. Thirty grains of a soft extract introduced between the skin and muscles of the back killed a rabbit in five minutes, and a five months' puppy in twenty minutes.§

The root is much less energetic than is represented by some authors, and probably varies in this respect at different seasons. I have found that four ounces and a half of juice, the produce of twelve ounces of roots collected in November, had no effect on a dog when secured in its stomach by a ligature on the gullet; and that four ounces obtained from ten ounces of roots in the middle of June, when the plant was coming into flower, merely caused diarrhœa and languor. Orfila had previously observed that three pounds

---

* Geiger's Magazin für Pharmacie, xxxv. 72, 259.
† Edin. Medical and Surgical Journal, xxxix. 383.
‡ Geiger, in Magazin für Pharmacie, xxxv. 284.
§ Edinburgh Roy. Soc. Transactions, xiii. 398, 415.

of roots had no effect in the month of April; but that two pounds in the end of May, when the plant was in full vegetation, killed a dog in six hours.* The alcoholic extract of the juice obtained from six ounces of roots on the last day of May, I have found to kill a rabbit in thirty-seven minutes, when introduced in a state of emulsion between the skin and muscles of the back; and the effects were analogous to those obtained with the extract of the leaves. The differences depending on season will probably account for various persons having found the juice of the root harmless. Gmelin quotes an instance where four ounces of the juice were taken without injury. He adds another where three ounces of the juice of the herb were swallowed daily for eight days with as little effect. But, as he judiciously observes, other less active plants have probably been sometimes mistaken for hemlock.†

The alkaloid, conia, seems to be the active principle of hemlock, and is a poison of extraordinary virulence. On investigating this subject in 1835,‡ I found that it is a local irritant, possessing an acrid taste, and capable of exciting redness or vascularity in any membrane to which it is applied; but that these topical effects are readily overwhelmed by its swift and intense narcotic action. This action consists of swiftly spreading palsy of the muscles, which affects first those of voluntary motion, then the respiratory muscles of the chest and abdomen, and lastly the diaphragm, so as to terminate by causing asphyxia. The paralytic state is usually interrupted from time to time by slight convulsive twitches of the limbs and trunk at the beginning. The muscular contractility is impaired or annihilated by the topical action of the poison, but not by its indirect action through absorption. The heart is not appreciably affected; for it contracts vigorously long after all motion, respiration, and other signs of life are extinct; and it contains after death, not florid but dark blood in its left cavities. The blood undergoes no alteration. The external senses are little, if at all impaired, until the breathing is almost arrested; and volition too is retained. But a contrary inference may be drawn by a careless observer, in consequence of the paralytic state taking away the means, by which in animals sensation is expressed and volition exercised. The action of conia, in short, is confined to the spinal cord; and it acts as a sedative, by exhausting the nervous energy.

Conia is probably a deadly poison to all orders of animals: at least I found it to be so to the dog, cat, rabbit, mouse, frog, fly, and flea; and Geiger killed the kite, pigeon, sparrow, slow-worm, and earth-worm with it. It acts through every texture where absorption is carried on readily, through the stomach, eye, lungs, cellular tissue, peritonæum, or veins; and its activity is in proportion to the speed with which absorption is carried on in the part. It acts therefore through absorption. Its activity is increased by neutralization with an acid, by which it is rendered much more soluble in water. Few

---

* Toxicologie Gén. ii. 303.   † Pflanzengifte, S. 605.
‡ Transactions of the Royal Soc. of Edinburgh, xiii. 383.

poisons equal it in subtilty and swiftness. A single drop, applied to the eye of a rabbit, will kill it in nine minutes; and three drops in the same way will kill a strong cat in a minute and a half. Five drops, introduced into the throat of a little dog, began to act in thirty seconds, and proved fatal in one minute. And when two grains, neutralized with thirty drops of weak hydrochloric acid, were injected into the femoral vein of a young dog, it died before there was time to note the interval, so that only two or three seconds at most had elapsed, before all internal signs of life were extinct. This extraordinary rapidity of action seems incompatible with its operation taking place by conveyance of the poison with the blood to the spinal cord. Mr. Blake, as formerly mentioned (p. 15), denies that its action in this way was ever so swift in his hands, and alleges that he could never observe the interval to be shorter than fifteen seconds. If the reader, however, will consult the original account of my éxperiment,* which was made along with Dr. Sharpey, he will see that we could scarcely be mistaken as to the interval in that instance.

Symploms in Man.—M. Haaf, a French army surgeon, has described a fatal case of poisoning with hemlock, which closely resembled poisoning with opium. The subject of it, a soldier, had partaken along with several comrades of a soup containing hemlock leaves, and appeared to them to drop asleep not long after, while they were conversing. In the course of an hour and a half they became alarmed on being all taken ill with giddiness and headache; and the surgeon of the regiment was sent for. He found the soldier, who had fallen asleep, in a state of insensibility, from which, however, he could be roused for a few moments. His countenance was bloated, the pulse only 30, and the extremities cold. The insensibility became rapidly deeper and deeper, till he died, three hours after taking the soup.† His companions recovered.

Dr. Watson has briefly described two cases which were fatal in the same short space of time. The subjects were two Dutch soldiers, who, in common with several of their comrades, took broth made with hemlock leaves and various other herbs. Giddiness, coma, and convulsions were the principal symptoms. The men who recovered were affected exactly as if they had taken opium.‡

When the dose is not sufficient to prove fatal, there is sometimes paralysis, attended with slight convulsions, as in a case noticed by Orfila.§ More commonly there is frantic delirium. Matthiol has related an instance of this last description, occurring in the cases of a vine-dresser and his wife, who mistook the roots for parsneps. Both of them became in the course of the night so delirious that they ran about the house, knocking themselves against every object which came in their way.‖ Kircher, as quoted by Wibmer, tells a parallel story of two monks who became so raving mad after eating

* Transactions, &c. xiii. 393, 315.   † Corvisart's Journal de Méd. xxix. 107.
‡ Philos. Transactions, xliii. No. 473, p. 18.   § Toxicol. Gén. ii. 311.
‖ Gmelin's Pflanzengifte, p. 604.

the roots, that they plunged into water, imagining that they were turned into geese, and they were affected for three years with incomplete palsy and neuralgic pains.* These and some other cases of the like kind, recorded by the older medical authors, must be received with reserve. Independently of other considerations, there is often no certainty that the poison was really the hemlock of modern botanists, and not some other umbelliferous vegetable.

Morbid Appearances. — In Haaf's case the vessels of the head were much congested ; and the blood must have been very fluid, for on the head being opened a quantity flowed out, which twice filled an ordinary chamber-pot. This state of the blood likewise occurred in a case which I examined here some years ago along with Dr. C. Coindet of Geneva. A hypochondriacal old woman took by advice of a neighbour two ounces of a strong infusion of hemlock leaves with the same quantity of whisky, which she swallowed in the morning fasting. She died in an hour, comatose and slightly convulsed. The vessels within the head were not particularly turgid ; but the blood was everywhere remarkably fluid. Dr. Coindet subsequently found that a small portion of the infusion prevents fresh drawn blood from coagulating ; but I suspect there must have been some mistake here, for a carefully prepared alcoholic extract of very great power, which was used in my experiments alluded to above, had no such effect on blood fresh drawn from rabbits and dogs. On account of this extreme fluidity of the blood, it often flows from the nose, but the skin is much marked with lividity.† The fluidity of the blood is nothing more than the result of the proximate cause of death, — slowly formed asphyxia.

Of Poisoning with Water-Hemlock.

Another plant of the order Umbelliferæ, the water-hemlock or *Cicuta virosa*, possesses also great energy as a poison ; and in its effects it appears to resemble considerably the hydrocyanic acid. The plant is indigenous. It is easily known from other umbelliferous species inhabiting watery places by the peculiar structure of its root-stock, which is not fleshy, but hollow, and composed of a number of large cells with transverse plates.

From a numerous set of experiments with the root of the cicuta performed by Wepfer, it appears to cause true tetanic convulsions in frequent paroxysms, and death on the third day.‡ Simeon ascertained that the alcoholic extract of the root is very poisonous.§ Schubarth found that an ounce of the juice of the stems and leaves, collected after the flowers had begun to blow, produced no effect on the dog.‖ It is probably inert, or at all events feebly poisonous in this climate, although it grows luxuriantly in many localities. I have

* Die Wirkung der Arzneimittel und Gifte, i. 172.
† Gmelin's Pflanzengifte, p. 603.
‡ Cicut. Aquaticæ Hist. et Noxæ, 134. § Annalen der Pharmacie, xxxi. 258.
‖ Archiv für Medizin. Erfahr. 1824, i. 84.

found that twelve ounces of juice, expressed from sixteen ounces of roots in the beginning of August, merely caused some efforts to vomit, when secured in the stomach of a dog by a ligature on the gullet; that the alcoholic extract of twelve ounces of leaves gathered at the same time had no effect when introduced in the form of emulsion between the skin and muscles of the back of a rabbit; and that the alcoholic extract of two ounces of unripe seeds proved equally inert when imployed in the same way.

Symptoms in Man. — Wepfer has likewise related several instances which occurred in the human subject. Among the rest he has described the cases of eight children who ate the roots instead of parsneps. Of those who were seriously affected, one, a girl six years old, who ultimately recovered, had tetanic fits, followed by deep coma, from which it was impossible to rouse her for twenty-four hours. Two of them died. The first symptoms in these two were swelling in the pit of the stomach, vomiting or efforts to vomit, then total insensibility, with involuntary discharge of urine, and finally severe convulsions, during which the jaws were locked, the eyes rolled, and the head and spine were bent backwards, so that a child might have crept between the body and the bed-clothes. One of them died half an hour after being taken ill, and the other not long after.[*] Mayer of Creutsburg mentions four cases, which were occasioned by the roots. One of the individuals, a child three years old, was attacked with colic, vomiting, and convulsions, and died in a few hours. The three others, the eldest of whom was six years of age, had coldness, paleness of the features, dilated immoveable pupils, violent colic, general spasms, and insensibility. The action of the heart was intermitting and the breathing oppressed. After the remains of the roots were brought up by emetics, and infusion of gall was administered, they gradually recovered. They had eaten between them no more than a single root weighing about two ounces, as they had in their possession another of that weight, which they said was not so large. This accident happened in the middle of March.[†]

According to Guersent, poisoning with the cicuta commences with dimness of sight, giddiness, acute headache, anxiety, pain in the stomach, dryness in the throat, and vomiting.[‡]

Mertzdorff has related the particulars of the inspection of three cases which proved quickly fatal with convulsions and vomiting. Nothing remarkable seems to have been found except great gorging of the cerebral vessels.[§]

Of Poisoning with Hemlock Dropwort.

The *Œnanthe crocata* of botanists, the hemlock-dropwort, five-finger-root, or dead-tongue of vernacular speech in England, a species of the same family with the last two, and an abundant plant in some localities throughout this country, has usually been held one

* Cic. Aquat. &c. 80, and 107.   † Journal de Chimie Médicale, 1842, 877.
‡ Article Ciguë, Diction. des Sciences Méd.
§ Journal Complementaire, xvii. 361.

of the most virulent of European vegetables. It seems well entitled
to this character in general ; but climate, or some other more obscure
cause, renders it inert in some situations.

It is said to be liable to be confounded with common hemlock, or
Conium maculatum, — a mistake which can happen only in very ignorant hands. It has smooth, dark-green leaves, more fleshy, and
much less minutely divided, than those of hemlock; it presents a
purplish appearance at the joints only of the stem, and no diffused
purple spots ; its fruit is oblong and black, not round, rough, and
light brown ; and its root, instead of being single, long, tapering, and
little branched, consists of from two to ten tubers, like fingers, which
are white, and terminate in a few rootlets. These tubers are formed annually in summer from the flowering stem of the season, and send
out flowering stems the subsequent year. During the first autumn,
winter, and spring they are firm, white, and amylaceous ; but in their
second summer they become more pulpy, less amylaceous, and grayer.
At all times they emit, when broken across, an oleo-resinous juice,
which quickly becomes yellow; this juice abounds most when the
plant, which is growing at their expense, is about to flower ; and it
abounds much more at this period in localities in the south of England, than in Scotland, especially in the neighbourhood of Edinburgh.

Brotero and some others have attempted to subdivide the species
into two, the *Œnanthe crocata* proper, and the *Œ. apiifolia*. But the
best authorities deny that these can be distinguished ; and from what
I have now seen in sundry localities, it appears to me that the distinctions pointed out by Brotero, confessedly obscure enough in
themselves, are the result of differences in climate, soil, and situation.

The only analysis of this plant with which I am acquainted is one
executed in 1830 by MM. Cormerais and Pihan-Dufeillay, who found
in the root a resinoid matter, which adheres obstinately to the solid
portion of it, and which seems to be the active ingredient.* I have
subjected the roots to various processes, and among the rest to that
by which Geiger detected conia in hemlock, but without discovering
any indication of the existence of an alkaloid. My materials, however, were not well fitted for a chemical analysis ; because the
œnanthe root of this neighbourhood is inert or nearly so. The whole
plant contains a heavy-smelling volatile oil, which may be obtained
by distillation in the usual way, and most abundantly from the ripe
seeds. This oil is yellowish, viscid, and inert.

It is strange that a plant, so universally considered a potent poison,
and so frequently the cause of fatal accidents, has not yet been made
the subject of physiological investigation. A few imperfect experiments by M. Cormerais and his companion, made with the resinoid
matter of the roots, show that this substance produces in animals dulness, convulsions of the voluntary muscles, a semi-paralytic state of
the hind legs, and sometimes shortness of breath, vomiting, and fluid
evacuations by stool. All the animals experimented on recovered.
On repeating these experiments with larger quantities I found the
resin of the root, grown near Woolwich, and kindly sent to me by

* Journal de Chimie Médicale, 1830.

Dr. Pereira, to be a poison of great energy and singular properties:. Twenty-four grains obtained from eight ounces of roots in the middle of December, when introduced in the form of emulsion between the skin and muscles of the rabbit, caused in half an hour depression, uneasiness, and hurried breathing, — then twitches of the ears, neck, and fore-legs, — next combined spasm and convulsive starting of the head and limbs, — then, after a quiet interval, a more violent fit of the same kind, affecting the whole body with a singular combination of tetanus and convulsive starting, — finally, after several such fits, a paroxysm more violent than before, ending in immoveable tetanic rigidity, which speedily proved fatal, 78 minutes after the application of the poison. No morbid appearance could be detected in the body. The heart contracted vigorously for some time after death. These phenomena correspond in the main with what has been recorded of the symptoms caused by the roots in man. — Dr. Pereira informs me he had found the juice both of the root and leaves to act as a poison, either when introduced into the peritonæum, or when injected into the veins; and in the latter way it was so energetic as to prove fatal in one minute.

Symptoms in Man. — Since Lobel first took notice of the poisonous properties of the œnanthe root in 1570, an uninterrupted series of observations has been published, down to the present day, showing that in France, Germany, Holland, Spain, and various parts of England as far north as Liverpool, it is at all seasons of the year, even in October and in the beginning of January, a poison of great activity. In several of the cases death has been occasioned by a single handful of the roots, in one instance by a piece no bigger than the finger, or even in consequence of the individuals merely tasting them. A girl seems to have had a narrow escape after eating, with an interval of three hours, two pieces of the size of a walnut. Very seldom has death been delayed beyond four hours, and on some occasions a single hour has been sufficient. Sometimes the symptoms have been slow in making their appearance, an hour and a half having occasionally elapsed before the effects were evident; but in every instance their progress was rapid, once the symptoms had fairly set in; and some died in convulsions almost immediately after being taken ill.

The particular effects have been variable. Most generally the first symptoms have been giddiness and staggering, as if from ordinary intoxication, occasionally headache, and often extreme feebleness of the limbs. Stupor has then generally succeeded, sometimes with the intervention of efforts to vomit, sometimes too with an interval of delirium. Convulsions have also commonly made their appearance in the next place; and ere long a state of insensibility has ensued attended in every instance with occasional violent convulsive fits like epilepsy, and with permanent locked-jaw; which symptoms have continued till near death. In one or two cases the individual has suddenly, without any premonitory symptoms, fallen down convulsed, and died almost immediately. In one or two instances again, the effects have rather been those of irritant poisoning, namely, inflammation of the mouth and throat, spasms of the muscles.

of the throat, vomiting, and excessive weakness and faintness, without any convulsions or insensibility. — It appears then that this plant is a true narcotico-acrid poison. The emanations from the plant are said on some occasions to have proved injurious ; but the effect here was probably the work of the imagination.

Aware of these singular properties being generally ascribed to the *Œnantl e crocata*, I was anxious to make a methodical examination of the subject, physiologically as well as chemically, — especially as the plant grows in great abundance and very luxuriantly in a locality not far from Edinburgh. But I have found it in that situation, to all appearance, quite inert. The juice of fourteen ounces of the root in the end of October had no effect on a little dog when secured in the stomach by a ligature on the gullet. The juice of sixteen ounces in the middle of June was also without effect. An alcoholic extract of four ounces of the full grown leaves in the end of June, introduced into the cellular tissue in the form of emulsion, had no effect on a rabbit. An alcoholic extract of three ounces of the ripe seeds was administered in the same way with the same result. Finally, the resinoid extract of eight ounces of the root, analogous to that which had proved so deadly in my hands when obtained from Woolwich plants, had also no effect whatever, when prepared from those growing in the neighbourhood of Edinburgh. Relying upon these results, I ate a whole tuber weighing an ounce, without observing any effect, except its disagreeable taste ; which was the only circumstance that prevented me from trying a larger quantity. — It may be well to add, that, amidst the numerous cases of poisoning with œnanthe now on record, there is not one that has occurred in Scotland. At the same time, the common people in Scotland are not at all given to rash experiments in cookery, or to make use of vegetables not produced by the care of the gardener or farmer.*

The only other locality from which I have been hitherto able to obtain plants for examination is the neighbourhod of Liverpool, where a fatal case of poisoning with it occurred near the close of last century. When the juice of sixteen ounces of this root in the beginning of September was secured in the stomach of a dog, efforts to vomit were produced, followed by several fits of violent convulsions and spasm of the voluntary muscles, a paralytic state of the fore-legs, and a constant tendency to fall backwards ; but the animal recovered.

No morbid appearances of any note have been observed after death in any of the fatal cases which are recorded. — The most appropriate treatment consists in the prompt employment of emetics, and diffusible stimulants.

Of Poisoning with Fool's Parsley.

Another umbelliferous plant of great activity is fool's parsley, or

---

* Instead of quoting special facts on the subject of poisoning with Œnanthe, I have thought it better to give in the meantime a short analysis of a long investigation, which I have from time to time made on the subject, and which was read in the Royal Society of Edinburgh last year. This paper will be published ere long ; and the references and experiments will then be supplied, which, if introduced here, will lead to disproportionate details.

Æthusa cynapium. It has occasioned several accidents by reason of
its resemblance to parsley, — from which, however, it is at once
distinguished by the leaves being dark and glistening on their lower
surface, and by the nauseous smell they emit when rubbed. It contains an alkaloid, which crystallizes in rhombic prisms, and is soluble
in water and alcohol, but not in ether. It was discovered by Professor
Ficinus of Dresden.*

Orfila found that six ounces of the juice, when retained in the
stomach of a dog, by a ligature, caused convulsions and stupor, and
death in an hour.†

Symptoms in Man. — Some interesting information on the characters and properties of this plant is contained in the Medical and
Physical Journal. Among other cases the writer relates those of
two ladies who ate a little of it in a sallad instead of parsley, and who
were soon seized with nausea, vomiting, headache, giddiness, somnolency, pungent heat in the mouth, throat, and stomach, difficulty in
swallowing and numbness of the limbs.‡ Gmelin has related the
case of a child, who died in eight hours in consequence of having
eaten the æthusa. The symptoms were spasmodic pain in the stomach, swelling of the belly, lividity of the skin, and difficult breathing.§ In two children who recovered, the chief symptoms at the
height of the poisoning were complete insensibility, dilated, insensible
pupil, and staring of the eyes. In one of them there was also frequent vomiting, in the other convulsions. The treatment consisted
in the administration of milk, sinapisms to the legs, and cold spunging
with vinegar.||

CHAPTER XXXV.

OF THE NARCOTIC RANUNCULACEÆ.

THE greater part of the poisons belonging to the Natural Family
Ranunculaceæ are acrid only in their action, and have been already
taken notice of among the irritants. Two only are yet known to possess narcotic properties, namely, *monkshood*, and *black hellebore*. The
latter is a true narcotico-acrid. The former has till lately been always
considered so ; but its acrid properties seem doubtful or feeble, while
its action on the nervous system is most intense.

Of Poisoning with Monkshood.

Monkshood, the *Aconitum napellus* of botanists, is an active poison, and has commonly been considered a true narcotico-acrid. But
its effects have been hitherto much misunderstood. It has been used
for criminal purposes in Ireland ; and in 1841, a woman, M‘Conkey,

---

* Lond. Philos. Magazine, N. S. ii. 392.
† Toxicol. Gén. ii. 323.   ‡ London Med. and Phys. Journal, xiv. 425.
§ Geschichte der Pflanzengifte, 571.
|| Wittke in Magazin für Pharmacie, xxxii. 228.

who was executed there for poisoning her husband, was proved to have administered this substance [see p. 61]. The root of another species, the *A. ferox*, is well known to be in common use as a poison, under the name of Bikh, in Bengal, and Nabee, in the Madras Presidency.

The toxicological history of the genus, and of this species in particular, has been rendered complex and obscure, by the extreme difficulty of distinguishing accurately the several species from one another. The whole genus, now a numerous one, is generally conceived to be eminently poisonous. But from some observations of my own, as well as an elaborate inquiry, not yet made public, by Dr. Alexander Fleming,* a recent graduate of this university, I am inclined to think that this is a mistake, that the poisonous species are not numerous, and that many aconites are inert, at least in this climate.

The *A. napellus*, a doubtful native of Britain, and the most common species in our gardens, shoots up annually a leafy stem from a black, tapering, spindle-shaped root. The stem, which is from two to five feet high, ends in a long dense spike of fine blue flowers; and when the seeds ripen in autumn, it dies down, and the root also shrivels and perishes. But in the spring, while the stem is rising, one or more tubers form near the crown of the root; each tuber quickly assumes the spindle-shaped form of its parent, but has a light brown, instead of a brownish-black tegument; and when the plant is in flower, the new tuber, destined for the root of next year's plant, is as large as the parent one, firmer, more amylaceous, and not so apt to shrivel in drying. This mode of propagation has led some to describe the root erroneously as sometimes palmated. Dr. Fleming considers the young, full-grown tuber to be the most active part of the plant; but the root of the existing plant, the leaves, and also the seeds, are highly energetic; and every part is more or less so.

Every part of the *A. napellus*, but especially the root, affects remarkably the organs of taste, producing a very singular sense of heat, numbness, and tingling of those parts of the mouth to which it is applied. Dr. Fleming has ascertained, that this peculiar taste, or rather sensation, is a property belonging to the narcotic principle of monkshood, and that in all probability it is a measure of the activity of the plant as a poison. It is most intense in the root, next in the seeds, and next in the leaves before the flowers blow. Geiger first ascertained, and I have since observed, that the sensation thus occasioned by the leaves diminishes in intensity as the flowers expand, and almost disappears when the seeds ripen. Contrary to what has been often stated, it is not diminished by drying the leaves, even with the heat of the vapour-bath. Nor is it materially lessened by time, if the dried leaves be preserved with care; for I have found it intense after six years. Geiger observed some years ago, that several species or varieties do not possess it. I have ascertained that *A.*

* Prize Thesis, on the Physiological and Medicinal Properties of the Aconitum napellus. Edinburgh, 1844.

napellus, *sinense*, *tauricum*, *uncinatum*, and *ferox*, possess it intensely, *A.* *schleicheri* and *nasutum* feebly, *A.* *neomontanum* very
feebly ; all of which are therefore probably poisonous, in proportion
to the intensity of their taste. *A. ferox*, well known as a deadly
poison in the East, and undoubtedly the most virulent of all the species, produces by far the most intense and persistent effect on the
mouth of all the species I have had an opportunity of examining.
Those which do not produce it at all, at least in this climate, are *A.*
paniculatum, lasiostomum, vulparia, variegatum, nitidum, pyrenaïcum,
and *ochroleucum*. It would be premature to say that all these species are inert ; but I suspect they are : and, at all events, I have
ascertained that the leaves of *A. paniculatum*, although the officinal
species recognised in the London Pharmacopœia, are quite inactive
in this climate ; and Dr. Fleming has found the root inert in medicinal doses of considerable magnitude.

The properties of monkshood have been traced by Geiger and
Hesse to a peculiar alkaloid, named aconitina : which is white,
pulverulent, fusible, not volatile, soluble in ether and alcohol,
sparingly so in water, and capable of forming crystallizable salts
with acids. It produces most intensely the peculiar impression
caused by the plant on the mouth, tongue, and lips ; and it is a
poison of tremendous activity, probably indeed the most subtle of
all known poisons. Although not a volatile principle, it has been
supposed peculiarly liable to decomposition by heat, at least in its
natural state of combination in the plant or its pharmaceutic preparations. This opinion is founded on the uncertainty of the medicinal
action of the common extract of the shops, and on the results of experiments on animals by Orfila.[*] In one experiment he found that
half an ounce of the extract of the Parisian shops had no effect at
all on a dog, while a quarter of an ounce killed another within two
hours. Careless preparation may account for such differences ; but
at the same time an error in choosing the species of plant is an
equally probable explanation. The properties of monkshood appear
to me to resist a heat of 212°, either in drying the plant or in preparing an extract from it.

The medico-legal chemistry of monkshood has not been studied.
If any of the suspected matter be obtained in a pure state, its best
character is its remarkable taste ; to which I have found nothing
exactly similar in the numerous trials I have made with other narcotic and acrid plants. A complex substance, such as the contents
of the stomach, or vomited matter, should be evaporated over the
vapour-bath to the consistence of thin syrup, and agitated with absolute alcohol. The filtered alcoholic solution being then evaporated,
the extract may be subjected to the sense of taste.

Action. — The action of monkshood is a subject of great interest,
but has hitherto been much misunderstood. Sir B. Brodie, who
was the first to examine it in recent times, found that the leading
phenomena in animals, were staggering, excessive weakness, slow

* Toxicologie Gén. 1827, ii. 211.

laborious respiration, and slight convulsive twitches before death.* Had these observations been followed up by his successors with a discriminating eye, toxicologists would not have been so much misled as they have been. Orfila, who was the next to examine the subject experimentally, failed to appreciate the phenomena with exactness.† He thinks monkshood acts peculiarly upon the brain, causing delirium, and that it is a local irritant, capable of developing more or less intense inflammation. A single experiment made in 1836 convinced me that the former statement is incorrect, and led me to consider that the symptoms depend in a great measure on gradually-increasing paralysis of the muscles, which terminates in immobility of the chest and diaphragm, and consequent asphyxia. Dr. Pereira, in some experiments with an alcoholic extract, published in 1842, took notice of two remarkable phenomena, — an extraordinary diminution of common sensation, evidenced by the animal being insensible to pinching and pricking, — and the total absence of stupor, as shown by the animal following its owner, and recognizing him when called.‡ Similar observations have been made in poisoning with monkshood in man. The ablest investigation yet undertaken into the actions of this substance is contained in the unpublished Inaugural Dissertation of Dr. Fleming.

He found that the most remarkable symptoms are weakness and staggering, gradually increasing paralysis of the voluntary muscles, slowly increasing insensibility of the surface, more or less blindness, great languor of the pulse, and convulsive twitches before death. He farther observed that the pupil becomes much contracted ; that the irritability of the voluntary muscles is impaired ; that the veins are congested after death, the blood unaltered, and the heart capable of contracting for some time after respiration has ceased. Lastly, he maintains that this poison has not, as is generally thought, any irritant properties, that neither the plant, nor its extract, nor its alkaloid occasions vascularity in any membrane to which it is applied, even, for example, in the lips or tongue while burning and tingling from its topical action ; that this peculiar effect is therefore merely a nervous phenomenon ; and that he never could observe either the diffuse cellular inflammation described by Orfila to arise from the application of monkshood to a wound, or the inflammatory redness of the alimentary canal noticed by others as one of its effects when swallowed.

Orfila ascertained that monkshood exerts its action through the medium of the blood ; for its effects are greater when it is introduced into a wound, than when it is swallowed, and they are still greater when it is injected directly into a vein. It is a poison of very great activity. I have found that thirty grains of an alcoholic extract, the produce of three-quarters of an ounce of fresh leaves, will kill a rabbit in two hours and a quarter, if introduced between

* Philosophical Transactions, 1811, p. 183.
† Toxicologie Gén. 1827, ii. 211, and 1843, ii. 361.
‡ Elements of Materia Medica, 1842, ii. 1804.

59

the skin and muscles of the back.   Five drachms of the root in one of Orfila's experiments with the dog, occasioned death in twenty-one minutes, when swallowed.

The alkaloid, aconitina, seems to produce in animals precisely the same effects as the plant or its extract.   Orfila and Dr. Pereira agree in this ; and my own observation, limited to a single experiment, is to the same effect.   It is probably the most subtile of all known poisons.   Dr. Pereira mentions that the fiftieth part of a grain has endangered life when used medicinally.*   In my experiment the tenth of a grain, introduced in the form of hydrochlorate into the cellular tissue of a rabbit, killed it in twelve minutes.

Symptoms in Man. — A perplexing discrepance exists in the accounts that have been published of the effects of monkshood on man ; which seems to have arisen, less from any actual contrariety in the phenomena, than from loose observation, or a misunderstanding of the facts ; for most of the recent statements of competent observers are consistent with one another.

Dr. Fleming says that in medicinal doses it occasions warmth in the stomach, nausea, numbness and tingling in the lips and cheeks, extending more or less over the rest of the body, diminution in the force and frequency of the pulse, which sometimes sinks to 40 in the minute, great muscular weakness, confusion of sight or absolute blindness ; and if the dose be unduly large, there is a sense of impending death, sometimes slight delirium, and a want of power to execute what the will directs, but without any loss of consciousness.   The warmth which is excited is unattended with any elevation of temperature, vascularity of the skin, or acceleration of the pulse.   No true hypnotic effect is produced ; but by inducing serenity, or deadening pain, it may predispose to sleep.   The highest degree of these effects is not unattended with danger.

When it is administered in doses adequate to occasion death, it seems in general to operate by inducing extreme depression of the circulation.   Dr. Fleming recognizes two other modes of death in animals, — first, by an overwhelming depression of the nervous system, proving fatal in a few seconds, without arresting the action of the heart, — and secondly, by asphyxia, or arrestment of the respiration, the result of paralysis gradually pervading the whole muscular system, respiratory, as well as voluntary.   But these effects, he thinks, cannot be recognized in the cases which have been published of poisoning in man, because the dose required to produce either of them is very large.   The least variable symptoms in the human subject are, first, numbness, burning, and tingling in the mouth, throat, and stomach, — then sickness, vomiting, and pain in the epigastrium, — next, general numbness, prickling, and impaired sensibility of the skin, impaired or annihilated vision, deafness, and vertigo, — also frothing at the mouth, constriction at the throat, false sensations of weight or enlargement in various parts of the body, — great muscular feebleness and tremor, loss of voice, and laborious breathing,

* Elements of Materia Medica, 1842, ii. 1811.

— distressing sense of sinking and impending death, — a small, feeble, irregular, gradually-vanishing pulse, — cold, clammy-sweat and pale bloodless features, — together with perfect possession of the mental faculties, and no tendency to stupor or drowsiness, — finally, sudden death at last, as from hemorrhage, and generally in a period varying from an hour and a half to eight hours. The symptoms may begin in a few minutes, as in a case observed by Dr. Fleming, which was occasioned by the tincture of the root; or they may be postponed for three-quarters of an hour, as in an instance recorded by Dr. Pereira,* which arose from the root being used by mistake for horse-radish. Two or three drachms of the root are sufficient to kill a man ; and Dr. Fleming mentions one instance where two grains of the alcoholic extract occasioned alarming effects, and another where four grains proved fatal. I may observe, however, that I have given six grains of a carefully prepared alcoholic extract (the same of which thirty grains killed a rabbit in little more than two hours), to a female suffering from rheumatism, without being able to observe any effect whatsoever.

If all the reports of cases now on record are to be trusted, the following anomalies have occurred. Some persons are said to have presented convulsions. Slight spasmodic twitches of the muscles are not uncommon, and probably depend, as Dr. Fleming suggests, on venous congestion, the result of incomplete asphyxia. Stupor and even apoplectic insensibility are also sometimes represented to have been observed. If really ever present, they must depend on the same cause ; but there is reason to apprehend, that extreme nervous depression and faintness have been mistaken for stupor and coma. Delirium of the frantic kind, mentioned by some of the older authors, is justly considered by Dr. Fleming to be of doubtful occurrence, as it has never been observed in recent times. Irritation in the alimentary canal is distinctly mentioned as indicated by prominent symptoms, even in some cases observed but a few years ago, and apparently with care. Dr. Fleming properly objects to nausea, vomiting, or pain in the epigastrium as evidence of irritation in the stomach ; for these symptoms may all depend on the same local nervous impression which is produced on the organs of taste. And he denies that purging is ever produced in any genuine case of poisoning with monkshood. The following, however, seem unequivocal examples of irritation in the alimentary canal. M. Pallas† mentions, that three out of five persons, who took a spirituous infusion of the root by mistake for lovage [*Ligusticum levisticum*], died in two hours with burning in the throat, vomiting, colic, swelling of the belly and purging. A similar set of cases is described by M. Degland.‡ Four persons took the tincture of the root by mistake for tincture of lovage ; and three of them were seized with burning pain from the throat to the stomach, a sense of enlargement of the

* Elements of Materia Medica, 1842, ii. 1806.
† Thèse Inaugurale, Paris, 1822, quoted by Orfila, Toxic. Gén., 1827, ii. 221.
‡ Journal de Chimie Médicale, iii. 344.

tongue and face, colic, tenderness of the belly, vomiting, and purging. One of these, who ultimately recovered, had frantic delirium for some time after the other symptoms went off. The two others died, one in two hours, the other half an hour later. Dr. Pereira* and Dr. Fleming doubt the authenticity of these cases ; and it may be, that such unusual symptoms may have arisen either from some other root mistaken by the narrators for monkshood, or from irritant substances given along with or after it. At the same time I may mention, that in the first trials I made with monkshood as a medicine, using a carefully-prepared extract of the root, I was deterred from proceeding by two patients being attacked with severe vomiting, griping, and diarrhœa.

It may be well to conclude these general statements by the particulars of a few well authenticated cases. Dr. Pereira describes two that were occasioned by the root having been dug up in February by mistake for horse-radish.† The parties, a gentleman and his wife, ate, the former about a root and a half, the latter not much more than half a root. Both of them in three-quarters of an hour had burning, and numbness in the lips, mouth, and throat, extending to the stomach and followed by vomiting. The husband had subsequently violent and frequent vomiting, partly owing to an emetic. His extremities became cold, the lips blue, the eyes glaring, and the head covered with cold sweat. There was no spasm or convulsion, but some tremor. He had no delirium, or stupor, or loss of consciousness, but complained of violent headache. The respiration was not affected ; and although he felt very weak, he was able to walk with a little assistance only a few minutes before death ; which took place, as if from fainting, about four hours after the poison was swallowed. — His wife, in addition to the early symptoms already mentioned, had such weakness and stiffness of the limbs that she was unable to stand ; and she could utter only unintelligible sounds; but she had no spasms or convulsions. She experienced a strange sensation of numbness in the hands, arms, and legs, diminution of sensibility over the whole integuments, especially of the face and throat, where the sense of touch was almost extinguished. She had also some dimness of vision, giddiness, and at times an approach to loss of consciousness, but no delirium, sleepiness, or deafness. She recovered, under the use of emetics, laxatives, and stimulants. In neither of these cases was there any diarrhœa. — A patient of Mr. Sherwen,‡ five minutes after taking a tincture of the root, suffered from the same incipient symptoms as above, but without actual vomiting. The face seemed to her to swell, and the throat to contract; she became nearly blind, and excessively feeble, but did not lose her consciousness. The eyes were fixed and protruded, and the pupils contracted, the jaws stiff, the face livid, the whole body cold, the pulse imperceptible, the heart's action feeble and fluttering, and the breathing short and laborious. An emetic was followed first by violent convulsions, and then by vomiting; after

* Elements of Materia Medica, ii. p. 1807.   † Ibidem, p. 1806.
‡ Lancet, 1836-37, ii. 13.

which she slowly recovered. At all times she was so sensible as to be able to tell how the accident happened. — Dr. Ballardini of Brescia met with twelve simultaneous cases of poisoning with the juice of the leaves, used by mistake for scurvy-grass [*Cochlearia officinalis*]. Each person had three ounces of juice. Three of them died in two hours ; but the rest were saved. The chief symptoms were extreme weakness and anxiety, paleness and distortion of the features, dilatation of the pupils, dulness of the eyes, giddiness, headache, chiefly occipital, some distension and pain of the belly, vomiting of a green matter, and in some diarrhœa. The whole body was cold, the nails livid, the limbs cramped, the pulse small and scarcely perceptible. In the fatal cases there were convulsions.* — MM. Pereyra and Perrin mention, that, while using the alcoholic extract in the Hospital of St. André at Bordeaux, the sample of the drug happened to be changed when the dose had been raised so high as ten grains ; and that the patients who were taking it were then all seized with burning in the mouth and throat, vomiting, pungent pains in the extremities, cold sweating, anxiety, extreme general prostration, great slowness and irregularity of the pulse, convulsions, and congestion in the venous system. One patient died ; the others recovered under no other treatment than stimulant friction along the spine.† An infant at Suippe, in the French Department of the Marne, ate a few leaves and flowers of monkshood, while walking in a garden. Soon afterwards he began to stagger as if tipsy, and to complain of pain in the belly. In two hours an emetic was given ; but a few minutes afterwards, the eyes became convulsed, the jaws locked, the trunk bent rigidly backward, and the limbs convulsed ; and death ensued in five minutes more.‡

Morbid Appearances. — In Ballardini's fatal cases the pia mater and arachnoid were much injected ; there was much serosity under the arachnoid and in the base of the cranium ; the lungs were considerably gorged with blood ; the heart and great vessels contained but a little black fluid blood : the villous coat of the stomach was spotted with red points ; and the small intestines presented inwardly red patches and much mucus. In the Bordeaux case there was venous congestion in the head and chest, the lungs particularly being much gorged with blood. The right side of the heart was full of blood, of gelatinous consistence. In Pallas's cases the gullet, stomach, small intestines and rectum were very red, the lungs dense, dark, and gorged, and the cerebral vessels turgid.

Few trustworthy observations have been made on the effects of the other species of aconite. Dr. Pereira found the A. ferox of the East Indies to be a much more deadly poison to animals than common monkshood ; but its effects were otherwise identical.§ Three grains of the root put into the throat of a rabbit, killed it in nineteen mi-

* Annali Universali di Medicina, 1840, iii. 635.
† Buchner's Repertorium für die Pharmacie, lxviii. 199.
‡ Journal de Chimie Medicale, 1840, 94.
§ Edinburgh Journal of Natural Science, 1830, 235.

nutes ; one grain of the alcoholic extract, introduced into the peritonæum, proved equally deadly. Nine grains will kill a cat in four
hours.* —— Of the other aconites the A. cammarum, and A. ly-
coctonum are said to have proved fatal frequently in Germany ; but
no accurate facts on the subject are on record. — It was stated above
that the A. paniculatum, supposed by De Candolle to have been the
true aconite of Baron Störck, is inert in this country. I introduced
the alcoholic extract of three ounces of the fresh leaves collected near
the end of June, into the cellular tissue between the skin and muscles
of a young rabbit, having previously converted the extract into an
emulsion with mucilage and water.   This was four times the dose of
A. napellus, which I had found sufficient to kill a strong adult rabbit
in two hours and a quarter ; but no effect whatever was produced. —
Mr. Ramsay of Broughty Ferry has described a case of fatal poisoning
with a handful of aconite leaves which were mistaken for parsley, and
which he supposes to have been those of A. neomontanum.   The subject, a boy of fourteen, was attacked with a sense of burning in the
mouth, throat, and stomach, afterwards with vomiting and convulsions, and died considerably within five hours.†   The very feeble
taste of this species — which besides is little cultivated in Scotland,
— inclines me to doubt whether it was the species that produced such
violent effects.

Of Poisoning with Black Hellebore.

Black hellebore, or Christmas-rose, the *Helleborus niger* of botanists,
is a true narcotico-acrid poison.   It is a doubtful native of this country.   It produces a large white ranunculus-like flower about mid-
winter.   The root, the only part used in medicine, or to be found in
the shops, consists of a short root-stock and numerous, long, black
undivided rootlets.   The fresh root in January is not acrid to the taste.
Its active principle appears from the researches of MM. Feneulle and
Capron, to be an oily matter containing an acid.‡
   Its action has not yet been examined with particular care.   Two
or three drachms of the root killed a dog in eighteen hours, when
swallowed ; two drachms killed another in two hours, when applied
to a wound ; and six grains in a wound caused death in twenty-three
hours.   In all cases the leading symptoms are efforts to vomit, giddiness, palsy of the hind-legs, and insensibility.§   Ten grains of the
extract introduced into the windpipe killed a rabbit in six minutes.‖
Orfila found redness of the rectum, when the animals survived a few
hours.   But none of these experiments show the powerful irritant
action exerted by the root upon man.
   The Bulletins of the Medical Society of Emulation mention two
cases of poisoning with hellebore, which arose from the ignorance of

* Dr. Hunter. Calcutta Med. Phys. Transactions, ii. 410.
† Northern Journal of Medicine, 1844, i. 120.
‡ Journal de Pharmacie, vii. 503.   § Orfila, Tox. Gén. ii. 225.
‖ Schabel, Diss. Inaug. be Effectibus Veratri albi et Hellebori nigri, p. 8, Tubing.

a quack-doctor. Both persons, after taking a decoction of the root were seized in forty-five minutes with vomiting, then with delirium, and afterwards with violent convulsions. One died in two hours and a half, the other in less than two hours.* Morgagni has related a case which proved fatal in about sixteen hours, the leading symptoms of which were pain in the stomach, and vomiting. The dose in this instance was only half a drachm of the extract.† In a case not fatal, related by Dr. Fahrenhorst, the symptoms were those of irritant poisoning generally, that is, burning pain in the stomach and throat, violent vomiting, to the extent of sixty times in the first two hours, cramps of the limbs, and cold sweating. The most material symptoms were at this time quickly subdued by sinapisms to the belly and anodyne demulcents given internally; and in four days the patient was well. The dose here was a table-spoonful of the root in fine powder.‡ In small doses of ten or twenty grains, it is well known to be a powerful purgative to man. I have known severe griping produced by merely tasting the fresh root in January.

The morbid appearances in Morgagni's case were the signs of inflammation in the digestive canal, particularly in the great intestines. In the case described in the French Bulletins, there was gorging of the lungs, and the stomach had a brownish-black colour as if gangrenous.

The other species of hellebore have not been carefully examined; but it is probable that they all possess similar properties. The *H. hyemalis* and *viridis* are said by Buchner to be weaker than the *H. niger;* and the *H. fœtidus* is the most poisonous of all.§

CHAPTER XXXVI.

OF POISONING WITH SQUILL, MEADOW-SAFFRON, WHITE HELLEBORE, AND FOXGLOVE.

THE natural family *Liliaceæ,* and the allied family, *Melanthaceæ,* contain many species which possess narcotico-acrid properties. Those which are best known in Europe are squill, meadow-saffron, cevadilla, and white hellebore. To these may be added foxglove, as possessing properties in some measure analogous, and also rue and ipecacuan.

Of Poisoning with Squill.

The root of the squill, or *Squilla maritima,* possesses the properties of the narcotico-acrids. Orfila's experiments on animals, indeed, assign to it only an action on the nervous system. He found that

* Bullet. de la Soc. Méd. d'Em. Avril. 1818.
† De Sedibus et Causis Morborum, Epist. lix. 15.
‡ Wibmer, die Wirkung der Arzneimittel und Gifte, iii. 10.
§ Buchner's Toxicologie, 272.

two ounces and a half of the fresh root, when secured in the stomach of a dog by a ligature on the gullet, excited efforts to vomit, dilated pupil, and lethargy; and in two hours the animal suddenly fell down in a violent fit of tetanus, and expired. From thirty-six grains injected into the jugular vein no effect followed for sixteen hours; when at last, as in the former case, the animal dropped down convulsed and died immediately.*

The effects, however, caused by squill on man leave no doubt that it is also an active irritant; for it causes sickness, vomiting, diarrhœa, gripes, and bloody urine, when given in over-doses. It has likewise produced narcotic symptoms in man. Lange mentions an instance of a woman, who died from taking a spoonful of the root in powder to cure tympanitis. She was immediately seized with violent pain in the stomach; and in a short time expired in convulsions. The stomach was found every where inflamed, and in some parts eroded.† — A woman, whose case is mentioned in a French journal, after taking from a female quack a vinous tincture made with seventy-five grains of extract of squill, was seized with nausea and severe colic, to which were added in twenty-four hours a small contracted pulse, extreme tenderness of the belly, and cold extremities; and she died in the course of the second day.‡ Twenty-four grains of the powder have proved fatal.§ I have seen a quarter of an ounce of the syrup of squills, which is a common medicinal dose, cause severe vomiting, purging, and pain.

An acrid principle, named scillitin, has been discovered in the squill. A difference of opinion prevails as to its nature. Some chemists consider it to be a resin; but Landerer has obtained it in the crystalline form, with alkaline properties. A grain of it will kill a dog.

Of Poisoning with White Hellebore and Cevadilla.

White hellebore, the rootstock of *Veratrum album,* and cevadilla, the seed and capsules of *Asagræa officinalis,* and possibly of *Veratrum sabadilla,* seem to be characteristic examples of the narcotico-acrid poisons. They both possess a strong bitter taste, followed by acridity. The cevadilla-seed in particular has an intensely disagreeable and persistent bitter taste, and produces at the same time a combination of acridity and numbness of the lips, tongue, and cheeks. They owe their active properties chiefly to an alkaloid of great energy, termed veratria.

White hellebore root is familiarly known to be a virulent poison. The best account of its effects is contained in a Thesis by Dr. Schabel, published at Tübingen in 1817. Collecting together the experiments previously made by Wepfer, Courten, Viborg, and Orfila, and adding a number of excellent experiments of his own, he infers

* Toxicol. Gén. ii. 202.
† Tentamen Physico-medicum de Remediis Brunsvicensibus, 176.
‡ Journal de Chimie Médicale, 1842, p. 651.
§ Vogel — Journal de Physique, lxxv. 194.

that it is poisonous to animals of all classes, — horses, dogs, cats, rabbits, jackdaws, starlings, frogs, snails, and flies; — that it acts in whatever way it is introduced into the system, — by the stomach, rectum, windpipe, nostrils, pleural membrane of the chest, an external wound, or the veins; — that it produces in every instance symptoms of irritation in the alimentary canal, and injury of the nervous system; — and that it is very active, three grains of the extract applied to the nostrils of a cat having killed it in sixteen hours.*

Symptoms in Man. — Its effects on man are similar. A singular account of several cases of poisoning with the root is contained in Rust's Journal. A family of eight people, in consequence of eating bread for a whole week, in which the powder of the root had been introduced by mistake instead of cumin seeds, were attacked with pains in the belly, a sensation as if the whole intestines were wound up into a clue, swelling of the tongue, soreness of the mouth, and giddiness; but they all recovered by changing the bread and taking gentle laxatives.†

Another set of cases of a more aggravated nature, though still not fatal, is given in Horn's Archives.‡ Three people took the root by mistake for galanga. The symptoms that ensued were characteristic of its double action. In an hour they all had burning in the throat, gullet, and stomach, followed by nausea, dysuria, and vomiting; weakness and stiffness of the limbs; giddiness, blindness, and dilated pupil; great faintness, convulsive breathing, and small pulse. One of them, an elderly woman, who took the largest share, had an imperceptible pulse, stertorous breathing, and total insensibility even to ammonia held under the nose. Next day she continued lethargic, complained of headache, and had an eruption like flea-bites. A fatal case is quoted by Bernt from Schuster's Medical Journal. A man took twice as much as could be held on the point of a knife, was attacked with violent and incessant vomiting, and lived only from morning till night. The gullet, stomach, and colon were here and there inflamed.§

No detailed inquiry has yet been made respecting the properties of cevadilla; but there can be no doubt that it will prove an energetic poison, similar in its effects to white hellebore, and probably more active. Wibmer quotes Villemet for the fact, that half a drachm of the seeds excites vomiting and convulsions in the cat and dog, and Lentin for the case of a child, who died in convulsions in consequence of the powder having been used inwardly and outwardly.‖

The alkaloid, veratria, has been made the subject of experiment by various physiologists. The most complete investigation yet undertaken is that of Dr. Esche;¶ who found that it causes in a few minutes restlessness, anxiety, salivation, slowness and irregularity of the pulse, slow respiration, nausea, violent vomiting, borborygmus,

* De Effectibus Ver. alb. et Hell. nigri. Tubingæ, 1817.
† Mag. für die gesammte Heilkunde, xiv. 547.
‡ Archiv für Mediz. Erfahrung, 1825.　　§ Beiträge zur Gerichtl. Arzneik. iv. 47.
‖ Die Wirkung der Arzneimittel und Gifte, v. 437.
¶ Diss. Inaug. De Veratriæ Effectibus, Lipsiæ, 1836, quoted by Wibmer, v. 434.

spasms of the abdominal muscles and brisk purging of watery mucus, often tinged with blood; — that by and by the muscles become extremely feeble, so that the animal cannot support itself; — that coldness of the surface succeeds, together with spasmodic contractions of the throat, face, and extremities, but without any stupor; — and that finally the respiration and pulse gradually become extinguished, extreme prostration ensues, and death takes place in a fit of tetanic spasm. No particular morbid appearance was found in the dead body, and especially no sign of inflammation. Magendie found, that one grain in the form of acetate killed a dog in a few seconds when injected into the jugular vein, and in nine minutes when injected into the peritonæum; and that the principal symptom in such rapid cases was tetanic spasm.

Of Poisoning with Meadow-Saffron.

The *Colchicum autumnale*, meadow-saffron, or autumn-crocus, is a more familiar poison in this country than white-hellebore, and seems to possess very similar properties. Two parts of the plant are met with in the shops, the *cormus* or bulb, and the seeds; both of which are poisonous. Both have a strong, disagreeable, persistent, bitter taste. The seeds, and probably the bulb also, contain a bitter crystalline principle, called colchicina, which is soluble in water, neutralizes acids, and possesses intense activity as a poison.

A good physiological investigation into the action of colchicum as a poison is still wanting. Baron Störck found that two drachms of the dried bulb caused in dogs violent diarrhœa and diuresis, ending fatally.* Sir Everard Home observed that the active part of about two drachms dissolved in sherry, caused in a dog, when injected into the jugular vein, slow respiration, languor of the pulse, vomiting, diarrhœa, extreme prostration, and death in five hours.† — Geiger and Hesse, the discoverers of colchicina, gave a cat a tenth of a grain, which occasioned salivation, vomiting, purging, staggering, extreme languor, colic, and death in twelve hours.‡

The effects of colchicum on man, like those observed in animals, rather associate it with the acrid than with the narcotic poisons.

In the Edinburgh Journal a case is briefly noticed of a man who took by mistake an ounce and a half of the wine of the bulb, and died in forty-eight hours, after suffering much from vomiting, acute pain in the stomach, colic, purging, and delirium.§ — Chevallier has described a similar case arising from the wine of the bulb having been given intentionally as a poison. In a few minutes burning pain, urgent thirst, and frequent vomiting of mucus ensued; and death took place in three days.‖ — Three American soldiers, who drank by mistake a large quantity of colchicum wine prepared from

* Libellus de Colchico, 1763, p. 17.   † Philosophical Transactions, 1816.
‡ Annalen der Pharmacie, vii 275.
§ Edin. Med. and Surgical Journal, xiv. 262.
‖ Journal de Chimie Médicale, viii. 351.

the bulb, died with similar symptoms. One of them, who took eighteen ounces, and died in two days, presented the leading symptoms of malignant cholera, namely, frequent vomiting, copious rice-water stools, cramps of the abdominal muscles and flexion of the extremities, coldness of the skin, tongue, and breath, blueness of the nails, dull, sunken eyes, contracted pupils, and collapse of the features. The two others had at first similar symptoms, which passed into those of chronic dysentery, and proved fatal in a few weeks.[*] — M. Caffe has related the case of a young lady who destroyed herself by taking five ounces of the wine containing the active matter of rather more than the fourth part of one bulb. She was soon seized with acute pain in the stomach, then with frequent vomiting, general coldness and paleness, a sense of tightness in the chest and oppression of the breathing, a slow thready pulse, and extreme prostration, — and subsequently with severe and constant cramps in the soles of the feet. In eleven hours she had less frequent efforts to vomit, but was excessively exhausted ; in twenty hours the pulse was imperceptible ; and in two hours more she died. There was no suppression of urine, no purging, no diminution of sensibility, delirium, convulsions, or change in the state of the pupils.[†] About a twelvemonth afterwards the sister of this patient put an end to herself with the same preparation, of which she took the same quantity ; and she died, with precisely the same symptoms, in twenty-eight hours.[‡] M. Ollivier met with two cases of death within twenty-four hours, in consequence of a tincture being taken which contained the active part of forty-eight grains of the dry bulb ; and a third case of death in three days caused by three doses of a watery decoction made each time with 46 grains of the bruised bulb collected in July. Severe purging and prostration followed each dose. There was no symptom of any affection of the brain.[§] — Mr. Henderson describes a case occasioned by an ounce of the tincture. No injury accrued for three hours. The patient then had gnawing pain in the stomach followed by vomiting, and then by purging, at first bilious, afterwards watery, and attended with numbness in the feet, and subsequently a sense of prickling. In the course of the second day there was intense gnawing pain in all the joints of the extremities, profuse acid sweating, tightness in the head, and pain in the hindhead and nape of the neck. Blood-letting, laxatives, and hyoscyamus were employed with success ; but the case seems very nearly to have proved fatal.[||]

The seeds produce similar effects. Bernt has noticed the cases of two children who were poisoned by a handful of colchicum seeds, and who died in a day, affected with violent vomiting and purging.[¶] Mr. Fereday of Dudley relates a carefully detailed case of a man who died in forty-seven hours after swallowing by mistake two

[*] Repertorium für die Pharmacie, lxxi. 131.
[†] Annales d'Hygiène Publique, xvi. 394.
[‡] Ibid. xii. 397.
[§] Journal de Chimie Médicale, 1839, 589.
[||] London Medical Gazette, 1838-39, ii. 763.   [¶] Beiträge, &c. iv. 246.

ounces of the wine of the seeds, and in whom the symptoms were acute pain, coming on in an hour and a half, then retching, vomiting, and tenesmus, feeble pulse; anxious expression, afterwards incessant coffee-coloured vomiting, suppression of urine, excessive weakness of the limbs and feeble respiration, and, for a short period before death, profuse, dark, watery purging. There was neither insensibility nor convulsions.* — Blumhardt relates a similar case caused by an infusion of a large tablespoonful of the seeds. In three-quarters of an hour the man was seized with griping, and then profuse diarrhœa and vomiting. Next morning, twelve hours after the poison was taken, his physician found him still affected with vomiting and purging, but not with pain. He seemed, indeed, to suffer so little, and to improve so much under the use of emollients, that he was thought to be fairly recovering. But next day the pulse was almost imperceptible, the countenance and extremities were cold, the voice hoarse, the breathing hurried, the eyes sunk, the pupils dilated, the epigastrium tender, and the forehead affected with pain; and he died at twelve the same day.†

The leaves, too, are poisonous. Dr. Bleifus has related a case in proof of this. A man gathered the leaves in the middle of May, and, after cooking them, ate about two ounces for supper. In six hours he was seized with violent colic, vomiting, and purging. In fifteen hours, when his physician first saw him, the countenance was ghastly as in malignant cholera, the pupils dilated and scarcely contractile, but the mind entire. He complained of rheumatic pains in the neck, and burning pain in the pit of the stomach. He had frequent vomiting and purging, spasms of the muscles of the belly, coldness of the skin, a slow, small, wiry pulse, and cramps of the fingers and the calves of the legs. Coffee and lemon-juice allayed the vomiting, and a temporary amendment ensued. But early on the third morning he became worse, and soon afterwards the narrator of the case found him dying.‡

The flowers are not less poisonous than the bulbs, leaves, and seeds. A case is noticed in Geiger's Journal of poisoning with a decoction of some handfuls of the flowers, where death occurred within twenty-four hours, under incessant colic, vomiting and purging.§

Doubts exist as to the degree of activity of colchicum. Some practitioners direct half an ounce of the tincture of the seeds to be given as a medicinal dose,‖ even four times a-day.¶ Others administer from one to two drachms night and morning. According to more general experience, these are dangerous doses. Dr. Lewins, junior, has seen dangerous symptoms from a drachm given thrice a day for a week;** a fatal case occurred a few years ago in the Edinburgh Infirmary, from this amount having been given for a few days

* London Medical Gazette, x. 160.
† Repertorium für die Pharmacie, lxix. 382.   ‡ Ibidem, 377.
§ Magazin für Pharmacie, xxv. 237.
‖ Dr. Duncan's Dispensatory, 953.   ¶ Spillan, quoted by Lewins.
** Edinburgh Medical and Surg. Journal, lvi. 186

only ; I have known very violent effects produced by half an ounce taken by mistake, although most of it was brought away by emetics in an hour ; and, in medical practice, I have seldom seen the dose of a sound preparation gradually raised to a drachm thrice a day, without such severe purging and sickness ensuing as rendered it prudent to diminish or discontinue the remedy. There is no doubt, however, that larger doses have occasionally been taken without any ill effect. Constitutional peculiarity can alone account for such differences in the instance of the tincture of the seeds. As to the preparations of the bulb, an additional source of diversity of effect is a difference in the activity of the bulb according to season. On this point no accurate facts have yet been brought forward. The bulb is usually directed to be gathered in July, when it is most plump and firm, and most charged with starch. Orfila, however, says that three bulbs, collected at this time, had no effect whatever on a dog ;[*] and Buchner maintains that it is most energetic in the autumn, when the flowering stem is rising.[†] I suspect, on the other hand, that it is very energetic in the spring, when it is watery, more membranous, and shrivels much in drying; for it is then very bitter.

The morbid appearances are chiefly those of inflammation of the alimentary canal.

In the bodies of the children mentioned by Bernt there was considerable redness of the stomach and small intestines ; in Geiger's case inflammation of the stomach and duodenum only ; in the case mentioned in the Edinburgh Journal, and in that related by Chevallier, there was no morbid appearance at all to be found. In Mr. Fereday's case the omentum was curled and folded up between the stomach on the one hand, and the liver and diaphragm on the other ; the stomach and intestines were coated with much mucus ; there was no appearances of inflammation there but on two points, one in the stomach, the other in the jejunum, where a red patch appeared, owing to blood effused between the muscular and peritoneal coats ; the bladder was empty, the pleura red, the lungs much gorged, their surface, as well as that of the diaphragm and heart, covered with ecchymosed spots ; and the skin over most of the body presented patches of a purple efflorescence. — In Blumhardt's case the muscles were rigid twenty-three hours after death ; the heart and great vessels contained coagulated blood ; the cardiac end of the gullet was internally dark-violet ; the stomach externally of a clear violet hue, and its veins turgid ; the gall-bladder turgid with greenish-yellow bile ; and the inner membrane of the whole small intestines chequered here and there with red, inflamed-like spots.[‡]— In one of M. Caffe's cases there was congestion of the cerebral vessels, coagulated blood in the heart, uniform grayness, softness, and brittleness of the mucous coat of the stomach, and enlargement of the muciparous follicles of the small intestines, as well as unusual distinctness and lividity of the

[*] Toxicologie Gén. 1827, ii. 257.   [†] Toxikologie, 349.
[‡] Repertorium für die Pharmacie, lxix. 384.
60

Peyerian glands. In the other case putrefaction was so far advanced in forty-eight hours as to make the appearances equivocal.

The treatment consists in evacuation of the stomach and bowels by emetics and oleaginous laxatives in the early stage, and afterwards in the employment of opium, stimulants, the warm-bath, and occasionally bloodletting.

Of Poisoning with Foxglove.

Foxglove, or *Digitalis purpura,* a plant which is common in this country both as a native and in gardens, possesses powerful and peculiar properties. The leaves are considered its most active part. They contain an alkaloid ; but chemists have not fixed its nature with precision. M. Le Royer of Geneva procured a pitchy, deliquescent, uncrystallizable substance ;[*] but more lately M. Pauguy obtained a principle in fine acicular crystals, soluble in alcohol and ether, but insoluble in water, alkaline in its reaction, and of a very acrid taste. This principle is called digitalin.[†] It seems to be the same substance, which has also been detected by Radig, as quoted by Dr. Pereira.[‡] The leaves, like those of other narcotic vegetables, yield by destructive distillation an empyreumatic oil similar in chemical qualities and physiological effects to the empyreumatic oil of hyoscyamus.[§]

From an extensive series of experiments on animals by Orfila with the powder, extract and tincture of the leaves, foxglove appears to cause in moderate doses vomiting, giddiness, languor, and death in twenty-four hours, without any other symptoms of note ; but in larger doses, it likewise produces tremors, convulsions, stupor and coma. It acts energetically both when applied to a wound, and when injected into a vein.[‖] Mr. Blake has inferred from his researches, that when injected into the jugular vein, it occasions both obstruction of the pulmonary capillaries, and direct depression of the heart's action. In the dog an infusion of three drachms of leaves arrested in five seconds the action of the heart ; which was motionless after death, turgid, inirritable, and full of florid blood in its left cavities. An infusion of an ounce, injected back into the aorta from the axillary artery, caused in ten seconds great obstruction of the systemic capillaries, indicated by sudden increase of arterial pressure in the hæmadynamometer ; the heart was unaffected for forty-five seconds, when it became slow in its pulsations, and the arterial pressure diminished ; and in four minutes the heart ceased to beat, although for a little longer it continued excitable by stimulation. As no affection of the brain or spine was apparent before the heart became affected, the author infers that the action depends on the poisoned blood being circulated through the substance of the heart, and not on any intermediate influence upon the nervous centre.[¶]

[*] Bibliothèque Universelle de Génève, xxvi. 102.
[†] Duncan's Supplement to the Dispensatory, p. 49.
[‡] Elements of Materia Medica, 1842, p. 1208.
[§] Dr. Morries, Edin. Med. and Surg. Journal, xxxix. 377.
[‖] Toxicologie Gén. ii. 286.
[¶] Edinburgh Med. and Surg. Journal, li. 342.

Symptoms in Man. — Upon man its effects as a poison have been frequently noticed, partly in consequence of its being given by mistake in too large a dose as a medicine, partly on account of the singular property it possesses, in common with mercury, of accumulating silently in the system, when given long in moderate doses, and at length producing constitutional effects even after it has been discontinued. The effects of a dose somewhat larger than is usually given, are great nausea, frontal headache, sense of disagreeable dryness in the gums and pharynx, some salivation, giddiness, weakness of the limbs, feebleness and increased frequency of the pulse, in a few hours an appearance of sparks before the eyes, and subsequently dimness of vision, and a feeling of pressure on the eye-balls. These effects may be occasioned by so small a dose as two or three grains of good foxglove.* The symptoms arising from its gradual accumulation are in the slighter cases nausea, vomiting, giddiness, want of sleep, sense of heat throughout the body, and of pulsation in the head, general depression, great languor and commonly retardation of the pulse, sometimes diarrhœa, sometimes salivation, and for the most part profuse sweating. A good instance of this form of the effects of foxglove is mentioned in the Medical Gazette. A man took it at his own hand for dropsy during twenty days, when the pulse sank to half its previous frequency, he was seized with restless, want of sleep, incoherent talking with imaginary persons, dilated pupils, nausea, thirst, and increase of urine ; and these complaints did not materially subside for six days.† The depressed action of the heart may be the occasion of death in particular circumstances. Mr. Brande mentions from the experience of Dr. Pemberton the case of an elderly woman, who, while under the full influence of foxglove, fell in a fainting fit on walking across the floor ; after which, although she at first got better, there were frequent attacks of fainting and vomiting till she died.‡ In other instances convulsions also occur ; and it appears from a case mentioned by Dr. Blackall, that the disorder thus induced may prove fatal. One of his patients, while taking two drachms of the infusion of the leaves daily, was attacked with pain over the eyes and confusion, followed in twenty-four hours by profuse watery diarrhœa, delirium, general convulsions, insensibility, and an almost complete stoppage of the pulse. Although some relief was derived from an opiate clyster, the convulsions continued to recur in frequent paroxyms for three weeks ; in the intervals he was forgetful and delirious ; and at length he died in one of the convulsive fits.§

A case which exemplifies the effects of a single large dose is related in the Edinburgh Journal. An old woman drank ten ounces of a decoction made from a handful of the leaves in a quart of water. She grew sick in the course of an hour, and for two days

* Wibmer, Die Wirkung, &c. ii. 312, from Schroek, de Digit. Purpurea, 1829.
† London Med. Gazette, 1842-43, i. 270, from Schmidt's Jahrbucher, Aug. 1842.
‡ Dictionary of Mat. Med. and Pharmacy, 1839, 219.
§ Blackall on Dropsy, p. 173.

she had incessant retching and vomiting, with great faintness and cold sweats in the intervals, some salivation and swelling of the lips, and a pulse feeble, irregular, intermitting, and not above 40. She had also suppression of urine for three days.*

A somewhat similar instance may be found in the Journal de Médecine. A man, fifty-five years old took by mistake a drachm instead of a grain for asthma, and was attacked in an hour with vomiting, giddiness, excessive debility, so that he could not stand, loss of sight, colic, and slow pulse. These effects continued more or less for four days, when the vomiting ceased; and the other symptoms then successively disappeared, the vision, however, remaining depraved for nearly a fortnight.†

A very interesting fatal case, which arose from an over-dose administered by a quack doctor, and which became the ground of a criminal trial at London in 1826, is shortly noticed in the same Journal. Six ounces of a strong decoction when taken as a laxative early in the morning. Vomiting, colic, and purging, were the first symptoms; towards the afternoon lethargy supervened ; about midnight the colic and purging returned; afterwards general convulsions made their appearance ; and a surgeon, who saw the patient at an early hour of the succeeding morning, found him violently convulsed, with the pupils dilated and insensible, and the pulse, slow, feeble, and irregular. Coma gradually succeeded, and death took place in twenty-two hours after the poison was swallowed.‡

This is the only case in which I have seen an account of the appearances in the dead body, and they are related imperfectly. It is merely said that the external membranes of the brain were much injected with blood, and the inner coat of the stomach red in some parts.

The affections induced by poisoning with digitalis are often much more lasting than the effects of most other vegetable narcotics. Dr. Blackall's case is one instance in point, and another no less remarkable in its details is described in Corvisart's Journal. The usual local and constitutional symptoms were produced by a drachm of the powder being taken by mistake ; and the slowness of the pulse did not begin to go off for seven days, the affection of the sight not for five days more.§

The preparations of foxglove are very uncertain in strength. From what I have observed in the course of their medicinal employment, I conceive few powders retain the active properties of the leaves, and even not many tinctures. Two ounces of the tincture of the London College have been taken in two doses with a short interval between them, yet without causing any inconvenience.‖ This assuredly could not happen with a sound preparation.

* Edin. Med. and Surg. Journ. vii. 149.
† Bidault de Villiers, Journal de Médecine, Novembre, 1817.
‡ Edin. Med. and Surg. Journ. xxvii. 223, from Morning Chronicle, Oct. 30 and 31, 1826.
§ Journal de Méd. xl. 193.
‖ Williams in Medical Gazette, i. 744.

Of Poisoning with Rue.

The *Ruta graveolens*, or rue, although its wild variety is expressly declared by Dioscorides to be mortal when taken too largely, has attracted little attention as a poison in recent times, and is indeed scarcely considered deleterious. Orfila seems to have found it by no means active ; for the juice of two pounds of leaves, secured in the stomach of a dog by tying the gullet, did not prove fatal till the second day, the symptoms were not well marked, and the only appearances in the dead body were the signs of slight inflammation in the stomach. Even when the distilled water was injected into a vein, the only effects were a temporary nervous disorder similar to intoxication.*

According to the late experimental inquiry, however, by M. Hélie,† rue is possessed of peculiar and energetic properties. All parts of its organization, especially the roots and leaves, produce the effects of the narcotico-acrid poisons ; and although he never met with any instance of a fatal result, its activity is such as to render this event not improbable, even when the dose is by no means very large. His attention was drawn to the subject in consequence of finding, that it was often employed in his neighbourhood for producing abortion, — a property ascribed to it immemorially by the country-people of France ; and all the instances he has seen of its poisonous action were cases in which it had been given with this object. Sometimes the juice of the leaves is given, sometimes an infusion of them, sometimes a decoction of the root ; and in one instance a woman took a decoction of two roots, each about as thick as the finger. The effects were, severe pain in the stomach, followed by violent and obstinate vomiting, drowsiness, giddiness, confusion, dimness of sight, difficult articulation, staggering, contracted pupils, convulsive movements of the head and arms, like those of chorea, retention of urine, slowness of the pulse, and great prostration. There was never any purging. In the course of two days or a little more miscarriage took place, preceded by the usual precursors, and followed by abatement of the symptoms of poisoning. At the period of the milk-fever, however, these symptoms again increased, and the patient was also attacked with swelling and pain in the tongue and copious salivation. In about ten days the pulse began to increase in frequency ; and a mild typhoid fever commonly succeeded, from which recovery took place slowly. In another case the symptoms throughout their whole course were so mild, that, although miscarriage occurred, the subject of it was not confined to bed, and in fifteen days recovered her health completely. M. Hélie adds, that with full knowledge of the doubts entertained by eminent authorities, whether any substance whatever possesses a peculiar property of inducing miscarriage, he is strongly persuaded that rue is really a substance of

* Toxicologie Gén. 1843, ii. 442.
† Annales d'Hygiène-Publique, 1838, xx. 180.

the kind, and that it will take effect even when there is no natural tendency to miscarriage, or any particular weakness of constitution.

Notwithstanding these statements, it may be suspected that M.
Hélie has overrated both its poisonous properties and its virtues as a
drug capable of inducing miscarriage.

Of Poisoning with Ipecacuan.

Ipecacuan is well known as an emetic. It is procured from a plant
of the natural family Rubiaceæ, the *Cephaëlis ipecacuanha*. It contains
a peculiar principle, not yet crystallized, which is white, permanent in
the air, sparingly soluble in water, easily soluble in alcohol and ether,
fusible about 122° F., capable of forming crystallizable salts with
acids, and possessing an alkaline reaction on litmus. It was discovered by M. Pelletier.*

Ipecacuan itself is not known to be a poison; because in consequence of its emetic properties it is quickly discharged from the
stomach. But in doses of considerable magnitude it would probably
be dangerous. In some constitutions the odoriferous effluvia from
the powder induce difficult breathing, anxiety, and imperfect convulsions. I have met with several instances of this singular idiosyncrasy, and one in particular where the subject of it, a surgeon's apprentice, suffered so often and so severely as to be induced to abandon
the medical profession. A German physician, Dr. Prieger, has published a remarkable case of a druggist's servant, who, in consequence of incautiously inhaling the dust of ipecacuan powder, was
attacked with a sense of tightness in the chest, vomiting, and soon
after an alarming sense of suffocation from tightness of the throat.
When these symptoms had continued several hours the uneasiness in
the throat was removed after the use of a decoction of uva-ursi and
rhatany-root ; but the dyspnœa remained several days.†

Its active principle, emeta, is a powerful poison. Two grains of
the pure alkaloid will kill a dog; and the symptoms are frequent vomiting, followed by sopor and coma, and death in fifteen or twenty-four
hours. In the dead body the lungs and stomach are found inflamed.
The same effects result from injecting it into a vein, or applying it to
a wound.‡ It appears, then, to be a narcotico-acrid. But its irritant properties are so prominent that it might be properly arranged
with the vegetable acrids.

CHAPTER XXXVII.

OF POISONING WITH STRYCHNIA, NUX VOMICA, AND FALSE ANGUSTURA.

The next group of the narcotico-acrids includes a few vegetable

---

* Recherches Chim. et Physiol. sur l'Ipecacuanha. Journal de Pharmacie, iii. 145.
† Rust's Magazin für die gesammte Heilkunde, xxxii. 182.
‡ Magendie. Formulaire pour la Préparation, &c. de plusieurs Nouv. Médicamens.
5eme ed. 67.

poisons that act in a very peculiar manner. They induce violent spasms, exactly like tetanus, and cause death during a fit, probably by suspending the respiration. But they do not impair the sensibility. During the intervals of the fits the sensibility is on the contrary heightened, and the faculties are acute.

Death, however, does not always take place by tetanus. In some cases the departure of the convulsions has been followed by a fatal state of general and indescribable exhaustion.

Besides thus acting violently on the nervous system, they also possess local irritant properties; but these are seldom observed on account of the deadliness and quickness of their remote operation on the spine and nerves.

They exert their action by entering the blood-vessels. The dose required to prove fatal is exceedingly small. The organ acted on is chiefly the spinal cord; but sometimes they seem also to act on the heart.

They seldom leave any morbid appearances in the dead body. Like the other causes of death by obstructed respiration, such as drowning and strangling, they produce venous congestion; but this is frequently inconsiderable. Sometimes, however, they leave signs of inflammation in the alimentary canal.

Their energy resides in peculiar alkaloids. The only poisons included in this group, are derived from the genus *Strychnos*. The bark of *Brucea antidysenterica* was long supposed also to possess similar properties; but it is now known that the bark of *Strychnos nux-vomica* was mistaken for the bark of that tree.

Several species of *Strychnos* have been examined, namely, the *S. Nux-vomica*, the *S. Sancti Ignatii* or St. Ignatius bean, the *S. colubrina*, or snake-wood, the *S. tieuté*, which yields an Indian poison the Upas tieuté, the *S. Guianensis*, and likewise the *S. potatorum* and *Pseudo-kina*; and all have been found to possess the same remarkable properties, except the last two, which are inert.

All of them, except the *S. pseudo-kina*, and probably the *S. potatorum*,* contain an alkaloid to which their poisonous properties are owing. This is *strychnia* or strychnin, a substance which has lately been made the subject of many experiments by chemists and physiologists.

Of Poisoning with Strychnia.

Strychnia was discovered by Pelletier and Caventou soon after the discovery of morphia.† For an account of the best process for preparing it, the reader may consult a paper by M. Henry in the journal quoted below.‡

Its leading properties are the following. Its crystals when pure are elongated octaedres. It has a most intensely bitter taste, perceptible, it is said, when a grain is dissolved in 80 pounds of water.§

* Plantes Usuelles des Braziliens, Livraison, i. 3.
† Ann. de Chim. et de Phys. x. 142. ‡ Journal de Pharmacie, viii. 401.
§ Ann. de Chim. et de Phys. x. 153.

It is very sparingly soluble in water, but easily soluble in alcohol and the volatile oils. Its alcoholic solution has an alkaline reaction. It forms neutral and crystallizable salts with the acids. In its ordinary form it is turned orange-red by the action of nitric acid ; which tint becomes violet-blue on the gradual addition of hydrosulphate of ammonia. The action of nitric acid is owing to the presence of a yellow colouring matter, or of another alkaloid, brucia, which is also contained in nux vomica, but exists in larger quantity in the false angustura bark. Pure strychnia is not turned orange-red by nitric acid.*

No poison is endowed with more destructive energy than strychnia. I have killed a dog in two minutes with a sixth part of a grain injected in the form of alcoholic solution into the chest ; I have seen a wild-boar killed in the same manner with the third of a grain in ten minutes ; and there is little doubt that half a grain thrust into a wound might kill a man in less than a quarter of an hour. It acts in whatever way it is introduced into the system, but most energetically when injected into a vein. The symptoms produced are very uniform and striking. The animal becomes agitated and trembles, and is then seized with stiffness and starting of the limbs. These symptoms increase till at length it is attacked with a fit of violent general spasm, in which the head is bent back, the spine stiffened, the limbs extended and rigid, and the respiration checked by the fixing of the chest. The fit is then succeeded by an interval of calm, during which the senses are quite entire or unnaturally acute. But another paroxysm soon sets in, and then another and another, till at length a fit takes place more violent than any before it ; and the animal perishes suffocated. The first symptoms appear in 60 or 90 seconds, when the poison is applied to a wound. When it is injected into the pleura, I have known them begin in 45 seconds, and Pelletier and Caventou have seen them begin in 15 seconds.† M. Bouillaud has recently found that it has no effect when directly applied to the nerves.‡ The experiments of Mr. Blake tend to show, that its action is exerted solely on the nervous system, and that it has no direct action on the heart, even when directly admitted into the blood by the jugular vein.§ It appears to act peculiarly by irritating the spinal cord.

Dangerous effects have often been occasioned by an accidental over-dose in ordinary medical practice. These are well exemplified by a case communicated to Dr. Bardsley by Dr. Booth of Birmingham. A man of 46, affected with hemiplegia for nearly four weeks, began to use strychnia, and had been affected by it for eleven days without particular inconvenience. During this period he took twice a day gradually increasing doses, till the amount of one grain was attained ; when the usual physiological effect having ceased to occur,

* Pelletier and Caventou, Ibidem, xxvi. 56.
† Annales de Chim. et de Phys. xxvi. 44.
‡ Archives Gén. de Méd. xii. 463.
§ Edinburgh Medical and Surgical Journal, li. 338.

the quantity was increased to a grain and a half. But the first dose caused anxiety and excitability, in three hours stupor and loss of speech, and at length violent tetanic convulsions, which proved fatal in three hours and three-quarters.* A fatal case, occasioned by the large dose of two scruples, has been recorded by a German physician, Dr. Blumhardt. In fifteen minutes, imperfect vomiting was brought on by emetics. At this time, the patient, a lad of seventeen, lay on his back, quite stiff, and with incipient fits of locked-jaw. The spasms gradually extended to the rest of the body, till at last violent fits of general tetanus were established, under which the whole body became as stiff as a board, the arms spasmodically crossed over the chest, the legs extended, the feet bent, so that the soles were concave, the breathing arrested, the eyeballs prominent, the pupils dilated and not contractile, and the pulse hurried and irregular. In the second severe fit he died, one hour and a half after taking the poison.† I have known very dangerous tetanic spasm induced by so small a dose as two-thirds of a grain of the ordinary impure strychnia of the shops; and Dr. Pereira describes a case, communicated by a friend, where death was occasioned by a dose of half a grain administered three times a day.‡ As each fit of spasm went off, respiration, which was found to have ceased, was maintained artificially; but no sooner did natural breathing return, than the paroxysm of tetanus returned also; and at length artificial inflation of the lungs failed to restore life.

The only accounts I have seen of the morbid appearances after death from strychnia are in the cases of Dr. Booth and Dr. Blumhardt. In the former, the muscles were in a rigid state, the fingers contracted, the vessels of the brain gorged, the membranes of the spinal cord highly injected; and four patches of extravasated blood were found between the spinal arachnoid and the external membrane. In the latter, twenty-four hours after death, there was general lividity of the skin, and extraordinary rigidity of the muscles. Fluid blood flowed in abundance from the spinal cavity, where the veins were gorged, the pia mater injected, the spinal column softened at its upper part, and here and there almost pulpy. There was also congestion and softening of the brain. The head and great vessels were flaccid, and contained scarcely any blood. The inner membrane of the stomach and intestines presented some redness, but not more than is often seen independently of irritation there.

Strychnia has been found by Pelletier and Caventou in four species of *Strychnos,* the *S. nux vomica, Sancti Ignatii, Colubrina,* and *Tieuté;* and from the researches of MM. Martius and Herberger on the composition and properties of the American poison Wourali, it is also probably contained in the *S. guianensis.*§ Vauquelin could not find it in the *S. pseudo-kina,* which is destitute of bitterness.

* Transactions of Provinc. Med. and Surg. Association, ii. 215.
† Journal de Chimie Médicale, 1837, 481.
‡ Elements of Materia Medica, ii. 1310.
§ Buchner's Repertorium für die Pharmacie.

Of Poisoning with Nux Vomica.

Tests of Nux Vomica. — Nux vomica, the most common of these poisons, is a flat, roundish seed, hardly an inch in diameter, of a yellowish or greenish-brown colour, covered with short silky hair, and presenting a little prominence on the middle of one of its surfaces. In powder it has a dirty greenish-gray colour, an intensely bitter taste, and an odour like powder of liquorice. It inflames on burning charcoal, and when treated with nitric acid acquires an orange-red colour, which is destroyed by the addition of protochloride of tin. Its infusion also is turned orange-red by nitric acid, and precipitated grayish-white with tincture of galls.

Orfila and Barruel have made some experiments on the mode of detecting it in the stomach, and the following is the plan recommended by them. The contents of the stomach, or the powder, if it can be separated, must be boiled in water acidulated with sulphuric acid. The liquid after filtration is neutralized with carbonate of lime, and then evaporated to dryness. The dry mass is then acted on with successive portions of alcohol, and evaporated to the consistence of a thin syrup. The product has an intensely bitter taste, yields a precipitate with ammonia, becomes deep orange-red with nitric acid, and will sometimes deposit crystals of strychnia on standing two or three days.* By this process Dr. R. D. Thomson, in a case which proved fatal in three hours, detected nux-vomica, although vomiting had been induced by emetics.†

These experiments it is important to remember, because, contrary to what takes place in regard to vegetable poisons generally, nux vomica is often found in the stomachs of those poisoned with it.

Its Mode of Action and Symptoms in Man. — The poisonous properties of nux vomica are now well known to the vulgar ; and in consequence it is occasionally made the instrument of voluntary death, although no poison causes such torture. It is difficult to conceive, considering its intensely bitter taste, how any one could make it the instrument of murder. But a fact is stated in Rust's Journal, which shows that it may be used for that purpose. At a drinking party one man wagered with another, that if he took a little *Cocculus indicus* in beer, he would be compelled to walk home on his head. The wager was taken and the potion drunk ; but nux vomica was substituted for the Cocculus indicus, itself too a virulent poison ; and the man went home and died in convulsions fifteen minutes afterwards.‡

Many experiments have been made on animals with nux vomica ; but the first accurate inquiry was that of Magendie and Delille read before the French Institute in 1809. The symptoms they remarked were precisely the same with those produced by strychnia. Half a drachm of the powder killed a dog in forty-five minutes, and a grain

* Archives Gén. de Méd. viii. 22.
† British Annals de Medecine, i. 106.
‡ Magazin für die gesammte Heilkunde, xvii. 119.

and a half of the alcoholic extract thrust into a wound killed another in seven minutes. The animals uniformly experienced dreadful fits of tetanic spasm, with intervals of relaxation and sensibility, and were carried off during a paroxysm.

The cause of death appears to be prolonged spasm of the thoracic muscles of respiration. The spasm of these muscles is apparent in the unavailing efforts which the animals make to inspire. The external muscles of the chest may be felt during the fits as hard almost as bone ; and, according to an experiment of Wepfer, the diaphragm partakes in the spasm of the external muscles.*

On account of the singular symptoms of irritation of the spinal cord, uncombined with any injury of the brain, this poison is believed to act on the spinal marrow alone. This is farther shown by the experiments of Mr. Blake with strychnia alluded to above. But from some experiments by Segalas it appears also to exhaust the irritability of the heart : for in animals he found that organ could not be stimulated to contract after death, and life could not be prolonged by artificial breathing.† A similar observation was made long ago by Wepfer, who found the heart motionless and distended with arterial blood in its left cavities ;‡ and a case of poisoning in the human subject to the same effect will be presently related. The pulse is always very weak, often wholly suppressed during a paroxysm ; and in the case alluded to it was found on dissection pale, flaccid and empty, having been apparently affected with spasm. The action exerted through the medium of the spinal cord on the muscles is wholly independent of the brain ; for Stannius found that in frogs the removal of the brain does not interfere with the effects.§

Of late poisoning with nux vomica has been common. The most characteristic example yet published is a case related by Mr. Ollier, of a young woman, who in a fit of melancholy, took between two and three drachms of the powder in water. When the surgeon first saw her, half an hour afterwards, she was quite well. But going away in search of an emetic, and returning in ten minutes, he found her in a state of great alarm, with the limbs extended and separated, and the pulse faint and quick. She then had a slight and transient convulsion succeeded by much agitation and anxiety. In a few minutes she had another, and not long afterwards a third, each about two minutes in duration. During these fits, " the whole body was stiffened and straightened, the legs pushed out and forced wide apart ; no pulse or breathing could be perceived ; the face and hands were livid, and the muscles of the former violently convulsed." In the short intervals between the fits she was quite sensible, had a feeble rapid pulse, complained of sickness with great thirst, and perspired freely. " A fourth and most violent fit soon succeeded, in which the whole body was extended to the utmost from head to foot. From

* Cicutæ Aquat. Hist. Noxæ, p. 295.
† Magendie, Journal de Physiol. ii. 361.
‡ Cicutæ Aquat. Hist. et Noxæ, p. 198.
§ Archives Gén. de Médecine, xlvi. 365.

this she never recovered : she seemed to fall into a state of asphyxia, relaxed her grasp, and dropped her hands on her knees.   Her brows, however, remained contracted, her lips drawn apart, salivary foam issued from the corners of the mouth, and the expression of the countenance was altogether most horrific.''   She died an hour after swallowing the poison.* — A case precisely similar, produced by three pence worth of the powder, and fatal in little more than an hour, is related by Mr. Watt of Glasgow.† — Another apparently also similar but fatal in three hours, is related by Dr. R. D. Thomson.‡   There is in fact very little variety of symptoms in different cases, where death occurs in the primary stage. — Occasionally even in such rapid cases there is a little vomiting in the first instance.   This was remarked in Mr. Watt's case, and also in another described by MM. Orfila and Ollivier.§

When death does not take place thus suddenly in a fit of spasm, the person continues to be affected for twelve or sixteen hours with similar, but milder paroxysms ; and afterwards he may either recover without farther symptoms, or expire in a short time apparently from exhaustion, or suffer an attack of inflammation of the stomach and intestines, which may or may not prove fatal.

M. Jules Cloquet has described a case, where the patient seemed to die of the excessive exhaustion produced by the violent, long continued spasms.   The tetanic fits lasted about twenty-four hours, the sensibility in the intervals being acute.   Slight signs of irritation in the stomach succeeded ; and death ensued on the fourth morning.‖

In the Bulletins of the Medical Society of Emulation another case is related, which arose from an over-dose of the alcoholic extract being taken by an old woman who was using it for palsy.   She took three grains at once.   Violent tetanus was soon produced ; and afterwards she had a regular attack of inflammation of the stomach and intestines, which proved fatal in three days.

The last instance to be noticed exemplifies very well the effects of the poison when the quantity is insufficient to cause death.   A young woman swallowed purposely a drachm mixed in a glass of wine.   In fifteen minutes she was seized with pain and heat in the stomach, burning in the gullet, a sense of rending and weariness in the limbs succeeded by stiffness of the joints, convulsive tremors, tottering in her gait, and at length violent and frequent fits of tetanus.   Milk given after the tetanus began excited vomiting.   She was farther affected with redness of the gums, inflammation of the tongue, burning thirst, and pain in the stomach.   The pulse also became quick, and the skin hot. Next day, though the fits had ceased, the muscles were very sore, especially on motion.   The tongue and palate were inflamed, and there was thirst, pain in the stomach, vomiting, colic and diarrhœa.   These

* Lond. Med. Repository, xix. 448.
† Glasgow Medical Journal.   August, 1830.
‡ British Annals of Medicine, i. 103.
§ Archives Gén. de Méd. viii. 17.   ‖ Nouv. Journ. de Méd. x. 157.

symptoms, however, abated, and on the fourth day disappeared, leaving her exceedingly weak.*

This and the previous case show clearly the double narcotico-acrid properties of the poison.

With regard to the dose requisite to prove fatal, the smallest fatal dose of the alcoholic extract yet recorded is three grains, which was the quantity taken in the case from the Parisian bulletins : Hoffmann mentions a fatal case caused by two fifteen grain doses of the powder ;† and in Hufeland's Journal there is another caused by two drachms, which was fatal in two hours.‡—A dog has been killed by eight grains of the powder, and a cat by five.§ It is even said that a dog has been killed by two grains.‖

It has been thought, from some observations by Mr. Baker on the medicinal use of nux vomica in Hindostan that, by the force of habit, the constitution may become to a certain extent accustomed to large doses of this poison, in the same manner as it acquires the power of enduring large doses of opium. The natives of Hindostan, often take it morning and evening for many months continuously, beginning with an eighth part of a nut, and gradually increasing the dose to an entire nut, or about twenty grains. If it is taken either immediately before or after meals, it never occasions any unpleasant effects; but if this precaution be neglected, spasms are apt to ensue.¶ As it is found unsafe, however, to increase the dose beyond one nut, and the poison is taken in the form of coarse powder, in which state it must be slowly acted on by the fluid in the stomach, it is probable that the modifying influence of habit is inconsiderable. Habit certainly does not familiarize the system to strychnia used medicinally. The same dose, which has once excited its peculiar physiological action, will for the most part suffice to excite it again, however frequently the dose may be repeated. — The facts mentioned by Mr. Baker show that nux vomica is not a cumulative poison ; and European experience, in the instance of strychnia, is to the same effect.

Morbid Appearances. — The morbid appearances differ according to the period at which death occurs. In Mr. Ollier's case, where death took place in an hour, the appearances were insignificant. The stomach was almost natural, the vessels of the brain somewhat congested, the heart flaccid, empty, and pale. In the case in Hufeland's Journal there was general inflammation of the stomach, duodenum and part of the jejunum. In Cloquet's case, a slower one, there was very little appearance of inflammation. In that from the Parisian bulletins, on the contrary, the stomach was highly inflamed, the intestines violet-coloured, in many places easily lacerated and apparently gangrenous. In an interesting dissection of a case, which

* Tacheron, London Med. Repository, xix. 456.   † Med. Rat. System, ii. 175.

‡ Journ. der Practischen Heilkunde, iv. 492.

§ Hillefeld, Exp. quædam circa venena. Gott. 1760. Quoted by Marx, die Léhre von den Giften, i. ii. 26.

‖ Rossi, Exp. de nonnullis plantis quæ pro venenatis habentur. Pisis, 1762. See Marx, i. ii. 29.

¶ Trans. of the Calcutta Med. and Phys. Soc. i. 138.

was quickly fatal, — that related by Orfila and Ollivier, there was found much serous effusion on the surface of the cerebellum, and softening of the whole cortical substance of the brain, but especially of the cerebellum.   Blumhardt too, found softening of the cerebellum and congestion of the cerebral vessels, together with softening of the spinal cord and general gorging of the spinal veins.   This is some confirmation of an opinion advanced not long ago in France by Flourence and others, that nox vomica acts particularly on the cerebellum.*   In Dr. R. D. Thomson's case, which was examined by Mr. Taylor, there was found much congestion of the whole membranes and substance of the brain and cerebellum, and even some extravasation of blood within the cavity of the arachnoid over the upper surface of the former.   Mr. Watt remarked in his case (sixty hours, however, after death in summer) softening of the substance of the brain and the lumbar part of the spinal cord.—In Orfila and Ollivier's case the lungs were found much gorged with black fluid blood. — In Blumhardt's case the heart and great vessels were entirely destitute of blood. — There is sometimes seen, as in Dr. R. D. Thomson's case, a brown powder lining the stomach, even although vomiting may have occurred.

The body appears sometimes to retain for a certain period after death the attitude and expression impressed on it by the convulsions during life.   In the instance mentioned by Orfila and Ollivier the muscles immediately after death remained contracted, the head bent back, the arms bent, and the jaws locked.   This state may even continue for some hours, so that the body appears to pass into the state of rigidity which precedes decay, without also passing through the preliminary stage of flaccidity immediately after death.   In the case related by Mr. Ollier, the body five hours after death " was still as stiff and straight as a statue, so that if one of the hands was moved the whole body moved along with it ;" and in Blumhardt's case the rigidity twenty hours after death was unusually great.   This state of rigidity, however, does not invariably occur.   On the contrary, in animals the limbs become very flaccid immediately after death; but the usual rigidity supervenes at an early period.†   In Dr. R. D. Thomson's case flaccidity immediately followed death.

Treatment. — Little is known of the treatment in this kind of poisoning.   But it is of the greatest moment to evacuate the stomach thoroughly, and without loss of time.   Hence emetics are useful ; but if the stomach-pump is at hand it ought to be resorted to without waiting for the operation of emetics.   Torosiewicz describes the case of a young woman who, after the usual symptoms had begun to appear in consequence of the administration of a tea-spoonful of powder, recovered under the action of an emetic followed by rhatany-

* Arch Gén. de Méd. viii. 18.

† I have not altered the statement as to this point in the former editions.   Yet I strongly suspect that authors, who describe the spasm which precedes death to continue as it were into the rigidity which occurs after death, must have observed inaccurately. For in the numerous experiments I have made and witnessed in animals, flaccidity invariably took place at the time of death, and continued for a moderate interval.

root.* When nux vomica is taken in powder, — the most frequent form in which it has been used, — it adheres with great obstinacy to the inside of the stomach. Consequently whatever means are employed for evacuating the stomach, they must be continued assiduously for a considerable time. If the patient is not attacked with spasms in two hours, he will generally be safe.

M. Donné of Paris has stated that he has found iodine, bromine, and chlorine to be antidotes for poisoning with the alkaloid of nux vomica, as well as for the other vegetable alkaloids. Iodine, chlorine, and bromine, he says, form with the alkaloids compounds which are not deleterious, — two grains and a half of the iodide, bromide, and chloride of strychnia, having produced no effect on a dog. Animals which had taken one grain of strychnia or two grains of veratria, did not sustain any harm, when tincture of iodine was administered immediately afterwards. But the delay of ten minutes in the administration of the antidote rendered it useless. In the compounds formed by these antidotes with the alkaloids, the latter are in a state of chemical union, and not decomposed. Sulphuric acid separates strychnia, for example, from its state of combination with chlorine, iodine, or bromine, and forms sulphate of strychnia, with its usual poisonous qualities.† It remains to be proved that the same advantages will be derived from the administration of these antidotes in the instance of poisoning with the crude drug, nux vomica, as in poisoning with its alkaloid.

In general little difficulty will be encountered in recognizing a case of poisoning with nux vomica. *Tetanus* or locked-jaw is the only disease which produces similar effects. But that disease never proves so quickly fatal as the rapid cases of poisoning with nux vomica; and it never produces the symptoms of irritation observed in the slower cases. Besides, the fits of natural tetanus are almost always slow in being formed; while nux vomica brings on perfect fits in an hour or less. It is right to remember, however, that nux vomica may be given in small doses, frequently repeated, and gradually increased, so as to imitate exactly the phenomena of tetanus from natural causes. Medical men will be at no loss to discover, on reflection, how the preparations of this drug may be rendered formidable secret poisons.

Of Poisoning with the St. Ignatius Bean and Upas Tieuté.

The *Strychnos Sancti Ignatii*, or St. Ignatius bean, contains about three times as much strychnia as nux vomica, namely, from twelve to eighteen parts in the 1000. It is very energetic. Dr. Hopf has mentioned an instance of a man, who was attacked with tetanus of several hours' duration after taking the powder of half a bean in brandy, and who seems to have made a narrow escape.‡

* Repertorium für die Pharmacie, lxv. 80.
† Le Globe, vii. 525. — Août 19, 1829.
‡ Henke's Zeitschrift für die Staatsarzneikunde, ii. 169.

The *Strychnos tieuté* is the plant which yields the Upas tieuté, one of the Javanese poisons. This substance has been analyzed by Pelletier and Caventou, and found to contain strychnia.* From the experiments of Magendie and Delille, the Upas tieuté appears to be almost as energetic as strychnia itself.† Mayer found that the bark of the plant which yields it, when applied in the dose of fifty grains to a wound, killed a rabbit in two hours and a half.‡ Dr. Darwin has given an account of its effects on the Javanese criminals, who used formerly to be executed by darts poisoned with the tieuté. The account quoted by him is not very authentic; yet it accords precisely with what would be expected from the known properties of the poison. He says, that a few minutes after the criminals are wounded with the instrument of the executioner, they tremble violently, utter piercing cries, and perish amidst frightful convulsions in ten or fifteen minutes.§

Of Poisoning with False Angustura Bark.

Besides these poisons of the genus Strychnos, the present group comprehends another, of the same properties, which was once supposed to be derived from a plant of a different family, the *Brucea antidysenterica.*

A species of bark, commonly called the false angustura bark, was introduced by mistake into Europe instead of the true angustura, cusparia, or bark of the *Galipea officinalis.* It was long supposed to be the bark of the *Brucea antidysenterica;* but it is now known to be the bark of *S. nux vomica.*‖ It is a poison of great energy. It gave rise to so many fatal accidents soon after its introduction, that in some countries on the continent all the stores of angustura were ordered to be burnt. It contains a less proportion of strychnia, but more of the alkaloid brucia than nux vomica, the seed of the plant.

According to Andral, brucia is twenty-four times less powerful than strychnia;¶ but the bark itself is as strong nearly as nux-vomica, for Orfila found that eight grains killed a dog in less than two hours.**

The symptoms it induces are the same as those caused by nux vomica. They are minutely detailed in a paper by Professor Emmert of Bern.†† It appears that during the intervals of the fits the sensibility is remarkably acute: a boy who fell a victim to it implored his physician not to touch him, as he was immediately thrown into a fit. Professor Marc of Paris was once violently affected by this poison, which he took by mistake for the true angustura to cure ague.

* Ann. de Chim. et de Phys. xxvi. 44.   † Orfila, Toxicol. Gén. ii. 364.
‡ Journal de Chim. Méd. vi. 593.   § Botanic Garden, ii. 256.
‖ See my Dispensatory, p. 395. Orfila adheres to the old error in the last edition of his Toxicology, in 1843.
¶ Magendie, Journ. de Physiologie, iii. 267.   ** Toxicol. Gén. ii. 377.
†† Ueber die giftige Wirkungen der unächten Angustura. — Hufeland's Journal, xl. iii. 68.

He took it in the form of infusion, and the dose was only three-quarters of a liqueur-glassful; yet he was seized with nausea, pain in the stomach, a sense of fulness in the head, giddiness, ringing in-the ears, and obscurity of vision, followed by stiffness of the limbs, great pain on every attempt at motion, locked-jaw, and impossibility of articulating. These symptoms continued two houts; and abated under the use of ether and laudanum.*

Some interesting experiments were made by Emmert with this poison to show that it acts on the spine directly, and not on that organ through the medium of the brain. If an animal be poisoned by inserting the extract of false angustura bark into its hind-legs after the spinal cord has been severed at the loins, the hind-legs as well as the fore-legs are thrown into a state of spasm; or if the medulla oblongata be cut across and respiration maintained artificially, the usual symptoms are produced over the whole body by the administration of it internally or externally, — the only material difference being that they commence more slowly, and that a larger dose is required to produce them, than when the medulla is not injured. On the other hand, when the spinal cord is suddenly destroyed after the symptoms have begun, they cease instantaneously, although the circulation goes on for some minutes.†

The true angustura bark has a finer texture than the other, and is darker coloured, aromatic, pungent, and less bitter. The ferrocyanate of potass causes in a muriatic infusion of the false bark a precipitate, which is first green ahd then becomes blue; and the same reagent converts into blue the reddish powder which lines the bark. No such effects are produced on the true angustura bark. Nitric acid renders the rusty efflorescence of the spurious bark deep dirty blue, but has no such effect on the true bark; which, besides, never exhibits a yellow efflorescence.

With the preceding poisons Orfila has arranged also some poisons used by the American Indians; but, as in Europe they are mere objects of curiosity, it is scarcely necessary to treat of them particularly here.

The most interesting and best known of them is the *woorali-poison* of Guiana, variously called woorara, urari, or curare, by different authors. It is believed to have been traced by Martius to a new species of strychnos, the *S. guianensis*, and more recently by Dr. Schomburg to a different species, the *S. toxicaria* of that traveller. But the action it exerts does not correspond exactly with what would be expected of a plant belonging to that genus.

The effects of woorali have been investigated by Sir B. Brodie in the Philosophical Transactions for 1811-12, in Orfila's Toxicology, in Magendie's Memoir on Absorption, and in Fontana's Traité des Poisons. But the most detailed inquiry is that by Emmert, published in 1818. It produces, not convulsions or spasm of the mus-

* Journal de Pharmacie, ii. 507.
† Meckel's Archiv für Anatomie und Physiologie, i. 1.

cles, but on the contrary paralysis, and probably occasions death in this way by suspending the respiration, in the same way as hemlock and conia. According to Emmert's experiments the spine only is acted on, and not the brain also.* Some remarkable experiments were made in 1839 by Mr. Waterton, to show the power of artificial respiration in accomplishing recovery from its effects. After the animals had fallen down motionless from the action of the poison introduced through a wound, and when the action of the heart had become so feeble as not to affect the pulse, artificial respiration, continued in one instance for seven hours and a half, and in another for two hours, had the effect of restoring the animals to health.†

CHAPTER XXXVIII.

OF POISONING WITH CAMPHOR, COCCULUS INDICUS, ETC.

THE third group of the narcotico-acrids resemble strychnia in their action so far, that they occasion in large doses convulsions of the tetanic kind. But they differ considerably by producing at the same time impaired sensibility or sopor. They are camphor, Cocculus indicus, its active principle picrotoxin, the Coriara myrtifolia, the Upas antiar, a Java poison, and perhaps also the yew-tree.

Of Poisoning with Camphor.

Camphor dissolved in oil soon causes in dogs paroxysms of tetanic spasm. At first the senses are entire in the intervals ; but by degrees they become duller, till at length a state of deep sopor is established, with noisy laborious breathing, and expiration of camphorous fumes ; and in this state the animal soon perishes. A solution of twenty grains in olive oil will kill a dog in less than ten minutes when injected into the jugular vein. When camphor is given to dogs in fragments, it does not excite convulsions, but kills them more slowly by inducing inflammation of the alimentary canal. These are the results of numerous experiments by Orfila.‡

They are confirmed by others performed more lately by Scudery of Messina ; but this experimentalist likewise remarked, that the convulsions were attended with a singular kind of delirium, which made the animals run up and down without apparent cause, as if they were maniacal. He also found the urinary organs generally affected, and for the most part with strangury.§ Lebküchner discovered camphor in the blood of animals poisoned with it.∥

Symptoms in Man. — The symptoms caused by camphor in man

* Ueber das Americanische Pfeilgift. Meckel's Archiv für Anatomie und Physiologie, iv. 65.

† Reported by Dr. Reid Clanny in Lancet, 1838-39, ii. 285.

‡ Toxicol. Gén. ii. 400.   § Annali Univ. di Med. xxxvi. 102.

∥ Diss. Inaug. Tubingæ, 1819, p. 9.

may not have been observed; but so far as they have been witnessed, they establish its claim to be considered a narcotic and acrid poison. Its effects appear to be singularly uncertain: at least they are very discrepant; and the reason for this is not apparent.

Its narcotic effects are well exemplified in an account given by Mr. Alexander from personal experience, and by Dr. Edwards of Paris, as they occurred in a patient of his who received a camphor clyster.

Mr. Alexander, in the course of his experiments on his own person with various drugs, was nearly killed by this poison, and has left the best account yet published of its effects in dangerous doses on man. After having found, by a previous experiment, that a scruple did not cause any particular symptom, he swallowed in one dose two scruples mixed with syrup of roses. In the course of twenty minutes he became languid and listless, and in an hour giddy, confused, and forgetful. All objects quivered before his eyes, and a tumult of undigested ideas floated through his mind. At length he lost all consciousness, during which he was attacked with strong convulsive fits and maniacal frenzy. These alarming symptoms were dispelled, on Dr. Monro, who had been sent for, accidentally discovering the subject of his patient's experimental researches, and administering an emetic. But a variety of singular mental affections continued for some time after. The emetic brought away almost the whole camphor which had been swallowed three hours before.*

In Dr. Edwards's patient, the symptoms were excited by an injection containing half a drachm of camphor. In a few minutes he felt a camphrous taste, which was followed by indescribable uneasiness. On then going down stairs for assistance, he was astonished to feel his body so light, that he seemed to himself to skim along the floor almost without touching it. He afterwards began to stagger, his face became pale, he felt chilly, and was attacked with a sense of numbness in the scalp. On then taking a glass of wine, which he asked for, he became gradually better; but for some time his mind was singularly affected. He felt anxious, without thinking himself in danger; he shed tears, but could not tell why; they flowed in fact involuntarily. For twenty-four hours his breath exhaled a camphrous odour.†

Hoffmann has related a case analogous to those of Alexander and Edwards. The dose was two scruples taken in oil; the symptoms vertigo, chilliness, anxiety, delirium, and somnolency.‡

These cases would seem to indicate very considerable activity; yet there can be little doubt that even larger doses have been at times taken with much less effect. Thus, from an account given by Dr. Eickhorn of New Orleans, of its operation on himself, when incautiously swallowed to the amount of two drachms in frequent small doses within three hours, it would appear that the only result was great heat, palpitation, hurried pulse, and pleasant intoxication,

* Experimental Essays, 128.   † Orfila, Toxic. Gén. ii. 406.
‡ Ibid., 407.

then moisture of the skin, next profound sleep for some hours, attended with excessive sweating, and finally no ultimate ill consequence except great debility.* I am assured by a correspondent, Dr. Jennison of Cambridge, U. S., that a medical friend of his has given 90 grains of camphor four times a day in phrenitis, with safety and advantage.

Professor Wendt of Breslau has related an instance, which proves the irritant action of camphor on man, and likewise the uncertainty of the dose required to act deleteriously. In the case of Mr. Alexander, two scruples would in all probability have proved fatal, had they not been discharged in time by vomiting. In the case now to be noticed, 160 grains were taken in a state of solution in alcohol, and were not vomited ; yet the individual recovered. He was a drunkard, who took four ounces of camphorated spirit, prescribed for him as an embrocation. Soon afterwards he was attacked with fever, burning heat of the skin, anxiety, burning pain in the stomach, giddiness, flushed face, dimness of sight, sparks before the eyes, and some delirium. He soon got well under the use of almond oil and vinegar, but did not vomit.†

Morbid Appearances. — The morbid appearances caused by camphor have not, so far as I know, been witnessed in man. In dogs examined immediately after death, the heart is no longer contractile, and its left cavities contain arterial blood of a reddish-brown colour. When the poison has been given in fragments, it leaves marks of inflammation in the stomach and intestines. Orfila found these organs much inflamed in such circumstances.‡ Scudery found the membranes of the brain much injected, and the brain itself sometimes softened ; the inner membrane of the stomach either very red, or checkered with black, gangrenous-like spots of the size of millet-seeds ; the duodenum in the same state ; the ureters, urethra, and spermatic cords inflamed ; and every organ in the body, even the brain, impregnated with the odour of camphor.§

Of Poisoning with Cocculus Indicus.

The *Menispermum cocculus, Cocculus suberosus,* or *Anamirta cocculus* of botanists, is a creeping plant which grows in the island of Ceylon, on the Malabar coast, and in other parts of the East Indies. Its fruit, which is the only part of the plant hitherto particularly examined, is like a large, rough, grayish-black pea, and is known in the shops by the name of Cocculus indicus. It has a rough, ligneous pericarp, enclosing a pale grayish-yellow, brittle kernel, of a very strong lasting bitter taste. The medical jurist should make himself well acquainted with its external characters, because, besides being occasionally used in medicine, it is a familiar poison for destroying fish, and has also been extensively used by brewers as a substitute

* London Med. Gazette, xi. 772. From American Journal of Med. Science.
† Rust's Magazin für die gesammte Heilkunde, xxv. 88.
‡ Toxicol. Gén. ii. 400.   § Annali, &c. xxxvi. 106.

for hops, — an adulteration which is prohibited in Britain by severe statutes. It has been analyzed by M. Boullay of Paris,* who found in it besides other matters, a peculiar principle termed picrotoxin. This principle constitutes, according to Boullay, about a fifth part of the kernel ; according to Nees von Esenbeck, only a hundreth part :† and my own experiments agree with the results of the latter. It is moderately soluble in water, and crystallizes readily from a hot acidulous watery solution. It is more soluble in hot alcohol, from which it crystallizes in granular masses. Ten grains of it killed a dog in twenty-five minutes in the second paroxysm of tetanus.

The seeds themselves occasion vomiting soon after they are swallowed ; so that animals may often swallow them, if not without injury, at all events without danger. But if the gullet be tied, the animal soon begins to stagger ; the eye acquires a peculiar haggard expression, which is the sure forerunner of a tetanic paroxysm ; and the second, third, or fourth fit commonly proves fatal. Three or four drachms will kill a dog when introduced into the stomach ; less will suffice when it is applied to a wound ; and still less when it is injected into a vein.‡ Wepfer has related a good experiment, from which he infers that Cocculus indicus acts by exhausting the irritability of the heart. In the intervals of the fits the pulse could not be felt ; and on opening the chest immediately after death, he found the heart montionless and all its cavities distended.§ Orfila also sometimes found the heart motionless, and its left cavities filled with reddish-brown blood.‖

This poison does not seem to possess distinct acrid properties in regard to animals. M. Goupil indeed found that it produced vomiting and purging,¶ but Orfila could not observe any such effect. According to Goupil it possesses the singular property of communicating to the flesh of animals, more particularly of fish, that have been killed with it, some of the poisonous qualities with which it is itself endowed. The accuracy of this statement may be doubted, the alleged fact being contrary to analogy. Besides, this poison has been used immemorially in the East for taking fish ; and it is familiarly used for the same purpose in some parts of France, though prohibited by statute. Chevallier mentions that in a particular parish the inhabitants live half the year on fish caught with this poison ; and that a friend of his made trial of fish so caught, without the slightest injury.**

Symptoms in Man. — Although it is well known that malt liquors have often been adulterated with Cocculus indicus for the purpose of economizing hops, cases of poisoning in the human subject are rare, because the quantity required to communicate the due degree of bitterness is small. Professor Bernt has shortly noticed a set of cases, which arose in consequence of an idiot having seasoned soup with it

---

* Ann. de Chimie, lxxx. 109.
† Buchner's Repertorium für die Pharmacie, xxiv. 55.
‡ Orfila, Toxicol. Gen. ii. 411.   § Cicut. Aquat. Hist. p. 186.
‖ Toxicol. Gén. ii. 412, 414.   ¶ Ibidem, ii. 410.
** Annales d'Hygiène Publique, xxix. 346.

by mistake. Nine people were taken ill with sickness, vomiting, pain in the stomach and bowels; and one died in twelve days.* The symptoms under which this person died are not stated; but the account of the accident sent to Bernt imputed death to the poison, — which is improbable, considering the length of the interval before death.

In the same group with camphor and Cocculus indicus Orfila has arranged *Upas antiar*, a Javanese poison. This poison is a very bitter milky juice or extract, which is known in Europe only as an article of curiosity. It has been sometimes confounded with the Upas tieuté. It owes its properties to a neutral principle called antiarin.† From the experiments of MM. Magendie and Delille,‡ as well as from those of Sir B. Brodie§ and of Emmert‖ it appears to act in the same manner, and to produce the same effects, as camphor and Cocculus indicus. In small doses it acts as an irritant; in large doses it causes convulsions and coma.

It is here noticed principally because it is one of the poisons which act violently on the heart. If the body of an animal be examined immediately after death from the Upas antiar, the heart is found to have lost its irritability, and the left ventricle to contain florid blood: Schnell found, that, like many other active poisons, it has no effect when applied to the divided end of a nerve.¶

The *Coriaria myrtifolia* is also supposed by some to possess the properties of the present group, and is sufficiently important from its energy, and its occasional injurious effects on man, to claim some notice here.

Its toxicological action has been investigated by Professor Mayer of Bonn, who found that it excites in most animals violent fits of tetanus, giving place to apoplectic coma; and that in the dead body the brain is seen gorged with blood, the blood in the heart and great vessels fluid, the heart not irritable immediately after death, and the inner membrane of the stomach yellowish and shrivelled. A drachm of the extract of the juice killed a cat in two hours when swallowed; half a drachm applied to a wound killed another in eighty-five minutes; and six grains in the same way killed a kitten in three hours and a half. A drachm swallowed by a young dog killed it in two hours and a half. Ten grains of the extract of the infusion applied to a wound killed a kitten in six hours; and three grains another in three hours. A buzzard was killed in three-quarters of an hour by half a drachm of the extract of the juice. Frogs are also soon killed by it. Rabbits, it is remarkable, are scarcely affected by this poison, either administered internally, or applied to a wound, — a drachm in the former way, and half as much in the latter, having produced no effect at all. A grain, however, injected into the jugu-

* Beitrage zur Gerichtl. Arzneikunde, iii. 241.
† Mulder in Pharmaceutisches Central-Blatt, 1838, p. 511.
‡ Orfila Toxicol. Gén. ii. 396.   § Philos. Trans. 1811.
‖ Diss. Inaug. sistens historiam Veneni Upas antiar, &c. Tubingæ, 1815.
¶ Diss. Inaug. de Veneno Upas antiar, Tubingæ, 1815, p. 27.

lar vein occasioned in about five hours a single convulsive paroxysm, which proved immediately fatal.*

Instances of poisoning with this substance have occurred in the human subject, — generally in consequence of its having been taken in various parts of the continent with senna, which it is employed to adulterate. Sauvages has recorded two cases of death occasioned by the berries. In one, a child, death took place within a day under symptoms like epileptic convulsions; and in the other, an adult, who swallowed only fifteen berries, convulsions, coma, and lividity of the face were produced, ending fatally the same evening, though the greater part of the berries were discharged by emetics.† In recent French journals various similar cases are recorded.. M. Fée describes five cases, one of them fatal. In this instance, a male adult, death occurred within four hours after he took an infusion of senna adulterated with the coriaria; and the symptoms were violent convulsions, locked-jaw and colic.‡ M. Roux has noticed a great number of cases in the fullest paper yet published on its effects on man, and gives the details of three which came under his own notice, and of which one proved fatal. In the fatal case, that of a child three years and a half old, who took between eighty and a hundred berries, the symptoms were heat and pricking of the tongue, sparking and rolling of the eyes, loss of voice, locked-jaw, and convulsions recurring in occasional fits of eight or ten minutes in duration. Death ensued in sixteen hours and a half.§ Roux refers also among other instances to those of no fewer than ten soldiers, who were attacked at the same time in consequence of eating the berries, and of whom two died. In Roux's fatal case there was injection of the membranes of the brain, and no other particular appearance; in that mentioned by Fée, there was inflammation of the stomach and bowels; and in one of Sauvages's cases no morbid appearance at all was discovered.

Considering these very pointed proofs of the poisonous qualities of the coriaria, it is not a little singular that doubts have lately arisen whether it is a poison at all. Peschier of Geneva says he has ascertained that tanners, who use it in their trade on account of the powerful astringency of the leaves, also take it internally for gleet, and that he gave a decoction of an ounce to chickens, dogs, and men, without witnessing any ill effect.||

Of Poisoning with Yew.

The leaves and berries of the *Taxus baccata*, or yew, are known to be poisonous; but their effects have not been investigated with care. I have arranged it in the meantime with the present group.

M. Grognier, as quoted by Orfila, ascertained that a decoction of eight ounces of berries without seeds had no effect on a dog; that a

* Buchner's Repertorium, xxxi., and Hufeland's Journal, lxviii. iv. 43.
† Mém. de l'Acad. des Sciences, 1739, p. 47.
‡ Journal de Chim. Méd. iv. 528.
§ London Medical and Physical Journal, April, 1829.
|| Mémoires de la Soc. de Phys. et d'Hist. Nat. de Génève, v. 194.

pound and a half of seeds had no effect on a horse ; that three
ounces of the juice of the leaves given to a large dog merely caused
vomiting ; and that a decoction of twelve ounces of leaves, confined
in the stomach of a dog by a ligature on the gullet, had also no effect.   But two ounces of the juice of the leaves killed a small dog ;
and Orfila himself ascertained, that thirty-six grains of extract of the
leaves, injected into the jugular vein, caused giddiness, stupor, and
death.*

Accidents have repeatedly happened to children in this country
from yew-berries.   Mr. Hurt of Mansfield has given the particulars
of an interesting case.   A child, three years and a half old, two
hours after eating the berries, was observed to look ill at dinner,
and became affected with lividity and heaviness of the eyes, as if he
was about to fall asleep.   Vomiting followed, without any pain ; and
he died before a medical man, who was sent for, could arrive.   Four
other children, somewhat older, who had eaten the seeds, were made
to vomit by emetics, and got well.   The dead body of the first child
presented many livid spots, redness of the villous coat of the stomach,
and gorging of the brain and membranes with blood.   A mass of
berries, seeds, and potatoes was found in the stomach.† — Dr. Hart-
mann of Frankfort mentions that a girl, who took a decoction of the
leaves to produce abortion, died in consequence, but without having miscarried.‡ — Dr. Percival has related other cases in his essays.§

CHAPTER XXXIX.

OF THE POISONOUS FUNGI.

A FOURTH group of poisons possessing narcotico-acrid properties, includes the poisonous *fungi* or mushrooms.

Accidents arising from the deadly fungi being mistaken for eatible
mushrooms are common on the continent, and especially in France.
They are not uncommon, too, in Britain ; but they are less frequent
than abroad, because the epicure's catalogue of mushrooms in this
country contains only three species, whose characters are too distinct
to be mistaken by a person of ordinary skill ; while abroad a great
variety of them have found their way to the table, many of which
are not only liable to be confounded with poisonous species, but are
even also themselves of doubtful quality.

The present subject cannot be thoroughly studied without a knowledge of the appearance and characters of all the fungi which have
been ascertained to be esculent, as well as of those which are known
to be deleterious.   This information, however, I cannot pretend to
communicate, as it would lead to great details.   In what follows,

* Lancet, 1836-37, i. 394.   † Ibid.
‡ Rust's Magazin für die gesammte Heilkunde, xxiii. 374.
§ Essays, &c. iii. 257.

therefore, a simple list will be given of the two classes, with references to the proper source for minute descriptions of them, and some general observations on the effects of the poisonous species.

List of the wholesome and poisonous Fungi. — The only good account yet published of the innocent or eatable fungi of Great Britain is contained in an elaborate essay on the subject by Dr. Greville of this place. He enumerates no fewer than twenty-six different species, which grow abundantly in our woods and fields, and which, although most of them utterly neglected in this country, are all considered abroad to be eatible, and many of them delicate. They are the following: *Tuber cibarium,* or common truffle; *T. moschatum* and *T. album,* two species of analogous qualities; *Amanita cæsarea* or *aurantiaca,* the Oronge of the French, a species which is often confounded by the ignorant with a very poisonous one, the *A. muscaria,* or *pseudo-aurantiaca; Agaricus procerus; A. campestris,* the common mushroom of meadows; *A. edulis,* or white caps; *A. oreades,* or Scotch bonnets; *A. odorus; A. uburneus; A. ulmarius; A. ostreatus; A. violaceus; A. deliciosus; A. piperatus;* and *A. acris; Boletus edulis;* and *B. scaber; Fistulina hepatica; Hydnum repandum; Morchella esculenta,* the common morelle; *Helvella mitra,* and *H. leucophæa.* Of these the *Agaricus acris, procerus,* and *piperatus* are probably unwholesome; and the *Amanita cæsarea* is very rare in this country, if indeed it is indigenous at all. The *A. muscaria,* with which it is apt to be confounded, is common enough. The species to which our cooks confine their attention are the *Tuber cibarium* or truffle, the *Agaricus compestris,* or common mushroom, and the *Morchella esculenta,* or morelle. The *Agaricus edulis* is also to be met with in some markets, but is not in general use.[*]

The best description of the poisonous species is to be found in Orfila's Toxicology. He enumerates the *Amanita muscaria, alba, citrina,* and *viridis;* the *Hypophyllum maculatum, albocitrinum, tricuspidatum, sanguineum, crux-melitense, pudibundum* and *pellitum;* the *Agaricus necator, acris, piperatus, pyrogalus, stypticus, annularis,* and *urens.*[†] To these may be added the *Agaricus semiglobatus,* on the authority of Messrs. Brande and Sowerby,[‡] the *A. campanulatus,*[§] the *A. procerus,* on the authority of a case by Dr. Peddie of this city,[||] the *A. myomica,* on the authority of Ghiglini,[¶] the *A. panterinus* on that of Dr. Paolini of Bologna,[**] the *A. bulbosus* of Bulliard, or *Amanita venenata,* on that of Pouchet,[††] the *Agaricus vernus, insidiosus, globocephalus, sanguineus, torminosus* and *rimosus,* on that of Letellier,[‡‡] and the *Hypophyllum niveum* on the authority of Paulet.

Circumstances which modify their qualities. — The qualities of the

[*] On the Esculent Fungi of Great Britain. Mem. Wernerian Society, iv. 339.
[†] Toxicol. Gén. 417-428.
[‡] London Med. and Phys. Journal, iii. 41.   [§] Ibid. xxxvi. 451.
[||] Edinburgh Med. and Surg. Journal, xlix. 192.
[¶] Journal de Chimie Médicale, 1835, 488.
[**] Annali Universali di Medicina, 1842, i. 549.
[††] Journal de Chimie Médicale, 1839, 325.
[‡‡] Journal de Pharmacie, 1837, 369.

fungi as articles of food are liable to considerable variety. Some, which are in general eaten in safety, occasionally become hurtful; and some of the poisonous kinds may under certain circumstances become inert, or even esculent. But the causes which regulate these variations are not well ascertained.

It has been thought by some that most fungi become safe when they have been dried ;* and there may be some truth in this remark, as their poisonous qualities appear to depend in part on a volatile principle. But it is by no means universally true. Foderé mentions that the *Agaricus piperatus* continues acrid after having been dried.†

Climate certainly alters their properties. The *Agaricus piperatus* is eaten in Prussia and Russia ;‡ but is poisonous in France. The *Agaricus acris* and *A. necator*, also enumerated above as meriting their names, are used freely in Russia.§ The *Amanita muscaria* in France and Britain is a violent poison, and is considered so even in Russia ;‖ but in Kamschatka it yields a beverage which is used as a substitute for intoxicating liquors.¶

There is some reason to believe also that the weather or period of the season influences some of the esculent species. Thus Foderé has mentioned instances of the common morelle having appeared injurious after long-continued rain.**

Even the *Agaricus campestris* or common mushroom is generally believed to become somewhat unsafe towards the close of the season, or as it turns old. Its external characters at that time are sensibly altered ; the margin of the cap is more acute, its white colour less lively, and the fleshy hue of its lamellæ is changed to brown or black. In this state, however, I have often eaten it freely and with impunity.

Cooking produces some difference on their effects. The very best of them are indigestible when raw ; and some of the poisonous species may lose in part their deleterious qualities when cooked, because heat expels the volatile principle ; but, on the whole, I believe the effect of cooking has not been satisfactorily shown to be considerable. Dr. Pouchet of Rouen seems to have clearly proved, that the poisonous properties of two of the most deadly fungi, the *Amanita muscaria* and *A. venenata*, may be entirely removed by boiling them in water. A quart of water, in which five plants had been boiled for fifteen minutes, killed a dog in eight hours, and again another in a day ; but the boiled fungi themselves had no effect at all on two other dogs ; and a third, which had been fed for two months on little else than boiled amanitas, not only sustained no harm, but actually got fat on this fare.†† Pouchet is inclined to think that the whole poisonous plants of the family are similarly circumstanced. — On the other hand some cryptogamous botanists have maintained that the

* Foderé, Médecine Légale, iv. 61, and 58.   † Ibidem.
‡ Haller, Hist. Stirp. Helv. Indig. ii. 328.
§ Bongard, London Medical Gazette, 1838, i. 414.   ‖ Ibidem.
¶ Greville, p. 344, from Langsdorf's Annalen der Wetterrauischen Gesellschaft.
** Foderé, Médecine-Légale, iv. 59.
†† Journal de Chimie Médicale, 1839, 322.

qualities of the esculent mushrooms are injured by cooking, and that when used in the raw state they may be taken for a long time as a principal article of food without injury. This statement, as to the effect of mushrooms when used for a length of time as food, will be more fully considered presently. It is easy to understand how boiling may remove their active properties, although other modes of cookery may not do so. Roasting had no effect in impairing the activity of *Agaricus procerus* in the case observed by Dr. Peddie.

On certain persons all mushrooms, even the very best of the eatable kinds, act more or less injuriously. They cause vomiting, diarrhœa, and colic. In this respect they are on the same footing with the richer sorts of fish, which by idiosyncrasy act as poisons on particular constitutions. It is probably under this head that we must arrange an extraordinary case mentioned by Sage of a man who died soon after eating a pound of truffles. He was seized with headache, a sense of weight in the stomach, and faintness ; and he lived only a few hours.[*]

Lastly, it is not improbable from a singular set of cases to be related presently, that, contrary to what some botanists have alleged, the best mushrooms when taken in large quantity, and for a considerable length of time, are deleterious to every one.

Foderé,[†] Orfila,[‡] Decandolle,[§] and Greville,[‖] have laid down general directions for distinguishing the esculent from the poisonous varieties ; but it is extremely questionable whether their rules are always safe ; and certainly they are not always accurate, as they would exclude many species in common use on the continent. It appears that most fungi which have a warty cap, more especially fragments of membrane adhering to their upper surface, are poisonous. Heavy fungi, which have an unpleasant odour, especially if they emerge from a *vulva* or bag, are also generally hurtful. Of those which grow in woods and shady places a few are esculent, but most are unwholesome ; and if moist on the surface they should be avoided. All those which grow in tufts or clusters from the trunks or stumps of trees ought likewise to be shunned. A sure test of a poisonous fungus is an astringent, styptic taste, and perhaps also a disagreeable, but certainly a pungent, odour. Some fungi possessing these properties have indeed found their way to the epicure's table ; but they are of very questionable quality. Those whose substance becomes blue soon after being cut are invariably poisonous. Agarics of an orange or rose-red colour, and boleti which are coriaceous or corky, or which have a membranous collar round the stem, are also unsafe ; but these rules are not universally applicable in other genera. Even the esculent mushrooms, if partially devoured and abandoned by insects, are avoided by some as having in all probability acquired injurious qualities which they

  * Edin. Med. and Surg. Journal, ix. 379.
  † Médecine Légale, iv. 55, *et passim.*   ‡ Toxicol. Gén. ii. 445.
  § Essai Sur les Propriétés Médicales des Plantes, 320.
  ‖ Mem. Wernerian Soc. iv. 342.

do not usually possess; but this test I have often disregarded. —
These rules for knowing deleterious fungi seem to rest on fact and
experience; but they will not enable the collector to recognise every
poisonous species. The general rules laid down for distinguishing
wholesome fungi are not so well founded, and therefore it appears
necessary to specify them.

On the Poisonous Principle of the Fungi. — Few attempts have
been hitherto made to discover by chemical analysis the principles
on which the effects of the poisonous mushrooms depend. M. Braconnot analyzed a considerable number both of the esculent and
poisonous species, and found in some a saccharine matter, in others
an acrid resin, in others an acrid volatile principle, and in all a
spongy substance, which forms the basis of them, and which he has
denominated fungin.* The last ingredient is innocuous, and it
does not appear that M. Braconnot could trace the peculiar powers
of the fungi to any of the acrid principles. The subject was afterwards resumed by M. Letellier, who says he found in some of them
one, in others two poisonous principles. One of these is an acrid
matter so fugacious, that it disappears when the plant is either dried,
or boiled, or macerated in weak acids, alkalis, or alcohol. To this principle he says are owing the irritant properties of some fungi. The
other principle is more fixed, as it resists drying, boiling, and the
action of weak alkalis and acids. It is soluble in water, has neither
smell nor taste, and forms crystallizable salts with acids; but he
did not succeed in separating it in a state of purity. To this principle he attributes the narcotic properties of the fungi. He found
it in the *Amanita bulbosa, muscaria,* and *verna;* and he therefore
proposed to call it amanitine. Its effects on animals appear to resemble considerably those of opium.† — Chansarel found that the
poisonous principle resides in the juice, and not in the fleshy part
after it is well washed.‡

Of the Symptoms produced in Man by the Poisonous Fungi. — The
mode of action of the poisonous fungi has not been particularly examined; but the experiments of Paulet long ago established that they
are poisonous to animals as well as to man.§

The symptoms produced by them in man are endless in variety,
and fully substantiate the propriety of arranging them in the class of
narcotico-acrid poisons. Sometimes they produce narcotic symptoms
alone, sometimes only symptoms of irritation, but much more commonly both together. It is likewise not improbable, that fungi, even
though not belonging to the varieties commonly acknowledged as poisons, induce, when taken for a considerable length of time, a peculiar depraved state of the constitution, leading to external suppuration and gangrene. Each of these statements will now be illustrated
by a few examples.

* Ann. de Chimie, lxxix. 265; lxxx. 272; lxxxvii. 237.
† Archives Gén. de Méd. xi. 94.   ‡ Repertorium für die Pharmacie, lxvi. 117.
§ Traité des Champignons. — Also Mém. sur les Champignons coëffés. Mem. de la
Soc. Roy. de Méd. i. 431.

The following is a good instance of pure narcotism. A man gathered in Hyde Park a considerable number of the *Agaricus campanulatus* by mistake for the *A. campestris*, stewed them, and proceeded to eat them ; but before ending his repast, and not above ten minutes after he began it, he was suddenly attacked with dimness of vision, giddiness, debility, trembling, and loss of recollection. In a short time he recovered so far as to be able to go in search of assistance. But he had hardly walked 250 yards when his memory again failed him, and he lost his way. His countenance expressed anxiety, he reeled about, and could hardly articulate. The pulse was slow and feeble. He soon became so drowsy that he could be kept awake only by constant dragging. Vomiting was then produced by means of sulphate of zinc ; the drowsiness gradually went off ; and next day he complained merely of languor and weakness.*
— An equally remarkable set of cases of pure narcotism, which occurred a few years ago in this city, has been related by Dr. Peddie. Half an hour after eating the *Agaricus procerus*, an elderly man and a boy of thirteen were attacked with giddiness and staggering, as if they were intoxicated ; and in an hour they became insensible, the man indeed so much so that for some time he could not be roused by any means. Emetics having little effect, the stomach was cleared out by the pump, and powerful stimulants were employed both inwardly and outwardly, by means of which sensibility was in some degree restored. Occasional convulsive spasms ensued, and afterwards furious delirium, attended with frantic cries and vehement resistance to remedies, and followed by a state like delirium tremens. The pupils were at first much contracted, afterwards considerably dilated as sensibility returned, and in the boy contracted while he lay torpid, but dilated when he was roused. In neither instance was there any pain felt at any time ; nor were the bowels affected. Another boy who took a small quantity only had no other symptom but giddiness, drowsiness, and debility.† — A singular form of the narcotic effects of the fungi occurred in the case of a boy of fourteen, who had eaten the *Agaricus panterinus* near Bologna. In the course of two hours he was seized with delirium, a maniacal disposition to rove, and some convulsive movements. Ere long these symptoms were succeeded by a state resembling coma in every way, except that he looked as if he understood what was going on : and in point of fact really did so. He recovered speedily under the use of emetics.‡

In the next set of cases the symptoms were those of almost pure irritation. Several French soldiers in Russia ate a large quantity of the *Amanita muscaria*, which they had mistaken for the *Amanita cæsarea*. Some were not taken ill for six hours and upwards. Four of them, who were very powerful men, thought themselves safe, because while their companions were already suffering, they them-

* London Med. and Phys. Journal, xxxvi. 451.
† Edinburgh Medical and Surgical Journal, xlix. 192.
‡ Annali Universali di Medicina, 1842, i. 549.

selves felt perfectly well; and they refused to take emetics. In the evening, however, they began to complain of anxiety, a sense of suffocation, frequent fainting, burning thirst, and violent gripes. The pulse became small and irregular, and the body bedewed with cold sweat; the lineaments of the countenance were singularly changed, the nose and lips acquiring a violet tint; they trembled much; the belly swelled, and a profuse fetid diarrhœa supervened. The extremities soon became livid, and the pain of the abdomen intense; delirium ensued; and all four died.*

Such cases, however, do not appear to be very common; and much more generally the symptoms of poisoning with the fungi present a well-marked conjunction of deep narcotism and violent irritation, as the instances now to be mentioned will show.

Besides the four soldiers whose cases have just been described, several of their comrades were severely affected, but recovered. Two of these had weak pulse, tense and painful belly, partial cold sweats, fetid breath and stools. In the afternoon they became delirious, then comatose, and the coma lasted twenty-four hours.

A man, his wife, and three children, ate to dinner carp stewed by mistake with the *Amanita citrina*. The wife, the servant, and one of the children had vomiting, followed by deep sopor; but they recovered. The husband had true and violent cholera, but recovered also. The two other children became profoundly lethargic and comatose, emetics had no effect, and death soon ensued without any other remarkable symptom. The individuals who recovered were not completely well till three weeks after the fatal repast.† This set of cases shows the tendency of the poisonous fungi to cause in one person pure irritation, and in another pure narcotism.

The last set of cases to be mentioned were produced by the *Hypophyllum sanguineum*, a small conical fungus of a mouse colour, well known to children in Scotland by the name of *puddock-stool*. This species seems to cause convulsions as well as sopor. A family of six persons, four of whom were children, ate about two pounds of it dressed with butter. The incipient symptoms were pain in the pit of the stomach, a sense of impending suffocation, and violent efforts to vomit; which symptoms did not commence in any of them till about twelve hours after the poisonous meal, in one not till twenty hours, and in another not till nearly thirty hours. One of the children, seven years of age, had acute pain of the belly, which soon swelled enormously; afterwards he fell into a state of lethargic sleep, but continued to cry; about twenty-four hours after eating the fungi the limbs became affected with permanent spasms and convulsive fits; and in no long time he expired in a tetanic paroxysm. Another of the children, ten years old, perished nearly in the same manner, but with convulsions of greater violence. The mother had frequent bloody stools and vomiting; the skin became yellow; the muscles

---

* Corvisart's Journ. de Méd. xxxi. 323, from Vadrot. Diss. Inaug. sur l'empoisonnement par les Champignons.
† Orfila, Toxicol. Gén. ii. 433. .

of the abdomen were contracted spasmodically, so that the navel was drawn towards the spine; profound lethargy and general coldness supervened ; and she too died about thirty-six hours after eating the fungus. A third child, after slight symptoms of amendment had shown themselves, became worse again, and died on the third day with trembling, delirium, and convulsions. This patient, who had taken very little of the poison, was not attacked till about thirty hours after the meal. The fourth child, after precursory symptoms like those of the rest, became delirious, and had an attack of colic and inflammation of the bowels, without diarrhœa ; but he eventually recovered. The father had a severe attack of dysentery for three days, and remained five days speechless. For a long time afterwards he had occasional bloody diarrhœa ; and, although he eventually recovered, his health continued to suffer for an entire year.[*] The cases now mentioned illustrate clearly the simultaneous occurrence of narcotic and irritant symptoms in the same individuals.

A striking circumstance in respect to the symptoms of poisoning with the fungi, is the great difference in the interval which elapses before they begin. In the first case the symptoms appear to have commenced in a few minutes ; but, on the contrary, an interval of twelve hours is common ; and Gmelin has quoted a set of cases, seventeen in number, in which, as in one of those related by Picco, the interval is said to have been a day and a half.[†] The tardiness of the approach of the symptoms is owing to the indigestibility of most of the fungi. Their indigestibility is in fact so great, that portions of them have been discharged by vomiting so late as fifty-two hours after they were swallowed.[‡]

Another circumstance, worthy of particular notice, is the great durability of the symptoms. Even the purely narcotic effects of some fungi have been known to last above two days. In the instance just alluded to, the vomiting of the poison was the first thing that interrupted a state of deep lethargy, which had prevailed for fifty-two hours. The symptoms of irritation, after their violence has been mitigated, might continue, as in the instance quoted from Orfila, for about three weeks.

It was stated above, that some people are apt to suffer unpleasant effects from eating even the best and safest of the esculent mushrooms. These effects, which depend on idiosyncrasy, are confined chiefly to an attack of vomiting and purging, followed by more or less indigestion. Some persons have been similarly affected, even by the small portion of mushroom-juice which is contained in an ordinary ketchup seasoning. This accident, however, may very well be often unconnected with idiosyncrasy; as I have seen those who gather mushrooms near Edinburgh, for the purpose of making ketchup, picking up every fungus that came in their way.

There is some reason for suspecting that even the best mushrooms,

* Picco — Mém. de la Soc. Roy. de Méd. 1780-81, p. 355.
† Geschichte der Pflanzengifte, 639.
‡ Aymen, in Hist. de la Soc. Roy. de Méd. i. 344.

when taken as a principal article of food for a considerable length of time, will prove injurious, and that they then induce a peculiar depraved habit, which leads to external suppuration and gangrene. The only cases which have hitherto appeared in support of this statement, were lately published in Rust's Journal. A family, consisting of the mother and four children, were seized with a kind of tertian fever, and the formation of abscesses, which discharged a thin, ill-conditioned pus, passed rapidly into spreading gangrene, and proved fatal to the mother and one of the children. No other cause could be discovered to account for so extraordinary a conjunction of symptoms in so many individuals, except that for two months they had lived almost entirely on mushrooms; and the probability of this being really the cause, was strengthened by the fact, that the father who slept always with his family, and who alone escaped, lived on ordinary food at a place where he worked not far off.* In opposition, however, to the natural inference from this narrative, some have believed, that mushrooms may be safely eaten to a large amount and for a long time, provided they be used raw. A botanist of Persoon's acquaintance, while studying the cryptogamous plants in the vicinity of Nuremberg, says he found that the peasants ate them in large quantities as their daily food ; and, in imitation of their custom, he ate for several weeks nothing but bread and raw mushrooms ; yet at the end he experienced an increase rather than a diminution of strength, and enjoyed perfect health. He adds that they lose their good qualities by cooking; but he has supplied no facts in support of that statement.† It is said that eatable fungi, used for a considerable time as a principal article of food, as in Russia, cause greenness of the skin.‡ There is no reason for supposing, as some have done,§ that wholesome mushrooms may produce the effects of the poisonous kinds, if eaten in large quantity.

Of the Morbid Appearances. — The morbid appearances left in the bodies of persons poisoned by this deleterious fungi have been but imperfectly collected.

The body is in general very livid, and the blood fluid; so much so sometimes, that it flows from the natural openings in the dead body.‖ In general, the abdomen is distended with fetid air, which, indeed, is usually present during life. The stomach and small intestines of the four French soldiers (p. 705), presented the appearance of inflammation passing in some places to gangrene. In two of them especially, the stomach was gangrenous in many places, and far advanced in putrefaction. The same appearances were found in Picco's cases. In these there was also an excessive enlargement of the liver. The lungs have sometimes been found gorged or even inflamed. The vessels of the brain are also sometimes very turgid. They were par-

* Rust's Magazin für die gesammte Heilkunde, xvi. 115.
† Persoon, Traité sur les Champignons comestibles, 157.
‡ Journal de Pharmacie, Sept. 1836.
§ Edwards in Lancet, 1836-37, ii. 512.
‖ Picco — Hist. de la Soc. &c. pp. 357, 359.

ticularly so in a case related by Dr. Beck, where death was occasioned in seven hours by an infusion of the *Amanita muscaria* in milk. The whole sinuses of the dura mater, as well as the arteries were enormously distended with blood ; the arachnoid and pia mater were of a scarlet colour ; the vessels of the membrane between the convolutions, together with the plexus choroides, were also excessively gorged ; and the substance of the brain was red. Lastly, a clot of blood, as big as a bean, was found in the cerebellum.[*]—The stomach, unless there had been vomiting or diarrhœa, will usually contain fragments of the poison, if it has not been taken in a state of minute division ; and this evidence of the cause of death may be obtained, even although the individual survived two days or upwards. Sometimes fragments are found in the intestines. In one of Picco's patients who lived twenty-four hours, there was found in the neighbourhood of the ileo-cæcal valve, which was much inflamed.[†]

Of the Treatment.—The treatment of poisoning with the fungi does not call for any special observations. Emetics are of primary importance ; and after the poison has been by their means dislodged, the sopor and inflammation of the bowels are to be treated in the usual way. No antidote is known. Several have at different times been a good deal confided in ; but none are of any material service. Chansarel found acids useless, but thought infusion of galls advantageous.[‡]

In concluding the present chapter it is necessary to take notice of a variety of poisoning, not altogether unimportant in a medico-legal point of view. A person may seem to die of poisoning with the deleterious fungi, from eating esculent mushrooms intentionally drugged with some other vegetable or mineral poison. It must be confessed, that if the murderer is dexterous in the choice and mode of administering the poison, such cases might readily escape suspicion, and even when suspected might not be cleared up without difficulty. The ascertaining the species of mushroom, by finding others where it has been gathered, will not supply more than presumptive proof of the wholesomeness of that which has been eaten ; because the esculent and poisonous species sometimes grow near one another, and have a mutual resemblance, so that a mistake may easily occur. The presumption may be somewhat strengthened by evidence derived from the interval which elapses before the symptoms begin, from the nature and progress of the symptoms themselves, and from the morbid appearances. Some one or other of these circumstances may establish the fact of poisoning with a deleterious fungi. It is impossible, however, that they shall ever establish satisfactorily that the fungus was naturally wholesome ; and, on the whole, the only decided evidence of poisoning by some other means will be the actual discovery of another poison.

The case now under consideration is not a mere hypothetical one.

* Hist. de la Soc. &c. p. 357.   † Ibidem.
‡ Repertorium für die Pharmacie, lxvi. 117.

Ernest Platner has related a very interesting example, which proves how easily poisoning of the kind supposed may be accomplished without suspicion. A servant-girl poisoned her mistress by mixing oxide of arsenic with a dish of mushrooms. She died in twenty hours, after suffering severely from vomiting and colic pains. On dissection there were found inflammation of the stomach, gangrenous spots in it, clots of blood in its contents, and redness of the intestines. Her death, however, was ascribed to the mushrooms having been unwholesome ; and the real cause was not discovered till thirteen years after, when the girl was convicted of murdering a fellow-servant in a somewhat similar way by mixing arsenic with her chocolate, and then confessed both crimes.*

Poisonous Mosses. — It is not improbable that some of the mosses possess poisonous properties similar to those of the deleterious fungi. Dr. Winkler of Innsbruch mentions that the *Lycopodium selago* is used in the Tyrol in the way of infusion for killing vermin on animals ; and that unpleasant accidents have been produced in man by its accidental use. Its effects appear to be sometimes irritant, but more generally narcotic in their nature.†

CHAPTER XL.

OF THE EFFECTS OF POISONOUS GRAIN AND PULSE.

The different sorts of grain are subject to certain diseases, in consequence of which meal or flour made from them is apt to be impregnated with substances more or less injurious to animal life. It is likewise believed, that unripe grain possesses properties which render it to a certain extent unfit for the food of man.

It is for the most part difficult to trace satisfactorily the operation of the poisons now alluded to, because they are seen acting only in times of famine and general distress, when it is not always easy to make due allowance for the effect of collateral circumstances. There is one poison of the kind, however, whose baneful influence has been so frequently and unequivocally witnessed, that no doubt now exists regarding its properties, I mean *spurred rye*, or *ergot*. It is a poison of no great consequence, perhaps, to the English toxicologist; for indeed I am not aware that a single instance of its operation has hitherto been observed in Britain.‡ But its effects are so singular, and the ravages it has often committed on the continent have been so dreadful, that a short account of it cannot fail to interest even the English reader. Besides, it has lately been introduced into the ma-

* Quæstiones Medicinæ Forenses, 1824, p. 206.
† Repertorium für die Pharmacie, xiv. 311.
‡ In the Philosophical Transactions for 1762 an account is given of a family of eight people in Suffolk, who had the gangrenous form of the disease induced by spurred rye. They had lived on damaged wheat, but never used rye meal. See Dr. Wollaston's paper, lii. 523, and Mr. Bone's Letter, Ibid. 526.

teria medica, as possessing very extraordinary medicinal qualities; and since its use is gaining ground, every medical jurist ought to be conversant with its properties as a poison. I have also met with an instance where it was administered for the purpose of procuring miscarriage.

Of Poisoning with Spurred Rye.

Spurred Rye, or *Secale cornutum*, the *Seigle ergoté*, or *Ergot* of the French, and *Mutterkorn*, or *Roggenmutter*, of the Germans, is a disease common to various grains, in consequence of which the place of the pickle is supplied by a long, black substance, like a little horn or spur. It has been known to attack many plants of the order Graminaceæ;[*] and among those used as food by man, it has been observed on barley, oats, spring-wheat, winter-wheat, and rye. But the rye seems peculiarly subject to it, almost all the poison which has caused epidemics, as well as what is now used in medicine, being produced by that grain.

Of the Cause and Nature of the Spur in Rye. — The spur attacks rye chiefly in damp seasons, and in moist clay soils, particularly those recently redeemed from waste lands in the neighbourhood of forests. Of all the places where the spur has been hitherto observed none combines these conditions so perfectly, and none has been so much infested with the disease, as the district of Sologne, situated between the rivers Loire and Cher, in France. According to the statistical researches of the *Abbé Tessier*, who in 1777 was deputed by the Parisian Society of Medicine to investigate the causes of the extraordinary prevalence of the ergot in that district, the country was then so much intersected by belts of wood around the fields, that the traveller in passing along might imagine he was constantly approaching an immense forest; the arable land was so poor, that, although it lay fallow every third season, it was exhausted in nine or twelve years at farthest, and then remained a long time in pasture before it could again bear white crops; the surface was so level, and consequently so wet, that crops were obtained only when the seed was sown on the tops of furrows a foot high; and the climate is so moist, that from the month of September till late in spring the whole country is overhung by dense fogs.[†] Here the rye, the common food of the peasantry, appears to have been in Tessier's time more liable to be attacked by the spur than in any other part of the continent. Tessier found, that after being thrashed it contained on an average about a forty-eighth part of ergot, even in good seasons; but in bad seasons, and taking into account a considerable propor-

[*] The Phalaris canariensis and aquatica, Panicum miliaceum Phleum, pratense, Alopecurus pratensis and geniculatus, Agrostis stolonifera, Aira cristata, Poa fluitans, Festuca duriuscula, Arundo arenaria and cinnoides, Lolium perenne, Elymus arenarius and europæus, Triticum spelta, junceum and repens, Holcus avenaceus and lanatus, Dactylis glomerata, besides those mentioned in the text. — See Robert, Erläuterungen und Beiträge zur Geschichte des Mutterkorns. — Rust's Magazin für die gesammte Heilkunde, xxv. 8.

[†] Mémoire sur la Sologne, in Hist. de la Soc. Roy. de Méd. i. 61.

tion which is shaken out of the ears and sheaves before they reach the barn, the proportion of ergot in the whole crop has been estimated so high as a fourth or even a third. In Sologne the disease was farther observed by Tessier to be always most prevalent in the dampest parts of a field, and to affect above all the first crop of fields redeemed from waste land, or from land which had previously been for some time in pasture.* The same connexion between moisture and the development of the ergot has been repeatedly traced in other parts of France, as well as in Germany.† And according to the experiments of Wildenow, it may be brought on at any time, by sowing the rye in a rich damp soil, and watering the plants exuberantly in warm weather.‡

Opinions are much divided as to the cause and nature of the spur. It had been conceived by some that nothing else is required for its production but undue moisture combined with warmth; and that under these circumstances the spur is formed simply by a diseased process from the juices of the plant.§ By others, such as Tillet, Fontana, and Réad, who also consider it to be simply a diseased formation, it has been held to arise from the germen being punctured when young by an insect;‖ and in support of this statement, General Field says he saw flies puncture the glumes in their milky state where spurs afterwards formed, and imitating the operation with a needle obtained the same result.¶ On the other hand, Decandolle, reviving a previous doctrine that the spur is a kind of fungus, conceived he had given strong grounds for believing this excrescence to be a species of *sclerotium*, which he terms *S. clavus*. Wiggers supports this doctrine by chemical analysis; for he endeavours to show that the basis of the structure of the spur is almost identical in chemical properties with the principle fungin.** Lastly, the most recent researches, those of Smith,†† Queckett,‡‡ and Bauer,§§ founded chiefly on microscopical observations, tend to a union and modification of these two views, — namely, that the great mass of the spur is a peculiar morbid formation, and that the whitish bloom which covers fresh specimens consists of a multitude of microscopic fungi in the form of *sporidia*, which thickly envelope and impregnate the parts of fructification in the nascent state of the embryo, and are in all probability the exciting cause of the morbid degeneration of the pickle.

* Mem. sur la mal. du Seigle appellée Ergot. Hist. de la Soc. Roy. de Méd. i. 427.

† Robert's paper, *passim*.

‡ Hecker's Jahrbücher der Staatsarzneikunde, i. 240.

§ Robert, in Rust's Magazin, xxv. 20. Tessier seems to have been of the same way of thinking.

‖ Tillet, Dissertation sur la cause qui corrompe les blés —Fontana, Lettre sur l'Ergot. Journ. de Phys. vii. 42. — Réad, Traité sur le Seigle Ergoté. 1771.

¶ Annals of Philosophy, N. S. xi. 14.

** Flore Française, VI. — Robert's paper, p. 15.

†† Inquisitio in Secale cornutum, &c. Commentatio præmio regio ornata, Gottingæ, 1831. Analyzed in Annalen der Pharmacie, i. 129.

‡‡ Linnæan Transactions, 1840, xviii. 449.

§§ Ibidem, 453.   ‖ Ibidem, 475.

Various opinions have been formed as to the mode of propagation of the spur. Fontana has alleged that one variety of it may spread from plant to plant over a field; and that he has expressly transmitted it by contact from one ear to another.* His opinion and statement of facts are at variance with experiments lately made by Hertwig, a German physician, who found that even when the ear while in flower was surrounded for twelve days with powder of spurred rye, the healthiness of the future grain was not in the slightest degree affected.† The same results have also been obtained by Wiggers, and more recently by Dr. Samuel Wright.‡ Wiggers, however, although he could not produce spurs in the way indicated by Fontana, observed that the white dust on the surface of the spurs will produce the disease in any plant, if sprinkled in the soil at its roots, appearing therefore to be analogous to the sporules or spawn of the admitted fungi. Mr. Queckett has made the most precise experiments on the mode of reproduction of the disease. He succeeded in infecting rye repeatedly with ergot by means of the sporidia developed on the spurs; but it is remarkable that he could not in the same way infect wheat or barley.§

Description and analysis of Spurred Rye. — The spur varies in length from a few lines to two inches, and is from two to four lines in thickness. If it is long, there is seldom more than one or two on a single ear, and the remaining pickles of the ear are healthy. But the ears which have small spurs have generally several, sometimes even twenty; and when there are many, few of the remaining pickles are altogether without blackness at the tips.‖ The substance of the spur is of a pale grayish-red tint; and externally it is bluish-black or violet, with two, sometimes three, streaks of dotted gray. It is specifically lighter than water, while sound rye is specifically heavier, so that they are easily separated from one another.¶ It is tough and flexible when fresh, brittle and easily pulverized when dry. The powder is disposed to attract moisture. It has a disagreeable heavy smell, a nauseous, slightly acrid taste, and imparts its taste and smell both to water and alcohol. Bread which contains it is defective in firmness, liable to become moist, and cracks and crumbles soon after being taken from the oven.** — It is easily known, when entire, by its external characters. Its powder, which is of an obscure grayish-red hue, is best known by the action of solution of potash, which immediately disengages a powerful odour of ergot, and forms a lake-red pulp; and this pulp yields by filtration a splendid lake-red solution, which gives a beautiful lake-red flaky precipitate, when either neutralized by nitric acid, or treated with an excess of solution of alum.

Spurred rye has been repeatedly subjected to analysis. The earlier

* Lettre sur l'Ergot. Journal de Physique, vii. 42.
† Lorinser, Beob. und Vers. über die Wirkung des Mutterkorns, 1824, noticed in Robert's paper, p. 28.
‡ Edinburgh Medical and Surgical Journal, lii. 306. Harveian Prize Essay.
§ Linnæan Transactions, xix. 140.
‖ Tessier, 421.   ¶ Ibid. 428.   ** Robert, 28

researches of Vauquelin* and of Pettenkofer† do not lead to any pointed results. The presence of hydrocyanic acid indicated by Robert,‡ would not account for the very peculiar effects of ergot, and has besides been denied by Wiggers. Winkler obtained various principles from it, and among the rest a thick, rancid, slightly acrid oil, and a nauseous, sweetish, acrid fluid ; but he did not determine, any more than his predecessors, in which of these principles the active properties of the spur reside.§ Wiggers supplied more definite information on the subject. He denies the presence of hydrocyanic acid, and says he found ergot to consist chiefly of a heavy-smelling fixed oil, fungin, albumen, osmazôme, waxy matter, and an extractive substance of a strong, peculiar taste and smell, in which, from experiments on animals, he was led to infer that its active properties reside. I have obtained all his chief results, except the most important of them ; for the substance which ought to have been his ergotin was destitute of marked taste or smell of any kind.‖ Dr. Wright too could not obtain the ergotin of Wiggers, and concludes from his own experiments, that the spur consists of fungin, modified starch, mucilage, gluten, osmazôme, colouring matter, various salts, and thirty-one per cent. of fixed oil, in which the active properties of the poison seemed to him to reside.¶ Buchner, however, thinks that the oil is not itself active, but owes its apparent energy to an acrid principle which alcohol removes from it, and which is not removed from the crude substance in separating the oil in the usual way by sulphuric ether, unless the ether be somewhat alcoholized.** However this may be, it seems ascertained by the experiments of Dr. Wright, that the fixed oil, obtained by means of common ether, concentrates in itself the peculiar properties possessed by ergot, either in small doses as a medicine, or in a single large dose as a poison.

Effects of Spurred Rye on Man and Animals. — Before proceeding to relate the effects of this poison on man, it should be mentioned, that at different times doubts have been entertained, whether the baneful effects ascribed to it might not really arise from some other cause. But independently of the connexion which has been frequently traced between the poison and the diseases imputed to it in the human subject, the question has been set at rest by the experiments which have been tried on animals, and which indeed were instituted with a view to settle the point in dispute.

The experiments hitherto made on animals are variable in their results, yet sufficient to show that spurred rye is an active poison of a very peculiar kind. According to the observations collected by Dr. Robert from a variety of authors, it follows that it is injurious

* Bulletins de la Soc. Philomatique, 1817, 58.

† Buchner's Repertorium für die Pharmacie, iii. 65.

‡ Rust's Magazin, xxv. 43, also Keyl, Dissertatio de Secali Cornuto ejusque vi in corpus humanum salubri et noxia.

§ Rust's Mag. für die gesammte Heilk. xxv. 47.

‖ Annalen der Pharmacie, i. 159.

¶ Edinburgh Medical and Surgical Journal. lii. 302, and liv. 51.

** Repertorium für die Pharmacie, lxxv. 168.

and even fatal to all animals which are fed for a sufficient length of time with a moderate proportion of it, unless they escape its action by early vomiting; that dogs and cats, in consequence of discharging it by vomiting, suffer only slight symptoms of irritant poisoning; — but that swine, moles, geese, ducks, fowls, quails, sparrows, as well as leeches and flies, are sooner or later killed by it; — and that the symptoms it causes in beasts and birds are in the first instance giddiness, dilated pupil, and palsy, and afterwards diarrhœa, suppurating tumours, scattered gangrene throughout the body, and sometimes dropping off of the toes. Wiggers ascertained that nine grains of the substance he has considered its active principle occasioned in a fowl dulness, apparent suffering, gradually increasing feebleness, coldness and insensibility of the extremities, and in three days a fit of convulsions, ending in death.* Taddei lately found, that sparrows were killed by six grains of it in six or seven hours, with symptoms merely of great weakness, torpor, and indisposition to stir.†

Dr. Wright, whose experiments are the most extensive and precise yet made on this subject, found that a single dose, consisting of a strong infusion of between two drachms and a half and six drachms of ergot, if introduced into the jugular vein of a dog, occasions death, sometimes in a few minutes, sometimes not for more than two hours, with symptoms of alternating spasm and paralysis, occasionally a tendency to coma, and often depressed or irregular action of the heart, or even complete arrestment of its function; — that, when introduced into the cellular tissue, it produces inflammation and suppuration, sometimes circumscribed, sometimes diffuse, and always attended with an unhealthy discharge and great exhaustion; — and that, when admitted into the stomach, it excites irritation of the alimentary canal, excessive muscular prostration, at first excitability, but afterwards singular dulness or even complete obliteration of the senses, and occasional slight spasms; but that it is not a very active poison through this channel, as above three ounces are required to prove fatal to a dog. When it was administered in frequent small doses, he could not observe the effects remarked by Robert, but found that it induced a peculiar cachectic state, indicated by extreme muscular emaciation and weakness, loss of appetite, frequency of the pulse, repulsive fetor of the secretions and excretions, congestion of the alimentary mucous membrane, excessive contraction of the spleen, enlargement of the liver and absorbent glands, and non-formation of callus at the ends of fractured bones.‡

With regard to its effects on man, it has been found by express experiment, that a single dose of two drachms excites giddiness, headache, flushed face, pain and spasms in the stomach, nausea, and vomiting, colic, purging, and a sense of weariness and weight in the limbs.§ But it is not in this way that it has been usually introduced into the system; nor are these precisely the symptoms already hinted

* Annalen der Pharmacie, i. 180. † Annali Universali di Medicina, 1839, iv. 12.
‡ Edinburgh Medical and Surgical Journal, lii. 119, liii. 1.
§ Robert's paper, p. 223, also Lorinser's Versuche, &c. of which there is an analysis in Edinb. Med. and Surg. Journal, xxvi. 453.

at as particular in its action.   The effects now to be mentioned form
a peculiar disease, which has often prevailed epidemically in different territories on the continent, and which arises from the spur being
allowed to mix with the grain in the meal, and being taken as food
for a continuance of time in rye-bread.   The affection produced differs much in different epidemics and even in different cases of the
same epidemic.   Two distinct disorders have been noticed; the one
a nervous disease, characterized by violent spasmodic convulsions;
the other a depraved state of the constitution, which ends in that remarkable disorder, dry gangrene; and it does not appear that the two
affections are apt to be blended together in the same case.

The first form of disease, the *convulsive ergotism* of the French
writers, has been very well described by Taube, a German physician,
as it occurred in the north of Germany in 1770-1.   In its most acute
form, it commenced suddenly with dimness of sight, giddiness and
loss of sensibility, followed soon by dreadful cramps and convulsions
of the whole body, *risus sardonicus*, yellowness of the countenance,
excessive thirst, excruciating pains in the limbs and chest, and a
small, often imperceptible pulse.   Such cases usually proved fatal in
twenty-four or forty-eight hours.   In the milder cases the convulsions
came on in paroxysms, were preceded for some days by weakness
and weight of the limbs, and a strange feeling as of insects crawling
over the legs, arms, and face; in the intervals between the fits the
appetite was voracious, the pulse natural, the excretions regular; and
the disease either terminated in recovery, with scattered suppurations,
cutaneous eruptions, anasarca or diarrhœa, or it proved in the end
fatal amidst prolonged sopor and convulsions.*   Another more recent
and very clear account of this form of the disease has been given by
Dr. Wagner of Schlieben from his experience of an epidemic which
prevailed in the neighbourhood of that place so lately as the years
1831 and 1832.   In consequence of unusual moisture and late frosts
in the summer of 1831, the rye was so much spurred in many fields
that a fifth at least of the pickles was diseased.   As soon as the country people proceeded to use the new rye, convulsive ergotism began
to show itself, and it recurred more or less till next midsummer,
when the diseased grain was all consumed.   The usual symptoms
were at first periodic weariness, afterwards an uneasy sense of contraction in the hands and feet, and at length violent and permanent
contraction of the flexor muscles of the arms, legs, feet, hands, fingers and toes, with frequent attacks of a sense of burning or creeping
on the skin.   These were the essential symptoms; but a great variety of accessory nervous affections occasionally presented themselves.   There was seldom any disturbance of the mind, except in
some of the fatal cases, where epileptic convulsions and coma preceded death.   Every case was cured by emetics, laxatives, and frequent small doses of opium, provided it was taken in reasonable time,
and the unwholesome food was completely withdrawn.†

The other form of disease, which has been named *gangrenous er-*

---

* Taube — Geschichte der Kriebelkrankheit, quoted in Robert's paper, p. 209.
† Journal der Praktischen Heilkunde, lxxiii. iv. 3, and lxxiv. v. 71, vi. 3.

gotism, by the French writers, and is known in Germany by the vulgar name of creeping-sickness (*kriebelkrankheit*), has been minutely described by various authors. In the most severe form, as it appeared in Switzerland in 1709 and 1716, it commenced, according to Lang, a physician of Lucerne, with general weakness, weariness, and a feeling as of insects creeping over the skin; when these symptoms had lasted some days or weeks, the extremities became cold, white, stiff, benumbed, and at length so insensible that deep incisions were not felt; then excruciating pains in the limbs supervened, along with fever, headache, and sometimes bleeding from the nose; finally the affected parts, and in the first instance the fingers and arms, afterwards the toes and legs, shrivelled, dried up, and dropped off by the joints. A healthy granulation succeeded; but the powers of life were frequently exhausted before that stage was reached. The appetite, as in the convulsive form of the disease, continued voracious throughout.[*] In milder cases, as it prevailed at different times in France, nausea and vomiting attended the precursory symptoms, and the gangrenous affection was accompanied with dark vesications.[†] In another variety, which has been witnessed in various parts of Germany, the chief symptoms were spasmodic contraction of the limbs at first, and afterwards weakness of mind, voracity and dyspepsia, which, if not followed by recovery, as generally happened, either terminated in fatuity or in fatal gangrene.[‡]

These extraordinary and formidable distempers were first referred to the operation of spurred rye in 1597 by the Marburg Medical Faculty, who witnessed the ravages of the poison in Hessia during the preceding year. Since then repeated epidemics have broken out in Germany, Bohemia, Holstein, Denmark, Sweden, Lombardy, Switzerland, and France.[§] About the close of last century, partly in consequence of the attention of the respective governments being turned to the subject, partly by reason of the improved condition of the peasantry in these countries, and the greater rarity of seasons of famine, the epidemics became much less common or extensive. Nevertheless the creeping-sickness has been several times noticed in Germany since the present century began.[‖]

Spurred rye is now generally believed to possess another singular quality, in consequence of which it has been lately introduced into the materia medica of this and other countries, — a power of promoting the contractions of the gravid uterus. This property seems to have been long familiar to the quacks and midwives of Germany; and towards the close of last century it rendered ergot so favourite a remedy with them, that several of the German states prohibited the use of it by severe statutes.[¶] It was first fairly brought under the

---

[*] Descriptio morborum ex usu clavorum secalinorum cum pane, 1717. A full extract is given of this work in Acta Eruditorum, An. 1718. Lipsiæ, p. 309.

[†] L'Abbé Tessier, Mém. sur les effets du Seigle Ergoté. Hist. de la Soc. Roy. de Méd. ii. 611.

[‡] Robert, in Rust's Magazin, xxv. 205.

[§] Ibid. 200.   [‖] Ibid. 204.

[¶] Ibid „ 231, 232.

63*

notice of regular accoucheurs by the physicians of the United States between the years 1807 and 1814.*   There appears little reason for doubting that it possesses the power of increasing the contractions of the uterus when unnaturally languid ; and consequently it has been employed, apparently with frequent good effect, to hasten languid natural labour, to promote the separation of the placenta, and to quicken the contraction of the womb after delivery.   These facts, however, are mentioned chiefly as preparatory to the statement, that it has been also supposed to possess the power of producing abortion, and has been actually employed for that purpose in some foreign countries, and even in this city.   Accurate information is still much wanted on this subject.   No other poison seems so likely to possess a peculiar property of the kind.   Nevertheless it is the opinion of the best authorities, that spurred rye has no such power, except in con-nexion with violent constitutional injury produced by dangerous doses ; and that it is endowed with the property only of accelerating natural labour, not of inducing it, particularly in the early months of pregnancy.

It seems from the experiments of Dr. Wright to have no power whatever of inducing miscarriage in the lower animals.†   Notwith-standing the improbability, however, of its possessing the property of bringing on abortion, it is one of the substances at present occasion-ally employed with the view of feloniously causing this accident. In a case of attempt to procure abortion, which occurred not long ago in this city, one of the articles repeatedly employed, but without success, was powder of spurred rye, — as I had occasion to ascertain by chemical analysis.

Of Spurred Maize. — It has been already observed, that many other plants of the Natural Family of Grasses are subject to the ergot be-sides rye.   But the only other species in which the disease has been particularly examined is Indian corn or maize [*Zea Mays*].   It ap-pears from the inquiries of M. Roullin that maize is very subject to the spur in the provinces of Neyba and Maraquita in Colombia ; that the spur forms a black, pear-shaped body on the ear in place of the pickle ; and that in this state the grain, which is known by the name of *maïs peladero*, possesses properties injurious to animal life.   Its effects, however, are somewhat different from those of spurred rye. Men who eat the ergotted maize lose their hair and sometimes their teeth, but are never attacked with dry gangrene or convulsions. When swine eat it, which after a time they do with avidity, the bristles drop off, and the hind-legs become feeble and wasted.   Mules likewise lose their hair, and the hoofs swell.   Fowls lay their eggs without the shell.   Apes and parrots, which frequent the fields of spurred maize, fall down as if drunk ; and the native dogs and deer experience similar effects.‡

* Stearns in New York Med. Rep. 1307. — Bigelow in New England Journal of Med. and Surg. v. — Prescott in Lond. Med. and Phys. Journ. xxxvi.
† Edinburgh Medical and Surgical Journal, liii. 29.
‡ Revue Médicale, 1829, iii. 332.

Of the Rust of Wheat.

There are several other diseases to which grain is liable, and which are much more common in this country than the ergot. But very little is known of their effects on the animal body ; which circumstance, since the wheat of this and other countries often suffers from them, is probably sufficient to show that their influence must be trifling, or at all events very seldom called forth. Wheat is liable to three diseases. One is a disease of the stalk and leaf rather than of the ear, and has the effect of preventing the development of the ear or its pickles, and of covering the plant with a brown powder. Of the two other diseases, which both attack the pickles of the ear, one consists in the substitution of a brown dry powder for the farina of the pickle, and the other of a deposition of black moist matter in the fissure of the pickle, the substance of which it also invades and partially destroys. One of these is called in Scotland *brown rust*, the other *black rust*.

Of the three diseases the only one which is apt to infect the flour is the black rust. The others, as they consist of a light dry powder, are almost entirely separated in thrashing and winnowing the grain. But the black rust being damp and adhesive, it is carried along with the pickles. Such pickles are almost invariably separated by the farmer if they are abundant ; for otherwise, on account of the dark colour and disagreeable odour of the matter deposited on them, the flour possesses external qualities which would be at once recognized by a dealer of ordinary experience.

It is not improbable, that a moderate impregnation of bread with the powder formed by the diseases in question may take place, without leading to any unpleasant effect on the human body. Experiments to this effect were made by Parmentier with one of them, termed in France *carie*, or caries of wheat, which from his description appears to be the black rust of of Scottish farmers. He gave two dogs each two drachms daily of the powder for fifteen days, without remarking any sign of ill health. Bread made with wheat flour containing a 64th of the powder, when eaten by various people, and Parmentier among the rest, to the amount of a pound daily for several days, caused slight headache and pain in the stomach the first day only ; and in larger proportion it had as little effect.[*]

It appears, then, that the introduction of any deleterious ingredient into wheat bread is hardly to be dreaded from the common diseases to which wheat is liable in this country.

Of Unripe Grain.

Wheat and other grains have been supposed to acquire qualities detrimental to health, from being cut down while unripe, or used immediately after being cut down, although ripe. I am not aware that accidents have ever been traced or even imputed to such causes

[*] Hist. de la Soc. Roy. de Méd. i. 346.

in this country ; and, on the whole, I believe it is generally considered here, that imperfect ripening of the pickle rather lessens the
quantity, than impairs the quality, of the flour. But several times
epidemics have been ascribed in France to unripe wheat. In 1801
M. Bouvier read a memoir to the Society of Medicine at Paris, ascribing to new and unripe wheat an epidemic dysentery, which laid
waste several districts of the department of the Oise in the autumn of
1793.   These districts abound in small farms of a few acres, on the
produce of which the cultivators depend in great measure for their
subsistence.   Hence in unfavourable seasons the corn was commonly
cut down before it was ripe, and made into bread soon after being
reaped.   It was accordingly among the peasantry of these farms
only, and not among the agriculturists in large farms, which were
under better management, that the epidemic prevailed.   Bouvier remarks, that at all times when the long continuance of wet weather
has compelled the inhabitants of a district to cut down the wheat
before it is ripe, or a previous dearth has forced them to use it when
newly cut, epidemic disorders of the bowels have been observed to
rage in the latter months of autumn.   And as an instance of this he
refers to the year 1783, when the crops around Paris were believed
to have been injured by the extraordinary prevalence of fogs, and
were cut down unripe and used immediately.   Various epidemics
broke out in the metropolis, and still more in the surrounding country.*   This is an important subject for farther inquiry ; but at present
I cannot help thinking that M. Bouvier exaggerates the effects of the
immaturity of the grain.   At all events, the grain is often cut down
in an unripe state in various districts of this country ; and I have
never heard that any epidemic diseases were produced.   When M.
Bouvier witnessed the epidemic of 1793 in the department of the
Oise, he instructed the inhabitants of his own parish to dry the unripe corn before thrashing it, to repeat the process before the grain
was converted into flour, and to mix with the flour a larger quantity
than usual of yeast in making it into bread ; and he states that in the
succeeding yeer, which was even more unfavourable to the crops,
they were enabled, by following these directions, to use unripe corn
with safety.

Of Spoiled Bread.

This is the fittest opportunity for noticing certain injurious effects
sometimes observed from the use of spoiled or mouldy bread.   On
the continent repeated instances have occurred of severe and even
dangerous poisoning from spoiled rye-bread, barley-bread, and even
wheat-bread.   Several instances have been observed of horses having been killed in a short space of time with symptoms of irritant
poisoning after eating such bread with their ordinary food.†   And
Dr. Westerhoff has given an account of its effects on two children
and several adults.   In children the symptoms were redness of the

---

* Sedillot's Journ. Gén. de Méd. xiv. 200.
† Journal de Chimie Médicale, viii. 558.

features, dry tongue, frequent weak pulse, violent colic pains, urgent thirst and headache, and subsequently vomiting and diarrhœa, alternating with great exhaustion and sleepiness. The bread in these instances was made of rye.* It appears that in bread so spoiled a variety of mucedonous vegetables are developed, especially the *Penicillium glaucum* and *P. roseum ;* and it is imagined by some, that this circumstance may account for the deleterious effect of the bread.†

Of the Effects of Darnel-Grass.

Grain is also rendered more or less injurious by the accidental or intentional admixture of a variety of foreign substances, by which, in common speech, it is said to be adulterated. The subject of the adulteration of grain is a very important topic in medical police. But as this practice seldom imparts to the grain qualities decidedly poisonous, the consideration of it would be misplaced here. One variety, however, the accidental adulteration of flour with the seeds of the *Lolium temulentum* or darnel-grass calls for some notice ; for it may occasion not only symptoms of poisoning, but even also death itself.

This is the only poisonous species of the natural order of the grasses. The seeds appear to be powerfully narcotic, and at the same time to possess acrid properties. Seeger gave a dog three ounces of a decoction of the flour, and observed that it was seized in five hours with violent trembling and great feebleness, which were succeeded in four hours by sopor and insensibility ; but it recovered next day.‡

When mixed with bread and taken habitually by man, darnel-grass has been known to cause headache, giddiness, somnolency, delirium, convulsions, paralysis, and even death. M. Cordier found by experiment on himself, that very soon after eating bread containing darnel-grass flour, he felt confusion of sight and ideas, languor, heaviness, and alternate attacks of somnolency and vomiting. The bread was commonly vomited soon after he ate it.§ Seeger has related some cases in which the somnolency was much more deep ; and states that general tremors are almost always present.‖ A few years ago almost the whole inmates of the Poor's House at Sheffield, to the amount of eighty, were attacked with analogous symptoms after breakfasting on oatmeal porridge ; and it was supposed that the meal had been accidentally adulterated with the lolium. The chief symptoms were a piercing stare, violent agitation of the limbs, quivering of the lips, frontal headache, confusion of sight, dilated pupil, small tremulous pulse, twitches of the muscles, and palpitation. In twelve hours all of the persons attacked were well but two, who had strong convulsions in the subsequent night, but also eventually recovered.¶

* Journal de Chimie Médicale, vii. 122.
† Guérard in Annales d'Hygiène-Publique, xxix. 35.
‡ Orfila, Toxic. Gén. ii. 466, from Seeger, Diss. Inaug. Tubingæ, 1760.
§ Sur les Effets de l'Ivraie. — Nouv. Journ. de Méd. vi. 379.
‖ Orfila, Toxicol. Gén. ii. 466.
¶ London Med. and Phys. Journal, xxviii. 182.

A similar accident is mentioned by Perleb, as having happened at Freyburg in the House of Correction. The inmates, soon after eating bread made with new flour, were attacked to the number of forty, with loss of speech and somnolency ; and for some days afterwards they complained of sickness.[*] The accident was ascribed to darnel-grass. In a recent instance which happened in the workhouse of Beninghausen, and which was traced to the lolium, seventy-four people were attacked with giddiness, tremor, convulsions, and vomiting. Those who had led a dissipated life suffered most, and children least of all.[†]

Sometimes this poison appears to excite symptoms of intestinal irritation, without acting as a narcotic. A small farmer near Poicters in France saved five bushels of the seed from a field of wheat, — had it ground with a single bushel of wheat, and afterwards made bread with the mixture for his own family. He himself, with his wife and a servant, began to eat the bread on a Thursday ; but the two last were so violently affected with vomiting and purging, that they refused to continue taking it. He persevered himself, however, till on the Sunday evening he became so ill that his wife wished to send for medical aid. This he refused to allow, and next day he expired after suffering severely from fits of colic.[‡]

Bley of Bemburg has examined chemically the grain of lolium. He obtained from it a bitter extractive matter, without any characteristic chemical properties, but which killed a pigeon. The seed has a very feeble bitterish taste. Bley maintains that its poisonous properties are essential to it, and not incidental, as some think.[§]

Of the Effects of certain Poisonous Leguminous Seeds.

Among the injurious substances with which various grains are apt to be accidentally mixed from their growing together, two leguminous plants may be here shortly mentioned, as they have often been the source of disagreeable accidents on the continent.

In the department of the Cher and Loire in France, severe effects have been traced to bread made partly with flour of the *Lathyrus cicera*. M. Desparanches, in a report to the Prefect of the Department, says this flour occasionally forms one-half of that of which bread is made in some parishes; that it produces sometimes sudden incapability of walking, sometimes imperfect paraplegia and pain, with a draggling gait and turning in of the toes, and sometimes also slight convulsive movements of the thighs and legs.[‖] Similar effects have been traced to this substance formerly. Virey says it has been known to produce in particular a singular stiffness and state of semiflexion of the knee-joint, compelling the individual to move the limbs in one rigid mass.[¶]

The *Ervum ervilia*, or Bitter-vetch, which is not a native of this

* Buchner's Toxikologie, 174.
† Annalen der Pharmacie, xvi. 318.   ‡ Hist. de la Soc. Roy. de Méd. ii. 297.
§ Repertorium für die Pharmacie, xlviii. 160.
‖ Nouvelle Bibliothêque Méd. iii. 439.
¶ Journal de Pharmacie, ii. 397.

country, has also been found in France to possess analogous properties. In 1815, according to Virey, a great variety of herbs grew up with the grain, in consequence of the wetness of the summer; and their seeds were thus subsequently mixed with the wheat and rye. Among these he particularizes the bitter-vetch as peculiarly noxious, because it produces so great weakness of the extremities, but especially of the limbs, that the individual trembles while standing, and totters when he walks, or even requires the help of stilts; and he adds, that horses are similarly affected, so as to become almost paralytic.*

The *Cytisus laburnum*, or laburnum tree, is another plant of the same family, which yields poisonous seeds. The whole plant is more or less deleterious. But it is chiefly the seed that has attracted attention hitherto.

I am not acquainted with any experiments relative to the action of the seeds on animals. — Its effects on man present considerable variety, and show that it is a true narcotico-acrid. In some instances they seem to have been purely narcotic. My colleague Dr. Traill has communicated to me two cases of this nature. In one of these, that of a child two years old, the first evident effects were sudden paleness and a fit of screaming, followed immediately by insensibility, and then by coldness of the whole body and lividity of the face; but vomiting having been induced by warm water and mustard, the seeds were discharged, the symptoms abated, and next day he was quite well. The other case was that of a boy who was left by his companions at Dr. Traill's door in a state of complete insensibility, with froth at the mouth and a feeble pulse. An emetic, administered immediately, brought up a large quantity of laburnum seeds; after which the pulse became firmer, and sensibility quickly returned. — Mr. North has briefly noticed a similar case of a child, who after eating laburnum flowers, was seized with paleness and twitches of the face, coldness of the skin, laborious breathing, efforts to vomit, and great feebleness of the pulse. But recovery took place after the flowers were vomited.†— In other instances the effects have been chiefly limited to an irritant action on the stomach and bowels. Dr. Bigsby of Newark informs me that a few years ago a little girl in his neighbourhood, in consequence of eating the seeds, was attacked with violent vomiting and purging, and became in other respects very ill, but recovered in forty-eight hours. — Most generally, however, the effects are partly irritant, partly narcotic. In 1839 Dr. Annan of Kinross communicated to me the case of a little boy, who in an hour after swallowing a small quantity of unripe seeds, was attacked with violent vomiting and ghastly expression of countenance, and then fell into a very drowsy state, from which he was constantly roused by shaking him and dashing cold water on his body. But for a month afterwards he continued subject to vomiting and diarrhœa. — Mr. Bonney of Brentford has related the particulars of eleven cases, which presented all the varieties of poisoning with the seeds. The

* Journ. de Pharm., ii. 397.   † London Medical and Physical Journal, lxii. 86.

subjects were children from seven to nine years of age; and they took, some of them one seed, and none more than five. Three scarcely suffered at all. One vomited the poison and got well at once. Of the others, some had only nausea and feebleness of the pulse, another had also dilatation of the pupils, some had vomiting and purging, others great drowsiness, others again both sets of symptoms. In all the pulse was weak and generally rapid. Emetics, laxatives and ammonia were administered with success.[*]

The leaves of this plant are stated by Vicat, a good authority, to possess the property of acting violently as an emetic and purgative;[†] and Cadet says the unripe pods have been known to produce in small quantities severe vomiting, and profuse, protracted diarrhœa.[‡]

My attention was lately turned by a criminal trial in this country to the effects of the bark, which is not alluded to as a poison by any author, although its properties seem well known to the peasantry in the north of Scotland. A lad Gordon was tried lately at Inverness for administering poison to a fellow-servant, and it was proved that he gave her laburnum-bark in broth. She immediately became very sick, and was soon attacked with incessant vomiting and purging, pain in the belly, rigor, and extreme feebleness; and several days elapsed before she could return to her work. The sickness, vomiting, purging and pain continued afterwards to recur more or less; great emaciation ensued; in six weeks she was so much reduced as to be compelled to quit service; and even six months afterwards, she continued so ill with a chronic dysenteric affection, that fears were entertained for her life, although eventually she did recover. Being consulted in the case, I was inclined to rely in the general properties of the plant and the peculiar, intense, nauseous bitterness of the bark, even more intense there than in the seeds, as adequate proof that the bark was capable of producing the effects observed in this case. I was scarcely prepared, however, to find it so deadly a narcotic poison, as it proved to be on careful experiment. Dr. Ross of Dornoch, who saw the woman and was also consulted on the part of the crown in the case, found that from twenty to seventy grains of dried laburnum-bark caused speedy and violent vomiting when administered to dogs, but no other marked effect. I found that when an infusion of a drachm of dried bark was injected into the stomach of a strong rabbit, the animal in two minutes began to look quickly from side to side, as if alarmed and uncertain in which direction to go, then twitched back its head two or three times, and instantly fell on its side in violent tetanic convulsions, with alternating opisthotonos and emprosthotonos so energetic that its body bounded with great force upon the side up and down the room. Suddenly in half a minute more all motion ceased, respiration was at an end, and, excepting that the heart continued for a little to contract with some force, life was extinct. No morbid appearance was visible anywhere. The heart was gorged, but irritable. Dr. Ross subsequently repeated this experiment, and obtained analo-

* Lancet, 1840-41, 552.   † Hist. des Plantes Ven. de la Suisse, 1776, p. 49.
‡ Bulletins de la Société de Pharmacie, 1809, p. 48.

gous results; but the animals he operated on did not die for half an hour or upwards.*

MM. Chevallier and Lassaigne have discovered in the seeds an active principle called cytisin, a nauseous, bitter, brownish-yellow, neutral, uncrystallizable substance, of which small doses killed various animals amidst vomiting and convulsions, and eight grains taken by man in four doses brought on giddiness, violent spasms, and frequency of the pulse, lasting for two hours, and followed by exhaustion.†

A great number of Brown's division Papilionaceæ of the present natural family probably possess similar properties.

CHAPTER XLI.

OF POISONING WITH ALCOHOL, ETHER, AND EMPYREUMATIC OILS.

THE last group of the narcotico-acrids comprehends *alcohol, ether,* and the *oleaginous products of combustion.*

Of Poisoning with Alcohol.

Of its Action on Animals, and Symptoms in Man. — Alcohol has been generally believed, since the experiments of Sir B. Brodie,† to act on the brain through the medium of the nerves, and to do so without entering the blood. This may be doubted. At least in some experiments performed several years ago by Dr. C. Coindet and myself it appeared not to act so swiftly, but that absorption might easily have taken place before its operation began. At all events, through whatever channel it may operate, there is no doubt that it enters the blood; for in man the breath has a strong smell of spirit for a considerable time after it is swallowed; and it has been found in the tissues and secretions after death from large doses. Professor Orfila found that alcohol is a violent poison when injected into the cellular tissue ; and that it produces through that channel the same effects as when taken into the stomach.‡ In the course of our experiments Dr. C. Coindet and I found that it acted with great rapidity when injected into the cavity of the chest.

Authors who have treated of the action of alcohol and spirituous liquors on man, have distinguished three degrees in its immediate effects.

1. When the dose is small, much excitement and little subsequent depression are produced.

2. When the effect is sufficiently great to receive the designation of poisoning, the symptoms are more violent excitement, flushed face,

---

* Cases and Observations in Medical Jurisprudence. — Edinburgh Medical and Surgical Journal, 1843, lx. 303.

† Journal de Pharmacie, iv. 340, 554.

‡ Philosophical Transactions, ci. 118. § Toxicol. Gén. ii. 451.

giddiness, confusion of thought, delirium, and various mental affections, varying with individual character, and too familiar to require description here.   These symptoms are soon followed by dozing and gradually increasing somnolency, which may at length become so deep as not to be always easily broken.   After the state of somnolency has continued several hours, it ceases gradually, but is followed by giddiness, weakness stupidity, headache, sickness, and vomiting.

This degree of injury from alcohol may prove fatal, either in itself, by the coma becoming deeper and deeper, — or from the previous excited state of the circulation causing diseases of the brain in a predisposed habit, — or more frequently from the occurrence of some trifling accident, which in his torpid state the individual cannot avoid or remedy, such as exposure to cold, falling with the face in mud or water, suffocation from vomited matters getting into the windpipe, and the like.

Of simple poisoning by the gradual increase of coma the following judicial case in which I was consulted is a characteristic example. Two brothers drank in half an hour three bottles of porter, with which three half-mutchkins (24 ounces) of whisky had been secretly mixed by a companion, whose object was to fill them drunk by way of joke.   In the course of drinking both became confused.   In fifteen minutes after finishing the last bottle one of them fell down insensible, and had no recollection of what happened for twelve hours; but he recovered.   The other staggered a considerable distance for an hour, and then became quite insensible and unable to stand.   In four hours more consciousness and sensibility were quite extinct, the breathing stertorous and irregular, the pulse 80 and feeble, the pupils dilated and not contractile, and deglutition impossible.   In this state he remained without any material change till his death, which took place in fifteen hours after he finished his debauch.   A surgeon saw him when he had been five hours ill, but did little for his relief, as the case appeared hopeless.

There is a singular variety in the principal symptoms of this form of poisoning, even when completely formed.   From a careful tabular analysis of no fewer than twenty-six cases, chiefly of the present denomination, collected by Dr. Ogston of Aberdeen from the experience of the police-office there, it appears that when the stage of stupor is fully formed, the person is sometimes capable of being roused, sometimes immovably comatose for a long time, — that the pulse is sometimes imperceptible or very feeble, sometimes distinct or even full, generally slow or natural, seldom frequent, very seldom firm, — that the pupils are occasionally contracted, much more generally dilated, and in a few instances alternating between one state and the other, — that the countenance is commonly pale, sometimes turgid and flushed, — and that the breathing is for the most part slow, and also soft, yet not unfrequently laborious, but very rarely stertorous. Convulsions are rare, having been observed twice only, and on both occasions in young people of the age of twelve or fourteen.*   Dr.

* Edin. Med. and Surg. Journal, xl. 277.

Ogston has tried to group these several symptoms together in classified cases; but the general conclusions at which he arrives are subject to important exceptions. Neither do any of the special symptoms seem to bear a marked relation to the ultimate event. It is peculiarly worthy of remark, that very many cases got well where the pupils were much dilated, the coma profound, and the pulse imperceptible.

In the present form of poisoning with alcoholic fluids, it usually happens that if the stage of stupor be completely overcome, recovery speedily ensues, without any particular symptom except headache, giddiness, sickness, and the customary consequences of a debauch. But on some occasions the comatose stage is succeeded by one which indicates much cerebral excitement, — by flushed face, injected eyes, restlessness, a febrile state of the pulse, and delirium, even of the violent kind. In other cases this affection puts on very much the characters of a slight attack of typhoid fever.

In the second variety of the second degree of intoxication, an apoplectic disposition is called into action by the excited state of the circulating system; and death ensues from apoplexy or some other disease of the brain, rather than from simple poisoning. Thus in some instances, as will be more fully mentioned under the head of the morbid appearances, extravasation of blood is found within the head after death, preceded by the usual phenomena of ordinary intoxication. Since this is a rare effect of intoxication, it must be considered as the result of poisoning with spirits, exciting sanguineous apoplexy in a predisposed constitution. In other cases the stupor of intoxication, after putting on all the characters of apoplexy for two days and upwards, terminates fatally without extravasation. Here the poison operates by developing a constitutional tendency to congestive apoplexy. Again, this mode of action is still more clearly shown in some cases, where an interval of returning health occurs between the immediate narcotic effects of the poison and the ultimate apoplectic coma which is the occasion of death. Such a course of events, which, however, is of rare occurrence, is well exemplified in the following cases. A man drank 32 ounces of rum one afternoon, and was comatose most of the ensuing night. Next morning, though very drowsy, he was sensible when roused; and in the evening he was considered convalescent. But two days afterwards he became delirious; in two days more he died comatose; and congestion was the only appearance found in the brain.* Another instance, most remarkable in its circumstances, is the following, which has been related by Dr. Golding Bird. A workman in a distillery, after drinking eight ounces of rectified spirit by mistake for water, suddenly fell down senseless and motionless, and remained so for eleven hours. He then began to recover, and came round so far that he returned to his work next morning. After this he continued to pass dark, pitch-like evacuations. In three weeks he became drowsy, mistook one thing for another, answered questions sluggishly,

* Cooke on Nervous Diseases, i. 219.

and had a frequent pulse, and dilated sluggish pupils ; in which state he continued three weeks later when the account was published.* The following case, related by Dr. Chowne, also seems to belong to the same category, although it presents anomalies. A boy, eight years of age, soon after swallowing about eight ounces of gin, said he felt like a drunk man, and suddenly became motionless and insensible. In no long time he vomited a fluid of the odour of gin ; and in seven hours from the commencement a fluid was withdrawn from the stomach, possessing no longer any such odour. He was now motionless, insensible, pale, and cold ; the pupils were contracted, the pulse feeble and hurried, the breathing stertorous and slow ; and he made ineffectual efforts to vomit. Stimulants of all kind had little effect on him for a day and a half, when the breathing became more natural, and his look quite intelligent. Yet he could not answer questions, exhibited no sign of volition, and had a pulse so frequent as 160. In twenty-four hours more the breathing became laborious and rattling, and the lips livid ; and death took place near the close of the third day. The only appearances of any note in the dead body were general injection of the arachnoid membrane of the brain, and effusion of frothy mucus into the bronchial ramifications.† Similar to these is the following extraordinary case which has been communicated to me by Dr. Traill. A boy seven years of age, who was persuaded by two miscreants to take nearly five ounces of undiluted whisky, suffered for two days from the ordinary symptoms of excessive intoxication, which were then immediately followed by epileptic convulsions. These continued to recur with more or less violence, but always frequently, for two months down to the date of the judicial investigation to which the case gave rise. All these forms of the effects of drinking ardent spirits can scarcely be considered as simple poisoning, but as the result of poisoning developing a tendency to diseases of the head.

The third variety of poisoning with spirits in the second degree proves fatal, not in itself, but by some trivial accident happening, from which the individual cannot escape on account of his powerless insensibility. Thus, it is no uncommon thing for persons in a state of deep intoxication to fall down in an exposed place, where they perish from cold, or to tumble with the face in a puddle, and so be suffocated, or to be choked by inhaling the contents of the stomach imperfectly vomited, or by lying in such a posture that their neckcloth produces strangulation. These statements are so familiar, that it is unnecessary to illustrate them by special facts. The reader's attention was called to such accidents in the previous editions of this work. Two well-marked cases of the kind have been since published by Mr. Skae.‡

In cases of simple poisoning in the second degree the progress of the symptoms is on the whole remarkably uniform, gradual and uninterrupted. But there are likewise some anomalies which it may be well to notice. Thus, occasionally after the phenomena of ordinary intoxication have gone on gradually increasing without having attained a very great height, sudden lethargy supervenes at once, and may prove fatal with singular rapidity. My colleague, Dr. Alison, has communicated to me the particulars of a case of the kind where death took place from simple intoxication, twenty minutes after the state of lethargy began. The individual reached his home in a state of reeling drunkenness, but able to speak and give an indistinct account of himself. He then became lethargic, and died in the course of twenty minutes. On examining the body, Dr. Alison could not discover any morbid appearance, except some watery effusion on the surface of the brain and in the ventricles; but the contents of the stomach had a strong smell of spirits. Instances of such excessive rapidity, however, are rare, unless from the third form of poisoning. — An anomaly of a different kind, of which a remarkable example was brought judicially under my notice, is sudden supervention of deep insurmountable stupor, without the usual precursory symptoms, yet not till after a considerable interval subsequently to drinking. In May, 1830, a lad of sixteen, in consequence of a bet with a spirit-dealer, swallowed sixteen ounces of whisky in the course of ten minutes, and, pursuant to the terms of the wager, walked up and down the room for half an hour. He then went into the open air, apparently not at all the worse for his feat; but in a very few minutes, while in the act of putting his hand into his pocket to take out some money, he became so suddenly senseless as to forget to withdraw his hand, and so insensible that his companions could not rouse him. A surgeon, who was immediately procured, contented himself with giving several clysters and a dose of tartaremetic, which did not operate; and the young man died in the course of sixteen hours. The cause of the retardation of the symptoms was partly perhaps that he had taken supper only an hour before drinking the spirits, but chiefly, I presume, because the stupor was kept off for a time by the stimulus of determination to win his bet. — Several cases somewhat similar have been described by Dr. Ogston. In these sudden insensibility came on while the individuals had been drinking freely for some time, without showing any marked sign of approaching intoxication.* The cause of the postponement and sudden invasion of the stupor does not exactly appear; but a familiar cause of its abrupt invasion in ordinary cases of drunkenness is sudden exposure to cold.

It is impossible to fix the extremes of duration of the present form of poisoning in fatal cases. For, on the one hand, one or other of the accidents mentioned above may bring the case to a speedy close; and, on the other hand, the supervention of apoplexy may protract it to several days. The ordinary duration in fatal cases seems to be from twelve to eighteen hours.

3. The third degree of poisoning is not so often witnessed, because, in order to produce it, a greater quantity of spirits must be swallowed

* Edin. Medical and Surg. Journal, xl. 278.

64*

pure and at once, than is usually taken by those among whom poisoning in the second degree chiefly occurs.   When swallowed in
large quantity, as by persons who have taken foolish wages on their
prowess in drinking, there is seldom much preliminary excitement; coma approaches in a few minutes and soon becomes profound, as in apoplexy.   The face is then sometimes livid, more
generally ghastly pale; the breathing stertorous, and of a spirituous
odour; the pupils sometimes much contracted, more commonly
dilated and insensible; and if relief is not speedily procured, death
takes place, — generally in a few hours, and sometimes immediately.
According to Mr. Bedingfield, who witnessed many cases of poisoning with rum at Liverpool, which always follow the arrival of the
West India vessels, the patient will recover if the iris remains contractile; but if it is dilated and motionless on the approach of a light,
recovery is very improbable.*

A case is briefly alluded to by Orfila of a soldier, who drank eight
pints of brandy for a wager, and died instantly.†   A case of the
same kind is quoted by Professor Marx.‡   Another, which happened
in the person of a London cabman, is noticed in a French Journal.   The man, for a bribe of five shillings, drank at a draught a
whole bottle of gin; and in a few minutes he dropped down dead.§
Similar accidents occur not infrequently in this country; but I have
not met with any fully described by authors.   A case of the less
rapid variety of the present form occurred at the Infirmary here in
1820.   A man stole a bottle of whiskey; and, being in danger of
detection, took what he thought the surest way of concealing it, by
drinking it all.   He died in four hours with symptoms of pure coma.

Convulsions are not common in such cases.   I have seen a remarkable example, however, in which the coma was accompanied
with constant alternating *opisthotonos* and *emprosthotonos*.   The subject was a boy who had been induced to drink raw whisky by an
acquaintance, and had been two hours insensible before I saw him.
The stomach-pump, which was immediately applied, brought away
a large quantity of fluid with a strong spirituous odour; and he recovered his senses in fifteen minutes, but remained very drowsy for
the rest of the day.

Such are the forms of poisoning with spirits usually admitted by
authors.   But it also appears to act sometimes as an irritant.   After
its ordinary narcotic action passes off, another set of symptoms occasionally appear, which indicate inflammation of the alimentary canal.
Cases of this kind are exceedingly rare; yet they have been met
with, as the following extract shows.   "A young man at Paris had
been drinking brandy immoderately for several successive days,
when at length he was attacked with shivering, nausea, feverishness,
pain in the stomach, vomiting of everything he swallowed except

* Edinb. Med. and Surg. Journal, xii. 489, from Bedingfield's Compendium of Med.
Practice.
† Toxicol. Gén. ii. 454.   ‡ Die Lehre von den Giften, I. ii. 306.
§ Journal de Chimie Médicale, 1839, 129.

cold water, thirst, and at last hiccup, delirium, jaundice, and convulsions; and death took place on the ninth day. On examining the body the stomach was found gangrenous over the whole villous coat; the colon too was much inflamed; and all the small intestines were red."[*]

A case of great complexity, but probably of the same nature, has been related by Opitz in Pyl's Memoirs. The subject was a woman liable to epilepsy, and addicted to excessive drinking. After one of her drinking-bouts she was seized with vomiting and severe pain of the bowels, afterwards with delirium, then with convulsions, and she died in twenty-four hours after the first attack. The stomach and intestines were greatly inflamed, a table-spoonful of blood was effused into the ventricles of the brain, and the left lung was purulent.[†]

Besides the immediately fatal effects of spirituous liquors now described, there is still another variety of poisoning more common than any yet mentioned, and constituting a peculiar disease. People who fall into the unhappy vice of habitual intoxication, after remaining in a state of drunkenness for several days together, are often attacked with a singular maniacal affection, which is accompanied with tremors, particularly of the hands, and after enduring for several days, ends at last in coma. When the delirium is not so violent, the disease by proper treatment may be cured. But frequently, after the delirium and tremor have continued mildly for some time, they increase, and the delirium becomes furious, or coma rapidly supervenes; in either of which cases the disorder commonly proves fatal in two or three days more. This disease, which is now familiar to the physician, is called *delirium tremens*. It is supposed by some to depend on inflammation of the membranes of the brain, followed by effusion.

Other diseases, besides *delirium tremens*, are also slowly induced by the habitual and excessive use of spirituous liquors; but in general the habit of intoxication acts in inducing these diseases only as a predisposing cause. A particular variety of tuberculated liver probably arises from the habitual use of spirits without the co-operation of other causes. That variety of disease of the kidney, which was first brought under the notice of the profession by Dr. Bright,[‡] is also obviously often connected with the habit of drinking spirits. The following have been enumerated among the diseases where the same habit acts powerfully as a predisposing cause — indurated pancreas, — indurated mesenteric glands, — scirrhous pylorus, — catarrh of the bladder, — inflammation, suppuration and induration of the kidneys, — incontinence of urine, — aneurism of the heart and great vessels, — apoplexy of the lungs, — varicose veins, — mania, — epilepsy, — tendency to gangrene of wounds, — spontaneous combustion.[§]

Of the Morbid Appearances. — Some doubts exist as to the morbid appearances in the bodies of those poisoned by spirituous liquors.

[*] Corvisart's Journ. de Méd. xvii. 43. [†] Aufsätze, v. 94.

[‡] Bright's Reports of Medical Cases, i. 1.

[§] See on this subject, Grötzner, über die Truncksucht unde ihre Folgen. — Rust's Mag. für die ges. Heilkunde, xx. 522.

In animals killed by alcohol, Orfila says he found the villous coat of the stomach constantly of a cherry-red odour. I have several times remarked the same appearance. When the stomach was empty before the alcohol was introduced, I have always found the prominent part of its rugæ of a deep cherry-red tint, the margin of the patches being more florid, and evidently consisting of a minute network of vessels.

In man these signs of irritation have not been always observed. In the patient who died in the Infirmary here, the stomach was quite natural to appearance. Dr. Ogston notices injection of the small intestines and thickening of the mucous membrane of the stomach and intestines as common appearances in the cases he has examined; but he seems to consider these the effects not of the last fatal dose, but of the habit of frequent excessive drinking.*

The blood in the heart and great vessels is commonly fluid and very dark, and the lungs are sometimes more or less gorged with the same fluid.

The state of the brain differs much according to the mode of death. Sometimes great congestion and even actual extravasation of blood are found in the heads of persons who have died of excessive continuous drinking, — the excitement of such a debauch being apt, as already mentioned, to induce apoplexy in a predisposed habit. Accordingly extravasation was found by Professor Bernt of Vienna in no less than four cases of the kind, two of which happened in the persons of young men not above twenty-two years of age;† and Dr. Cooke quotes another in his work on nervous diseases.‡ I have myself met with another remarkable instance. A female out-pensioner of Trinity Hospital here, who was much addicted to drinking, and for fourteen days after the New-year of 1830 had been very little in her sober senses, soon after arriving at home one evening much intoxicated, fell down comatose, and died in ten or twelve hours. An enormous extravasation of clotted blood was found in the ventricles, producing extensive laceration of the right middle and anterior lobes of the brain. — In such cases it is natural to suppose that a predisposition to apoplexy must concur with the intoxication; otherwise it is not easy to see why death from extravasation is not more frequently produced by excessive drinking.

Extravasation is not apt to occur in the cases of rapid death brought on by a very large quantity swallowed at once. The circulation, indeed, is during life in a state quite the reverse of excitement; and accordingly the brain and its membranes are found quite healthy. They were particularly so in the man who died in the hospital here. It is right to mention, however, that one of Bernt's cases, although the symptoms and other particulars are not mentioned, possibly belongs to the present variety, as the man swallowed for a wager a quart of brandy at a draught.§ According to Dr. Ogston, who has given the best account of the appearances within the head

* Edin. Medical and Surg Journ. xl. 292.
† Beiträge zur Gerichtl. Arzneik. ii. 59, iii. 38.   ‡ On Nervous Diseases, i. 219.
§ Beiträge zur Gerichtl. Arzneik. iii. 38.

in the ordinary cases of this kind, there is usually serous effusion under the arachnoid membrane, occasionally minute injection of vessels, commonly more or less general gorging of the larger veins, and especially effusion of serosity to the amount of two or even four ounces in the ventricles.*

When delirium tremens proves fatal, effusion is commonly found among the membranes of the brain ; and occasionally to a great extent. In one instance, which proved fatal in two or three days, I have seen minute vascularity of the membranes, with effusion of fibrin, and without effusion of serosity ; but such cases are rare. There is also, according to Andral, very extensive softening of the mucous coat of the stomach.† In an instance mentioned in Rust's Journal, besides effusion into the cerebral membranes, there was found an enormous accumulation of fat in all the cavities, a conversion of the muscular substance into fat, and a nauseous sweet smell from the whole body.‡

In all cases of rapid poisoning with spirituous liquors some of the poison will be found in the stomach. For when the case is one of pure narcotic poisoning, unaided by the effects of blows, exposure to cold, or the like, and the person dies in a few hours, the poison cannot be all absorbed before death. — Although the spirituous liquors used in Britain have all very powerful odours, the inspector in a case of importance ought not to confine himself to this test alone. He must subject the suspected matter to distillation ; and then remove the water from what distils over by repeated agitation with dry carbonate of potass, till he procures the alcohol of the spirit in such a state of purity as to be inflammable.

Alcohol may also be in some circumstances detected in the tissues and secretions of the body. A spirituous odour has been remarked not infrequently in various parts, and especially in the brain. Dr. Cooke mentions a case in which the fluid in the ventricles of the brain had the smell and taste of gin, the liquor which had been taken ;§ Dr. Ogston adverts to an instance, in which after death by drowning during intoxication, he found in the ventricles nearly four ounces of fluid, having a strong odour of whisky ;‖ in the case which occurred in the hospital here the odour of whisky was said to have been perceived in the pericardium ; and in a man who died of long-continued intoxication from immoderate drinking Dr. Wolffe found that the surface, and still more the ventricles, of the brain had a strong smell of brandy, although the contents of the stomach had not.¶

The presumption afforded by such facts as these, in favour of the absorption of alcohol and the possibility of detecting it throughout the animal system, has been turned to certainty by the late experimental researches of Dr. Percy ; who found that in animals poisoned with

* Edin. Med. and Surg. Journal, xl. 282, 284, 293.
† Répertoire Gén. Anat. et de Physiol. Pathologique, i. 51.
‡ Magazin für die ges. Heilkunde, xxi. 522.
§ Treatise on Nervous Diseases, i. 222.
‖ Edin. Medical and Surgical Journal, xl. 293.
¶ Rust's Magazin für die gesammte Heilkunde, xxv. 126.

alcoholic fluids, as well as in the case of a man who died during the night after drinking a bottle of rum, alcohol could be detected, generally in the urine, and also in the brain, by cautious distillation, and removing the water from the distilled fluid by means of dry carbonate of potass.* Dr. Percy gave me an opportunity of verifying his results with the brain of the man; and I had no difficulty in obtaining from a few ounces of brain a sufficiency of spirit to exhibit its combustion on asbestus repeatedly.

It is hardly necessary to add, that when the individual has survived the taking of the poison a considerable length of time, an odour of spirits will not be perceived either in the stomach or elsewhere. In the out-pensioner of Trinity Hospital, for example, who survived about twelve hours, no spirituous odour could any where be perceived. In such cases the poison disappears during life by absorption. — A question may even be entertained, whether the odour may not sometimes be imperceptible at the inspection of the body, although the poison was really present immediately after death. It is probable that, as in the instance of hydrocyanic acid, the alcohol, on account of its volatility or fluidity, will evaporate or percolate away in a few days. In this manner only can be explained the occasional absence of the odour in persons who have been killed in the early stage of drunkenness. I could not perceive any odour of whisky in the stomach of the woman Campbell, who was murdered by the notorious resurrectionist Burke, although she had drunk spirits to intoxication half an hour before her death. The body was not examined till thirty-eight hours after.† It must be observed, however, that alcohol may exist in the contents of the stomach and be detected by chemical analysis, although it is not indicated by its odour. I have twice had occasion to observe this, where the bodies were disinterred some time after death.

From all that has been said, there ought seldom to be much difficulty in recognizing a case of poisoning with spirituous liquors.

But, before quitting the subject, a form of it must be noticed which may be extremely difficult to distinguish. It was formerly remarked that the eatable mushrooms have been sometimes poisoned with substances possessing effects on the system analogous to those caused by the deleterious fungi. In the same manner spirituous liquors may be poisoned with narcotics allied to them in action. Thus, in former parts of this work, it has been stated that a young man was killed during a debauch in consequence of his companions having mingled opium with his wine; that many persons have been poisoned and some killed by fermented liquors drugged in the same manner; that murder has been accomplished by poisoning wine with nightshade; and that several fatal accidents have occurred in consequence of liqueurs having been too strongly impregnated with hydrocyanic

* Prize Inaugural Dissertation, on the presence of alcohol in the brain after poisoning with it. Edinburgh, 1839, *passim.*

† Cases and Observations in Medical Jurisprudence. — Edin. Med. and Surg. Journal, xxxi. 239.

acid, to give them a ratafia flavour. Cases of this nature may be embarrassing. In general, they may be made out by attending strictly to the symptoms, the quantity of liquor taken, and the contents of the stomach. But, it must be admitted, that if a murderer, who chooses such a method, should season his guest's drink judiciously, and ply him well with it, a medical jurist might be puzzled to determine whether the liquor was to blame in point of quality or quantity.

Of the Treatment. — The treatment of poisoning with alcoholic fluids does not differ essentially from that of poisoning with opium. In the former, as in the latter, the chief objects must be to remove the poison from the stomach, and to rouse the patient from his state of stupor; but in poisoning with alcoholic fluids it is also frequently necessary to treat a secondary stage of reaction by local and even general antiphlogistic measures. As to the primary object, the removal of the poison from the stomach, it appears that in the present form of poisoning emetics are more seldom effectual than in the case of other narcotics, and that the stomach-pump should be promptly resorted to. It is remarkable that the operation of clearing out the stomach is likewise often a sufficient stimulus to dispel stupor immediately and even permanently. I have seen almost complete consciousness permanently restored with the discharge of the alcoholic fluid; and the same remark has been made by others. Where the senses are not thus restored, one of the most effectual stimulants, according to the practice of the police-office of this city, is the injection of water into the ears. Great advantage has been derived, as in poisoning with opium, from the cold affusion applied to the head. Dr. Ogston, who has appended to his paper formerly quoted a very useful summary of the treatment of poisoning with spirits, has found this a safe and effectual remedy where the heat of the head was unnaturally great and that of the body not too low.[*] Cases have been published where it proved successful although the pulse was gone at the wrist, the breathing scarcely perceptible, and the temperature of the whole body greatly reduced.[†] It is doubtless a powerful remedy: but where the general temperature of the surface is much lowered, I conceive it should be restricted to the head and neck, and conjoined with the application of warmth to the body. Dr. Ogston objects to the general use of blood-letting in cases of poisoning with spirits, as being often apt to be followed by sudden sinking. Where other remedies are judiciously used, it is probably seldom called for; and the purpose it is intended to serve, namely, the relief of cerebral congestion and determination, is better fulfilled by the local employment of cold, and local blood-letting. Ammonia and its acetate have been found useful as internal stimulants where the stupor is deep. The treatment of the secondary affections adverted to above does not require specific mention.

[*] Edin. Medical and Surgical Journal, xl. 295.
[†] Smith, London Medical Gazette, ix. 502.

Of Poisoning with Sulphuric and Nitric Ether.

Sulphuric ether and nitric ether are poisons of the same nature with alcohol. But the effects produced by them when taken in considerable doses are not very well known.

Orfila found that half an ounce of sulphuric ether introduced into the stomach of a dog and secured there by a ligature on the gullet, excited efforts to vomit, in ten minutes inability to stand, and in six minutes more, insensibility. In fifteen minutes more the animal revived a little, but soon became again comatose; and it died in three hours after the commencement of the experiment. The villous coat of the stomach was reddish-black, the other coats of a lively red colour.*

The effects of the ethers on man have not been accurately ascertained. From some observations published in the Journal of Science, sulphuric ether appears to act energetically even in small doses. In moderate quantity it produces a strong sense of irritation in the throat, a feeling of fulness in the head, and other symptoms like those excited by nitrous-oxide gas. A gentleman, in consequence of inhaling it too long, was attacked with intermitting lethargy for thirty-six hours, depression of spirits and lowness of pulse.† When long and habitually used, as by persons afflicted with asthma, its dose must be gradually increased; and it appears that considerable quantities may then be taken for a great length of time without material injury. I have been informed of an instance of an asthmatic gentleman about sixty years of age who consumed sixteen ounces every eight or ten days, and had been in the habit of doing so for many years. Yet, with the exception of his asthma, he enjoyed tolerable health.

An interesting case has been published which proves that nitric ether in vapour is a dangerous poison when too freely and too long inhaled. A druggist's maid-servant was found one morning dead in bed, and death had evidently arisen from the air of her apartment having been accidentally loaded with vapour of nitric ether, from the breaking of a three-gallon jar of the *spiritus etheris nitrici*. She was found lying on her side, with her arms folded across the chest, the countenance and posture composed, and the whole appearance like a person in deep sleep. The stomach was red internally, and the lungs were gorged.‡ The editor of the journal, where this case is related, says he is acquainted with a similar instance where a young man became completely insensible from breathing air loaded with sulphuric ether, remained apoplectic for some hours, and would undoubtedly have perished had he not been discovered and removed in time.

Of Poisoning with the Oleaginous products of Combustion.

The physiological effects of these substances have not yet been extensively investigated. It has been already mentioned, that the

---

* Toxicol. Gén. ii. 456.   † Journal of Science, iv. 158.
‡ Midland Med. and Surg. Reporter, i., or Edin. Med. and Surg. Journal, xxxv. 452.

empyreumatic oils of tobacco and other narcotic vegetables are active poisons; and that the emanations from candle snuffings and imperfectly consumed tallow probably owe their injurious properties to a peculiar oil. Many empyreumatic oils are known, and some are used in medicine, which act powerfully on the animal system as stimulants and antispasmodics. Among these may be enumerated naphtha, oil of galbanum, oil of guiaiac, oil of amber, oil of wax, and Dippel's oil. The last in particular, which is the rectified empyreumatic oil of hartshorn, but is prepared also from blood and various animal matters,* has been a good deal used of late on the continent for medical purposes, and has even been resorted to as a poison for the purpose of self-destruction.

The only one of these substances whose physiological properties have been examined with particular care, is the empyreumatic oil procured by the destructive distillation of lard. When freed of adhering acid by rectification from quicklime, this oil is limpid and very volatile, has an insupportable smell, and when diffused in the air, irritates the eyes and nostrils, and even excites giddiness. Buchner found it to possess simple narcotic properties. When a mouse was confined under a jar, into which a little of its vapour was introduced, it suddenly tried to escape, immediately fell down exhausted, and, although soon afterwards removed into the open air, expired in about fifteen minutes, without convulsions. It is much less powerful when introduced into the stomach, yet is still a dangerous poison through that channel; for five drops projected into the throat of a chaffinch very nearly proved fatal; and the only symptoms were excessive exhaustion, slow respiration, and insensibility.†

Similar effects have been occasionally observed in man. The late Professor Chaussier has related a case of poisoning in the human subject from the *oil of Dippel*, or rectified empyreumatic oil of hartshorn. It is merely mentioned, however, that the individual, on taking a spoonful by mistake, died immediately; and that no morbid appearance could be discovered in the dead body.‡ Another case has been more recently related, where the poison was the impure oil of commerce, from which the oil of Dippel is prepared by rectification. The subject was a woman, who took it intentionally in the dose of an ounce and a half. The symptoms induced could not be ascertained; but it appeared, that she had been attacked with vomiting, and, finding the action of the poison either less speedy, or less supportable than she expected, had thrown herself into a well and been drowned. The appearances in the body clearly showed that in this instance the poison had not acted as a pure narcotic. The whole body exhaled the peculiar fetid odour of the oil. The palate, tongue, throat, and gullet, were white and shrivelled. The stomach had outwardly a diffuse rose tint, crossed by gorged black veins, which here and there had burst and formed patches of extravasation. The contents of the stomach consisted of remains of food, a good

* Fechner's Repertorium für Organischen Chemie, i. 1078.
† Toxikologie, 395.   ‡ Diction. des Scien. Méd. xxi. 605.

65

deal of the oil, some water, and likewise some extravasated blood. Its villous coat was thick, covered with red points, corrugated into prominent rugæ, but not eroded. The intestines also presented signs of irritation, but in an inferior degree.* Dr. Kurtze, a German author, mentions that the impure oil [Oleum Animale Fœtidum] was given with malicious intention in repeated doses to an infant eighteen days old, whom he attended, and that it caused crying and vomiting; and he quotes Froriep's Notizen, for the case of a woman of thirty, who swallowed nearly two ounces, and, after repeated attacks of vomiting, threw herself into a well and was drowned.†

These facts seem to establish sufficiently the propriety of arranging the empyreumatic oils among the narcotico-acrids.

Oil of turpentine possesses somewhat similar properties; but is much less active. It was found by Professor Schubarth, that two drachms of this oil administered to a dog produced immediate staggering, cries, tetanus, failure of the pulse and breathing, and death in three minutes; and in the dead body he remarked flaccidity of the heart, gorging of the lungs, and redness of the stomach.‡ It is likewise well known to be a powerful poison for vermin, such as lice, fleas, and worms. — On man its effects are capricious. It is frequently used along with other laxatives against obstinate constipation of the bowels, and either in the same manner or alone as a remedy for intestinal worms. For these purposes it has been at times administered in very large doses, for example in the quantity of two, three, or four ounces, without any other effect than brisk purging. But on the other hand it has sometimes, in much inferior doses, induced violent hypercatharsis, or acted severely on the urinary organs, producing strangury and bloody micturition, or affected the brain, producing a state like intoxication, followed by trance for many hours.§ I am not aware that it has ever proved fatal.

Oil of tar, a composite substance obtained by the distillation of wood-tar, is another pyrogenous fluid of poisonous properties. Messrs. Slight of Portsmouth have related the case of a seaman, who, after taking nearly four ounces by mistake for spirits, was attacked with frequent vomiting of a matter having a strong odour of tar, attended with excessive pain in the bowels and loins. Nothing was done for his relief till about seven hours afterwards, when he was freely bled and purged, with immediate relief; and next morning he was so better as to be able to resume his work. The urine had a strong tarry odour, and for some time he suffered from heat in passing it.‖ A case occurred in the London Hospital, in which the symptoms were very different. A lad of eighteen, while intoxicated, took two or three draughts of oil of tar, although aware of its being poisonous. Not long afterwards he became insensible, and had laborious, rattling re-

* Journal Universel. Novembre, 1829.
† Henke's Zeitschrift für die Staatsarzneikunde, xxx. 425.
‡ Horn's Archiv für Med. Erfahrung, 1824, i. 89, 91.
§ Duncan's Dispensatory, 12th edition, p. 552.
‖ Lancet, 1832-33, ii. 598.

spiration, coldness of the extremities, suffusion of the conjunctiva, contraction of the pupils, and an exceedingly feeble pulse. The stomach-pump brought away a liquid with an overpowering smell of tar. Stimulants, external as well as internal, venesection, and turpentine clysters were of little avail; the insensibility continued, with only a short and imperfect interval; and he died about twenty-four hours after swallowing the poison. The pulmonary mucous membrane was highly injected, the lungs gorged with blood and of a tarry odour, the stomach and intestines natural, except that the whole *valvulæ conniventes* were yellow,—the brain and its membranes also natural.[*] It is mentioned in the paper of Messrs. Slight that a gentleman at Brighton died in consequence of a druggist using oil of tar by mistake for something else in making up a prescription.

Creasote is another pyrogenous substance possessing considerable activity as a poison. It is now extensively used in small doses as a medicine for a variety of purposes.

It has been made the subject of physiological experiment by various inquirers, and especially by Dr. Cormach; who found that doses of twenty-five or forty drops caused death in a few seconds when injected into the jugular vein of a dog, by arresting the heart's action, and without visibly altering the condition of the blood; that a quantity somewhat larger caused only sopor and spasmodic twitches of the muscles, if injected into the carotid artery, and without proving fatal; that thirty drops introduced into the stomach of a rabbit excited convulsions, acute cries, and death in one minute, apparently from arrestment of the action of the heart; and that the same dose given to a dog brought on salivation, giddiness, tetanic spasm, a feeble, fluttering, almost imperceptible pulse, and general insensibility, with dilated immovable pupils; but recovery took place under the employment of blood-letting.[†] — The effects of too large a medicinal dose in man are pain in the stomach and vomiting, and also, according to Dr. Elliotson, giddiness, headache, and stupor.[‡] Dr. Pereira alludes to a case, mentioned in the Times newspaper, of death caused in 36 hours by two drachms taken at once; and in this instance acute pain in the abdomen was a prominent symptom.[§] I presume this is the same case which is mentioned in the Edinburgh Medical and Surgical Journal as having occurred at Liverpool.[‖] — The results of Dr. Cormack's experiments on animals lead to the conclusion, that in poisoning with creasote, this substance may always be detected in the body, if it has not been removed by artificial means a considerable time before death.

* Lancet, 1833-34, i. 902.
† Natural, Chemical, Medicinal, and Physiological Properties of Creasote. Harveian Prize Essay, 1836, p. 66 to 99.
‡ Medico-Chirurgical Transactions, xix.
§ Elements of Materia Medica, 1842, i. 419.   ‖ lii. 291.

CHAPTER XLII.

OF COMPOUND POISONING.

HAVING now investigated the three great classes of poisons in their relations to physiology, practice of physic, and medical jurisprudence, it will be necessary to offer a few observations on a subject of considerable medico-legal importance, which has been almost overlooked in systems of Toxicology, — Compound Poisoning.

When two poisons of different or opposite properties are administered about the same time in poisonous doses, the effects of the one may overpower and prevent the operation of the other, or they may merely modify the action of one another. In this manner the usual symptoms produced by one or by both may be entirely or in a great measure wanting; and even in the dead body the usual appearances occasioned by one or both may be modified or perhaps altogether absent.

Although in the course of reading I have met with a sufficient number of cases of the kind to show that compound poisoning is an object of some consequence to the medical jurist, the facts hitherto made public are not so numerous as to render a systematic arrangement of them practicable. The most advisable course, therefore, seems to be merely to describe for the present the cases which have been brought under my notice. These are as follows:

1. *Poisoning with Arsenic and Alcohol.* — A man, after taking twelve ounces of whisky at a debauch, swallowed, an hour afterwards, while in a state of excitement, but not particularly drunk, a quantity of arsenic, the dose of which could not be ascertained. Fifteen minutes after the arsenic was taken medical aid was procured, upon which repeated attempts were made to produce vomiting by means of ipecacuan and sulphate of zinc, but to no purpose. The stomach-pump was therefore resorted to; and, after at least an hour had been spent in previous attempts by emetics, the stomach was cleared of a fluid in which arsenic was unequivocally detected. No symptom of poisoning with arsenic followed. As the man took the arsenic seven hours after a meal, when of course the powder would at once be brought freely in contact with the villous coat of the stomach, it must, I think, be inferred, that the operation of the arsenic was impeded or prevented by the narcotism previously induced by the ardent spirits. For this case I am indebted to a former pupil, Mr. King.

Poisoning with Arsenic and Alcohol.. — A case of the same description with the last, but which proved fatal in consequence of the large quantity of arsenic taken, has been related by Dr. Wood of Dumfries. A lad of seventeen, after a night's debauch, swallowed half an ounce of arsenic early in the morning. In two hours and a half, when Dr. Wood first saw him, there was no symptom of poisoning with arsenic, — no symptom at all indeed but languor and drowsiness. A few minutes afterwards he had slight vomiting, which was repeatedly renewed by artificial means. For some hours the pulse was but little elevated. In eighteen hours he began to sink, and presented the usual constitutional symptoms of poisoning with arsenic ; and in forty-one hours he expired. But from first to last he had scarcely any local symptom except vomiting, even although the stomach presented after death signs of violent irritation.*

3. *Poisoning with Tartar-Emetic and Charcoal Fumes.* — Under the head of poisoning with antimony, notice has already been taken of the case of a man who, after swallowing seventeen grains of tartar-emetic, attempted to commit suicide by suffocating himself with the fumes of burning charcoal. He recovered from both attempts, suffered severely from the usual narcotic effects of carbonic acid gas, but showed scarcely any symptom of the irritant action of tartar-emetic.†

4. *Poisoning with Alcohol and with Laudanum.* — Under the head of poisoning with opium, allusion has already been made to a remarkable case related by Mr. Shearman, where the usual effects of opium were much retarded in an individual who, at the time of swallowing the opium, was in a state of excitement from intoxication. For five hours there was no material stupor. But after that the usual narcotic symptoms supervened and eventually proved fatal.‡ The excitement of intoxication, however, has not always the effect of suspending the action of opium ; for in a case which came under my notice in the Infirmary of this city, — that of a woman, who swallowed an ounce and a half of laudanum while much intoxicated, — the usual narcotic symptoms were fully formed in an hour : and although the stomach-pump was applied soon afterwards, she expired in less than five hours from the time the laudanum was swallowed, — those who had charge of her before she was brought into the hospital having neglected to use the proper means for keeping her roused.

5. *Poisoning with Laudanum and Corrosive Sublimate.* — Of all the cases of compound poisoning I have met with, the most remarkable is an instance which occurred in Edinburgh Castle, a few years ago, of poisoning with laudanum and corrosive sublimate. In this case, the individual, a young soldier, swallowed about the same time two drachms of the latter and half an ounce of the former. He had at first no violent symptoms whatever, indicating the operation of corrosive sublimate ; which is an extremely rare occurrence. Afterwards he had frequent purging and tenesmus, with bloody stools and all the usual phenomena of violent dysentery, but no pain of belly, no tenderness even on firm pressure, no vomiting except under the use of emetics. On the fourth day a violent salivation set in ; and under this and the dysenteric affection he became quickly exhausted, yet not so much, but that on the day of his death, the ninth after he took the poison, he was able to walk a little in his room without as-

* Edin. Med. and Surg. Journal, xxxiii. 61.
† Journal Universel des Sc. Méd. xvii. 120.
‡ London Med. and Phys. Journal, xlix. 119.

65*

sistance. He died on the close-stool rather unexpectedly. I have unfortunately lost the original notes I had of this case, and have forgotten whether any narcotic symptoms were present at first ; but my impression is that they were present, though in a slight degree only. Most of the previous particulars were communicated to me by the late Dr. Mackintosh. The stomach, duodenum, ileum, colon, and rectum were found after death enormously inflamed, ulcerated, and here and there almost gangrenous. — In this instance some of the corrosive sublimate must have been decomposed by the laudanum, and an insoluble meconate of mercury formed. But the quantity thus decomposed could have been but a small proportion of the whole, — as was indeed proved by the extensive ravages actually committed in the whole alimentary canal. I conceive, therefore, that there is no other way of accounting for the slight apparent effects of the corrosive sublimate, at the commencement particularly, than by supposing that the narcotic operation of the opium veiled or actually retarded the irritant action of the corrosive sublimate.

6. *Poisoning with Opium and Belladonna.* — A lady, who used a compound infusion of opium and belladonna as a wash for an eruption in the vulva, took it into her head one day to use the wash as an injection ; and actually received three successive injections, containing each the active matter of a scruple of opium and half an ounce of belladonna leaves. Fortunately none of the three was retained above a few minutes, except the last, which was not discharged for ten minutes. In less than an hour, she was found in bed in a deep sleep, but the true cause was not suspected till three hours later. She was then completely insensible and motionless, with the face pale, the pupils excessively dilated and not contractile, the pulse frequent and small, and the breathing hurried. After the use of purgative injections, blood-letting, leeches to the head, and sinapisms to the legs, she began in five hours to show some sign of returning consciousness, which improved after a fit of vomiting. When thoroughly roused, her vision continued dim, the pupils excessively dilated, and the ideas somewhat confused. For three days the pulse continued frequent, and the pupils somewhat dilated.* Here the opium seems to have prevented the delirium usually induced by belladonna in the early stage, while on the other hand the belladonna prevented the usual effect of opium on the pupils, and actually produced the opposite action.

7. In the following cases, the active poisons to which the individuals were exposed were so numerous, that it is impossible to say which or how many of them occasioned the symptoms. A colour-maker was superintending a process in which cobalt, arsenic, mercury, sal-ammoniac, and nitric acid were subjected to heat in a mattrass, when the mattrass suddenly gave way, and a dense vapour was instantly discharged. The manufacturer, before he could escape, fell down insensible; and though speedily removed, he died in no long time, affected with enormous swelling of the abdomen. A

* Martin-Solon. Journal Hebdomadaire, viii. 73.

workman who was also present, escaped by a window; but was nevertheless immediately attacked with swelling of the belly, which speedily became very great, and was attended with pain in the jaws, and dimness of sight. These symptoms were very slowly dissipated under the use of cold bathing and purgatives, which brought away an enormous quantity of fetid gas.*

These are not the only examples of compound poisoning which have come under my attention. But others I have noticed are not detailed with sufficient exactness to make it worth while to quote them. The instances given, however, are sufficient to show that poisons of opposite qualities given about the same time in large doses will disguise one another's effects, or impede, or perhaps even prevent them, in a manner which renders such a combination of circumstances an important subject of inquiry for the medico-legal toxicologist.

It is probable that the modifying influence is established in one of two ways, — either by one poison producing a state of venous plethora or distension, which impedes, or for a time prevents, the absorption of the other, — or by one poison producing an insensibility of the membrane with which the other is in contact; so that not only the local injury actually done has not the usual remote effect on the constitution, or on distant organs, but likewise is at times substantially less extensive than in ordinary circumstances. These reflexions arise naturally from a review of the preceding cases; but of course farther facts are necessary to give them weight.

* Gueneau de Mussy. Archives Gén. de Med. Deuxiême Série, i. 594.

INDEX.

66

DESCRIPTION OF THE PLATE.

1. Small funnel-shaped tube for testing minute portions of liquids.
2. Apparatus for the distillation of fluids suspected to contain acids, one-seventh the natural size.
3. Tube for reducing very small portions of arsenic or mercury. The figure is of half the natural size. The ball may be blown larger, if the material to be reduced is bulky.
4. A small glass funnel for introducing the material into the tube Fig. 1, without soiling its inside.
5. The ordinary apparatus for disengaging sulphuretted-hydrogen. The funnel must be a little longer than the emerging tube. The fluid should not be at any time much higher than in the figure, in order to secure the operator against its effervescing up into the emerging tube. The figure is a fourth of the natural size.
6. Instrument for washing down scanty precipitates on filters. It is a thin bottle capable of standing heat — half-filled with water, which may be boiled on occasion,— and having its cork pierced with a small tube drawn at its outer end to a very fine bore. The breath is impelled into the bottle, and, the bottle being then reversed, a very fine stream issues with great force.

Fig. 1.   Fig. 2.   Fig. 5.

Fig. 3.   Fig. 4.   Fig. 6.

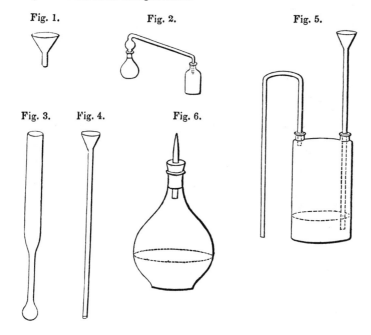

7. Tubes of natural size for collecting small portions of mercury by the process, p. 300.
8. Pipette, one-fourth the natural size, for removing by suction fluids lying over precipitates. Some have a rectangular bend in the upper part, by means of which the
operator sees better the point of the instrument when in action ; but such pipettes
are difficult to clean. That represented in the figure is easily cleaned with a
feather.
9. Apparatus for reducing the sulphurets of some metals by a stream of hydrogen. A,
the vessel with zinc and diluted sulphuric acid, the latter of which may be renewed
by the funnel B. C, a ball on the emerging tube to prevent the liquid thrown up
by the effervescence from passing forward. D, E, corks by which C and G are
fitted into F, the tube which contains the sulphuret at F. G, the exit-tube for the
sulphuretted-hydrogen, plying into a vessel containing acetate of lead. When the
hydrogen has passed long enough to expel all the air, the spirit-lamp flame is applied at F ; and when sulphuretted-hydrogen is formed, the lead solution is blackened. The figure is one-third the size of the apparatus.
For Description of Figures 10 and 11, see p. 212.

Fig. 7.   Fig. 8.   Fig. 9.

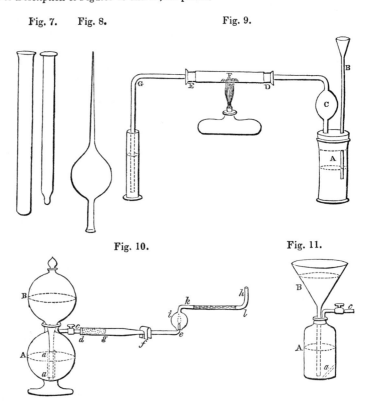

Fig. 10.   Fig. 11.

THE END.

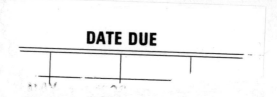

DATE DUE

MA